THE **AUPHA** MANUAL OF HEALTH SERVICES MANAGEMENT

Edited by

Robert J. Taylor, MHA, FACHE
Susan B. Taylor

AUPHA

AN ASPEN PUBLICATION®
Aspen Publishers, Inc.
Gaithersburg, Maryland
1994

Library of Congress Cataloging-in-Publication Data

The AUPHA manual of health services management / edited by Robert J.
Taylor, Susan B. Taylor.
p. cm.
Includes bibliographical references and index.
ISBN 0-8342-0363-4
1. Health services administration. I. Taylor, Robert J., 1940- .
II. Taylor, Susan B., 1941- .
[DNLM: 1. Health Services—organization & administration.
2. Leadership. 3. Management Information Systems. 4. Health
Resources. 5. Delivery of Health Care. W84.1 A926 1993]
RA971.A93 1994
362.1'068—dc 20
DNLM/DLC
for Library of Congress
93-7288
CIP

Editorial Resources: Barbara Priest

Library of Congress Catalog Card Number: 93-7288
ISBN: 0-8342-0363-4

Printed in the United States of America

2 3 4 5

*Dedicated to health service managers
who recognize that
a firm grounding in the fundamentals
frees us to innovate*

Table of Contents

Editors and Advisors xv

Contributors xvii

Consultants xxi

Preface xxvii

Part I   **Leadership** 1

Chapter 1   **Health: The Emerging Context of Management** 3
               Gary L. Filerman

               Introduction 3
               The Pressures for Change 5
               Resources and Health Systems 6
               Mandate for the Future: Primary Health Care-Centered Systems 8
               Mandate for Change: Organizations and Systems Respond 11
               The Challenge: From Administrators and Managers to
                  Leadership in Administration 14
               The Mission is Health: What It Means for You 15
               Education for Leadership in Administration 17

Chapter 2   **Management Effectiveness** 19
               David B. Starkweather and Donald G. Shropshire

               Introduction 19
               The Basics of Management 20
               Special Characteristics of Health Care Management 27
               Additional Special Characteristics 31

Effective Leadership 39
The Future of Management 42

Chapter 3   Managing Quality **45**
Daniel R. Longo and Donald W. Avant

Introduction 45
Management Principles 45
History 46
Program Management 49
The Future of Quality Management 57

**Chapter 4   Knowledge for the Leadership of Continual Improvement
in Health Care** **60**
Paul B. Batalden and Thomas W. Nolan

Traditional Improvement and Underlying Knowledge 60
Quality in Health Care 61
Prerequisites for Continual Improvement 63
Activities for Leaders 68
Conclusion 71

Chapter 5   Organizational Learning **73**
Barbara P. McCool

Introduction 73
Management Principles 74
Organizational Role and Function 75
Resource Requirements 80
The Future of Human Resource Development 81
Conclusion 83

Part II   Organization and Management **85**

Chapter 6   The Organization and Financing of Health Care Services **87**
Gerard F. Anderson and Stephanie L. Maxwell

Introduction 87
Management Principles 88
Health System Organization 88
Health System Financing 96
The Future of Health Care Organization and Financing 100

Chapter 7   Organizational Designs for Health Care **103**
G. Ross Baker, Lutchmie Narine, and Peggy Leatt

Introduction 103
Management Principles 104

Major Determinants of Organizational Design in Health Care 104
Choosing Organizational Designs 106
Functional and Divisional Organizational Designs 107
Matrix Organizations 111
Program Management 111
Conclusion 116

Chapter 8 **Managed Care's Evolving Role** **118**
Gordon D. Brown, Kenneth Bopp, and Michael R. Soper

Introduction 118
History and Background 119
Managed Care Organization Models 121
Organization and Management Structure 126
Managing Unit Costs 136
Managing Utilization 140
The Management of Quality 145
The Future of Managed Care 146

Chapter 9 **Multiunit Systems** **150**
Steven R. Orr

Introduction 150
Organizational Role and Function 150
Leveraging the Multiunit System 153
Common Focus and Directed Momentum 155
Asset Maximization 157

Chapter 10 **Governance** **160**
James E. Orlikoff

Governance Principles and Functions 160
Role of Governance in the Health System 160
Profile of Hospital Governing Boards 164
Governance Roles, Responsibilities, and Functions 167
Quality Management 172
Issues in Governance 174
The Future of Governance 178

Chapter 11 **Physician Organization and Management** **182**
Rockwell Schulz and Donald E. Detmer

Introduction 182
The Role of the Physician 183
Resource Requirements 188
Quality Management 192
The Future of Physician Organization and Management 194

Chapter 12   **Nursing Organization and Management** **204**
Joan Gygax Spicer and Diane E. Nitta

Introduction 204
Functions, Activities, and Processes 204
Management Principles 205
The Organizational Role and Function of Nursing 205
Organizational Structure 208
Resource Requirements 213
Managing Quality 219
Worldwide Challenges for Nursing Leaders 222
Conclusion 224

Part III   **Information Management and Planning** **227**

Chapter 13   **Information Systems Management** **229**
Charles J. Austin and Richard C. Howe

Introduction 229
Management Principles 230
Organizational Role 231
Organizational Relationships 235
Planning and Managing Information Systems 237
Resource Requirements 245
Quality Management 248
The Future of Information Systems Management 249

Chapter 14   **Clinical Data Systems** **252**
Edward J. Hinman

Introduction 252
Management Principles 253
Organizational Role 253
Functions of Clinical Data Systems 255
Clinical Information Applications 259
Quality Management 260
Legal and Ethical Issues 261
The Future of Clinical Data Systems 264

Chapter 15   **External Information Management** **267**
Homer H. Schmitz and Charles A. James

Introduction 267
Management Principles 268
Public Accountability 268
Monitoring the External Environment 271
Ethics and Confidentiality 275

| | Quality Management | 278 |
| | The Future of External Information Management | 280 |

Chapter 16 **Financial Planning and Mangement** **283**
David J. Fine and Rohn J. Butterfield

	Introduction	283
	Management Principles	283
	The Evolution of Health Care Financing	284
	Organizing the Finance Function	289
	The Finance Functions	290
	Quality Considerations: The Audit Function	304
	Managing and Planning for Capital Investment	305
	The Future of Financial Planning and Management	308

Chapter 17 **Strategic Planning and Marketing** **311**
Trevor A. Fisk

	Introduction	311
	Functions	311
	Management Principles	314
	Organizational Role and Function	314
	Planning Activities	316
	Marketing Activities	322
	Resource Requirements	326
	Quality Management	327
	The Future of Strategic Planning and Marketing	328

Part IV **Resource Management** **333**

Chapter 18 **Human Resource Management** **335**
Laura Avakian

	The Functions of the Human Resources Department	335
	Management Principles	336
	Organizational Role and Function	336
	Tasks and Responsibilities	338
	Legal and Contractual Responsibilities	345
	Organization and Employee Development	350
	Resource Requirements	353
	Quality Management	356
	The Future of Human Resource Management	358

Chapter 19 **Materials Management** **361**
Walter J. Wentz

| | Functions | 361 |
| | Management Principles | 362 |

Purchasing 363
Receiving and Stores 370
Distribution 373
Processing 374
Control 376
Organizational Function 378
Resource Requirements 380
Quality Management 382
The Future of Materials Management 384

Chapter 20   **Pharmacy Services** **386**
William A. Gouveia

Introduction 386
Management Principles 386
Organizational Roles and Functions 387
Drug Information and Education 388
Drug Procurement, Receiving, and Storage 392
Drug Preparation and Distribution 393
Clinical Pharmacy Services and Pharmaceutical Care 396
Teaching and Research 397
Resource Requirements 397
Quality Management 398
Performance Indicators 398
The Future of Pharmacy Services 400

Chapter 21   **Food and Nutritional Services** **405**
M. Rosita Schiller, Kay N. Wolf, and Judy L. Miller

Introduction 405
Major Functions 406
Management Principles 406
Organizational Structure 407
Resource Requirements 420
Quality Controls 424
The Future of Food Service Management 425
Conclusion 429

Chapter 22   **Facilities Planning and Construction** **433**
Robert Douglass

Introduction 433
Management Principles 434
The Role of Management 435
Planning and Design 437
Construction 454
Quality Management 463

Chapter 23 **Technology Assessment and Management** **470**
Thomas E. Skorup

Introduction 470
Technology Assessment 471
Strategic Technology Planning 474
Technology Acquisition 476
Technology Management 476
Technology Audits 484
The Future of Technology Assessment and Management 485

Chapter 24 **Housekeeping and Environmental Services** **487**
Paul A. Johnson

Introduction 487
Management Principles 488
Organizational Role and Function 488
Resource Management 492
Quality Management 496
The Future of Housekeeping and Environmental Services 496

Chapter 25 **Safety and Security** **501**
Allan McLean and Fredrick G. Roll

Introduction 501
Safety 502
Security 510
The Future of Safety and Security Management 521

Chapter 26 **Risk and Insurance Management** **523**
Aaron Liberman

Introduction 523
Management Principles 524
Health Services Organizations and Litigation 525
Implications for the Delivery of Health Services 526
Management of Risk 527
Preventive Measures 528
The Insurance Marketplace 529
Quality Management of Risk 535
Risk Management Involvement in Evaluating Clinical Records 537
The Role of the Risk Manager in Establishing Contractual Relationships ... 538
The Role of the CEO in Establishing a Risk Management Program 538
The Future of Risk and Insurance Management 538

Chapter 27 **Legal Services** **540**
David Warren and Douglas Hastings

Introduction 540
Management Principles 540

The Role of Lawyers and Legal Services in Health Services Management 541
Legal Issues in Health Services Management 544
Resource Requirements 553
Quality Management and Legal Services 556
Managing Legal Resources in the Future 557

Part V   Health Service Access and Delivery **559**

Chapter 28   Accessing Health Care **561**
              Stephen J. Williams

              Introduction 561
              Measuring Access 562
              Access and System Structure 567
              Mechanisms to Inhibit and Encourage Access 569
              Access, Integration of Services, Financing, and Government 571
              Access: The Policy and Management Concerns 574
              Access in the Future 577

Chapter 29   Primary Care Services **579**
              Frederick J. Wenzel

              Introduction 579
              Organization of Primary Care Services 580
              Primary Care Group Practice Clinics 582
              Quality Management 584
              The Future of Primary Care 585
              Conclusion 587

Chapter 30   Acute Care Services **589**
              John H. Westerman and Robert J. Taylor

              Introduction 589
              Foundations of Acute Care 590
              Impact on Acute Care and Hospitals 593
              The Future of Acute Care 595
              Quality Management 595

Chapter 31   Specialty Diagnostic and Therapeutic Services **597**
              Michael B. Shirk

              Introduction 597
              The Organizational Role of Specialty Services 598
              Managing Human Resources 601
              Management of Technological Resources 605
              The Future of Specialty Services 607

Chapter 32   **Mental Health Services** **611**
Saul Feldman and Eric N. Goplerud

    Introduction 611
    Inpatient Mental Health Services 614
    Alternatives to Inpatient Treatment 616
    Personnel 618
    Characteristics of Mental Health Administration 619

Chapter 33   **Continuum of Care** **623**
Kenneth D. Bopp, Gordon D. Brown, and Robert H. Daugherty

    Introduction 623
    Management Principles 623
    The Changing Context of Illness 624
    Organizationa and Managment Implications 626
    Network Coordination and Financing 633
    The Continuum of Care in the Future 635

Index **641**

Editors and Advisors

Editor

Robert J. Taylor, MHA, FACHE
President
Taylor Associates International
Washington, DC

Assistant Editor

Susan B. Taylor
Vice President
Taylor Associates International
Washington, DC

Associate Editor

Gary L. Filerman, PhD
The Pew Health Professions
    Commission
Washington, DC

Contributing Editor

John T. Foster, MHA, FACHE
Keene, New Hampshire

Advisors

Mary L. Berg, MHA
Area Administrator
Kaiser Permanente Health Care
    Program
Kensington, Maryland

Manuel A. Bobenreith, MD
Senior Faculty, Andalucin School of
    Public Health
University of Granada
Granada, Spain

Thomas W. Chapman, MHA,
    FACHE
President and Chief Executive
    Officer
Greater Southeast Healthcare System
Washington, DC

William A. Gravely, Jr., MHA,
    FACHE
President
Culpeper Memorial Hospital
Culpeper, Virginia

William M. Moss, MHA, FACHE
President
Potomac Hospital
Woodbridge, Virginia

Fred C. Munson, PhD
Professor, Organizational Theory
    and Analysis
Department of Health Services
    Management and Policy
University of Michigan
Ann Arbor, Michigan

Charles O. Pannenborg, MD
Division Chief, Population and
    Human Resources, African
    Region
Occidental and Central Africa
    Department
The World Bank
Washington, DC

Robert Patterson, MD
Baxter Health Care Corporation
Deerfield, Illinois

Jorge Peña, MPH
Regional Advisor
Health Development Technology
Pan American Health Organization/
    World Health Organization
Washington, DC

Bernardo Ramirez, MD
Vice President
Association of University Programs
    in Health Administration
Arlington, Virginia

Cornell Scott
Executive Director
Hill Health Corporation
New Haven, Connecticut

Kent Stevens, MS, MPH
President
Berkeley Medical Group
Percellville, Virginia

Contributors

Gerard F. Anderson, PhD
Director, Johns Hopkins Center for
 Hospital Finance and Management
Baltimore, Maryland

Charles J. Austin, PhD
Professor and Chairman, Department
 of Health Services Administration
School of Health Related Professions
University of Alabama at
 Birmingham
Birmingham, Alabama

Laura Avakian, MA
Vice President, Human Resources
Beth Israel Hospital
Boston, Massachusetts

Donald W. Avant, MSPH
Health Care Consultant
McKinleyville, California

G. Ross Baker, PhD
Assistant Professor, Department of
 Health Administration
University of Toronto
Toronto, Ontario

Paul B. Batalden, MD
Vice President for Medical Care
Head of Quality Research Group
Hospital Corporation of America
Nashville, Tennessee

Kenneth D. Bopp, PhD
Assistant Professor, Health Services
 Management
University of Missouri
Columbia, Missouri

Gordon D. Brown, PhD
Professor and Director, Health
 Services Management
University of Missouri
Columbia, Missouri

Rohn J. Butterfield, MBA
Vice President for Operations and
 Chief Operating Officer
St. Francis Medical Center
Monroe, Louisiana

Robert H. Daugherty, MSSW
Clinical Professor, Health Services
 Management Program
University of Missouri
Columbia, Missouri

Donald E. Detmer, MD
Vice President and Provost for Health
 Sciences
University of Virginia
Charlottesville, Virginia

Robert Douglass, FAIA
Founder, Robert Douglass
 Associates, Healthcare
 Consultants
Cambridge, Massachusetts

Saul Feldman, PhD
Chairman of the Board and Chief
 Executive Officer
U.S. Behavioral Health
Emeryville, California

Gary L. Filerman, PhD
The Pew Health Professions
 Commission
Washington, DC

David J. Fine, MHA
Professor and Chairman, Department
 of Health Systems Management
School of Public Health and Tropical
 Medicine

Tulane University
Vice Chancellor and Chief Executive
   Officer
Tulane University Clinic
New Orleans, Louisiana

Trevor A. Fisk
Vice President of External Relations
   (deceased)
Thomas Jefferson University
Philadelphia, Pennsylvania

Eric N. Goplerud, PhD
Director, Division of Planning, Policy
   and Evaluation
Substance Abuse, Mental Health
   Services Administration
U.S. Department of Health and
   Human Services
Rockville, Maryland

William A. Gouveia, MS
Director of Pharmacy
New England Medical Center
Associate Scientist
The Health Institute
Clinical Professor
Massachusetts College of Pharmacy
   and Allied Health Sciences
Assistant Professor
Tufts University School of Medicine
Boston, Massachusetts

Douglas Hastings, JD
Associate, Epstein, Becker & Green,
   PC
Attorneys at Law
Washington, DC

Edward J. Hinman, MD, MPH
Medical Director
Total Health Care, Inc.
Baltimore, Maryland

Richard C. Howe, PhD
Associate Senior Vice President
University of Cincinnati Medical
   Center
Cincinnati, Ohio

Charles A. James, PhD
Professor, Department of Finance
School of Business Administration
Saint Louis University
St. Louis, Missouri

Paul A. Johnson, BA, REH
Director of Housekeeping Services
Cape Fear Valley Medical Center
Fayetteville, North Carolina

Peggy Leatt, PhD
Professor and Chair, Department of
   Health Administration
Faculty of Medicine
University of Toronto
Toronto, Ontario

Aaron Liberman, PhD, FACHE
Consultant
Midlothian, Virginia

Daniel R. Longo, PhD
Professor
University of Missouri School of
   Medicine
Columbia, Missouri

Stephanie L. Maxwell, ScD (cand.)
Research Associate
Johns Hopkins Center for Hospital
   Finance and Management
Baltimore, Maryland

Barbara P. McCool
President
Strategic Management Services, Inc.
Washington, DC

Allan McLean
Director of Safety (retired)
University of Chicago Hospitals
Chicago, Illinois

Judy L. Miller, PhD, MBA, RD
Professor and Department Head
Hotel, Restaurant, Institution
   Management, and Dietetics
University of Kansas
Manhattan, Kansas

Lutchmie Narine, MSc
Doctoral Candidate, Department of
   Health Administration
University of Toronto
Toronto, Ontario

Diane E. Nitta, MA, RN, CNAA
Associate Administrator of Patient
   Care Services
Director of Nursing
Valley Medical Center
Fresno, California
Assistant Clinical Professor, School
   of Nursing
University of California, San
   Francisco
San Francisco, California

Thomas W. Nolan, PhD
Associates in Process Improvements
Silver Spring, Maryland

James E. Orlikoff, MA
President, Orlikoff & Associates
Chicago, Illinois
Trustee, South Suburban Hospital
Hazel Crest, Illinois

Steven R. Orr
President
Lutheran Health Systems
Fargo, North Dakota

Fredrick G. Roll, MA
Director of Security
Hospital Shared Services
   of Colorado
Denver, Colorado

M. Rosita Schiller, PhD, RD, LD
Professor and Director, Medical
   Dietetics Division
The Ohio State University
Columbia, Ohio

Homer H. Schmitz, PhD
Associate Professor, Department of
   Finance
School of Business Administration

Saint Louis University
St. Louis, Missouri

Rockwell Schulz, PhD
Professor, Department of Preventive
  Medicine
University of Wisconsin-Madison
Madison, Wisconsin

Michael B. Shirk, MBA, BS
President, Boone Hospital Center
Member, Christian Health System
Columbia, Missouri

Donald G. Shropshire, PhD
President and Chief Executive Officer
TMCare Corporation
Tucson, Arizona

Thomas E. Skorup
Healthcare Consultant
ERCI
Plymouth Meeting, Pennsylvania

Michael R. Soper, MD
National Medical Director and Senior
  Vice President
National Medical Department
CIGNA Healthplan, Inc.
Bloomfield, Connecticut

Joan Gygax Spicer, MSN, MBA, RN, CNAA
Assistant Director, Department of
  Nursing
Assistant Clinical Professor
School of Nursing
University of California, San
  Francisco
San Francisco, California

David B. Starkweather, PhD
Professor of Health Services
  Management
School of Public Health
University of California, Berkeley
Berkeley, California

Robert J. Taylor, MHA
President
Taylor Associates International
Washington, DC

David G. Warren, J.D.
Professor, Health Law and Ethics
Department of Health
  Administration
Duke University
Durham, North Carolina

Walter J. Wentz, PhD
University Professor of Health
  Administration
Governors State University
University Park, Illinois

Frederick J. Wenzel, MBA
Executive Director
Marshfield Clinic
Marshfield, Wisconsin

John H. Westerman
Interim President
Association of University
  Programs in Health
  Administration
Arlington, Virginia

Stephen J. Williams, ScD
Professor and Head, Division of
  Health Services Administration
Graduate School of Public Health
San Diego State University
San Diego, California

Kay N. Wolf, MS, RD, LD
Instructor, Medical Dietetics Division
The Ohio State University
Columbus, Ohio

Consultants

The editors and contributors gratefully acknowledge the assistance and advice of the following individuals in the preparation of this book.

William E. Aaronson, PhD
Associate Professor of Health
 Administration
School of Business and Management
Temple University
Philadelphia, Pennsylvania

Gary Aden
Executive Vice President
American Healthcare System
San Diego, California

Barbara Arrington, PhD, FACHE
Department of Public Health and Health
 Administration
St. Louis University School of Public
 Health
St. Louis, Missouri

William Bain
Dun Britton Enterprises, Inc.
Toronto, Ontario, Canada

Steven D. Baron
President and Chief Executive Officer
The Miriam Hospital
Providence, Rhode Island

Walter E. Barton, MD
Professor of Psychiatry (Active
 Emeritus)
Department of Psychiatry
Dartmouth Medical School
Lebanon, New Hampshire

Thomas E. Batey, AIA
Hospital Corporation of America
 (retired)
Nashville, Tennessee

Jay S. Bauer, FAIA
Bauer and Wiley
Newport Beach, California

Christina Bethell
Senior Policy Analyst
Voluntary Hospitals of America
Chicago, Illinois

Glenn J. Black, Jr.
Vice President, Financial Services
Kennestone Regional Health System
Marietta, Georgia

Hildo Bryan Bolley, MSc
Assistant Professor
Health Management Research Unit
University of Toronto
Toronto, Ontario, Canada

Howard Book, MD
Psychiatrist-in-Chief
Women's College Hospital
Toronto, Ontario, Canada

Steve Brickner
Hospital Corporation of America
Quality Resource Group
Nashville, Tennessee

Carmhiel Brown, MED
Associate Vice President, Marketing and
 Public Relations
Thomas Jefferson University
Philadelphia, Pennsylvania

Montague Brown, DrPH
Chairman
Strategic Management Services, Inc.
Washington, DC

Thomas Allen Bruce, MD
W.K. Kellog Foundation
Battle Creek, Michigan

John J. Buckley, Jr., MBA, FACHE
President
Southern Illinois Healthcare Enterprises,
 Inc.
Carbondale, Illinois

Barbara E. Burke, RN, MSc, CHE
Vice President, Patient Services
St. Paul's Hospital
Vancouver, British Columbia, Canada

Patricia L. Burkett, MSPH
Regional Director of Hazardous
 Materials Compliance
Kaiser Permanente Medical Care
 Program
Oakland, California

George Caldwell
President Emeritus
Lutheran General Health Care System
Park Ridge, Illinois

Roger Camplin
President
Camplin, Bartels & Associates
Chandler, Arizona

Patrick Carroll
Vice President of Consulting Services
McJaul & Lyons, Inc.
Irvine, California

Iain F. Clayre, PhD
CMG Professional Services Corporation
Edmonton, Alberta, Canada

William O. Cleverley, PhD
The Ohio State University
Graduate Program in Hospital and Health
    Service Administration
Columbus, Ohio

Hirsch Cohen
President
University Health Plan
Cincinnati, Ohio

Edward Connors
President
Mercy Health Services
Farmington Hills, MI

Charles P. Conole, MBA, FACHE
Fellow, American College of Healthcare
    Executives
E.J. Noble Hospital
Gouverneur, New York

Neil Crane
Toronto Hospital Corporation
Toronto, Ontario, Canada

Kenneth Cummings, MD
Vice President for Medical Affairs
Saint Joseph Health Center
Kansas City, Missouri

Willy DeGeyndt, PhD
Principal Public Health Specialist
The World Bank
Washington, DC

Dennis Deniger
Vice President, Education Development
The ServiceMaster Company
Downers Grove, Illinois

Bernard Dickens
Professor, Health Law
University of Toronto
Toronto, Ontario, Canada

James R. Diaz, FAIA
Kaplan/McLaughlin/Diaz
San Francisco, California

Kathy Divis
Director of Marketing
University of Pennsylvania Medical
    Center
Philadelphia, Pennsylvania

Mark Doyne, MD
Nashville, TN

Neil Dworkin, PhD
Associate Director
United Hebrew Geriatric Center
New Rochelle, New York

Truman Esmond
President and Chief Executive Officer
Rush-Presbyterian-St. Luke's Health
    Plan
Chicago, Illinois

David Leslie Everhart
Chicago, Illinois

James Falick, FAIA
Falick Klein Partnership
Houston, Texas

Eli S. Feldman, MBA
Executive Vice President and Chief
    Executive Officer
Metropolitan Jewish Geriatric Center
Elderplan, Inc.
Brooklyn, New York

Seri Ferguson, RN, MN
Hospital Corporation of America
Nashville, Tennessee

Peter Fine
Senior Vice President, Operations
Northwestern Memorial Hospital
Chicago, Illinois

Howard Furtaw
Director of the National Board
National Executive Housekeepers
    Association
Westerville, Ohio

Paul Gamble
Director
Hospital Council of Metropolitan
    Toronto
Toronto, Ontario, Canada

Paul Geukers
Vice President and Assistant Executive
    Director
St. Joseph's Hospital
Nashua, New Hampshire

David L. Ginsberg, FAIA
Presbyterian Hospital
New York, New York

Glen H. Gray, MHA
Glendive, Montana

Barry Green, PhD
Professor and Chairman
Graduate Program in Health and Hospital
    Administration
University of Florida
Gainesville, Florida

Edgar A. Hager, MHSc
Occupational and Environmental Health
    and Safety
University Hospital
London, Ontario, Canada

George Harlow
Marshfield Hills, Massachussetts

James Hart
Health Resources Northwest
Seattle, Washington

Sally Hart
District Manager
Marriott Corporation Health Care
    Services
Washington Crossing, Pennsylvania

James E. Hartfield, MD
Associate Vice President
Associate Dean for Clinical Affairs
University of South Florida Health
    Sciences Center
Tampa, Florida

Gretchen Jane Hartman, MS, RD, LD
Food Service Consultant
Towson, Maryland

George T. Heery, FAIA
The Brookwood Group, Inc.
Atlanta, Georgia

John Henry
Administrator
Crawford Long Hospital
Emory University
Atlanta, Georgia

Jane Hirsch
Associate Director of Nursing
University of California Medical Center-
  San Francisco
San Francisco, California

Scott Hoffman, CPA
Genesis Healthcare International
Houston, Texas

Paul Hofmann
Executive Vice President and Chief
  Operating Officer
Alta Bates Corporation
Emeryville, California

Edward Hollowell
Hollowell, Eldridge & Ingersoll
Raleigh, North Carolina

John Horty
Horty, Springer & Mattern
Pittsburgh, Pennsylvania

Edith Hughes
Edmonton, Alberta, Canada

B. Jon Jaeger, PhD
Department of Health Administration
Duke University
Durham, North Carolina

Richard Jelinek, PhD
Chairman of the Board
Medicus Systems Corporation
Evanston, Illinois

Beth Johnson
Director, Quality Assessment and Risk
  Management
Sunnybrook Medical Centre
North York, Ontario, Canada

L.R. Jordan, MA, FACHE
President Emeritus
Miami Valley Hospital
Professor of Health Services
  Administration
University of Alabama at Birmingham
Birmingham, Alabama

Mohamed A. Karmali, MB.ChB,
  MRCP, FRCP, FRCP (C)
Microbiologist-in-Chief
The Hospital for Sick Children
Professor, Department of Microbiology
University of Toronto
Toronto, Ontario, Canada

Jack Kasten, JD, MPH
Lecturer, Department of Health Policy
  and Management
Harvard School of Public Health
Boston, Massachusetts

Paul Kennon, FAIA
Houston, Texas

John Kress
Director, Long Term Health
Association of University Programs in
  Health Administration
Arlington, Virginia

William Kreykes
President and Chief Executive Officer
Rhode Island Hospital
Providence, Rhode Island

Andrew A. Lasser, DrPH
Adjunct Professor
Oklahoma Medical Center
College of Public Health
Oklahoma City, Oklahoma

Merlin Lickhalter, AIA
Stone, Marracini, and Patterson
St. Louis, Missouri

Emmett Lorey, MD
Associate Medical Director (retired)
Permanente Medical Group
Oakland, California

Donald Lovasz
Divisional Vice President
SSM Health Care System
St. Louis, Missouri

Jeff Lozon
President
Glenrose Rehabilitation Hospital
Edmonton, Alberta, Canada

Murray Mackenzie
President
North York General Hospital
North York, Ontario, Canada

Joseph Mapa, DHA, FACHE, CHE
Executive Vice President and Chief
  Operating Officer
Mount Sinai Hospital
Toronto, Ontario, Canada

James McCarthy
Vice President for Human Resouces
Tucson Medical Center
Tucson, Arizona

Ron McQueen
Associate Professor
University of Toronto
Toronto, Ontario, Canada

Gary Mecklenburg
President
Northwestern Memorial Hospital
Chicago, Illinois

Norman Metzger, MA
Edmond A. Guggenheim Professor
  Emeritus
The Mount Sinai School of Medicine
New York, New York

Vytas Mickevicius
Vice President and Chief Operating
  Officer
The Toronto Hospital
Toronto, Ontario, Canada

John Miller
Chief Executive Officer
Alabama Quality Assurance Fund
Birmingham, Alabama

James Moon, PhD
Executive Assistant to the Vice President
University of Alabama-Birmingham
Birmingham, Alabama

William M. Moss, MHA, FACHE
President
Potomac Hospital
Woodbridge, Virginia

Eugene C. Nelson, DSc, MPH
Director, Quality Care Research,
  Measurement and Education
Dartmouth-Hitchcock Medical Center
Lebanon, New Hampshire

Clifford A. Nordal, BSc, MBA, FCCHSE
President
The Queen Elizabeth Hospital
Toronto, Ontario, Canada

Preface

Health services management is a unique profession, differing significantly from the field of general management—with its own challenges, approaches, and techniques. More than ever before, health service managers work under financial constraints and in a dynamic political environment that challenge the limits of their understandings and knowledge. Familiar managerial approaches fall short, historic relationships are altered, and new approaches threaten traditional organizational structures and the manager's role.

As a result, health service managers are continually seeking information on how to address, organize, and resolve a wide array of contemporary managerial issues. While a vast health management literature exists, it is difficult for the practitioner to filter through the overwhelming volume of information to find answers to management questions. *The AUPHA Manual of Health Services Management* has already done much of this job. The Manual is a single, comprehensive source of information on a broad range of health management issues, functions, and activities. It provides practical information on leadership, organizational approaches, functional activities, and management principles that are integrated into a comprehensive, meaningful whole. By

emphasizing basic managerial concepts, the Manual reinforces the essence of the manager's purpose—community service, accessible quality health care, and financial responsibility.

Those who aspire to managerial positions in hospitals, clinics, nursing homes, and other health service organizations will be well served by the Manual's comprehensive view and stress on fundamentals. The book will be especially helpful for students in health management and others entering the managerial ranks who wish to gain a quick grasp of the profession. In addition, board members, auxilians, and regulatory agency personnel will find the Manual a useful reference. Those who have received formal training in management will find the Manual a concise refresher.

The Manual is divided into five parts: Leadership, Organization and Management, Information Management and Planning, Resource Management, and Health Service Access and Delivery. Each chapter has been written to address a core subject or issue in health services management. For ease of reference all chapters are structured similarly. In addition, to illustrate continuity among subject areas, a few important themes are reflected in all chapters. Chapters begin with a statement of purpose or thesis and a synopsis of the chapter's content. Early in each chapter fundamental managerial principles are introduced—concepts that are universally applicable and helpful reminders of what is really important to managerial understanding. Each chapter also includes a discussion of quality management—as it fits into the organization's overall quality management program and the specifics of how it applies in the chapter's subject area. Each chapter also looks to the future—identifying trends that will shape the subject or issue in the years ahead. Chapters conclude with a list of suggested additional resources (organizations, books, and periodicals) that expand on themes introduced in the Manual. For easy reference a comprehensive topical index is provided at the end of the book.

We anticipate that *The AUPHA Manual of Health Services Management* will be a growing and evolving resource. Future editions will build on the beginning offered in this volume. As the practice of health service management changes, we expect our understanding of managerial concepts and principles to evolve as well. The Association of University Programs in Health Administration (AUPHA) welcomes your suggestions on how future editions can be shaped and expanded to meet your needs.

The Manual was developed over a period of four years, through a lengthy process of development and review, involving the contribution and critique of numerous experts. It would not be possible to acknowledge the nature and extent of each individual's contribution, but preceding this preface we have listed the many advisors, contributors, and consultants whom we wish to thank for their energy, hard work, and support.

The concept and contents of the Manual were developed under the direction of an AUPHA Editorial Advisory Committee composed of representatives of academia and management practice. Authors were selected for their demonstrated knowledge, management experience, and their communications ability. Each author's chapter outline was reviewed by selected authorities for currency and completeness. Draft manuscripts were reviewed by additional consultants, as well as by the editorial staff, for practicality, comprehensiveness, and clarity of thought. Most chapters went through several revisions. When completed, the entire manuscript was reviewed, resulting in further refinements. Still, in a work of this magnitude, there is much of value that has been excluded, and other points which we did not get quite right. For these omissions and errors we take full responsibility.

One organization in particular played a central role in the Manual's creation and preparation. The need for the Manual emerged from the work of the AUPHA as the world's leading organization devoted to improving the quality of health managerial education and practice. The AUPHA occupies a unique vantage point from which to observe the challenges faced by health service managers worldwide.

Robert J. Taylor
Susan B. Taylor
Washington, DC

Part I

Leadership

Gary L. Filerman

Health: The Emerging Context of Management

1

INTRODUCTION

Managing health services is one of the most challenging, consequential, and complex roles in modern society. The challenge is to provide affordable, appropriate, and high-quality services in the face of many obstacles. It is a consequential role because many management decisions ultimately affect the quality of life of individuals and of the community. The manager's role is especially complex because of the unique characteristics of the process of producing and providing health services, the relationship of the principal provider (the physician) to that process, and the difficulty of assessing the quality of the services rendered.

Professional health services administrators are successfully meeting the challenge every day. They have mastered the personal skills and developed the organizational capacity necessary to manage the internal and external forces impacting their organizations. Many are also providing organizational and community leadership. That is, they are managing (maintaining their organizations and achieving organizational objectives) and also leading (getting everyone in their organizations and communities behind a vision of a preferred future).

For health services administrators to become leaders, it is essential they understand the challenges facing health services, the strengths and the weaknesses of their organizations, and how their organizations relate to the changing health services system and to the social and political forces shaping the system. Leaders grow in effectiveness by assessing their own strengths and weaknesses. They continuously expand their knowledge and enhance their skills. This manual is a concise guide to how the health services delivery challenge is changing and to the administrators' mandate for leadership.

There are ten interrelated challenges facing today's health services managers, and all of them are embodied in society's conflicting health and medical care objectives. In the next decade, health services managers must do the following:

1. Embrace the concept of community-oriented (primary) health care and redirect the missions and roles of health organizations and professionals toward supporting this concept.
2. Improve the process of making public policy on health issues through the appropriate application of objective health services research.

3

3. Guide curative care services toward maximizing their potential contribution, as part of a comprehensive health care system, to the achievement of the global mission of health for all.

4. Lead the effort to establish broad support and commitment to continuous improvement in the quality of all health services.

5. Establish universal accessibility to appropriate and affordable quality health care services.

6. Organize the provision of proven, cost-effective solutions, such as clean water, immunization, and nutrition, to known health problems and risks.

7. Invest in technologies that are cost-effective for the community as well as the organization.

8. Design and implement programs promoting changes in individual behavior that lead to improved personal health.

9. Develop and implement improved managerial methods and techniques that maximize the productivity of the human, material, and financial resources devoted to improving health.

10. Improve methods and technologies for using information for decision making.

The organization and financing of health services are changing rapidly as leaders in government, business, and health care try to accommodate conflicting technical, social, and economic pressures. All of the familiar health services organizations have been swept into the process of change, and new kinds of organizations are emerging. Through all of the change there is one constant—the increasing recognition that competent management is essential in every organization and program and at every level. As a result, there is a global trend toward strengthening management resources and expanding managerial influence in organizing and operating health services. Health services in the twenty-first century will clearly be managerially driven (see Figure 1-1).

Managerial decisions directly affecting the quality of life in the community include decisions regarding (1) which services are *available* and which are not available, (2) the *cost* of services, (3) their *quality*, (4) the *effectiveness* with which the services are coordinated, and (5) the *humaneness* with which the services are provided. It is increasingly clear that expensive resources must be managed so that there is a direct relationship between how much is invested and the community benefit (as measured by the improved health status of the community).

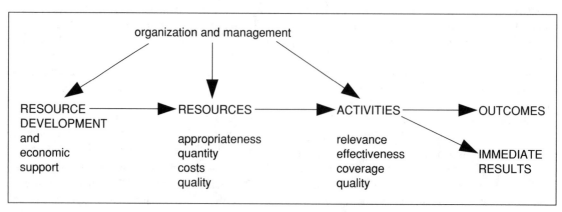

Figure 1-1 The Managerially Driven Health System. *Source:* Adapted from *Quality Assessment and Assurance in Primary Care* by M.I. Roemer and C. Montoya-Aguilar, p. 5, with permission of The World Health Organization, © 1988.

The definition of community benefit involves values. Health services administrators can focus attention on the social values that are at stake in health services decision-making processes and have the managerial skills that organizations need to realize those values. This chapter examines

- the pressures for fundamental changes in how health resources are invested
- how the universal recognition of the need for more emphasis on primary health care services is shaping the future of all health services
- the emerging role of health services administrators in ensuring that quality primary health care is available to everyone
- how health services administrators can develop the skills and values necessary to successfully manage change and influence its direction

THE PRESSURES FOR CHANGE

Every country is attempting to rationalize its investment in health services, and a clear consensus is emerging to try to achieve "health for all by the year 2000." Regardless of where a country is on the scale of economic development, the goal of "health for all" embodies the philosophy that, in a just society, access to affordable health services is a right, that health services must serve all citizens, and that quality must be continually improved.

In the industrialized countries, the progress of medical science has generated expectations that translate into public support for a continuously increasing flow of resources to health- and medical care–related activities. However, the rate of increase in the cost of providing care is now surpassing the rate of increase in the ability to pay for it. As a result, all countries are facing the fact that resources to purchase health and medical care are limited and that the objective of achieving health for all as a right is a complex challenge. This point is made by Margaret Catley-Carlson in the following quotation:

Once people understand how many factors determine an individual's health status, they will more readily accept that spending additional funds on health care may not be the best way to improve our health status. We are probably in what economists call the "flat of the curve," where increases in health care spending no longer produce increases in the quality of our health.

Economists also talk about "opportunity costs." Every additional dollar we spend on health care is a dollar not spent on other determinants of our health. Spending those extra dollars on health care bothers me enormously because I worry a great deal about competitiveness. There is a 3 percent difference between the amounts of their GNPs that Canada and Japan devote to health care. Japan devotes that extra 3 percent to education, higher forms of technical training, research, and becoming more competitive. If we could redirect our resources in a similar manner, the resulting increase in our prosperity might well improve the health status of many.[1]

Health has been defined by the World Health Organization as "a state of complete physical, mental, and social well-being and not merely the absence of disease or infirmity."[2] Achieving that high level of health in any population depends on solving many problems that are outside of the traditional domains of health and medical care providers and service organizations. As research demonstrates how personal behavior, economic status, education, housing, and other social factors significantly affect health status, there is increasing support for improving the health of the community by investing directly in those sectors. There is also increasing competition for resources among these sectors. Leaders in health services must help communities invest their limited resources wisely and guide the efforts of the health sector to claim the share of resources proportional to its contribution to improving health status.

For purposes of discussion, it is helpful to distinguish between medical care and health services. Medical care services diagnose, provide treatment, rehabilitate, and hopefully cure individuals. Health services focus upon promoting healthy behavior and protecting health and preventing disease in communities. To the extent possible, medical care overcomes the effects of the failures of health services. Most providers of care and their support systems pursue health and medical care objectives through organizations that plan, regulate, provide, and finance services. In virtually all societies, most of the energies and resources of such organizations are devoted primarily to providing medical care, although they are typically described as health organizations.

The global dilemma is that no country has or will have sufficient resources to accomplish all of its health promotion, protection, and medical care objectives. In any society, health for all can be achieved only by increasing the resources directed to all of the social conditions that affect health and by improving the cost-effectiveness (productivity) of the resources devoted to health and medical care.

Health professionals have an important role to play in resolving the dilemma. It is increasingly clear that the education and training of physicians and other health practitioners is often out of balance with societal needs. The explosion of biomedical knowledge and the increasing availability of sophisticated technology have caused professional education to focus upon curative solutions at whatever cost. The intellectual satisfaction derived from improved diagnosis and treatment (the caregiver's perspective) and the desire to benefit from more effective medical interventions (the patient's perspective) have pushed the medical care system toward highly specialized, fragmented, technology-based tertiary care.

The reality of the limits of economic growth in the face of rising public expectations has increasingly focused attention on the dilemma of providing health and medical care. The hard investment choices facing societies are being clarified and their implications debated with unprecedented intensity. Increased public understanding of the seriousness and implications of these choices has made health services and medical care provision a major area of public policy. Managing the changes that will result from emerging public policy will be the most significant and consequential responsibility of health services administrators in the 1990s and beyond. It will require broad knowledge of issues and options, advocacy skills, and new approaches to management.

RESOURCES AND HEALTH SYSTEMS

The term *health system* loosely describes all the resources a country devotes to health promotion, disease prevention, and medical care, including health organizations and their relationships (see Figure 1-2). Health systems continually evolve in response to changes in the following:

- Demographic and disease patterns of populations.
- Public policies regarding medical care quality, equity, access, cost-effectiveness, concern for the health of the public (particularly the labor force), and public expectations. Policy is often driven by problems of unequal access based on finance, geography, and socioeconomic class.
- The distribution of the economic burden of providing medical care among indirect sources (e.g., taxation and insurance) and direct sources (e.g., the individual and the employer) and the relationship between the economic burden of services and their accessibility.

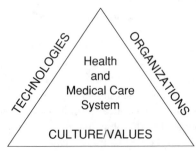

Figure 1-2 A national health and medical care system is the product of the country's culture, technology, and organizations.

- The political power of physicians relative to the power of governments, consumers, and, in some countries, hospitals and other service providers.
- Technical and biomedical developments that shape organizational roles; manpower definitions, roles, and needs; quality standards; resource investment patterns; and the costs of services.

One of the important characteristics of a health system is the degree to which it is centralized. Centralization is a function of the extent of government control or ownership of the system's resources. Many developing countries, whose citizens generally do not have the ability to pay for services, provide health and medical care through systems that are centrally owned and controlled. In such a system, the government defines the relationships among resources (such as physicians and hospitals). In some countries with centralized systems there are small (but growing), private, decentralized systems serving the relatively affluent urban populations.

At the other end of the continuum, the United States has the world's most decentralized system. It is characterized by diverse private and public ownership of health organizations, a wide variety of rapidly changing relationships among health resources, and competition. Laws discourage the interorganizational and resource planning usually associated with centralized systems. The Japanese and British systems and most other European systems are mixtures.

All health systems are shaped by public policies intended to achieve public health and medical care objectives. Developing countries struggle to increase the resources available to the health sector and to invest them wisely. As countries become more industrialized, expenditures for health and medical services tend to rise. They eventually reach a point at which governments struggle to contain the flow of resources to the health sector. In each country, that turning point is determined by political processes that balance priorities for allocating resources among such social objectives as health, education, housing, roads and other infrastructure, income support, and employment. It is essential that health services leaders contribute to that process a broad perspective on community benefit (see Figure 1-3).

Another key characteristic of health systems is the amount of money that countries spend directly on health and medical care. As Gerard Anderson points out in the next chapter, the United States devotes about 12.4 percent of its gross domestic product to health services, the highest percentage in the world.[3] Great Britain expends just over 6 percent with not very different health status results. There is little evidence that, beyond some undefined point, spending more money makes a proportional contribution to improving the health status of the community or to the public's satisfaction with services. Leaders in Great Britain argue that their country being at the low end of the industrial nation expenditure scale does not necessarily mean that its health services are underfinanced. The important question is what the money buys.

The optimal investment would move a country toward achieving health for all by preventing all preventable disease, finding all disease as early as possible, and providing treatment in the most cost-effective way known. Since some countries with relatively low expenditures have the same or better health status and public satisfaction as high-expenditure countries, it appears that resources are buying more health in the former countries (see Table 1-1).

The most significant managerial implication of these input-outcome discrepancies is that many of the objectives that health services administrators have pursued and the means employed to pursue them will not be appropriate for the future. Health and medical care organizations must make substantial changes, and the standards used for measuring their performance will change. The new objectives will focus on how to buy more health by improving living conditions, preventing disease, ensuring early detection, and providing cost-effective treatment. The criterion for successful organizational

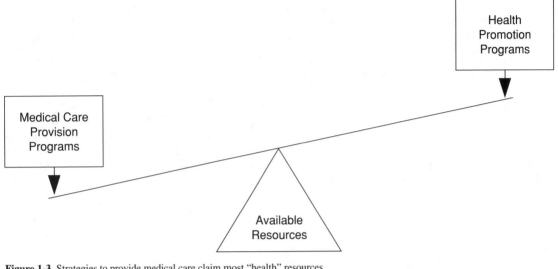

Figure 1-3 Strategies to provide medical care claim most "health" resources.

and managerial performance will be substantial improvement in the health status of the population served (i.e., community benefit).

MANDATE FOR THE FUTURE: PRIMARY HEALTH CARE–CENTERED SYSTEMS

How are the health and medical care needs of individuals to be met by a society that attempts to respond rationally to the resource allocation dilemma? There is increasing agreement that the answer is to ensure access to effective primary health care.

It is important to distinguish between primary care and primary health care. The term *primary care* usually refers to the front-line point of first contact with the medical care system. Most primary care is passive and reactive, designed to respond to the needs of sick people who come to the caregiver. The first step in improving the medical care system is to ensure access to high-quality, affordable primary care. Ideally, primary care services go beyond being merely reactive. They should reach out to the family, provide continuity, and promote prevention. Unfortunately, as of this writing, the incen-

tives in the American health finance systems do not encourage such an expanded mission.

There are many descriptions of what primary care services include and how they are organized, accessed, and related to secondary or tertiary services. This description is typical:

> In ideal primary care, an appropriately trained health professional or team provides most of the preventive and curative care for an individual or family over a significant period of time, coordinates any services that must be sought from other health professionals, and integrates and explains the patient's or family's overall health problems and care, giving adequate attention to their psychological and social dimensions.
>
> Today, a primary-care doctor or team can still provide most of the care that is necessary most of the time, but complications or new problems at times will require the expertise of others. Coordination can be assured if the primary provider assesses the situation, helps the patient with an appropriate referral, and then integrates the outcome of the referral into the patient's ongoing care."[4]

This primary care provider's role is the modern sequel to the role of the family general practitioner, although the primary care provider is more con-

Table 1-1 Three Health Systems: Comparative Facts at a Fingertip

Type of System	United States: Mixed Private/Public	Canada: Government Insurance	Great Britain: National Health Service
Population (000)	240,856	25,625	56,458
Per Capita Health Spending	$1,926	$1,370	$711
Health as % of GNP	11.1%	8.5%	6.2%
Life Expectancy, 1985 (years at birth)	74.7	76.5	74.8
Infant Mortality, 1985 (rate per 1,000 births)	10.6	7.9	9.4

Data are from 1986.

Source: Reprinted with permission from *Health Management Quarterly,* a publication of the Baxter Foundation, Vol. 11, No. 1, © 1989.

cerned with coordinating services and promoting health (see Exhibit 1-1).

In contrast, *primary health care* refers to a broader configuration of services reflecting different technology, philosophy, and values. The technology is appropriate to the resources of the society. The philosophy is that the interests of the individual are best served when the provider is close to and familiar with the individual's daily life and community. The value system holds that proactive preventive action, which reduces risks to the community, is more desirable than reactive curative action.

Primary health care has been defined as proactive: "A diversified health care team uses modern technology and resources to actively anticipate health damage and promote well being."[5] Figure 1-4 shows how a primary care (medical) system differs operationally from a primary health care system.

It is often argued that an effective primary health care system saves money in the long run by preventing or by treating illness before it becomes severe, complicated, and expensive. Others argue that the importance of effective primary health care lies in its contribution to improved quality of life, not in cost containment. Both claims are defensible.

The ideal primary health care system for each country depends upon the socioeconomic development and the health status of the population. How the system is organized and its priorities will depend upon the country's sickness patterns and resources. In industrialized countries, there has been rapid expansion of primary care organizations that focus more upon reducing high-cost hospital use than on promot-

Exhibit 1-1 Desirable Characteristics of Primary Care

- Services should be comprehensive (it was suggested that 85 to 95 percent of all services could be delivered by primary care providers) and should address problems of mental health, alcohol and other drug abuse, dental health, and chronic illnesses.
- Services should be coordinated by a primary care physician who assumes the role of case manager and should be linked to special community programs for problems such as HIV/AIDS, substance abuse, and mental illness.
- Services should be tailored to the health problems of the community, including members of the community who do not seek health services, and should be based on an epidemiological perspective, guided by community and patient data and research.
- Services should be sensitive to the community's cultural values, taking into consideration ethnic and racial diversity.
- Services should emphasize prevention and early intervention.
- Services should be provided in a manner that fosters a continuity of association between primary care providers and their clients; the primary care physician should receive feedback from medical specialists and other providers to whom he or she refers patients.

Source: Reprinted from *Observations of the Conferees, Executive Summary, The National Primary Care Conference 1992,* U.S. D.H.H.S., p. 7.

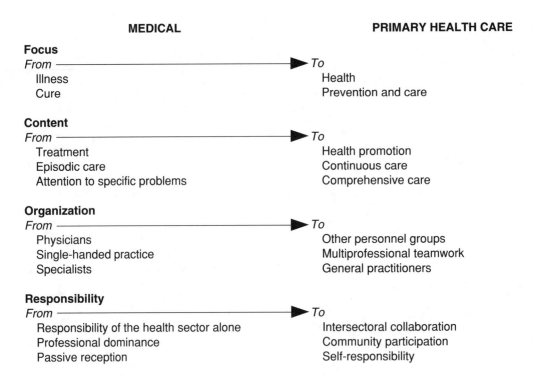

MEDICAL	PRIMARY HEALTH CARE

Focus
From ⟶ *To*

| Illness | Health |
| Cure | Prevention and care |

Content
From ⟶ *To*

Treatment	Health promotion
Episodic care	Continuous care
Attention to specific problems	Comprehensive care

Organization
From ⟶ *To*

Physicians	Other personnel groups
Single-handed practice	Multiprofessional teamwork
Specialists	General practitioners

Responsibility
From ⟶ *To*

Responsibility of the health sector alone	Intersectoral collaboration
Professional dominance	Community participation
Passive reception	Self-responsibility

Figure 1-4 The Change from a Medical-Centered to a Primary Health Care-Centered System. *Source:* Adapted from *Training for Primary Health Care* by H. Vouri, p. 2, with permission of the World Health Organization, © 1984.

ing community health status. In the United States, health maintenance organizations (HMOs) and neighborhood health centers are the best-known examples. They have the potential to evolve into providers of primary health care services. New primary care organizations (HMOs in particular) are also proliferating in some developing countries and entering into direct competition with the well-established hospital and specialty-centered medical systems. This is the case in Chile, Uruguay, Mexico, Brazil, and Indonesia, for example. The proliferation of these organizations is providing a basis for future primary health care systems.

In several countries, there is a substantial investment in managerial research to improve the organization of primary care, increase its impact on community health status, and enhance its relationship to the other parts of the health services system. The implications for management are tremendous be-

cause research is questioning the cost-effectiveness of current systems and generating new ways to plan, manage information, improve quality, organize personnel, use appropriate technology, and coordinate services in support of primary health care. New indicators of management and organizational performance are being developed. It is imperative that managers keep informed about health services research and how to apply its findings in support of organizational change.

The shortage of appropriately trained personnel is a significant barrier to the evolution from medical care to primary care and primary health care systems. The concept of quality held by physicians is a powerful determinant of the mission and priorities of organizations. Physicians' expectations are established by means of an education that is hospital, technology, and specialty centered. There is very little emphasis on primary care and virtually no exposure to the concept of primary health care. There is a pressing need for generalists who can span the boundaries of specialization and health. Education for medicine and the other clinical professions is under increasing pressure to support system reform. Management has the opportunity to contribute to the new perspective by creating incentives and clinical learning opportunities directed toward the primary health care needs of the community.

The American debate about how to solve the health and medical care dilemma is changing. It is moving away from a focus on access to and financing for the present system toward a discussion of fundamental reform. What the public needs and expects is a system that appropriately allocates resources to reduce risks while providing access to quality care at a reasonable cost. Professional, public, and political opinion is converging around the conviction that the best way to achieve that is through a primary health care–centered system. The mandate of leadership in administration is to facilitate change through adjusting organizational missions and roles in response to community needs and desires (see Exhibit 1-2).

Exhibit 1-2 Recommendations of the Sanitary Commission of Massachusetts (1850)

The need for a primary care–centered health system has been clear for over a century.

Recommendations

- Immunization and control of communicable disease
- Promotion of child health
- Improved housing
- Environmental sanitation
- Development of community health workers
- Public health education
- Promoting individual responsibility of health
- Community participation
- Establish multidisciplinary health boards to assess needs and plan programs based on epidemiologic evidence.

Source: Reprinted from *Report of the Sanitary Commission of Massachusetts: 1850* by L. Shattuck et al., Harvard University Press, 1948.

MANDATE FOR CHANGE: ORGANIZATIONS AND SYSTEMS RESPOND

A significant but often underestimated force driving the demand for change is the recurring competition for resources between hospitals and primary care organizations or between hospital-oriented specialists and primary care practitioners. Until the late 1960s, the conflict was muted. The dominant system model in most countries assumed that hospitals and primary care services were complementary elements of a single system, with community general hospitals at the center. It was assumed that family, primary care, or general practitioners would refer patients to the community hospitals. The core hospital offered at least the four major services (surgery, medicine, pediatrics, and obstetrics and gynecology). What the core hospital lacked in subspecialties and highly specialized services was provided by tertiary-level teaching institutions. Hospitals viewed comprehensiveness as essential to quality because it promoted easy collaboration among specialists. How closely the traditional model was approached in each country depended upon the resources and the degree of the system's centralization. In decentralized systems (e.g., the U.S. system), there have been few economic incentives to make the systems work.

Over the past 40 years, dissatisfaction with this model has been increasing. Unfortunately, the pursuit of institutional comprehensiveness is often independent of community need, driving duplication. Quality suffers when services established more for comprehensiveness or competition than need are underutilized and procedures are not performed frequently enough to maintain surgical, nursing, and laboratory skills. The development of new technologies fueled what some viewed as the insatiable appetite of hospitals for resources, an appetite reinforced by the political and financial power of hospital-based specialists. First-line primary care services, based upon general practitioners or nonphysician providers, cannot compete for resources even when the services are owned or controlled by a hospital. In practice, the hospital-centered model has not been implemented in most communities and where it has, it has not ensured distribution of resources according to the needs of most of the population. The majority of resources flow to acute care and benefit relatively few people.

The 1978 World Health Organization conference held in Alma-Ata, USSR, produced a worldwide consensus that expansion of primary care is essential for achieving "Health for All by the Year 2000." Furthermore, the conference called for three developments: "universal availability of essential health care to individuals, families, and population groups according to need; involvement of communities in planning, delivery, and evaluation of such care; and an active role from other sectors in health activities."[6] In retrospect, it was a turning point in setting global goals and expectations for health and medical care organizations. For the first time the effectiveness of the hospital- and specialty-centered model was openly challenged by medical and health leaders. One result of the Alma-Ata conference was that a number of countries initiated policies that separated the hospital component from the primary care component of their systems as a strategy to build up primary care programs. In most countries, the stature and priority of expanding primary care services was raised significantly.

In general, the relative amount of resources devoted to primary care has increased significantly in recent years. The relative resource flow to hospitals plateaued, particularly in developing countries. Instead there was an increase in the use of HMOs and other primary care organizations that provide incentives to contain hospital utilization. In all countries, cost-containment efforts have focused, with varied success, on controlling hospital utilization, replacement, and expansion. The impact of this continuing process is universal across industrialized and developing countries and across centralized and decentralized systems.

The response of medical care organizations (particularly hospitals) to intense public competition for resources, rising and often conflicting expectations, in-depth public scrutiny, and increasing demand for more effective primary care services has varied. Some institutions have moved quickly and creatively to become key primary care providers. Other well-established organizations are re-examining their missions and developing community service approaches that may significantly change their organizational design. Managers are introducing the concept of community benefit as an indicator of organizational performance. All are being challenged by new alternative service delivery organizations that are competing for public support. As stated by Richard J. Davidson, president of the American Hospital Association,

> Entrepreneurship for the 1990s . . . means nothing less than using savvy management to take charge of improving the health status of an entire community.
>
> . . . A hospital acting along can't accomplish this. But a hospital acting as a catalyst, nudger, cooperator, collaborator *and* competitor can do it. It will take a whole new set of management skills. Sometimes setting ego aside. Sometimes agreeing that the other provider can do something better. Sometimes working with schools, local government, foundations, business to maximize resources.[7]

One way to restructure the system is for the traditional provider institutions to form networks with organizations that respond more directly to the wants and needs of the general population, particularly people in underserved communities. Many well-managed hospitals and group practices recognize the social, economic, and cultural differences among communities, and they are developing partnerships with community-based organizations that provide primary care. Making use of community organization networks and entering into partnerships to improve community health are promising strategies. Mutual dependence and cooperation change the mission and roles of the partners and provide a foundation for building innovative organizations (see Exhibit 1-3).

From a global perspective it is evident that a new paradigm is emerging that is closing the gap between secondary care, tertiary care, and primary care. The post–Alma-Ata separation of hospitals from primary

Exhibit 1-3 American Hospital Association Policy on
Restructuring Health Care Delivery

Health care delivery should be fundamentally restructured by establishing community care networks that would provide patients with integrated care organized at the community level. Networks would be responsible for providing all of the services covered for their enrolled population and would coordinate patient care over time and across various provider settings. Patients would turn to their network for everything covered—from preventive care to acute care to long-term care services.

Community care networks are the keystone to universal access. They are designed to:

- *Focus on community health status.* Networks would be responsible for maintaining and improving the health status of their enrollees, giving them an incentive to reach out into their communities, and to work with public health, social service or other organizations that can help to measure and improve health status.
- *Focus on patients.* Networks would minimize patient hassles by truly managing and coordinating care, by making available a broad spectrum of care, and by giving patients a consistent point of access to the health care system.
- *Focus on prevention and primary care.* Networks would emphasize wellness in addition to the treatment of illness.
- *Focus on community-level solutions to community problems.* Networks would match local health care resources and strategies to local community needs and circumstances.

True managed care requires assessing patient health risks and needs. It means planning and organizing care so that problems are averted or treated early and all needed services are efficiently provided without unnecessary duplication of capacity. Within community care networks, patient needs would be returned to the focus of the delivery system and the management of care responsibility would be returned to the caregivers.

The primary caregiver would act as the care manager for that individual. It would be the primary caregiver's responsibility to ensure that an initial evaluation of health status is conducted, that appropriate primary care and preventive services are provided, and that services throughout the system are coordinated for the patient, particularly when specialty services are needed.

Source: Reprinted from *National Health Care Reform: Refining and Advancing the Vision* with permission of the American Hospital Association, © 1992.

care is being reversed. Many centralized systems are decentralizing, placing the responsibility on hospitals and primary care programs to cooperate at the community level and to allocate resources to improve community health status. Even the tradition of measuring hospital size by number of beds (measuring sickness) is giving way to measuring the size of an organization by the population or number of individuals served (measuring health).[8]

Alternative "delivery systems" are being developed as alternatives to fee-for-services private hospitals and doctors and to universal insurance systems with or without socialized (government-employed) providers. They include HMOs of all kinds, some forms of managed care, and other labels, none of which are clearly defined. They usually purchase or directly provide most of the acute care services an enrollee will need. A primary caregiver, usually a physician, acts as gatekeeper to the system, guiding and controlling the movement of the patient through the various services. That is supposed to ensure continuity of care and reduce costs. Ideally, alternative delivery systems emphasize disease prevention and health promotion, but that varies considerably among plans and models. The main purpose of most alternative systems is to encourage use of lower-cost services and to discourage physicians from using hospitals more for their own convenience than for the convenience of patients.

The growth of another alternative delivery system, the independent ambulatory care center, is a direct expression of the public's desire for access to primary care. Short-stay substitutes for traditional hospital services, such as day surgery, are also alternatives. Such services may gradually merge to form comprehensive health organizations (CHOs), adding preventive services. Canada is experimenting with CHOs paid for by the government on a capitation basis. Finland is developing community health centers that integrate primary care providers. The centers are coordinated with secondary and tertiary care, with appropriate divisions of labor.[9]

Alternative delivery systems, particularly HMOs that truly manage the patient's total care provide a foundation for the development of primary health care–centered systems. They usually serve defined populations, have a single point of entry through a primary care practitioner, and integrate primary, specialty, and hospital providers. One speaker at a national conference on primary care pointed out that "managed care organizations have the inherent interest, scale, and political independence to fundamentally reorder the priorities of medical care, including altering the role and status of primary care physicians."[10] Most are not yet being managed to proactively promote health, but in the future public policy and financial incentives are likely to encourage them to do so.

THE CHALLENGE: FROM ADMINISTRATORS AND MANAGERS TO LEADERSHIP IN ADMINISTRATION

In the near future many countries will define what "the right to health" means in practice and will try to allocate resources accordingly. The hard choices among desirable and essential social services will become even more of a personal issue for many people than it is today. Communities will be confronted with complicated, confusing, and competing health service organizations and financing options that must be explained and evaluated. The health services administrator is the professional best prepared and positioned to facilitate well-informed decision making by communities, governments, and employers as well as by health and medical care organizations.

In all kinds of health systems, assessing risks to health in the community and organizing resources optimally to control them requires data sharing and planning by service organizations. Competition is the antithesis of sharing responsibility for meeting community needs. As its limits as a cost containment strategy and its inability to meet community needs adequately become more clear, administrators will have to articulate just what are the driving values of their organizations. In the United States and in other countries with substantial private sec-

tors, health service administrators are in the key position to make or break efforts to implement effective, responsive, comprehensive health services.

The defining challenge of management will be the generation, articulation, and realization of a vision of health and medical care organization that recognizes the appropriate level of investment and is responsive to the needs of the community, the patients, and the organization.

The essential elements of a vision of the preferred future for any community are

- universal access to primary health care that encompasses health promotion and disease prevention as well as coordinated and comprehensive medical care
- redefined missions for most medical care institutions that emphasize their responsibility for developing and supporting the provision of quality primary health care services

A new breed of leaders in administration is needed, a breed that is philosophically committed to and competent to manage the change process. In order for health services organizations to attract and retain strong leadership, they must be prepared to make an appropriate investment in managerial capacity and in the continual development of managerial competencies. The kind of leadership they should seek can be characterized as follows:

1. Leadership that communities can look to for guidance and for visions of a preferred future in a time of unsettling change.
2. Leadership that is adept at educating owners, sponsors, community organizations, governments, and boards of directors to encourage and support management in its efforts to replace old visions with new visions.
3. Leadership that employs managerial epidemiology to assess population needs, measure the potential impact of options, and evaluate outcomes. Managerial epidemiology is the science of assessing a community's health ser-

vices needs from the perspective of health services resource management.

4. Leadership that has the political skills to build and maintain community support.
5. Problem solvers who employ a breadth of perspectives and a range of skills to enhance organizational flexibility.
6. Management and clinical leadership with skills in implementing continuous improvement and total quality management.
7. Leadership that has advocacy skills and the ability to assemble, interpret, and communicate complex information.
8. Leadership that has the necessary negotiating skills to manage the increasing conflict likely to emerge between and within professions and other stakeholders as new visions challenge old ones.
9. Leadership able to create an environment that encourages change and rewards managerial creativity.

The defining challenge of making the new vision real to communities moves the function of health management into a new paradigm. The professional dominance model is giving way to the acceptance of a dynamic equilibrium between professional and community interests. The equilibrium is dynamic because it is constantly changing. The type of leadership outlined above is needed to establish the equilibrium and to manage the continuous change process. The knowledge and skills essential for managing the change process are outcomes assessment and continuous quality improvement. As the two concepts converge, it has become clear that a profound change is occurring in the role of management in medical care and health services. They are increasing the validity of quality assessment and changing our concept of management's role in achieving quality improvement. Outcomes assessment and total quality management (TQM) have enormous implications, not only for how medical care is delivered but also for how to achieve improved health status in the community.

The basic philosophy of total quality management is that the quality of services provided can always be made better. The present level of quality, regardless of how good it actually is, is a benchmark against which to measure continuous improvement. The assessment of the outcomes of medical care clarifies the contribution of therapies or treatment patterns to the progress of patients. Outcome assessment makes it possible to specify what results are to be expected and helps explain short-term and long-term differences from the outcomes achieved by other providers. Obviously, outcome assessments are assessments of quality. Together continuous quality improvement and outcome assessment provide a new perspective on the effectiveness of health service organizations and their managers.

The science of outcome assessment and the experience of applying continuous quality improvement to health and medical care organizations are beginning to show us how to use them together to achieve integrated health improvement in the health status of the community (i.e., bring together improvements in the functional status of individuals and improvement in the health status of the community). The managers of primary health care organizations will have powerful tools with which to assess how effectively resources are being invested and to improve service quality. Service quality improvement will become the new criterion of managerial performance.

THE MISSION IS HEALTH: WHAT IT MEANS FOR YOU

The scope and accelerating pace of change in health and medical care services presents professional health services administrators with an unprecedented opportunity to demonstrate how managerial competence contributes to achieving health objectives. In the new paradigm, it is essential that managerial competence and clinical competence converge to refine the organizational mission continually and invest limited health resources optimally. The process of defining a new mission requires management to go beyond functional administration to provide a vision of the future that everyone understands and supports. This vision then functions as an integrating and forward-looking force in the organization. Successfully guiding organizations into the new paradigm is the essence of leadership.

The first challenge is to get unstuck from old managerial approaches, attitudes, and styles. The dominant managerial culture in health organizations has been static for years. Hospital management has been organized for central control rather than to foster adaptability and continuous change and improvement. Organizations adept at responding to changing community needs are not controlled tightly from the top in the new paradigm. Managerial responsibility and flexibility is widely dispersed, and the main emphasis is on what has been accomplished instead of how it was accomplished. It is the vision that guides the organization's behavior, not rigid rules. Leadership in administration is effective vision making, not rule making.

Similarly, the competencies and attitudes of successful management in the old system will not be sufficient for leadership in the future. The concept of successful management performance is changing. A currently successful manager who does not develop new competencies is unlikely to be considered successful in a few years. Competencies in diversification, mergers and expansion, marketing, financial management, and medical staff relations are useful but not sufficient. The new paradigm competencies include community and organizational assessment, integration of clinical and managerial perspectives, provision of leadership across multiple interests, guidance of governance toward new missions, appreciation of differences and cultures, and continuous organizational and personal improvement.

The central factor in the future of health services is change, and managerial competency and leadership require continual personal growth. A manager who does not continually improve him- or herself cannot lead an organization to continually improve

itself. As the leader helps define the vision of the future, colleagues look to the leader for an example of the managerial competencies and attitudes that are essential to achieve it. A manager who is self-satisfied and obviously stagnant cannot give dynamic leadership to organizational change.

The key question is, in light of the pressures for change facing health services in general and your organization in particular, what are your leadership strengths and weaknesses? Effective leaders assess themselves just as they assess others. The benchmark against which to measure personal growth and improvement is who you are now. Undertaking a personal assessment is a necessary first step in becoming strategically positioned for continued leadership. The best methods of assessment include using a self-assessment tool or an assessor who can serve as a mirror reflecting how other people see you. A trusted colleague outside of the organization might make a good assessor and might welcome a reciprocal arrangement.

The second step is to design a personal growth plan (Exhibit 1-4) that focuses on developing the competencies and attitudes that you will need in the future. The plan should have a two- or three-year time horizon. Most importantly, it must be demanding and doable. It is not difficult to draw up a plan that includes all the desirable things you would like to do, but you will probably never take three months off to visit foreign health care systems or two months off to visit different kinds of health and medical care organizations. It is not likely that you will set aside a month just to read the journals stacked up behind your desk. The development plan must be compatible with the reality of your life. At the same time, push back the boundaries of the time and energy you are investing in yourself. That will take discipline—and also support from spouse, family, organization, and colleagues. Your disciplined investment in continuous self-improvement will encourage all of those who are stakeholders in your competencies to do the same.

The plan will help you to invest your development time and money effectively. It will also give the manager a basis for negotiating with the organi-

Exhibit 1-4 A Three-Year Personal Development Plan Framework

Planning Stage

- Identify a colleague in another organization to be your self-assessment partner.
- Develop a first-year and long-term learning and growth objectives plan.
- Arrange for personal development time each year.
- Plan for professional college advancement.

Every Year

- Set aside three hours a week for developmental reading, which might include
  - one general opinion magazine (*Harper's, Atlantic,* or *The Economist*)
  - in-depth health policy journals (*Health Management Quarterly* and *Health Affairs*) and the policy articles in *The New England Journal of Medicine*
  - a book on general public policy, economics, or government
- Have lunch with your partner every two months to assess your progress.

Year 1

- Spend one week with a colleague in a different kind of health organization—something closer to the future.
- Attend a two- or three-day intense competency-building course.
- Revise your plan.

Year 2

- Attend a two- or three-day intense competency-building course.
- Spend four or five days with the senior management of a non-health-related service organization.
- Revise your plan.

Year 3

- Spend a week at a university health administration program as an "administrator in residence," working with a faculty advisor, attending classes, reviewing research activities, and meeting with faculty.
- Attend a two- or three-day intense competency-building course.
- Revise your plan.

---

zation for the resources necessary to implement the plan. Provision of such resources is an appropriate investment for any health or medical care organization. Personal development activities might include spending time as an executive in residence at a uni-versity health services administration program, expanding regular reading to include journals on public affairs and health services research, an exchange consultative visit to a colleague in another organization, taking an executive management program at a university, or going on a study tour of health services in another country.

EDUCATION FOR LEADERSHIP IN ADMINISTRATION

The complexity of the challenge and the consequences for the community mandate purposeful preparation for a career in health services management. Previous training in medicine, nursing, law, or business is useful but not sufficient. Individuals with clinical backgrounds need in-depth knowledge of management and the social sciences as they apply to health. Those with management training need systematic knowledge of medicine and health. Medical and nursing schools do not teach management, and management schools do not teach health. That is why programs in health services administration are specifically designed to combine the content that is essential to successful management and leadership in the health sector. Although a few gifted individuals may achieve successful administrative careers without such preparation, the way to optimize competence is to encourage everyone who aspires to the responsibility of health services administration to seek appropriate training.

Formal professional education for the management of health services is well established in most industrialized countries and in many developing countries. For example, in the United States, Canada, United Kingdom, Belgium, Mexico, Colombia, Brazil, Chile, the Philippines, and Australia, a master's degree is recognized as the ideal qualification for administrative practice. In several of those countries, and in many others, the growth of bachelor's degrees, certificates, and administrative specializations for clinicians reflects increasing efforts to ensure the competence of those who manage scarce and expensive community health resources.

The appropriate content of formal professional education has been validated by experienced successful administrators. It has been codified by the Accrediting Commission on Education for Health Services Administration which accredits graduate programs in health services administration in Canada and the United States (see Exhibit 1-5).

Professional education and continuous personal development are elements of a strategic framework for providing leadership to the organization as it moves toward the new paradigm. The following chapters provide up-to-date information on the environment and components of contemporary health and medical organizations. They describe the forces and the resources successful leaders will work with to achieve their visions of the future. But the first step for each leader is to design and implement a candid, personal self-analysis and development plan, which, although on a smaller scale, is as important as the assessment and strategic plan for the organization.

Exhibit 1-5 Criteria of the Accrediting Commission on Education for Health Services Administration

---

The curriculum of a program for professional health services administration must include:

- Understanding of the organization, financing, and delivery of health services, drawing on the social science disciplines (broadly defined to include economics, law, political science, psychology, sociology, and related disciplines).
- Assessment and understanding of the health status of populations; determinants of health and illness; and factors influencing the use of health services.
- Understanding of the values and ethical issues associated with the practice of health services administration and the development of skills in ethical analysis.
- Provision of opportunities for development of leadership potential, including stimulating creativity, and interpersonal and communication skill development.
- Understanding of and development of skills in economic, financial, policy, and quantitative analysis; positioning organizations favorably in the environment and managing these organizations for continued effectiveness; the management of human capital and information resources; assessing organizational performance; and methods to assure continuous improvement in the quality of services provided.

Source: Adapted from *Criteria for Accreditation of the Accrediting Commission on Education for Health Services Administration* with permission of the Accrediting Commission on Education for Health Services Administration.

NOTES

1. M. Catley-Carlson, Global Considerations Affecting the Health Agenda of the 1990's, *Academic Medicine* 67 (1992): 424.

2. P.F. Basch, *International Health* (New York: Oxford University Press, 1978), 204–205.

3. Organization for Economic Cooperation and Development 1991 Health Data File.

4. S. Jonas and S.N. Rosenberg, Ambulatory Care, in *Health Care Delivery in the United States,* ed. Steven Jonas (New York: Springer Publishing Company, 1986), 153.

5. J. Frenk et al., First Contact, Simplified Technology, or Risk Anticipation? Defining Primary Health Care, *Academic Medicine* 65 (1990):676.

6. E. Tarimo and A. Creese, eds., *Achieving Health for All by the Year 2000* (Geneva: World Health Organization, 1990), 1.

7. *AHA News* 28, no. 1 (1992):4.

8. Frenck et al., First Contact, Simplified Technology, or Risk Anticipation? 679. It is difficult to reverse the habit of using the number of beds per thousand population as a measure of health services availability. The ratio was popularized by the Hill-Burton hospital-building program in the United States in the 1940s and 1950s. It became an international standard and continues to endure long after it has ceased to have a credible place in U.S. health policy. Bed ratios have been used to justify hospital expansion, although there is no evidence that, beyond a minimum, achieving a particular ratio contributes to better community health status.

9. Tarimo and Creese, *Achieving Health for All by the Year 2000,* 104.

10. *Executive Summary: The National Primary Care Conference, 1992* (Washington, D.C.: Department of Health and Human Services, 1992), 16.

David B. Starkweather
Donald G. Shropshire

Management Effectiveness

2

Purpose: The effective health care manager brings together human and material resources in a manner that achieves favorable health-related outcomes consistent with the objectives of the organization.

INTRODUCTION

The above statement of purpose establishes two criteria for management effectiveness: that favorable outcomes should result and that these outcomes should be consistent with organizational objectives. But outcomes are hard to measure, and even if they are favorable, it is often unclear whether the results are due to managerial performance. Health care outcomes are especially difficult to determine, because they may occur a long time after the patients have been served. Further, organizational goals and objectives are often vague, making it difficult to determine whether particular outcomes are consistent with them. And for most health care organizations, objectives that relate to community service and public benefit are far more difficult to measure than the profit objectives of industrial organizations.

Despite the difficulties, it is crucial to maintain the underlying goals of health care management.

They set health care managers apart from most business executives. Without these goals, managers can become lost in activity without purpose.

This chapter presents the key elements of effective health care management. It does so by dividing the subject into specific components. The first categorization is by executive role: the different behavior associated with effective management. The second is by function: the various tasks performed by an executive. And the third is by management style: how an executive leads and influences others to perform for the organization.

These are generic elements: They are characteristic of effective management everywhere. But there are some special characteristics of health care management that call for different applications or emphases of these general elements. These have to do mostly with the professionalization of health care organizations. Many personnel are highly trained and experienced doctors, nurses, and so on. They are production workers in the enterprise, but they are also independent practitioners and demand autonomy. It follows that health care organizations cannot be managed by traditional top-down methods. Collaborative decision making must be substituted for hierarchic decision making.

Yet another feature of health care organizations is their complexity, which makes it necessary for them to have a high degree of coordination and integration. This calls for different management structures than are found in business and industry—or at least different applications of organizational designs known elsewhere.

A final distinguishing feature of health care enterprises is their propensity for conflict. Some managers view conflict as detrimental and to be avoided. The effective executive recognizes conflict as an important organizational dynamic, deals with it, and turns it to the benefit of the organization.

The chapter ends with an introduction to the moral leadership dimension of health care management: vision, commitment to the development of others, values, looking beyond, setting priorities, solving problems, balancing interests, and serving the public. These leadership qualities are developed further in other chapters.

THE BASICS OF MANAGEMENT

Current literature offers many new and valuable perspectives on managerial effectiveness, several or which are discussed in this and other chapters of this book, but the basics have not changed. Effective management can be discussed by focusing on three basic concepts. The first is the concept of a management *role:* the behavior associated with a management position in an organization. The second is the concept of a management *function:* any one of the varying tasks performed by executives. And the third is the concept of management *style:* the manner in which roles or functions are carried out. These three concepts can help illuminate the nature of effective management in virtually all organizations, but they also provide a basis for describing the special features of management in the health field.

Roles: The Nature of Managerial Work

Henry Mintzberg has offered a useful classification of executive roles.[1] Managers occupy three complementary roles: interpersonal, informational,

and decisional. The relative emphasis on each of the three varies among different organizations and even among different managers in the same organization.

The Interpersonal Role

The first role arises directly from an executive's formal authority and involves basic interpersonal relationships. The interpersonal role includes acting as a *figurehead*—performing the various ceremonial duties incumbent upon the head of any organized unit. While the CEO is lunching with an important visitor, a department head is attending an employee's retirement party. The role also involves *motivating* people to work and reconciling their individual needs with the goals of the organization. The approaches managers use to accomplish these objectives vary greatly (later in this chapter several options are discussed). The interpersonal role sometimes requires the executive to act as a *liaison* and to pursue or respond to contacts outside the normal hierarchy. This applies especially to top managers, whose contacts are primarily outside the organization, and to middle managers, whose contacts are with peers in other departments of the same organization. Early management theorists regarded contacts outside the hierarchy as dysfunctional,[2] but more recent observers describe such "networking" as essential to effective management.

The Informational Role

Through interpersonal contacts with subordinates and peers, a manager becomes the informational nerve center of his or her unit. The manager, although not knowing everything in detail, typically knows more than anyone else about the unit as a whole. Information, as well as the ability to provide or withhold it, is an important source of organizational power. Therefore, the processing of information is a key part of the effective manager's job.

There are three aspects of a manager's informational role. One is *monitoring:* scanning the environment for information, posing questions of subordinates and network contacts, and noting unsolicited information. Since not all data are useful or even valid, the effective manager filters out the trivial and retains a reservoir of pertinent information. Another informational role is as *disseminator,* since sooner or later a manager must share or distribute much of the information gathered. One way the manager does this is by acting as a *spokesperson* communicating information outside the organization or unit. Early observers considered the spokesperson role to be limited to top management, but it is now clear that organizations are "porous" at all levels.

The Decisional Role

This third broad role is the most popular and the one seen by managers as most central. Information is not an end in itself; it is used by successful managers to increase the quality of their decisions. The authority to make decisions is based on a manager's formal position; only the formal head of a unit can commit the unit to certain courses of action.

As shall be seen, health care organizations are peculiar as decision-making entities, since power is shared by managers and physicians. This means that decisions are seldom made alone by persons at the top of the units; instead they are usually made through the collaboration of several parties who share organizational power. Further, whenever decisions are made that lead to changes in behavior (which is a result of most decisions), effective managers obtain the participation of those affected. This secures their "buy in" and support for the actions required of them to implement the decision.

There are three aspects of a manager's decisional role. First, the manager must act like an *entrepreneur.* The successful manager seeks to improve his or her unit or adapt to changing conditions by developing new ideas and projects or pursuing new lines of activity. In prior times, managers felt that entrepreneurism was appropriate only for an organization's top executives. But recent studies of successful organizations make it clear that the capacity to be entrepreneurial should exist at all management levels. Later in the chapter there is a description of a management structure called service

line management. This structure is used by managers to create "small business units" capable of entrepreneurial activity. This same motivation—to create widespread entrepreneurism—lies behind the structure used for total quality management.

The decisional role also includes *disturbance handling.* Whereas entrepreneurism involves voluntary initiation of change, disturbance handling requires a manager to respond involuntarily to problems that are beyond his or her control (e.g., a sudden employee strike or an incident involving maltreatment of a patient). These disturbances are often rooted in underlying or latent organizational conflict, which is the focus of discussion later in the chapter.

Finally, the decisional role requires a manager to be a *resource allocator,* which means deciding who will get what. Resource allocation is probably the most important manifestation of organizational power. It is, in fact, a complex matter involving not only direct resource decisions but also decisions as to how to structure the enterprise so that others can make direct resource decisions. And note that even a manager's own time is an important resource to be distributed.

The three major managerial roles summarized above are not distinct or mutually exclusive. The effective manager integrates these roles and subroles and creates the right mix for his or her particular position.

Management Functions

The second way of describing effective management is to describe the functions performed by executives. The main functions are planning, organizing, staffing, directing, and controlling.[3] In practice these various functions are performed simultaneously, but they are discussed separately for the sake of clarity.

Planning

Managers are planning when they project a vision for the future and a course of action aimed at achieving certain declared objectives. At higher levels of management the focus is on determining an organizational mission and on determining appropriate goals and objectives, while at lower levels the important job is determining the way to achieve these ends. The former is strategic planning; the latter is operational planning. Likewise, the time frames of planning are different. Whereas top managers are devising long-range plans covering the next five or ten years, operations managers are planning for the shorter time frame of, say, an annual budget.

There is a tendency for managers to regard planning as a distinct task that must be completed before any actions are taken. Yet organizations that defer actions in this manner are likely to become stagnated. Planning, therefore, is a task that every manager must do every day. The object is to weave planning and action together. The concept of *strategic management* emphasizes the inclusion of implementation in planning as well as the ongoing integration of planning with other management functions.

Organizing

This function consists of grouping people and assigning activities so that tasks get done properly. The traditional management hierarchy is displayed in an organization chart, which presents the formal network of authority, accountability, communications, and relationships. Some management hierarchies promote decentralization of these features, while others promote centralization. Other features displayed in an organization chart include span of control (the number of subordinates reporting to a manager), type of authority relationship (line, staff, or functional), and levels of management. Typically, the smaller the span of control, the greater the number of levels of management. Likewise, the greater the number of levels, the more complicated the authority relationships.

As a practical matter, the criterion most often used for organizing departments is span of control. There is considerable variation in the number of subordinates that can be effectively managed. The factors include (1) the manager's ability to work

with people, (2) the capacity of subordinates to direct themselves instead of being directed by their supervisor, and (3) the complexity of the work to be done (simpler and more uniform tasks permit the reporting of more subordinates to a single boss).

Enterprises that face rapidly changing markets should redesign themselves frequently. This is because there are certain effective matches between the types of environment, types of organizational strategy, and types of management structure.[4] This fact is surprising or disconcerting to many managers, who perhaps would like to take comfort in the idea that a management structure, once set, is permanent.[5] In fact, an enterprise that does not alter its structure to match changing circumstances is destined to dwindle or fail. (As discussed later in this chapter, the management structures of health care organizations are currently undergoing important changes. See also Chapters 5 and 7.)

Staffing

This function includes the selection, placement, training, development, and compensation of subordinates. It also includes the evaluation of performance. In organizations of any size, there is a personnel or human resources department, and many managers feel that this department is responsible for performing most of these tasks. But personnel departments are staff departments: They operate only in a support or advisory role. Although line managers can be aided by their personnel departments, they cannot give up final responsibility for the main tasks of the staffing function.

In human resources management, the aim of every manager is to develop and realize the full potential of each person under his or her supervision. This is to the ultimate benefit of the organization.

Directing

This is the management function that initiates action. It obviously includes giving directions, assignments, and instructions. But it also includes building an effective group of subordinates who are motivated to perform. The amount of directing done by each manager varies a good deal; first-line supervisors do a great deal of detailed directing whereas top managers spend more time in other managerial functions.

Douglas McGregor has categorized managers as having two different sets of beliefs about subordinates, which he calls Theory X and Theory Y.[6] These theories influence their style of directing.

Theory X managers believe that people dislike work and will avoid it where possible. These managers see themselves as members of a small chosen group who want to lead and take responsibility, whereas the larger mass of people want to be directed and avoid responsibility. Theory X managers therefore see a need for strong controls and detailed directions. The behavior of subordinates is to be regulated through coercion and punishment if they do not perform properly and through monetary rewards if they perform well.

Theory Y managers believe that most people will work hard and assume responsibility provided they can satisfy personal needs and organizational goals at the same time. Therefore, these managers do not see the sharp division between leaders and followers that Theory X posits. They feel that performance is better regulated by internal controls (within the person) than external controls (see Table 2-1).

The best style of directing will vary depending on the employees to be directed and the situation. Theory X style calls for close supervision, detailed instructions, and exact deadlines. The manager is doing the planning of work and making the decisions. Some employees like this style and respond well to it, especially those with skill deficiencies, lack of experience, or personalities that want firm and structured direction. These employees feel Theory Y supervision is no supervision at all.

Other employees lose interest and initiative when working for a Theory X manager. In the extreme case, they will resist and even sabotage this sort of management. These employees respond well when consulted about their jobs and about changes in their work. They want to be delegated authority for job results and be provided with minimum directions, instructions, and deadlines. In this human resource approach, employees participate in setting the goals for work to be done, thus becoming committed and enthusiastic about its accomplishment. The manager assumes that untapped talents will become evident and maximize the contributions the employees can make toward the goals of the enterprise.

An important implication of this model is that managers need to examine carefully their personal assumptions about the motivations and behaviors of subordinates. This brings us to a serious problem. Since some employees in a unit are likely to respond to one style of direction and other employees to the other, how does a manager decide how to direct? The effective manager uses a *contingency approach*–varying the style of management according to the circumstances at hand. Contingency theory is discussed later in this chapter.

Controlling

This is the managerial function of checking to determine if employees are following the prescribed plan and correcting any problems that may have been discovered. Whereas planning, organizing, staffing, and directing are the steps required for implementing a job, controlling is concerned with making certain that the plan is correctly implemented. Although there may be extensive delegation of responsibility, managers need to carefully control what goes on because they always retain ultimate responsibility for whatever has been delegated.

Table 2-1 A Comparison of Theory X and Theory Y

Theory X	Theory Y
Production Centered	Employee Centered
Autocratic	Democratic
External Control	Internal Control
Close Supervision	General Supervision
Task Orientation	Relations Orientation
Directive	Supportive

In the traditional view, the process of controlling has four basic parts: (1) setting standards for time, quality, or quantity; (2) measuring results; (3) comparing results to standards; and (4) making necessary modifications. Standards should be measurable, easy to understand, and within the control of individuals. Too much measurement can be expensive and can alienate those being monitored. The core idea of control is to make modifications in behavior and performance when deviations from a plan are discovered. This means that an important part of the control process is feedback. If standards are not being met, then changes in objectives, standards, or performance should be undertaken.

In a more progressive view of control, as in total quality management, the assumption is made that the performance of any operating system can be improved and that measurement of system variation, coupled with feedback, will lead to higher performance or quality. In this way the techniques of management control become more promotive and less dependent on previously established standards.

Management Style

Thus far management has been discussed in terms of roles and functions. While management includes working with and through individuals and groups to accomplish objectives, leadership is the process of influencing individuals or groups. A person can exert leadership with or without an official title and whether or not he or she occupies a formal position. Most organizations have unofficial leaders, and it is unwise for managers to ignore or deny their existence.

Leadership is an illusive quality. Indeed, attempts to correlate effective leadership with various individual traits, backgrounds, or experiences have been unsuccessful. Some managers seem to lead naturally whereas others achieve leadership abilities through learning and development.

A number of concepts have been developed to help managers become effective leaders. Most of them are based on the following assumptions.[7]

1. The most important variant of leadership is the balance a manager achieves between a task-goal orientation (getting the job done regardless) and a relationship orientation (achieving good relations and morale regardless).

2. The circumstances and nature of the work are responsible for most of the factors that determine the best approach—as compared to the nature of the leader.

3. Managers should develop and alter their leadership approach depending on their analysis of the situation.

According to *contingency theory,* the best approach to leading others depends on (1) the circumstances the leader finds him- or herself in, (2) the nature of the followers, and (3) the nature of the work. Thus the effective manager is continually asking, "Which method will work here?" This approach contrasts with numerous models that assume there is one best way for a manager to lead. Managing an unskilled laborer is obviously different than managing a highly skilled doctor, and the approach that is effective in one case may be ineffective in the other.

Fiedler's contingency leadership model holds that a manager's effectiveness depends on two main factors: the leader's motivations and the extent to which the situation is favorable or unfavorable to the leader.[8] Leaders are motivated by satisfaction obtained from two sources: relationships with others (called consideration) and task-goal accomplishment (called structure). The relationship-motivated manager obtains satisfaction by maintaining good interpersonal relationships with subordinates. The task-oriented manager obtains satisfaction by accomplishing the goal. Most managers obtain satisfaction from both sources, but the relative importance of each varies widely. Importantly, Fiedler maintains that managers can vary their approach according to the situation.

The favorableness of a situation depends on three factors:

1. *The quality of the leader-subordinates relationship.* The friendlier the relationship, the more favorable the situation.

2. *The nature of the task.* The more structured and routine the task, the more favorable the situation.

3. *The power of the leader.* The more power, the more favorable the situation.

Contingency theory suggests that relationship-motivated leaders are more effective than task-motivated leaders in moderately favorable situations and that task-motivated leaders are more effective in either highly favorable or highly unfavorable situations (see Figure 2-1).

In intermediate situations, relationship-oriented managers take a nondirective approach, asking others in the group to share in the decision-making process and interacting with subordinates in a considerate, permissive fashion (Theory Y at work). For example, the head of the food service department enjoys good interpersonal relations with her subordinates. She is developing a new policy on food handling that will have a great impact on the work groups in the department. At this stage the situation is relatively vague

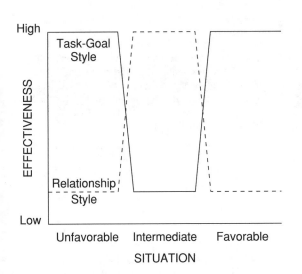

Figure 2-1 Effectiveness of Different Management Styles in Different Situations. *Source:* Reprinted from *A Theory of Leadership Effectiveness* by F.E. Fiedler, p. 146, with permission of McGraw Hill, © 1967.

and unstructured but moderately favorable, so the manager decides to consult with her subordinates and carefully considers their thoughts and ideas. Then, once the new policy is settled and approved, the situation calls for a more task-oriented style, since the main focus is on enforcing the food handling policy. Thus the food services manager has varied her style to fit the particular situation.

There are numerous other approaches for dealing with the issue of management style. A model developed by Vroom and Yetton focuses on how decisions are made and on the acceptance of decisions by subordinates.[9] The model also distinguishes between individual and group acceptance. Five decision styles are shown in Table 2-2. (Vroom and Yetton also provide a chart of different circumstances and situations that would call for one or another decision style.)[10]

In the path-goal model, a management style is considered effective if it makes rewards available to subordinates and makes these rewards contingent upon the subordinates' accomplishment of specific goals.[11] An important part of the manager's job is to clarify for subordinates the kind of behavior that is most likely to result in accomplishment; this is called path clarification. Again there are different decision-making styles: The directive leader lets subordinates know what is expected of them; the supportive leader treats subordinates as equals; the participative leader consults with subordinates and uses their suggestions and ideas; and the achievement-oriented leader sets challenging goals, expects subordinates to perform, and continually seeks improvement in performance.

Again, there are situational factors that dictate the choice of style. An example is the perception by an employee of his or her ability to accomplish the tasks at hand. The stronger the employee's belief in his or her ability to perform adequately, the less likely the employee is to accept a directive management style. Certain environmental variables are beyond the control of the employee but are important determinants of the employee's ability to perform, including the task, the formal authority system, and the work group. For example, the employee could

Table 2-2 Decision Styles for Leaders and Groups

Individual Level	Group Level
A1. You solve the problem or make the decision yourself, using information available to you at that time.	**A2.** You solve the problem or make the decision yourself, using information available to you at that time.
B1. You obtain any necessary information from the subordinate, then decide on the solution to the problem yourself. You may or may not tell the subordinate what the problem is in getting the information from him or her. The role played by your subordinate in making the decision is clearly one of providing specific information that you request rather than generating or evaluating alternative solutions.	**B2.** You obtain any necessary information from subordinates, then decide on the solution to the problem yourself. You may or may not tell the subordinates what the problem is in getting the information from them. The role played by your subordinates in making the decision is clearly one of providing specific information that you request, rather than generating or evaluating solutions.
C1. You share the problem with the relevant subordinate, getting ideas and suggestions. Then *you* make the decision. This decision may or may not reflect your subordinate's influence.	**C2.** You share the problem with the relevant subordinates individually, getting their ideas and suggestions without bringing them together as a group. Then *you* make the decision. This decision may or may not reflect your subordinates' influence.
D1. You share the problem with one of your subordinates, and together you analyze the problem and arrive at a mutually satisfactory solution in an atmosphere of free and open exchange of information and ideas. You both contribute to the resolution of the problem, with the relative contribution of each being dependent on knowledge rather than formal authority.	**D2.** You share the problem with your subordinates in a group meeting. In this meeting, you obtain their ideas and suggestions. Then *you* make the decision, which may or may not reflect your subordinates' influence.
E1. You delegate the problem to one of your subordinates, providing him or her with any relevant information that you possess but giving him or her responsibility for solving the problem alone. Any solution that the person reaches will receive your support.	**E2.** You share the problem with your subordinates as a group. Together, you generate and evaluate alternatives and attempt to reach agreement (consensus) on a solution. Your role is much like that of chairperson, coordinating the discussion, keeping it focused on the problem, and making sure that the critical issues are discussed. You do not try to influence the group to adopt "your" solution, and you are willing to accept and implement any solution that has the support of the entire group.

Source: Reprinted from Vroom, V.H., and Jago, A.G., On the Validity of the Vroom-Yetoon Model, *Journal of Applied Psychology,* April 1978, pp. 151–162, with permission of the American Psychological Association, © 1978.

be motivated by the work group and receive satisfaction from coworkers' expressed recognition that the job was done according to group norms. Research on this model indicates that the four decision-making styles can be used variously by the same manager in different situations.[12]

The models described above take into account the main principle of contingency management—that the best approach to leading others depends on the circumstances. The models help the manager "read" particular circumstances in order to come up with the approach that will be most effective.

SPECIAL CHARACTERISTICS OF HEALTH CARE MANAGEMENT

Thus far principles have been presented that would lead to effective management in virtually any organization. But there are special characteristics of health care organizations that call for modifications or differences in emphasis.

It has long been debated whether there are any real differences from a management point of view between health care organizations and general business enterprises. One difference has already been mentioned: the mission orientation of most health care organizations as community service enterprises versus the margin orientation of profit-seeking companies. The evolution of management education suggests that there are further differences. Special programs have developed at colleges and universities to develop health care managers. Also, the professional societies through which managers seek to maintain and enhance their skills are distinct. For example, organizations such as the American College of Healthcare Executives, the Canadian College of Health Services Executives, and the Medical Group Manager's Association are specifically for health care managers.

What are the features of health care organizations that call for special management? Four interrelated features are discussed in this section: complexity, power, the role of professionals, and decision making. An additional two, also interrelated, are presented in the section immediately following.

Complexity

Probably no other enterprise has the variety of "members" that health care organizations possess. Likewise, the span of education, skills, and experience is enormous. What other enterprise can claim the kind of educational gap that exists between the laborer who is put to work cleaning floors or washing dishes with virtually no training or orientation and the specialized brain surgeon whose formal education and professional certification include

15–25 years of post–high school training. And there is every variety between these extremes.

It is a characteristic of professionals to look to their own colleagues for direction, decisions, and evaluations. This is based on the belief that professional colleagues—not the organization—know what is right to do concerning professional matters. Take, for example, the struggle between hospital nursing directors and hospital administrators over who should determine proper nurse staffing levels. Nurses claim that such decisions can only be made by the profession of nursing—that only nurses are capable of making the analyses of and the judgments about patient care needs. Hospital administrators maintain that staffing of all personnel is their responsibility.

Health care organizations have been termed *professionalized* enterprises because of the variety of people licenced to perform one or another aspect of patient care. The earmarks of professionalization include extensive training and experience, norms of personal duty, responsibility for making judgments, and the need for individual and professional autonomy. Consider this list in light of the two theories of managerial leadership and control, Theory X and Theory Y.

The extensive training and experience that professionals must have reduce the need for the kind of close supervision and detailed direction associated with Theory X. Professionals' norms of personal duty are at odds with that theory's assumption that most persons do not wish to work and will get out of it whenever possible. Their acceptance of responsibility for making judgments and their need for autonomy do not square with the Theory X assumption that external control and direction are necessary. Indeed, professionals work best when the controls are internal. The effective executive of a professionalized organization, in other words, is a Theory Y manager.

Power

Authority is the right to command and exact obedience from others. It derives from the organization and is possessed by those who hold an official position. *Power* is the ability to get others to do what is desired of them. Authority allows managers to make decisions that guide the actions of others; power enables managers to carry out these decisions. According to Barnard's theory of acceptance, an official command will be followed only if it is accepted as legitimate and reasonable by those expected to respond.[13] Thus a manager can possess official authority but be incapable of getting anything accomplished. By contrast, a crazed or disgruntled employee can hold patients, nurses, or doctors hostage at gunpoint; the employee has power but no authority.

There are six different types of organizational power.[14] *Legitimate power* stems from implicit or explicit organizational rules and regulations. However, it still requires employees to accept that a manager has a legitimate right to control them and that they are bound to acceptance by virtue of having become employees.

Representative power is delegated to a leader by a group. The group implicitly agrees to follow as long as the leader consults the group and generally leads in the direction they want to go. This type of power plays an important role in most hospital medical staffs.

Expert power is the power of knowledge. It comes from specialized knowledge and skills that are crucial to getting the organization's jobs done. Expert power is also based on the perception of subordinates that their leader has special knowledge or expertise that can be useful in satisfying their needs. Thus experience gives credibility to a manager. Yet a manager often does not have expertise in every phase of the unit's work. It then becomes the manager's task to draw on the expertise of others, thus enhancing his or her own ability to influence.

Charismatic power is based on devotion—the admiration of one person for another. For example, a manager wields charismatic power to the extent that his or her subordinates feel a sense of devotion. Such a sense of devotion is often attended by a desire to identify with the charismatic leader. The follower basically says, "I want to be like the leader,

and thus I will act as the leader does or as I am told to do by the leader." To varying degrees, charismatic power causes the followers to operate on blind faith. In the extreme case, they identify so much with the leader that they act as they think or imagine the leader would want. Obviously, subordinates vary in their susceptibility to feelings of devotion and managers vary in their ability to generate devotion.

Coercive power is based on the perception of followers that the leader has the ability to punish. Tangible punishments include firing, demotion, a low rating, unsatisfying work assignments, and poor references. Psychological punishments include criticism, snubs, avoidance, and expressions of disapproval.

Reward power is based on the leader's ability to award something for worthy behavior—and the perception of followers that such is the case. Tangible rewards include promotions, raises, time off, satisfying work assignments, and preferred work space. Psychological awards include approval, praise, appreciation, and recognition.

Reward power is more effective in getting subordinates to *do* something, while coercive power is more effective in getting subordinates to *avoid* doing something. Coercive power is of less value in the long run because it reduces the self-esteem of those to whom it is applied, resulting in hostility, withdrawal, and rule breaking.

Clearly some types of power can be exercised by individuals or groups who possess no legitimate authority. A nurse supervisor with expertise power can challenge a staffing pattern and call in more nurses for a ward of very sick patients. An informal group leader can use his or her charismatic power to convince coworkers to go on a work slowdown or even perform acts of sabotage.

Work groups develop norms of behavior that regulate the activities of individual members of the group. Just as one member might be disciplined for laying back from work, another might be admonished for "beavering" or being overeager. Informal norms of conduct can be far more extensive and explicit than formal rules, regulating minutiae such as dress or hair style as well as the conduct of work. They can also constitute a powerful form of control that may be unknown to the formal manager. As an example, the staff of a large clinic's business office was angry at one coworker who produced fewer insurance billings and left uncompleted work for others to finish. When the staff went out for lunch, she was not included, and she was ignored at coffee breaks. The discipline was social isolation.

An effective manager strives to be both a formal and an informal leader, but this is sometimes not possible. A manager is unwise to deny the existence of informal leaders who can influence others. Employees are often influenced most by their work groups. Most effective managers learn to work with informal leaders in order to accomplish the objectives of their organization.

The Role of Professionals

There is little doubt in most organizations where the power lies: Legitimate power rests at the top. It is exercised by managers who hold various offices, and these offices are arrayed in a hierarchy surmounted by the chief executive officer. The CEO derives his or her authority from the owners of the enterprise, which may be an elected board, a corporation, or the government.

But in health care organizations, power is also derived from expertise and representation. In most U.S. and Canadian hospitals, physicians are formed into a quasi-independent organization called the medical staff. A certain amount of legitimate institutional power is exercised over physicians through the medical staff because it operates with bylaws approved by the board of the hospital. But in most North American hospitals, the power of doctors is derived from their expertise, and the medical staff operates by use of representative power.

Physicians are basically focused on providing patient care; the hospital is a workshop that enhances or detracts from the success of that care. The people who know most about the right kind of care are their medical colleagues, grouped formally or informally by specialty. The fundamental loyalty of physicians is to their patients, and their accountability is to their professional colleagues. This means that they are not concerned primarily with the success of the organization, nor do they acknowledge its legitimate power and authority. Yet physicians have enormous influence over hospital policies, operations, and employees.

In short, there are dual lines of authority in most hospitals. The same is true in other health care organizations, although the same formal structures may not exist. For example, in an established group practice the medical staff seldom exists as a formal entity; instead, the physicians own the enterprise and their representatives sit on its board of directors.

If physicians of the medical staff and executives of the institutional hierarchy constitute the polar extremes of power and decision making in health care organizations, nurses are positioned in the middle, at the point of transition. This is because nurses are both health care professionals and workers or managers in the institutional hierarchy.

As a result, nurses experience a good deal of ambivalence or role conflict. Part of their loyalty and accountability is to nursing as a profession, and consequently they strive for greater autonomy as health care practitioners. But they are simultaneously officials in the institutional hierarchy and have supervising, coordinating, and operational problem-solving responsibilities. They are often the implementors and enforcers of institutional rules, many of which do not directly concern nursing practice. When such rules are disregarded by doctors, nurses are put in the awkward position of demanding adherence from the doctors. This reverses the usual relationship of power, since in most of hospital medicine it is physicians who issue orders for nurses to follow.

Many nurses choose a career path that either emphasizes a branch of clinical nursing or leads to a position in nursing supervision and management. Few of the nurses, however, who desire to become clinical nurse specialists anticipate the extent to which their nursing careers will involve management, and thus many need management training as a part of their long-term career development. Indeed, almost all nurses have a dual role that comprises clinical practice and management.

Decision Making

The existence of the various health care professions requires health care organizations to use a coalitional rather than a bureaucratic approach to decision making (see Figures 2-2 and 2-3). The bureaucratic approach is the traditional top-down hierarchical approach. Coalitional decision making, by contrast, occurs when two or more groups each realize that they can accomplish more through long-term collaboration than by acting separately. In short, they recognize they are mutually dependent. For instance, a hospital needs doctors to bring it patients, but the doctors cannot care for their patients without the hospital.

The hospital and the medical staff are the two main coalition members. But there are usually others, such as various specialty groups within the medical staff, nurses, trustees representing the community or the stockholders, unions, and so on.

Decision making in a coalition involves a different process than in a bureaucracy. In the latter, virtually all decisions can be traced to a single individual who possesses legitimate authority. If there is a question about the legitimacy of the decision, the question is settled by "going up the chain of command."

In a coalition, the major decisions can be traced to an inner circle consisting of representatives of the various coalition members (in Figure 2-3, the most heavily shaded area). Unlike a bureaucracy,

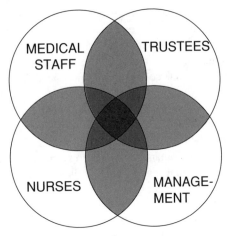

Figure 2-3 A Coalitional Structure for Organizational Decision Making

each member of the coalition has a veto (but is aware that regular exercise of the veto can bring operations to a halt). Also, each member is committed to reviewing major decisions with his or her coalition members before or after the inner circle takes action. Any question regarding the legitimacy of a decision is settled in a different way—by dispersal to the coalition members and return to the inner circle, since there is no higher authority.

Fundamentally, coalitional decision making occurs where organizational power is dispersed, as is usually the case in health care organizations. Coalitional decision making is often a messier and more confusing process than bureaucratic decision making, and indeed getting a decision finalized can be a slow and frustrating procedure.

Although bureaucratic and coalitional structures and processes are conceptually distinct, in fact they are combined in various ways in most hospitals. For example, the institutional portions of the hospital—building, supplies, finance, and so on—are usually organized along traditionally hierarchic lines, while those functions relating to patient care and professional affairs are frequently coalitional. Further, a professional department such as radiology may be run internally along hierarchic lines while key decisions about the department will be made using coalitional decision making. Thus, most health care

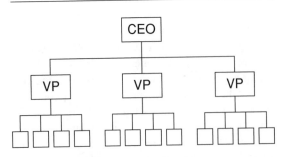

Figure 2-2 A Bureaucratic Structure for Organizational Decision Making

organizations can best be described as partial or quasi-coalitions.

The inner circle may be formal or informal. There are several examples of formal coalitional decision making in the literature,[15] but inner circles are typically informal. An inner circle, for instance, is rarely found on an organization chart, even when the various members represent formal hierarchies. In the inner circle, the hospital CEO or the vice-president for nursing might represent the institutional hierarchies, one or more physicians will represent the formal medical staff, and an officer of the board will represent the directors. These individuals, as well as representatives from the various patient care and professional departments, face a management challenge unique to the health field: managing simultaneously in the executive style characteristic of hierarchies and the political style characteristic of coalitions.

The inner circle is not a junta; it has a leader. But the leader of a coalition earns leadership rather than assuming it through power of office. Management skills and style are different from those appropriate for a bureaucracy, since the leader cannot make unilateral decisions. There is much emphasis on reasoning, persuasion, negotiating, conflict resolution, bargaining, and collective determination. Thompson has called the manager of a coalition the "superb politician."[16]

Although the most crucial inner circle operates at the top of a health care organization, there are numerous replications at lower levels—in surgical suites, emergency rooms, and intensive care units. A mechanism for decentralization being adapted by many hospitals in the 1990s, the service line or product line unit, incorporates many coalitional features. Such features are also characteristic of the methods used in total quality management. (See Chapter 7 for more on organizational models.)

ADDITIONAL SPECIAL CHARACTERISTICS

The previous section contained a description of four special and related features of health care organizations that call for different management: the great variety and spread of skills that call for contingency management, the high proportion of professionals who seek autonomy in their work and resist external control by the institution, the resulting proliferation of power, and the different approaches to decision making that flow from this unusual situation.

This section discusses two more special and related features of health care organizations. The first is the coordination and integration across many work groups that is required if the institution is to provide each patient with the right thing at the right time in the right place. Organizational coordination and integration is determined largely by management structure, but this very need for integration yields high levels of conflict, particularly when the parties involved have diverse backgrounds, expectations, and outlooks. This places conflict management high on the list of skills needed by a health care executive.

Coordination and Structure

Some organizations have parts that operate in relative isolation. A university, for instance, can have a history department that has virtually no connection with the mathematics department. In a hospital, on the other hand, almost every part must operate in coordination with the others. This puts a heavy burden on the enterprise: Its managers must ensure that adequate communication occurs between operating units, scheduling, and staffing for those tasks that need to be performed at precise times. In TQM terms, it is necessary to "break down the barriers" between departments.

Enterprises that function with operating units in relative isolation and with low requirements for coordination can function fairly well using *vertical communication:* Information passes up and down the hierarchy, and it is sufficient for coordination between units to take place at the top. By contrast, health care organizations, with their high coordination requirements, must have effective *horizontal communication:* Information must pass between parts at the operating level as well as at the top.

Take the example of a chemistry lab. As part of the research and design department of a firm manufacturing plastics, the chemistry lab can perform its tests and report the results in due time up the line to the research director. There is no ongoing operation that awaits the results of its tests. The same lab in a hospital must immediately perform tests upon specimens just drawn from patients, since doctors and nurses are waiting for the results. Indeed, sometimes testing must take place while a patient is undergoing surgery, and the procedure stops until the test results are known. To further heighten the need for coordination, it is often the case that the results of one set of tests determine another set that must be performed promptly. In short, there must be feedback as well as coordination.

The management structure of an organization determines not only the authority and accountability of various persons in the structure but also the pathways of communications and coordination between units—who does what for whom and when. The management structure assigns responsibility for effective coordination to certain points, usually called the points of integration.[17] (For additional discussion on organization structure, see Chapter 7.)

Management structures that enhance vertical communication take advantage of specialization. But the grouping together of specialists limits their ability to communicate and coordinate with other personnel in the organization; they are more likely to work with each other in order to improve their internal functioning. An example is the hospital pharmacy. If a large hospital is structured along vertical lines, all the pharmacists employed by the enterprise are placed in one department and one location, and the official in charge of that department deals with coordination between the pharmacy and other operating units. Thus, the point of integration is near the top of the enterprise and not at the operating level. An enterprise structured in this way is termed a functional organization.

Restructuring to enhance horizontal coordination results in a relatively flat hierarchy. The organization must abandon the efficient grouping of like specialists and instead establish points of integration at operating levels.

For example, each pharmacist might now serve a group of patient care units totalling, say, 75 beds. Each pharmacist, now called a clinical pharmacist, becomes immediately available to deal with all pharmaceutical and dispensing matters and can better integrate the pharmacy function with the rest of the patient care operation.

A number of other hospital functions and departments can similarly be restructured, including the laboratory, the business office, radiography, dietetics, budgeting, marketing, planning, admitting, social work, discharge planning, medical records, and information systems.

The final result is that the hospital is now a product organization: The management structure no longer groups like specialists together, the point of integration is at the operating level, and the new "mini-hospitals" (75-bed units) each contain a mix of people whose functions need to be coordinated and integrated. The term *product organization* is applicable because the basis of organizing is to provide patient care (a product) effectively rather than to perform certain specialized functions efficiently.

The kind of structure chosen—functional or product—depends on the size and complexity of the enterprise. A small organization must organize along functional lines because it would be too costly to duplicate all the specialists. But since it is small, the job of integration is done fairly well anyway. One reason is that the hierarchy does not have excessive levels, and thus top-level integration takes place near operations. Besides, most personnel see each other frequently and can coordinate naturally or informally. For instance, a small-hospital pharmacist is likely to see the head nurse in the cafeteria and solve the problem of a lost prescription.

By contrast, a large organization can afford to organize along product lines. In fact, this is a better alternative for it, because a large organization structured functionally does a poor job of integrating around its product. Production is likely to be slow and be plagued by many errors.

The general problem with a large functionally structured organization is that its lines of communication and accountability have become overlong, running through numerous vertical layers. Information is distorted and delayed, yielding either wrong responses to problems or responses that are too late. Further, the specialized units become more isolated and cease to understand or even care about their fit with the rest of the enterprise. Top management introduces more and more staff level coordination and control specialists, but without reorganization, they remain ineffective (and are expensive as well).

Returning to the pharmacy example, in a hospital made rigid by its functional structure, a nurse reports the lost pills to his head nurse, who feels she must go "up the chain" to the nursing director, where horizontal communication with the director of the pharmacy can take place. But the chief pharmacist is out of the hospital. He eventually checks his records and finds that there was some delay in filling the prescription because one pharmacist called in ill that morning. Further, the messenger department had delivered the prescription to the wrong nursing station because there were two patients in the hospital with the same name. This was eventually discovered and the pills were returned to the pharmacy. By the evening shift, the pills were redispatched to the correct nursing station, but the patient had in the meantime been transferred to a different room on the same nursing station. But another shift of nurses was now responsible; the trail of the missing pill got lost in the shift change.

In short, a major coordination snafu developed that could have been prevented if a clinical pharmacist had been on the ward and if there had been a manager responsible for coordination and integration at the operating level (as would be the case in a product structure).

As a general rule, high-volume, low-complexity activities can be decentralized, whereas low-volume, high-complexity activities must remain centralized. For example, routine lab tests can be performed on a decentralized basis by locating lab technologists and certain equipment within service line units, but complex procedures performed infrequently need to remain centralized. The same holds true for radiographs, dietary and food services, information systems, and so on.

The relationship between size, type of structure, and effectiveness is summarized in Figure 2-4. Hospitals organized along functional lines with 250–350 beds should consider reorganization; if they do not, they will be less effective and efficient and even dangerous to patients because of relatively large numbers of errors. Further, as the complexity of hospitals increases, the appropriate size for decentralization decreases. For this reason, medical care delivery will be pushed toward decentralized forms of management.

Another factor supporting decentralization is the importance of matching organizational environment, strategy, and structure. The decade of the 1980s saw competition emerge as a major force in U.S. health care delivery. While competition is being challenged by some as interfering with health care's community service orientation, it is likely to remain strong well into the future. Managers will need to restructure their organizations accordingly.

Much of the impetus for restructuring health care organizations has come from the study of other types of enterprises, especially those in high-tech production. These companies faced the need for quick product innovation, development, and marketing—and found they were unfit to meet the challenge. Formal and central planning had become a straitjacket, slowing down the development of new ideas and stifling the creative initiatives so much needed. Their vertical hierarchies further stifled the rapid development of new strategies and products. The larger and more established companies were being beaten in the marketplace by newer and smaller companies that were quicker and smarter.

The established firms restructured by creating "internal small business units." Each unit relates to a product or potential product, each contains the mix of functions necessary to advance the product, each is capable of integrating the personnel with the various skills needed, and, most importantly, each knows it can make the decision necessary to get its new product to the market. In the vernacular, these "skunk works" drive their strategies and products "through the knotholes" in the organizational walls of their own companies.

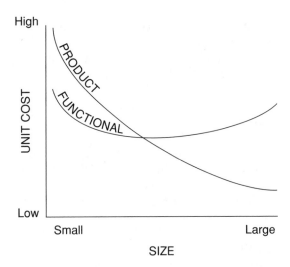

Figure 2-4 Relationship of Size, Structural Type, and Effectiveness. *Source:* Reprinted from Starkweather, D., The Rationale for Decentralization in Large Hospitals, *Hospital and Health Services Administration,* Spring 1970, pp. 27–45, with permission of Health Administration Press, Ann Arbor, Michigan, © 1970, Foundation of the American College of Healthcare Executives.

Hospitals that have implemented this type of structure call it service line management or product line management. The service line might be women's services, cancer treatments, or whatever. Although the restructuring is often a response to changed external conditions, especially increased competition, the result is similar to the "minihospital" structure implemented by hospitals to yield greater effectiveness in patient care delivery.

A service line or quality center spans inpatient and ambulatory care as well as prevention, treatment, and rehabilitation. Further, it incorporates planning, strategy, and marketing as well as ongoing operations. It is the principal unit of finance for purposes of budgeting, investment, and cost control. It is usually managed by a team of individuals with backgrounds appropriate to the need for integration. Nursing, medicine, and administration are three common backgrounds, although sometimes one person combines two of these backgrounds or has other talents, such as finance or marketing skills.

As outlined previously, a service line can incorporate a variety of other functional specialties. If the specialized personnel remain a part of their specialty units but are assigned to a particular service line, then the overall management structure is termed a matrix organization, since it retains the more traditional vertical form while encompassing product line units (see Figure 2-5). A matrix organization is complicated, and there is a potential for conflict due to tension between the service line managers and the heads of specialized departments. Also, most employees are accountable to two superiors: their service line boss and their specialty boss.

If the various specialized personnel are members of the service line unit and are not accountable to their specialty departments, the overall management structure is termed a unitary organization (see Figure 2-6). This form permits the highest level of integration at the operating level and the highest degree of decentralized decision making. However, this form can be expensive if the overall organization is not large enough to duplicate the various specialists without creating inefficiency.

Determining the proper structure for health care organizations will be one of the management challenges of the next century. This is because there must be a fit between a health care organization's structure and strategy and the environment in which it operates.

Conflict Resolution

Conflict can arise in any situation in which individuals or groups have incompatible goals or perceptions. There are several reasons why health care organizations are highly conflictive. Since it is hard to measure organizational effectiveness by outcomes, there is plenty of room for arguments over what is the right thing to do and how to do it. The wide variety of persons involved, especially professionals, gives rise to an equally wide variety of perspectives and expectations. These clash. In addition, the varied sources of power in health care organizations produce conflict over who has authority and who may decide what to do. Finally, the

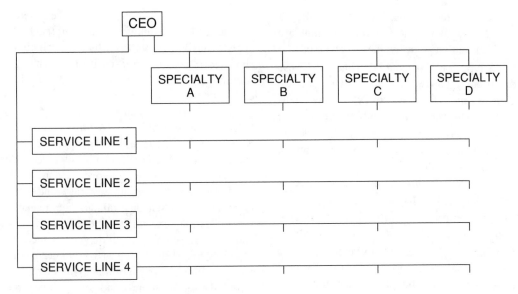

Figure 2-5 A Matrix Organizational Structure

sheer intensity of providing care can cause conflict: The unexpected is always arising, personnel are constantly dealing with life-and-death issues, most actions must be done at exactly the right time, and there can be no mistakes because there are seldom any second chances.

These factors combine and intensify one another. It is no wonder that observers of health care organi-

zations use phrases like "a built-in sense of rage," "conflict is endemic," and "most management is management by crisis."

Is conflict good or bad? It depends.

- Conflict can be good if it is recognized and not ignored. Conflict is usually the manifestation of some fundamental problem that needs ad-

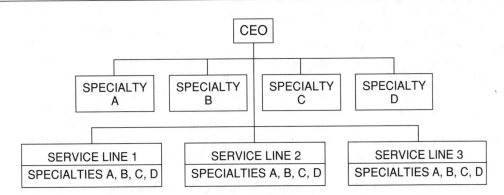

Figure 2-6 A Unitary Organizational Structure

dressing. Effective managers face conflicts rather than avoid them. Conflicts that are avoided seldom go away; they get worse.

- Some types of conflict are detrimental. These divert energy away from goal attainment, deplete resources (time or money), damage individuals, and make cooperation difficult.
- Some types of conflict are beneficial. Confict, for example, can lead to constructive problem solving, a search by people for ways of changing how they do things, and a greater acceptance of change in general.
- Too little expressed conflict leads to stagnation, but uncontrolled conflict invites chaos.
- Conflict is sometimes able to be handled by a conflict resolution process, and use of such a process can have benefits other than mere resolution of the conflict.

In short, it is not conflict per se that is good or bad but rather its management.

The effective health care manager must have skills and techniques to deal with conflict. One of the most important of these is diagnosis. Knowing the type of conflict and the level at which it is operating is crucial to its resolution.

There are three basic types of organizational conflict.

Goal conflict occurs when desired end states or preferred outcomes are incompatible. For instance, the dean of a medical school might want more clinical research support from the hospital laboratory, whereas the CEO of the hospital wants a quicker turnaround for tests in order to enhance diagnosis and treatment. Gains on one side are seen as losses on the other.

Cognitive conflict occurs when ideas or opinions are perceived as incompatible. This kind of conflict is due to a misunderstanding or misperception. The head nurse, to take an imaginary example, thought that the pharmacy department was slow to fill "stat" prescriptions, whereas the pharmacy department thought the nurses labeled some prescriptions "stat" unnecessarily. Once the cognitive dissonance was cleared up, the conflict could be resolved. Actually, the staff of the messenger department had been reduced, causing delays for which the pharmacists and nurses were blaming each other. The agreed solution was to stock commonly used drugs in unit doses at the nursing stations.

Affective conflict occurs when feelings or emotions are incompatible (i.e., people or groups become angry with one another). Suppose a hospital laundry manager had to deal with a high rate of turnover among her female employees. Many of those hired were also raising families and found the strict eight-hour work schedule taxing. The manager installed flextime scheduling, removed the time clocks, and taught the employees all the jobs on the laundry assembly line. The result was that women came and went at will from early morning to midnight, created informal assembly groups, and got the laundry out. In fact, the women began to feel it was "their" laundry and gradually assumed more responsibility for its successful operation. Turnover went down and laundry output per employee went up. Even so, it was hard to know who was working when, who was not working, and whether labor laws were being violated. A new vice-president was appointed whose supervisory duties included the laundry department. To her the laundry was sloppy, out of control, and in need of "managerial order." Here was the affective conflict: The new vice-president could not stand the laundry manager's management, and the laundry manager was irritated and threatened by the vice-president's rigidity. Whenever they met, there was heightened tension and open conflict. Soon they stopped meeting and distanced themselves. The laundry manager feared that her job was on the line.

These three types of conflict, as illustrated by the examples, appear to be interpersonal. However, they are really organizational, because the conflictive individuals represent organizational units and levels that are in contest over resources, how best to render care, or who has authority and power.

Organizational conflict occurs when there is discord caused by the way jobs are designed, the organization is structured, and formal authority is allocated.

Vertical conflict occurs between levels (e.g., the discord between the laundry manager and the vice-president). It often arises when subordinates resist attempts by superiors to restrict their autonomy. But it also arises from the other sources mentioned previously: misunderstandings, lack of consensus on goals, and so on.

Horizontal conflict occurs within the same hierarchic level (e.g., when each department strives for its own goals regardless of the effect on other departments). The nursing-pharmacy conflict over "stat" prescriptions is an example of horizontal conflict.

Line-staff conflict sometimes results when line managers feel that staff managers are using their technical knowledge to intrude upon the line managers' areas of legitimate authority. Open conflict is particularly likely when staff managers control resources used by line managers. For example, in a service line management structure, the implementation of a strategic plan for home health services for cancer patients might be held up by the staff-level marketing department, which has the authority to review such plans. Line managers usually feel that staff managers try to reduce their operational authority and autonomy, even though their line responsibility for obtaining results will remain unchanged.

Role conflict occurs when there is inconsistency or misunderstanding about the job a person is supposed to be doing. Such a misunderstanding can take place between a subordinate and a superior ("You told me to manage this laundry department efficiently; I thought I could put in flextime schedules and split shifts"), between different groups that depend on each other ("Admitting is supposed to stop elective admissions by 5:00 PM, but doctors keep calling at 7:00 PM saying a patient has just been sent to the hospital for admission"), or between an individual's notions of acceptable behavior and his or her job ("This admitting job requires me to stay after hours; it is wearing me out and I have no social life").

A classic model for dealing with conflicts is shown in Figure 2-7. Five styles (or methods) are

identified by their location on two dimensions: *concern for self* and *concern for others*. A person's desire to satisfy his or her own concerns depends on the extent to which the person is *assertive* in pursuing personal or unit goals. The person's desire to satisfy the concerns of others depends on the extent to which he or she is *cooperative.* The five styles thus represent different combinations of assertiveness and cooperativeness.

Avoidance involves behavior that is unassertive and uncooperative. People use this style to stay out of conflicts, ignore disagreements, or remain neutral. Sometimes conflict is avoided out of a calculation that "it will work itself out." Or avoidance might reflect an aversion to tensions or frustrations. In addition, although avoidance sometimes minimizes the possibility of escalation of conflict, ignoring issues is frustrating to others. Further, while the conflict at hand may seem to have gone away, there is usually a residue of feelings and relations that will impact future conflicts.

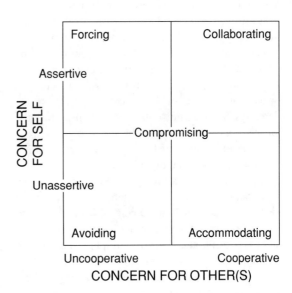

Figure 2-7 Conflict-Handling Styles. *Source:* Reprinted from *Handbook of Industrial and Organizational Psychology* by M.D. Dunnette, ed., p. 922, with permission of Marvin D. Dunnette.

In the example above, the laundry manager and the vice-president used the strategy of avoidance. They stopped meeting, communicated by memo, and effectively distanced themselves from each other and the issue of disagreement.

Forcing is an assertive and uncooperative method of dealing with conflict. It reflects a win-lose attitude: The forcing person feels that one side must win and the other must lose. This method usually helps a person achieve his or her goals, but its regular use by a manager develops fear, lack of respect, and hatred by those affected.

The vice-president could have used this method with the laundry manager and fired her. It is clear that the superior had the power in the situation and could have used it. This would have resolved the conflict.

Accommodating is a cooperative but unassertive method. Accommodating is often called the lose-win strategy. It may reflect unselfishness or simple submission. Accommodators are usually viewed favorably by others, although also being seen as weak and submissive.

Most interpersonal relationships in organizations are enduring (i.e., they have a past and a future). Therefore, accommodation in one conflict may have the purpose of buying reciprocal accommodation in the future, in which case accommodating would be part of a longer-term strategy of cooperation. The informal networks of most managers are laced with "chits" or "you owe me's." These are legacies from earlier conflicts that influence the process and outcome of subsequent ones. This is but one illustration of how informal organization helps to make formal organization work.

Collaborating is a highly cooperative and assertive method. It is a win-win method. It represents a desire to maximize joint outcomes. In order for it to work, both parties to a conflict have to be committed to the joint outcome. An example is the solution the laundry manager worked out with her employees; it met the employees' concerns as well as hers as the department manager.

The following tends to be true of managers who are effective at using the collaborative method[18]:

- They see conflict as natural and leading to a more creative solution if handled properly.
- They are trusting of others and exhibit candor.
- They believe that the parties at conflict have an equal role in resolving the issues and view the opinions of all parties as legitimate.
- They recognize that when conflict is resolved to the satisfaction of all parties, there results a greater commitment to the solution.
- They do not sacrifice any one person simply for the good of the group.

Compromising is an intermediately cooperative and assertive method. It is based on give and take and typically involves a series of negotiations and concessions. It is commonly used and widely accepted; indeed, many managers feel it is the only method available. Reasons for this include the following: (1) It can be seen primarily as a cooperative gesture even though it is also a holding back, (2) it is a practical approach and appeals to those who regard themselves as practical, and (3) it usually results in a legacy of good relations for the future. On the other hand, it can yield subsequent doubts about the fairness of the outcome and the equality of each party's concessions. Compared to the collaboration, compromise does not maximize joint satisfaction; rather, it results in moderate but partial satisfaction for each party.

Negotiation is based on the concept of interdependence: Both sides recognize that they mutually have needs and that they must work together after the conflict. The two parties are aware that each is trying to influence the other and that agreement is a function of (1) the power they bring to the situation and (2) their skill at bargaining. Party A's bargaining power depends on the attractiveness of party A's inducements to party B. It is measured in B's cost of disagreeing relative to B's cost of agreeing. The reverse is B's power.

As an illustration, the chief financial officer of a hospital (Party B) was charged with negotiating a contract price with the state (Party A) for all future

Medicaid patients. She knew there was a date by which a contract had to be signed, and she knew there would be no more than three bargaining sessions. She had a rough idea of the hospital's marginal costs of serving its Medicaid patients. She entered the first bargaining session with a price that was almost twice her hospital's marginal cost. The state negotiator rejected the bid; furthermore, he said he knew the hospital's costs and provided a figure that was almost exactly the same as the chief financial officer's estimate. Thus, not only did the state have substantial power deriving from the enticement of a very large contract, but it also had financial knowledge about the hospital that enhanced its bargaining position.

In general, there are four ways one party can gain bargaining power over another. Table 2-3 lists these four ways, along with examples based on the hospital-Medicaid price negotiation.

The chief financial officer concluded from her analysis of bargaining position that the hospital was in a weak position and faced either of two bleak futures: (1) It could contract at a price below marginal costs, thus losing money on more than a third of its business, or (2) it could refuse to contract, which would require it to downsize by more than a third. She calculated that two of the state's bargaining costs might be altered. The first was the state's long-term cost: It might want or need the hospital's future capacity to care for Medicaid patients and thus not wish to prevent the hospital from serving Medicaid beneficiaries in the future by failing to contract or contracting at a submarginal cost. Second, the state had an obligation to obtain contracts of sufficient volume to cover all Medicaid beneficiaries in the community. If the hospital did not contract, the state would need to contract with both of the other hospitals. Once these hospitals knew they had the state in this position, the state's cost of bargaining would go up because these hospitals would now "sharpen their pencils."

For this reason, the chief financial officer decided on this bargaining strategy: delay the second and third rounds of bargaining until just before the deadline. This would increase the state's calculation of its bargaining costs because it would have to take into account the option of contracting with two higher priced alternatives.

In the intervening time, a key event occurred that altered the balance of power. One of the two other hospitals calculated that a low-priced contract for 10 percent of its patients was "too great a cost to pay"; it advised the state privately that it was withdrawing from negotiations. The chief financial officer learned of this from a new accounting employee previously employed by the other hospital. This fact reduced her hospital's costs of disagreement and increased the state's costs of disagreement (by altering item 2 in Table 2-3).

Shortly before the deadline, the chief financial officer entered the second round of bargaining with a bid price of 20 percent above marginal costs. There were brief negotiations, during which the chief financial officer told the state negotiators that a price below marginal cost would "lead to the future elimination of the hospital as a Medicaid provider." The hospital and the state quickly agreed upon a price of 11 percent above marginal costs.

To summarize, managers of health care organizations face high levels of organizational conflict. How conflict is managed often determines whether it has beneficial or destructive effects upon the enterprise and the people involved. Effective conflict management starts with diagnosis, since conflict that is manifest may not be real. For conflict that is real, there is an array of techniques that can be brought to bear, each appropriate to different types and levels of conflict. The effective manager tries to find the resolution that lets all parties win.[19]

EFFECTIVE LEADERSHIP

As noted early in this chapter, the purposes of health care management are not identical to the purposes of management in other types of business. Likewise, health care leadership has certain unique elements.

Table 2-3 Sources of Bargaining Power

Party A Has Bargaining Power over Party B When:	Hospital-Medicaid Example
1. A can increase B's cost of disagreement.	The hospital will lose 35% of its patients if it does not contract.
2. A has alternatives that cost less than B.	The state can contract with two other hospitals in the same community.
3. B cannot increase A's cost of disagreement.	The hospital cannot prevent the state from negotiating a lower rate with another hospital.
4. B has no alternatives that cost less than A.	Lost Medicaid patients cannot be replaced by privately insured patients.

Health care organizations depend to an unusual extent on the service commitments of their employees, professionals, and volunteers. The satisfaction of serving and helping is psychic income that augments dollar income. It follows that setting the moral tone and reinforcing the values of service are important leadership tasks.

Health care organizations produce services, not things. Thus the precise measuring of performance, common in manufacturing is more difficult in health services delivery. While more sophisticated outcome measures are being developed, health services are less tangible. It follows that people in health care organizations are guided more by vision, goals, and values than by production targets and output payments. Leadership involves establishing and reinforcing a service-oriented morality.

Health care enterprises also do not possess tight corporate hierarchies where things get done because managers order them to be done. To a great extent, commands in health care enterprises will be followed only if they are accepted as legitimate and reasonable by those expected to respond. But what is reasonable and legitimate? This is what leadership establishes.

Finally, many health care enterprises (including most hospitals) are community benefit organizations relieved of the duty to pay taxes because they relieve poverty and suffering. Such organizations are part of a long tradition of private volunteerism and trusteeship. The values of service and community trust that underpin this tradition must be con-

stantly articulated and reinforced. Health care leadership must accept the main responsibility for setting community service goals and strategies.

In short, health care organizations are value driven, and their leaders establish and nurture the appropriate values. Below is a description of eight ways in which they can do this.

Vision

The effective manager must be able to articulate a clear vision for the organization or his or her unit and do it in such a way that others come to believe in that vision. Subordinates must buy into what the unit must do to advance the vision. They must become excited by the vision and develop a "can do" attitude.

Where is such a vision to come from? Perhaps from the history, tradition, and culture of the enterprise. Perhaps from its mission statement, which itself is an expression of vision. Perhaps from a strategic plan. Perhaps from the manager's own convictions about what is important to believe and do. Perhaps from discussion with those potentially affected by the vision. Whatever the source, the manager has to personally own the vision; otherwise, the manager will fail to inspire others.

Commitment to the Development of Others

The manager must encourage and support the efforts of individuals within the organization to maximize their understanding and skills and must create a working environment that motivates them to commit their personal energy and talents to the pursuit of organizational objectives.

Commitment to the development of others is an expression of trust in subordinates and in their initiative and creativity. This trust even encompasses permission to take risks and make mistakes, present alternative views, and offer dissent. In many ways, managing others means managing the development of others. In this role, the manager is more a mentor, educator, and coach than a boss (Theory Y at work). The focus will often be on finding and encouraging subordinates whose strengths compensate the manager's weaknesses. One result of developing others is that they come to feel a sense of loyalty—loyalty to the manager and loyalty to the organization.

But it all starts with trust. A leader has to be a trusting person (as well as trustworthy) and demonstrate trust by the way he or she manages. This is leadership by empowerment.[20] Subordinates will rise to the occasion when they feel trusted and empowered.

Establishing Values

It is the leader's job to discover and declare what his or her organization stands for, to establish a morality that becomes the standard for others, and to declare this in clear and inspiring terms. Organizations are strongly guided by culture; managing the evolution of organizational culture is the process of establishing values. It is important for the self-esteem and respect of subordinates to know that their actions are being evaluated in the context of a value system. They also are sensitive to these values and can be relied upon to reflect them in their behavior. The effective manager reinforces this system of values by personal example. This is "principled leadership."[21]

Learning

Health care organizations are public service organizations. The environment in which they oper-

ate is rapidly changing, and so they must be open to new knowledge. They must provide opportunities for their managers at all levels to go out beyond organizational boundaries in order to look, learn, and bring back.

Looking beyond includes the use of many formal methods: environmental assessment, long-range planning, SWOT (strengths, weaknesses, opportunities, threats) analysis, portfolio analysis, focus groups, and strategic management, to name a few. These methods are often of tremendous assistance in learning what to do and how to do it better, and they are frequently employed by the top managers responsible for the well-being of the entire organization.

Looking beyond, however, is a strategy other managers need to use as well. Department managers, for example, need to communicate with other department managers to determine whether the fit, integration, and contributions of their departments are proper and effective and whether changes, new directions, and new priorities are in order. Leading requires looking beyond, looking beyond leads to learning, and a learning organization is a more effective organization.[22] (See Chapter 5.)

Priorities and Direction

Establishing priorities adds focus. Setting the direction of the organization shows people what priorities are highest, how the organization's vision and values can be put into action, and where they should place their energies. Leadership establishes the strategic direction, and this focuses the organization's efforts on addressing its priorities. (See Chapter 17.)

Problem Solving

There is a difference between real problems and pseudoproblems. The effective manager knows how to identify the real ones. He or she also knows how to analyze the effects of possible solutions to problems and how to translate a plan into action. Problem solving is less difficult if the manager creates an atmosphere in which others feel empowered to solve problems. Problem solving is a shirt-sleeve management task.[23]

Balancing Interests

Health care organizations are comprised of and associated with myriad interest groups: employees, physicians, nurses, the community, patients, suppliers, insurers, lenders, politicians, the media, and so on. Often they do not have a specific group of owners (stockholders) whose interests should clearly be given the highest priority. The effective health care manager works to balance the interests of all the stakeholders, usually to the benefit of the largest good. This balancing often calls for skills in facilitation, negotiation, and conflict resolution.[24] It also requires consideration of ethical issues.

Public Benefit

Obviously organizational benefit is a goal of each manager. However, it should not be the only goal, and health care managers typically place community benefit and patient benefit at the top. This is the major difference between these executives and their business counterparts. The latter must "do no harm" and must "do well"; the former must "do good" for the public and patients they serve. Of course the commitment to doing good must become a major element of the enterprise's value system. The effective leader must not only have and demonstrate a commitment to the public benefit but know how and when organizational objectives and actions should be modified in order to meet broad community needs.

The commitment of health care organizations to the public benefit will be sorely tested in the years to come. In fact, the challenges to this commitment will increase as competition in the health care market becomes stronger and more widespread. This competition will stimulate health care institutions to be more business- and profit-oriented and encourage them to abandon their public benefit missions in favor of bottom-line margins.[25] In a market economy, it is true that no margin means no mission. It is not true that with margin comes mission. Health care executives have to determine the nature and depth of their commitment to community benefit. Those with a strong commitment will be better able to lead their organizations effectively.

THE FUTURE OF MANAGEMENT

The present provides clues about the needs and the characteristics of health care management at the beginning of the new century. Three fundamental and related features are discernible.

Decentralization

Centralized management and decision making do not provide the flexibility, discretion, and innovation needed by health care organizations facing changing environments and competitive markets. The new century will witness further decentralization of most health care enterprises. This decentralization will be structured along service and product lines, with operating units designed to provide a wide array of services and to be broadly managed. Increasingly, these units will be customer driven. They will provide more opportunities for health care managers but also make greater demands on them.

Focus on Patients

In the new century, managed programs, not departments, will be in the ascendancy, and these programs will be organized around defined patient types and patient needs. Support services will be decentralized to these program units, and a number of specialized staff members, such as pharmacists, nutritionists, and medical information specialists, will become part of the patient service team. Likewise, administrative work will be decentralized to program units (e.g., admitting, the business office, discharge planning, quality assurance, and utilization review). On these units and at the bedside, there will be full use of computers to process clinical and managerial information. Other miniaturized technologies will be in full use, reducing the dependency of these units on central, institution-wide diagnostic and therapeutic departments and increasing their flexibility and autonomy. The structure of the entire enterprise will thus become more flat, with fewer second- and third-level middle managers and supervisors.[26]

Focus on Quality Improvement

The new century will find effective health care managers placing an emphasis on continuous quality improvement. Their assumption will be that every operation can be improved through the use of systems studies based on process control charting and statistical quality control. Managers will improve operations employing a six-step process[27]:

1. Become aware that a problem exists.
2. Determine the specific problem to be solved.
3. Diagnose the causes of the problem:
   - Formulate hypotheses about possible causes.
   - Test the hypotheses using existing data or new experiments.
   - Continue until one or more causes are proven.
4. Determine remedies.
5. Implement remedies.
6. Implement controls to hold the gains.

These are the techniques of management science. Indeed, effective health care management in the new century will become less of an art and more of a science.

NOTES

1. H. Mintzberg, *Mintzberg on Management: Inside Our Strange World of Organizations* (New York: The Free Press, 1981).
2. H. Fayol, *General and Industrial Management,* trans. J.A. Conbrough (Geneva: International Management Institute, 1929).
3. H. Koontz et al., *Management,* 8th ed. (New York: McGraw-Hill, 1984).
4. R. Miles and C.S. Snow, Fit, Failure, and the Hall of Fame, in *Strategy and Organization,* eds. G. Carroll and D. Vogel (Marshfield, Mass.: Pitman Publishing, 1984).
5. P. Lawrence and J. Lorsch, *Organization and Environment: Managing Differentiation and Integration* (Boston: Harvard University Press, 1967).
6. D. McGregor, *The Human Side of Enterprise* (New York: McGraw-Hill, 1960).
7. J. Ivancevich et al., *Management* (Homewood, Ill.: Irwin, 1989).
8. F.E. Fiedler and M. Chemers, *Leadership and Effective Management* (Glenview, Ill.: Scott, Foresman, 1974).
9. V.H. Vroom and P. Yetton, *Leadership and Decision Making* (Pittsburgh: University of Pittsburgh Press, 1973).
10. V.H. Vroom, Can Leaders Learn to Lead? *Organizational Dynamics,* Winter 1976, pp. 17–28.
11. R.J. House, A Path-Goal Theory of Leadership Effectiveness, *Administrative Science Quarterly,* September 1971, pp. 321–339.
12. R.J. House and G. Dessler, The Path-Goal Theory of Leadership: Some Post-Hoc and A Priori Tests, in *Contingency Approaches to Leadership,* ed. J.G. Hunt (Carbondale, Ill.: Southern Illinois University Press, 1974).
13. C. Barnard, *The Functions of the Executive* (Cambridge, Mass.: Harvard University Press, 1938).
14. J.R.P. French and B. Raven, The Basis of Social Power, in *Studies in Social Power,* ed. D. Cartwright (Ann Arbor, Mich.: Institute for Social Research, University of Michigan, 1959).
15. D. Starkweather, The Rationale for Decentralization in Large Hospitals, *Hospital and Health Services Administration,* Spring 1970, pp. 27–45.
16. J. Thompson, *Organizations in Action* (New York: McGraw-Hill, 1967), 143.
17. J.G. March and H. Simon, *Organizations* (New York: Wiley, 1958).
18. M.A. Rahim, *Managing Conflict in Organizations* (New York: Praeger, 1986).
19. J.D. Stulberg, *Taking Charge: Managing Conflicts* (Lexington, Mass.: Lexington Books, 1987).

20. S. Covey, *The Seven Habits of Highly Effective People* (New York: Simon and Schuster, 1989).

21. S. Covey, *Principle-centered Leadership* (New York: Simon and Schuster, 1990).

22. P. Senge, *The Fifth Discipline* (New York: Doubleday, 1990).

23. T.J. Peters and R.H. Waterman, *In Search of Excellence: Lessons from America's Best Run Companies* (New York:

Harper & Row, 1982).

24. Stulberg, *Taking Charge.*

25. B. Gray, *The Changing Accountability of Doctors and Hospitals* (Cambridge, Mass.: Harvard University Press, 1992).

26. W.F. Jones and Ratcliff Architects, The Patient Centered Hospital (unpublished manuscript).

27. J.M. Juran, ed., *Quality Control Handbook,* 3rd ed. (New York: McGraw-Hill, 1974).

Daniel R. Longo
Donald W. Avant

Managing Quality

3

Purpose: The purpose of quality management is to establish a system that measures and manages patient care in a way that provides the best care for all patients. It identifies opportunities for improvement as well as system problems that require resolution. It ultimately fulfills a societal commitment of the health professions to the American public.

INTRODUCTION

This chapter provides a context in which to understand the evolution of quality management and its impact on the clinical and managerial activities of health care delivery organizations. The first section contains a list of management principles that apply to quality management. The second section explores the history and background of quality management from its origin to the present. In particular, it traces the major eras in this evolution, indicates the major trends of today, and predicts future trends. The last section explores the pragmatic implications of these trends for health care executives, whether clinical or administrative leaders.

MANAGEMENT PRINCIPLES

- Quality of care is a responsibility owed by health care professionals to those served.
- A knowledge of organizational systems, clinical medicine, general management, and statistics is vital to the management of quality.
- Quality of care measurement and management is a distinct body of knowledge with its own theories, concepts, methods, and techniques.
- Quality is both objective and subjective.
- A thorough knowledge of the health care delivery system is essential for understanding quality.
- Quality of care is not solely the domain of clinicians.
- Quality of care results from an interrelated system of processes.
- Quality management is an important management function.
- Good management theory applies to clinical quality management in the same way it applies to fiscal management.

- There is no "one" or "best" way to measure or manage quality.
- Quality of care can be continuously improved.
- A good quality management system is vital to organizational survival.

HISTORY

Today's managers of quality in health care are part of a long and colorful history. For example, this Babylonian cuneiform text from 2000 B.C. sets out billing guidelines for physicians as well as a penalty for incompetence:

> If the doctor shall treat a gentleman and shall open an abscess with the knife and shall preserve the eye of the patient, he shall receive ten shekels of silver. If the patient is a slave his master shall pay two shekels of silver. If the doctor shall open an abscess with a blunt knife and shall kill the patient or shall destroy the sight of the eye, his hand shall be cut off.[1]

Although our system of rewards and penalties has changed, society's interest in ensuring the best possible medical care has remained constant. The history of quality assurance is largely the history of physicians being asked for their best work by their regulators—the church, the state, or other members of their profession.[2]

However, the nursing movement led by Florence Nightingale deserves a great deal of credit for improving health care quality as well.[3] Nightingale wrote in *Notes on Nursing* that "the very first requirement of the hospital is that it do the patient no harm."[4] Her reforms included cleanliness, sanitation, and dietary improvements as well as the establishment of discipline and organization in the hospital routine. Her simple but humane approach greatly improved hospital mortality.

The twentieth century history of the quality of care evolution is outlined in Exhibit 3-1. After the 1910 Flexner Report, which upgraded medical education, the American College of Surgeons (ACS) began a similar project to improve hospitals. The minimum standard established by ACS is found in

Exhibit 3-1 Evolution of Quality Assessment

- 1910—Flexner Report
- 1918—American College of Surgeons
- 1951—Joint Commission on Accreditation of Healthcare Organizations
- 1965—Medicare
- 1972—PEP audit
- 1979—Problem-focused review
- 1981—Systematic monitoring and evaluation
- 1989—Integrated quality assessment
- 1990s—Total quality management/continuous quality improvement
- 1993+—Clinton health reforms

Exhibit 3-2. For about three decades beginning in 1920, the college developed criteria and promoted them in hospitals. Their goals included uniform organizations, regular review of records, adequate facilities, and regulation of practice.[5] In particular, ACS proposed the review of tissue removed in surgery and comparison of the findings with the preoperative diagnosis. This type of review is required by the Joint Commission on Accreditation of Healthcare Organizations today.

The growth in hospitals in the post–World War II through Hill-Burton (later Hill-Harris) funds further strengthened the role of hospital licensure laws and regulations, since meeting these regulations was a prerequisite for acquiring support for building projects.

Later, in 1952, the Joint Commission assumed the tasks of the hospital standardization program of the American College of Surgeons. In so doing, the Joint Commission initially took up Dr. E. A. Codman's method for evaluating patient care. Codman's system involved auditing medical records, assigning a favorable or unfavorable outcome, and following up one year later (see Exhibit 3-2). The Joint Commission used this system in its early Medical audit program. Quickly, Joint Commission accreditation became the "gold standard" sought after by the majority of U.S. hospitals. The accreditor's influence gained greater hold as it moved into the areas of mental health, long-term

Exhibit 3-2 The Minimum Standard

1. That physicians and surgeons privileged to practice in the hospital be organized as a definite group or staff. Such organization has nothing to do with the question as to whether the hospital is "open" or "closed," nor need it affect the various existing types of staff organization. The word "staff" is here defined as the group of doctors who practice in the hospital inclusive of all groups such as the "regular staff," "the visiting staff," and the "associate staff."

2. That membership upon the staff be restricted to physicians and surgeons who are (a) full graduates of medicine in good standing and legally licensed to practice in their respective states or provinces, (b) competent in their respective fields, and (c) worthy in character and matters of professional ethics; that in this latter connection the practice of the division of fees, under any guise whatever, be prohibited.

3. That the staff initiate and, with the approval of the governing board of the hospital, adopt rules, regulations, and policies governing the professional work of the hospital; that these rules, regulations, and policies specifically provide:

   (a) That staff meetings he held at least once each month. (In large hospitals the departments may choose to meet separately.)

   (b) That the staff review and analyze at regular intervals their clinical experience in the various departments of the hospital, such as medicine, surgery, obstetrics, and the other specialties; the clinical records of patients, free and pay, to be the basis for such review and analyses.

4. That accurate and complete records be written for all patients and filed in an accessible manner in the hospital—a complete care record being one which includes identification data; complaint; personal and family history; history or present illness; physical examination; special examinations, such as consultations, clinical laboratory, X-ray and other examinations; provisional or working diagnosis; medical or surgical treatment; gross and microscopical pathological findings; progress notes; final diagnosis; condition on discharge; follow-up and, in case of death, autopsy findings.

5. That diagnostic and therapeutic facilities under competent supervision be available for the study, diagnosis, and treatment of patients, these to include, at least (a) a clinical laboratory providing chemical, bacteriological, serological, and pathological services; (b) an X-ray department providing radiographic and fluoroscopic services.

Source: Minimum Standard of the American College of Surgeons' Hospital Standardization Program, 1918.

---

care, ambulatory care, hospice, and home care. Subsequent to the development of the Joint Commission, a variety of other accrediting organizations were organized by health groups. They tended to focus on programmatic accreditation, whereas the Joint Commission accredits an entire organization. Nonetheless, today the Joint Commission remains the premier voluntary accrediting body with Medicare-deemed status in the majority of states.

The Social Security Acts of 1965 and 1972, along with Joint Commission's shift in emphasis regarding peer and clinical review toward ongoing review of quality of care through patient care audits and studies, have had the greatest effect on quality of care issues since the Flexner Report.[6] Along with the establishment of Medicare and Medicaid in 1965 came the concept of utilization review, which began to integrate the concepts of quality of care and utilization management. Further, it tied together, at least from a payment and sanction perspective, the issues of cost and quality. It began a movement that has continued to this day. That is, as payers, whether they be federal, state, or employer groups, increasingly pay for the cost of health care, they increasingly demand accountability. They ask, Are the dollars expended resulting in a proportionate increase in good outcomes? Is the care appropriate? Is the care cost-effective? These questions will perhaps remain in the forefront of thinking on medical care for the foreseeable future. The 1972 act established professional standards review organizations (PSROs) that continued to strengthen the tie of quality and cost through government regulations by creating external review agencies for "peer review." The PSRO and related legislation place greater emphasis on retrospective audit or medical care evaluation as the definitive route for review and improvement of care quality.[7] After PSRO implementation, there were a variety of research efforts that aimed at improving methods for the review of medical care. Foremost among these is the work of Avedis Donabedian, who in numerous publications during this period articulated a conceptual model aimed at understanding quality of care. His model of structure, process, and outcome as the major components for reviewing quality of care is still valid today. From his 1966 article "Evaluating the Quality of Medical Care," published in the *Milbank Memorial Fund Quarterly,* through his 1985 text *The Methods and Findings of Quality Assessment and Monitoring,* Donabedian constructed a firm and comprehensive foundation and framework for understanding the complex concept of quality.

Other efforts during this period included a great deal of activity by the Joint Commission directed toward developing techniques for quality assurance and assessment. These efforts resulted in medical audits, in particular the performance evaluation procedure (PEP) audits. The next step was the development by Joyce Craddick and the California Medical Malpractice Experiment of a technique for the identification of problems through occurrence screening. This was followed by the systematic monitoring and evaluation approach of the Joint Commission. This approach was aimed at replacing periodic review of care with ongoing review. It set the stage for the later Joint Commission move in the late 1980s toward review of outcomes of care through quality improvement activities.

The mid-1980s were also characterized by increased public awareness and consumer concern about quality. The watershed event occurred in December 1986 when the Health Care Financing Administration (HCFA) publicly released its report on hospital mortality statistics. This was the first time in history that the public could read in the local newspaper about the experience of hospitals in treating Medicare patients. The release, hailed by consumers and consumer groups and denounced by providers, ushered in an era of public accountability. Once outcome data were released, there was no stepping back—the public's thirst for health care outcome data became insatiable. Other releases, in Iowa and Pennsylvania, included outcomes for non-Medicare patients.

Also of note is the history of public health departments in their inspection and licensure of health care facilities. While there is great variability in the nature and scope of such activities, what is clear is each state's need to monitor care in the interest of the public. The New York State Department of Health, under former commissioner of health Dr. David Axelrod and later under commissioner Mark Chassin, has often been in the vanguard. Although the New York State's reforms in the monitoring of resident hours and its comprehensive survey process were not always welcomed by the hospitals of the state, these clearly set the New York State Department of Health apart, at least in regards to hospital surveillance activities. Further, reforms under Dr. Chassin are aimed at linking outcomes with reimbursement. This is opening yet another chapter in the history of quality assessment and cost control.

The period from the mid-1980s to the early 1990s saw an explosion of quality of care initiatives and activities, ranging from research activities to demonstrations. These major initiatives were carried out by a variety of groups, including hospital associations, foundations, government agencies, business companies, accrediting bodies, and universities. Although they are too numerous to allow mention of each one, nine of the most notable during this time period are listed in Table 3-1.

Unlike in previous time periods, the great explosion of quality of care projects in the mid-1980s and 1990s set the stage for the presidential election of 1992, whose main focus was the domestic economy. Control of the rising cost of health care is viewed as the key to getting control of the national debt. Consequently, the reform of the health care system has been viewed as one of the major tasks for the Clinton administration. While the specifics of the Clinton plan and its implications will unfold over the coming years, it is clear that cost controls and quality monitoring will be major components of the reformed national health care system.

In summary, the history of quality assurance and management is rich and diverse. The recent initiatives, together with the prospects for substantial health care reform, make the challenges of the mid-

Table 3-1 Quality of Care Initiatives, Mid-1980s to Early 1990s

Organization	Initiative	Aims
Joint Commission on Accreditation of Healthcare Organization	Agenda for Change	To revamp accreditation to reflect outcomes of care
Hospital Association of New York State	Quality of Care Initiatives	To equip voluntary hospitals with state-of-the-art techniques in quality assessment
Hospital Research and Educational Trust	Quality Measurement and Management Project (QMMP)	To develop state-of-the-art tools and techniques to better measure and manage quality of hospital care
American Medical Association	Division of Quality of Care	To facilitate the development of practice guidelines
Robert Wood Johnson Foundation	Program to Improve the Quality of Hospital Care	To develop consortiums for the sharing of quality of care resources to improve hospital quality
Institute of Medicine	Study to Design a Strategy for Quality Review and Assurance in Medicine	Eight legislative charges consistent with study title
Agency for Health Care Policy and Research	Patient Outcome Research Teams (PORTs); practice guide	To develop and disseminate strategies that improve patient outcomes through identification of effective practices
Washington Business Group on Health	Quality of Care Initiatives for Employers	To contain the cost of health care while maintaining quality
Harvard Community Health Plan	Quality Improvement National Demonstration Project	To disseminate industrial quality improvement methods to health care settings

to late 1990s seem formidable. Perhaps even more formidable will be the political will of the American people to dramatically change the way in which care is provided, financed, and monitored. The 1990s are likely to usher in a century of tremendous progress, not only in the science of medicine but also in the science of quality measurement and management. As Bette Davis once said, "Buckle your seatbelts, we're in for a rocky ride."

PROGRAM MANAGEMENT

As indicated in the previous section, state, federal, and accrediting organizations have created an expanding web of regulations and standards that address the quality of patient care in health care organizations, especially those providing inpatient services. Crafting initiatives to meet these standards and the organization's own quality standards so that they form a cohesive program is a significant management challenge. The purpose of this section is to provide quality management program guidelines for selected management parameters. The parameters selected include program goals, structure, resources, basic policy content, quality assessment measures, operational considerations, and leadership.

Goals

Directing a quality management program requires setting goals. The first goal, of course, must be to establish an organized and contemporary program. Others are discussed below.

*Promoting Staff Acceptance, Participation, and
Training*

A quality management program is a complex undertaking. Without staff acceptance, the program
likely will drift aimlessly in the haze of daily operations. One strategy for engendering staff "buy in" is
to set meaningful goals for training and participation. For example, goals could be established that
address who undergoes initial orientation to an
organization's quality management program or that
are directed toward maintaining and stimulating
staff interest in the quality management program
(e.g., a quality management newsletter that informs
staff of changes in the program and recognizes outstanding quality management results).

*Advocating for Changes in Statutes, Regulations,
and Standards That Will Enhance Quality
Management*

Government and accrediting organizations, in
setting guidelines, often try to reach a consensus
that is broad and thoughtful. However, there is no
guarantee that the process will work. As a result,
organizations must be vigilant in monitoring regulations or standards to ensure they promote high-
quality patient care. One strategy might be to consistently advocate for changes in external standards
that would improve quality management. This requires the hospital leadership, including trustees,
administrators, and physician leaders, to track
changes in laws, standards, and regulations and also
to actively participate in local, state, and national
professional organizations that influence the setting
of requirements. Larger organizations may actually
have on staff individuals with expertise in quality of
care standards and regulations who will serve as liaisons to regulatory agencies.

Program Structure

Although organizational complexity may vary,
there are certain basic components that are common
to all quality management programs. Figure 3-1

shows the key components and their relationship in
a quality management program for an organization
with an organized medical staff.

Program Roles

Senior Leadership

The senior leadership encompasses the governing
body, senior organizational management, and medical staff officers. The involvement of the leadership
in quality assurance activities must be continuous,
and the quality management program must be given a
high priority for at least two reasons: First, the staff
and those closely associated with the organization
must understand that the program is of vital importance. Second, because of its scope and complexity,
the program will require extensive coordination and
direction by senior leaders. Supervising quality assurance is a new activity for many seasoned health care
managers, because it was not until the late 1980s that
health services management curricula consistently
addressed quality of care in a deliberate and systematic manner. Consequently, refocusing management
priorities and emphasizing continuing education for
current leaders may be required.

Medical Staff

In an organization with an organized medical
staff, there are several functions that are of particular importance to the quality management program:

- establishing patient care policies
- monitoring clinical activities
- conducting peer review
- meeting externally imposed or adopted regulations and standards
- conducting quality management evaluations
- making recommendations to the governing
  body regarding staff appointments, clinical
  privileges, and the medical staff's structure

Unfortunately, medical school and postgraduate
medical evaluation devotes very little time, if any,

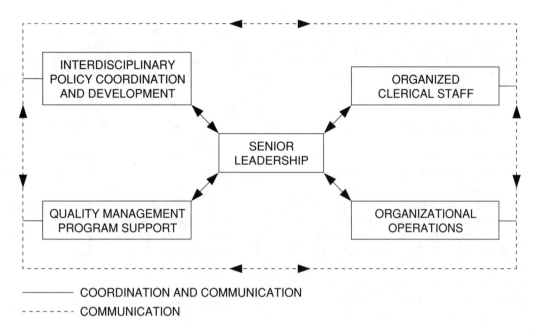

─────── COORDINATION AND COMMUNICATION

------- COMMUNICATION

Figure 3-1 Key Organizational Components of a Quality Management Program

to these topics. Perhaps a young student physician will be exposed through hospital quality or utilization management review activities. However, it is not until residency that a physician begins to experience the reality of practice and to confront the host of review requirements that must be met. Organizations such as the American College of Physician Executives have begun to meet the need for educating practicing physicians. However, further reform of medical education is required if medical students are to be truly prepared for the reality of practice. Students especially need to gain an understanding of quality of care concepts, measurement, and management. In the absence of formalized training, the task of education falls to the health care organization, which must provide carefully designed orientation and continuing education for physicians.

Departments and Services

Various departments and services establish patient care policies, monitor specified patient-related activities for compliance with internally or externally mandated standards, and conduct staff and program evaluations. Such policies and activities require coordination with the overall quality management program. They must be integrated in a manner that promotes cross-departmental reviews as well as review by all levels of the organization, from the department level up to the board of trustees. The success of the quality management program in the departments and services ultimately depends on the managers' taking ownership of the program in each department or service.

Program Support

The program's support staff implement and monitor policies regarding quality. The staff must be technically competent to advise and support departments in the management of their quality management activities. The support staff should have the capability to prepare reports and support the interdisciplinary policy coordination and development function, which is described below. Some estimates indicate that approximately 10 percent of an organization's budget should be spent on quality management support, including everything from computers to continuing education.

Interdisciplinary Policy and Coordination

Coordinating and developing policy should be the center of all quality management activities. The membership of the policy and coordination group should include representatives from senior leadership, the medical staff, appropriate support departments, and quality management support staff. Other organization-wide functions, such as infection control and safety, also should be represented.

In small organizations, representation may be combined, but the concept of interdisciplinary functions should be maintained to the greatest extent possible.

The coordination and policy group must ask probing questions regarding the program's activities and results. The following nine tasks are crucial responsibilities of this group:

- defining specific quality management goals
- developing a comprehensive quality management plan that sets the scope of activities for the program for a specified period
- conducting periodic program evaluations
- defining organization-wide functions and activities that are important to monitor
- regularly receiving and reviewing data from the quality management program
- identifying training needs
- recommending program policy changes to senior leaders
- reviewing and analyzing externally conducted quality assessments and making recommendations to appropriate organizational units and medical staff
- evaluating, integrating, and coordinating changing regulations and standards

This function requires the integration of activities from the patient's perspective. If properly conducted, it tracks patient care through the entire delivery system. While it needs to isolate specific problems, such as infections, there is a need to focus on the overall delivery system so that appropriate activities, such as the prophylactic administration of antibiotics two hours prior to surgery, can occur at the proper interval. Experience from industrial quality improvement and, most recently, from hospital quality improvement highlights the necessity for a systems perspective. James, in *Quality Management for Healthcare Delivery,* makes a compelling case for the view that quality improvement induces interdisciplinary coordination.[8]

Program Resources

Staffing

Although staffing needs will vary in accordance with organizational complexity, the following guidelines may prove helpful:

- Support the interdisciplinary policy coordination and development component.
- Support training, guidance, and advocacy activities.
- Assist the medical staff and the organization's departments and services in the management of their quality programs.

Data Systems

Increasingly, quality management requires handling and analyzing data. In *Integrated Quality Assessment,* Longo, Ciccone, and Lord devote two chapters to data system issues.[9] In the chapter "Using Information," they indicate the necessity of identifying internal and external information systems and integrating them into a comprehensive organizational quality management system. They also suggest methods for data verification, statistical analysis, and data display. In the chapter "Reporting for Quality," they devote considerable time to data presentation and reporting to committees, departments, medical staff, and the governing body. Experience suggests that quality management data systems serve as repositories for all quality management data, allow for integration of all aspects of patient care, promote easy retrieval, incorporate safeguards for confidentiality, and allow data to be stored in a manner that facilitates statistical analysis and interpretation. Further, graphic displays, such as pie charts, bar graphs, and the like, should be incorporated for ease in communication of results.

Current estimates are that data management accounts for 20–25 percent of an organization's quality management budget. (See Chapters 13, 14, and 15 for more on information systems.)

Training

Training staff, including the medical staff, at all levels of the organization is crucial. As previously mentioned, physicians receive little in the way of quality management education and training. The same can be said for most health care administrators, although recent changes in the curricula of health services management programs have begun to meet this need. The most neglected group of all are trustees, who are far more qualified to understand the fiscal performance of a health care organization than its quality of care performance.

As a result, the health care delivery organization faces a tremendous challenge to educate not only its staff members but also its leadership. Such training should encompass the following topics: quality of care theory and concepts; quality of care measurement, techniques, and systems; management of quality; interpretation of quality of care data; preparation and interpretation of quality management reports; implementation of quality management interventions; and components of quality management, including utilization management, risk management, infection control, patient satisfaction, and severity of illness methodology. In addition, time must be devoted to teaching quality assurance and

quality improvement. Finally, the requirements of accrediting bodies, regulatory agencies, and external review organizations must be understood.

Program Policies

Table 3-2 shows the key policy areas and policy documents for a quality management program. The policies are divided between patient care activities and programmatic aspects of the program.

Policies

Exhibit 3-3 outlines the major policies that should be incorporated in the organization's quality management plan.

With respect to credentialing, the bylaws should address the process for evaluating licensure, training, and experience. Training and experience information should be verified through primary sources only. Privileging is an important process whose steps should be clearly documented in the bylaws. Privileges should be

- based upon demonstrated current performance, including professional conduct and judgment and clinical and/or technical skills
- specific to the organization

Table 3-2 Key Quality Management Program Policies

Subject Area	Policy Document
Medical staff privileges	Medical staff bylaws
Organizational staff credentialing, appointment, and evaluation	Personnel policies
Patient care activities	Departmental policies and procedures
	Medical staff rules
Environment	Safety policies
Quality management programmatic activities	Quality Management plan

Exhibit 3-3 Policies To Be Incorporated in the Quality Management Plan

---

Medical Staff Bylaws
Membership eligibility
Credentialing
Appointment
Reappointment and privileging
Organizational structure of the medical staff
Patient care rules and monitoring

Patient Care Policies
Definition of an appropriate patient history and physical
Time limits on standing orders
Patient conditions that require consultation

Quality Management Plan
Program organization
Monitoring and quality improvement activities
Monitoring methods
Program goals
Time periods for evaluation

Personnel Policies
Requirement that an evaluation be done of each applicant's licensure and certification status, training, and experience
Requirement that the evaluation be done based on a job description that sets forth duties and performance criteria

Safety
Safety of the physical plant for employees
Maintenance of clinical equipment and utilities
Staff training
Internal emergency procedures
Fire safety

- clearly delineated, including the terms of temporary privileges
- based on peer recommendations

Bylaws should set time limits on privileges, and reprivileging should be based on data from the quality management program.

Also, the bylaws should require that the medical staff formulate recommendations regarding medical staff membership status and privileges and present them to the organization's governing body

for approval. A thoughtful review by the governing body will determine whether the medical staff has followed the procedures prescribed in the medical staff bylaws (see Chapter 11).

Each department's policies and procedures should address its full range of patient care services. The quality management program should establish basic organization-wide criteria that apply to each policy and procedure. Examples of criteria include the current validity of the authority that supports the patient care policy or procedure, patient satisfaction, organizational efficiency, and compliance with policy format requirements and organizational signatory requirements.

Program Assessment Measures

A quality management program must be able to assess the quality of patient care activities. Structure, process, and outcome are the three aspects traditionally assessed.

Structural standards concern the structure or arrangement of components in the organization's system of care provision. For example, a policy requiring all inpatients to have a comprehensive history and physical examination on a timely basis would qualify as a structural standard.

Process and outcome standards concern patient care procedures and their results. Ordinarily structural assessments alone are not sufficient to indicate quality of care reliably. Process and outcome measures also are needed. Programs generally employ a mix of process and outcome measures that varies by setting. Common measures include

- risk management screens (e.g., mortality, morbidity, and unplanned return to surgery)
- appropriateness and effectiveness of invasive procedures
- autopsy findings
- adverse drug reactions
- appropriateness of drug therapy
- utilization of health services by patients
- clinical guidelines

In addition to these common measures, a program may develop its own process and outcome measures for services in the organization.

The most useful process and outcome measures are developed systematically. The Joint Commission offers five approaches for developing a measure: (1) describing the scope of the measure, (2) defining terms, (3) explaining why an activity is important enough to be monitored and describing how the measure relates to the activity, (4) listing how and where the data will be collected, and (5) describing the evaluation methods and procedures.

The list of measures traditionally used by quality management programs is impressive. However, the list includes measures that concern relatively rare events, such as mortality, and tends to focus primarily on the provider. Recently, some have called for greater emphasis on measuring the more common, system-related features of care provision and on monitoring individual competence.

Remember that outcome and process measures do not in themselves indicate the quality of patient care. The measures flag potential adverse events or patterns. Once it has been established that a more intensive investigation is needed, a peer review should be conducted by qualified providers.

There should be ongoing assessment of the effectiveness of monitoring the process and outcome measures. The following criteria may prove useful in this task:

- The assessment measures are developed according to a protocol.
- Data are collected efficiently.
- Patient care has improved.
- The improvement has been maintained.

Key Operational Considerations

Medical Staff Integration

An organized medical staff often has significant latitude in determining its structure and processes. Traditionally, the staff expresses these decisions in its bylaws. However, the medical staff's independence does not negate the organization's responsibility for integrating medical staff activity into the quality management program. Here are several suggestions for achieving such integration:

- The medical staff should participate regularly in the program coordination and policy function.
- Quality management guidance from support staff should be available to the medical staff.
- Support staff also can aid in peer review by screening cases and summarizing data to identity trends in patient care.
- Reappointment and privileging depends on reviewing the performance of medical staff members. Many of the data essential to this process come from the medical record, which needs to be summarized by individual providers. This essential part of the quality management program must be supported by allocating sufficient budgetary resources and by making performance review an organizational priority.

Governance

A fully effective program requires an informed and involved governing body. The following kinds of information should be provided consistently to leadership:

- significant changes in program policies
- trends and patterns of key quality indicators used by the organization (benchmarked, if possible)
- findings from external evaluations by state, federal, and voluntary accrediting agencies
- changes in federal and state regulations and accreditation standards
- national developments in quality management

Management

The senior leadership of an organization needs to show evidence of its commitment to the quality management program. Here are some strategies to consider:

- Initiate communication regarding quality management activities. Communication could include announcements about improvements that have resulted from the quality management program, changes in standards or regulations and the implications for the organization, and recognition of exemplary work.
- During management rounds, visit with staff on an individual basis and discuss a timely aspect of the quality management program.
- Take appropriate care when delegating responsibility and authority. These suggestions might be helpful:
  —Define the scope of delegated activities to allow identification of relevant standards, regulations, and monitoring activities.
  —Set expectations for maintaining documentation and for identifying relative data sources.
  —Schedule periodic evaluations of department and service quality management activities.
  —Require that substantial reports be prepared for the quality management program.
  —Develop a protocol for scheduling follow-up meetings between the delegator and the delegatee.

Strategic Planning

Strategic planning, which addresses the future positioning of an organization, often requires analyzing data from several sources. The quality management program may highlight strengths or weaknesses that should be considered in planning. For example, repositioning of an organization might require expanding a service that the quality program has identified as problematic.

Leadership

A quality management program's effectiveness depends on a strong commitment by the organization's senior leadership. The kind of commitment that is necessary entails that the leadership gain expert knowledge about the standards, regulations, and methods of the program. Just as a photographer must know about light, film, and lenses, senior leaders must know about the uses and limitations of structure, process, and outcome measures (see Chapter 4).

For example, structural policies might include infection control policies, such as universal precautions for preventing bloodborne infections. These policies will likely define the operating parameters for a department or the entire organization. A leader ignorant of this could unknowingly establish conflicting policies. Sending mixed messages to the staff will make the quality management program less effective.

Similarly, senior leaders must understand process and outcome measures. Although these measures are often technical, they are applied in a management context that leaders must be able to articulate clearly.

Organizational policies and mechanisms are important to a program because they define roles, lend structure, and facilitate action. However, policies and mechanisms do not motivate people. Although a thorough discussion of motivating staff is beyond the scope of this chapter, managers can take the following steps in promoting quality.

Send a clear message. Senior leaders must believe in the importance of quality management. However, believing in the program is not enough. Managers must communicate their feelings to the staff. This is best done by deed, not words. Senior managers can support the program through ongoing involvement and by recognizing staff accomplishments.

Show how quality is useful. Managers must help individual workers see that the quality management program helps productivity. Motivation is dropping when workers say, "There is no reason for me doing it. It's just policy." In addition to creating a sense that the program is a high priority, senior leaders also must show how quality management can add to the staff's sense of productiveness.

Provide tools. It is difficult to do satisfying work without the right intellectual or physical tools. Failing to invest in good training and equipment can cause productivity to evaporate. What will remain will be a combination of frustration and cynicism about the integrity of senior leaders and their commitment to the quality management program.

Show support. Managers must tell staff explicitly that well-intended but failed efforts to improve quality will be considered "lessons learned." Increasing knowledge and skills has financial costs that, within reasonable limits, must be borne by the organization. Not supporting good-faith efforts, even if they do not succeed, risks encouraging a "bunker mentality"—staff members become defensive and seek only safe ground.

Accreditation

Accreditation is often optional for health care organizations. The cost of surveys and other considerations may tempt many organizations to forgo accreditation. However, the following arguments supporting accreditation should be considered prior to making a decision.

Accreditation reviews may seem like state or federal inspections because government inspectors and accreditors both observe the level of compliance with regulations and standards. But the similarity stops there. Government agencies generally limit their surveys to compliance, whereas the focus of accreditors is on testing and education. The education provided often includes onsite consultation as well as advice, publications, and seminars. There is sometimes instruction on state-of-the-art and emerging technologies. Accreditors also allow for onsite review, which can be more helpful than instructional courses.

Accreditation by a national accreditor gives a health care organization a national perspective for comparing survey results. For organizations with facilities in different states, this perspective can be helpful. For example, a multihospital system with

hospitals in various locations may utilize the Joint Commission's modified survey process for multihospital systems to identify trends across hospitals.

THE FUTURE OF QUALITY MANAGEMENT

As we approach the beginning of the twenty-first century, the following trends seem likely.

A variety of regulatory and voluntary approaches to quality management will develop. This blended approach will focus heavily on efficiency, effectiveness, and accountability.

The industrial methods of total quality management or continuous quality improvement will be incorporated into the quality management programs of most health care organizations. In most cases, these methods will be adapted rather than be implemented in their pure form.

Cost and quality will become more interconnected. Consequently, payment systems will reimburse based on demonstrated quality outcomes.

Outcome measurement and management will continue as total quality management and quality assurance become integrated and adopted as a "clinical quality improvement" system.

Public accountability will largely drive quality management. Data disclosures will become commonplace, and consumers will discuss quality outcomes with providers when discussing treatment, options, and prognosis. Tied to public accountability is the strengthening and refinement of the consumer movement.

Quality measurement systems will evolve into integrated systems that track and monitor the processes and outcomes of care across settings and providers.

Physician leaders will become more knowledgeable about cost issues, and lay health care leaders will become more knowledgeable about clinical quality issues.

Quality improvement methods will be applied increasingly in primary care as managed care systems expand.

Research into patient care guidelines and standards will continue and will become a major component of health services research.

The role of the board of trustees in quality measurement and management will continue because of increasing calls for public accountability. There will be a great deal of conflict between boards, administrators, and physician leaders, since the boards' tools and techniques will lag behind those of the other two groups. In some cases, trustees will request adoption of some industrial methods that may not be readily transferable to clinical settings.

All of the above trends will be greatly influenced by the Clinton health reforms of the 1990s, which will dramatically transform American medicine.

In summary, quality measurement and management will become an integral component of health care delivery organizations. It will transform many organizations, it will create conflict in others, but overall it will serve the interests of patients. After all, isn't that the main object of providing care?

ADDITIONAL RESOURCES

Organizations

American College of Physicians, Philadelphia, PA.

American Medical Association, Department of Quality Assurance, Chicago, IL.

Health Care Forum, San Francisco, CA.

Joint Commission on Accreditation of Health Care Organizations, Oakbrook Terrace, IL.

National Demonstration Program, Harvard Community Health Plan, Cambridge, MA.

Washington Business Group on Health, Washington, DC.

Books and Articles

Benson, D.S., and P.G. Townes, Jr. *Excellence in ambulatory care: A practical guide to developing effective quality assurance programs.* San Francisco: Jossey-Bass, 1990.

Berwick, D.M., et al. *Curing health care: New strategies for quality improvement.* San Francisco: Jossey-Bass, 1990.

Couch, J.B., ed. *Health care quality management for the 21st Century.* Tampa, Fla.: Hillsboro Printing, 1991.

Donabedian, A. *The criteria and standards of quality.* Ann Arbor, Mich.: Health Administration Press, 1982.

Donabedian, A. *The definition of quality and approaches to its assessment.* Ann Arbor, Mich.: Health Administration Plan, 1980.

Donabedian, A. *The methods and findings of quality assessment and monitoring: An illustrated analysis.* Ann Arbor, Mich.: Health Administration Press, 1985.

Freidson, E. *Profession of medicine.* New York: Harper & Row, 1970.

Graham, N.O. *Quality assurance in hospitals: Strategies for assessment and implementation.* Gaithersburg, Md.: Aspen Publishers, 1990.

Hospital Research and Educational Trust. *The Quality Measurement and Management Project,* 1991.

Joint Commission on Accreditation of Healthcare Organizations. *Primer on indicator development and application: Measuring quality in health care.* Oakbrook Terrace, Ill.: Joint Commission on Accreditation of Healthcare Organizations, 1990.

Joint Commission on Accreditation of Healthcare Organizations. *Striving toward improvement: Six hospitals in search of quality.* Oakbrook Terrace, Ill.: Joint Commission on Accreditation of Healthcare Organizations, 1992.

Lohr, K.N., ed. *Medicare: A strategy for quality assurance.* Vols. 1 and 2. Washington, D.C.: National Academy Press, 1990.

Longo, D.R., and D. Bohr. *Quantitative methods in quality management: A guide for practitioners.* Chicago: American Hospital Publishing, 1991.

Longo, D.R., et al. *Integrated quality assessment: A model for concurrent review.* Chicago: American Hospital Publishing, 1989.

Robert Wood Johnson National Program Office. *Program to improve the quality of hospital care.* Ithaca, N.Y.: Cornell University, 1991.

Rosen, G. The efficiency criterion in medical care, 1900–1920. *Bulletin of the History of Medicine* 50 (1976): 28–44.

Wenzel, R.P., ed. *Assessing quality health care: Perspectives for clinicians.* Baltimore: Williams & Wilkins, 1992.

NOTES

1. D.J. Fine and E.R. Meyer, Quality Assurance in Historical Perspective, *Hospital and Health Services Administration,* November–December 1983, 123–130.

2. Ibid.

3. D.R. Longo and R. Laubenthal, Compliance with Nursing Standards, *Quality Review Bulletin,* August 10, 1984, pp. 243–247.

4. F. Nightingale, *Notes on Nursing* (New York: Dover Publications, 1969).

5. Fine and Meyer, Quality Assurance in Historical Perspective.

6. Ibid.

7. Ibid.

8. B.C. James, *Quality Management for Healthcare Delivery* (Chicago: Hospital Research and Educational Trust, 1989).

9. D.R. Longo, K.R. Ciccone, and J.T. Lord, *Integrated Quality Assessment: A Model for Concurrent Review* (Chicago: American Hospital Publishing, 1989).

Paul B. Batalden
Thomas W. Nolan

Knowledge for the Leadership of Continual Improvement in Health Care

4

Continual quality improvement offers health care new opportunities for improvement. Managers will be prepared to lead the way if they master the knowledge that underlies this new approach.

TRADITIONAL IMPROVEMENT AND UNDERLYING KNOWLEDGE

In 1798, Edward Jenner demonstrated that smallpox could be controlled by vaccinating people with cowpox virus. Many decades later and with much additional knowledge of virology and immunology, we were able to embark upon the worldwide eradication of smallpox. By the early 1970s, the virus was limited to just a few countries, one of which was Bangladesh. Within Bangladesh, the disease was narrowed to just a few areas when a variety of civil disruptions, including the Muslim festival of Eid, occurred.[1] At that time, as was the custom, people returned to their birth homes for the celebration of the festival. This migration increased the range of smallpox infection within the country and added approximately three more years to the elimination of the infection in Bangladesh.[2]

The lack of knowledge of the system by which the smallpox virus produced disease in that setting

and the sources of variation that contributed to the production of the disease in that setting limited the speed and effectiveness of the application of existing virologic and immunologic knowledge.

Modern health care has been improved in many dramatic ways in the past century by the application of knowledge specific to a particular subject or discipline within health care. Beneficial innovations have included organ transplantation, joint replacement, elimination or substantial reduction of viral diseases such as smallpox and poliomyelitis, capitation and diagnosis-related payment arrangements, capital-building strategies such as debt financing and public equity offerings, and new types of practitioners, such as nurse-clinicians and physician assistants.

These improvements and many others have been significant. They have been brought about by the application of knowledge that has been developed by discipline-grounded experts. These experts have extended current knowledge and created new knowledge and incorporated it into existing and new practices in each of the specialties. The important twentieth-century tradition of training students and fellows in the core knowledge of each specialty has helped perpetuate a strong tradition of improvement through the application of subject matter knowledge and theory (see Figure 4-1).

The rate at which leaders have been able to improve health care and the nature of the improvements they have been able to make, however, are now held to be inadequate. Leaders in government, business, and other sectors of society suggest that health care leaders must be able to make different types of improvements and at a faster rate than they have been able to make by using the traditional subject/discipline-grounded knowledge that has helped them improve so much in the past. In short, health care leaders must look for better health care outcomes at lower cost.

During the last century, an approach to improvement has been developed outside of health care settings, but it is now available for use in health care. Some call this approach continual improvement. Others call it total quality management. Whatever term is used, the approach is different from traditional approaches because it makes use of additional and different knowledge than has traditionally been used. This chapter explores the foundations of the knowledge system underlying continual improvement.

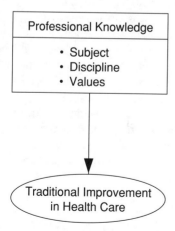

Figure 4-1 Professional Knowledge and Traditional Improvement in Health Care

QUALITY IN HEALTH CARE

Organization-wide continual improvement makes improvement of quality the main organizational focus. The key strategy is the matching of services and products to the needs in society or in the marketplace. In a health care organization, the object is to make the best match between patient needs and expectations and the services delivered so as to achieve maximum health benefits in an efficient and acceptable manner. The need served by health care organizations may be expressed simply as "health care" or by more specific descriptions such as the need to attain the highest level of well-being, the need to heal the sick, the need to limit the impact of illness on people's lives, to prevent illness and injury, or the need to reduce the burden of illness on society.

In fact, further specification of needs is at the heart of service design. However, the basic need (for health care) must always be kept in mind, and therefore care must be taken when further specifying needs. It is helpful to listen to and query the current and intended beneficiaries of health care services by asking questions such as these: "How do our services meet your needs?" or "What is the underlying need that our service or product addresses?" Because beneficiaries of care may be unable to state their exact needs, providers may be required to create a service or product prototype and ask, "Will this meet your needs?" The process of discerning, verifying, and clarifying needs is fundamental to health care systems design.

The closer the match between the services provided by an organization and the societal needs, the higher the quality of the services provided. How does one judge the closeness of the match? Answering this question requires having a definition of quality.

It is the responsibility of the provider of a service to define quality. Customers of the service (those who benefit from it) will generally not be willing to take the time to define quality, nor will their views necessarily represent the views of other customers. They will, however, assess the quality of the service when it is provided. It is the task of the producer of the service to define service quality in terms of measurable characteristics and to use these to evaluate the level of quality. The definition of service quality then becomes the basis for improvement of the service.

Exhibit 4-1 lists quality characteristics that have been found to be important to health care customers (e.g., patients, families, and purchasers). Different customers will weigh these characteristics differently. One of the most important goals of gaining knowledge about customers is to refine the definition of the quality of a service or product so that it takes into account the differences between groups of customers.

Another important aspect of matching services and needs is to offer each service at a price that the customers perceive as good value. With the current concern about the high cost of health care, cost has been thought of as a quality characteristic by many and as the only significant quality characteristic by some. In the present environment, there may be a need to prevent any further rise in cost using short-term fixes. However, in the long term, improving quality with methods that result in lower costs and that allow health services to be perceived as a better value is a more desirable solution. (Value is a function of quality and price. For example, the value of a service increases if its quality increases or its price decreases.)

That lower costs can be achieved through improving quality is being learned in industries outside of health care. (See, for example, the report of the Government Accounting Office on the companies that have won the Malcolm Baldrige National Quality Award or have been finalists for the award.)[3] Reduced costs from improved quality were fully documented by researchers at the Massachusetts Institute of Technology in their international study of the automotive industry.[4]

Equivalent evidence for the health care industry is mostly anecdotal at this time.[5] However, the list of quality characteristics in Exhibit 4-1 suggests that the same relationship of higher quality and lower cost can exist in health care.

The current emphasis on shortening lengths of hospital stay to reduce cost is needed because health care providers did not previously focus on duration of treatment as a quality factor. Most customers prefer shorter hospital stays to longer ones, and duration of treatment is one of the ways they judge quality.

Professionals who provide services based on expert knowledge—such as physicians, nurses, consultants, lawyers, and engineers—can overwhelm a problem using methods or resources that are out of balance with the magnitude of the problem. This does not provide value for the customer. Quality in professional services is achieved by providing the desired outcome while expending the minimum resources. The inspection and triage methods (e.g., appropriateness screening) now being employed in the name of cost reduction are examples of short-term remedies (which can add new sets of costs themselves). They are being resorted to because not enough attention was paid to improving quality by better matching diagnosis, prognosis, and treatment and by ensuring more appropriate durations of treatment. For example, inspecting against arbitrary limits of resources used (e.g., days in the hospital) to determine appropriateness of care after the cost has been incurred is a very expensive way to achieve cost reductions. Further, it adds a new step and new cost to care: inspection. A preferable alternative is to plan better and to design care using the

Exhibit 4-1 Quality Characteristics for Health Care

- Prevention of health problems
- Impact on physical, mental, social, and biological functioning (health outcomes)
- Ability to diagnose health problems
- Match between diagnosis, prognosis, and treatment
- Duration of treatment
- Access to care
- Interpersonal interaction (e.g., concern, caring, and professionalism)
- Level of anxiety concerning treatment
- Information useful for personal health care management

quality characteristics listed in Exhibit 14-1. For example, the cost-effectiveness of improving quality by preventing health problems should be obvious.

Progress in reducing the cost of health care depends on improving quality. The present focus on cost will not improve quality, and in some cases it may reduce quality and even increase total cost. As a result, health care administrators, third-party payers, and clinicians will become adversaries rather than collaborators—to the detriment of the beneficiaries of the services they provide.

PREREQUISITES FOR CONTINUAL IMPROVEMENT

Figure 4-2 shows the prerequisites for making continual improvement of quality a top priority in an organization. The four prerequisites are

1. leadership
2. investment in improvement
3. subject matter knowledge
4. knowledge for improvement

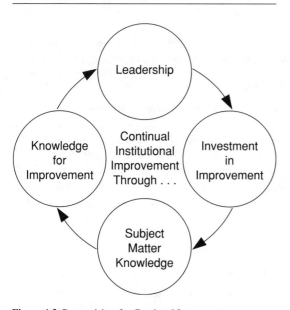

Figure 4-2 Prerequisites for Continual Improvement

Leadership

Leadership will be needed to aim any health care organization toward the improvement of quality. The first step in becoming a leader is to make the decision to lead. In the case of a top manager in a health care organization, this decision entails integrating the improvement of quality into his or her daily work as opposed to simply endorsing the concept of improving quality while delegating the actual work on improvement to others.

The areas of improvement knowledge and their implications provide a foundation for leadership. Acquiring this new knowledge will take time and study. However, there are specific characteristics of an organization that will enhance its ability to improve quality, and the leader can begin work on them immediately after making the decision to personally lead improvement.

First, the organization should function as a system. This requires that everyone know what the common purpose of the organization is and how his or her work helps fulfill that purpose. An integral part of establishing purpose is identifying and communicating the needs in the marketplace or in society that the services of the organization are intended to match.

People who need what the organization creates or delivers are potential customers or beneficiaries of the work of the organization. An important activity for the leader is to establish a customer focus for the organization. Having a customer focus means that benefits to the customers are the primary consideration when decisions are made, actions are taken, or investments are selected. The extent of customer focus in an organization is easy to measure. It simply requires reviewing the important decisions, actions, and investments of the last six months and uncovering the primary factors that were considered.

James Q. Wilson, in his book *On Character,* says that good character includes two important attributes: empathy and self-control.[6] *Empathy,* as he uses the term, means regard for the needs and feelings of others, and self-control means the ability to act with reference to the more distant consequences of current behavior. In terms of Wilson's definition, a leader of the improvement of quality must have good character. Lack of concern for people and a short-term view have been significant obstacles to improving quality in many organizations.

The leader must also build the system of improvement, the system by which knowledge of the customer is obtained, priorities are set, and aspects of the organization are designed or redesigned to improve the quality of its products and services.

Investment in Improvement

Improvement of quality requires investment. The primary investment is an investment of time—the time necessary for learning and making improvements. Everyone is so busy doing his or her job that there is little extra time to find new ways of doing things.

Other investments are also needed. Quality can be improved by enhancing the abilities of people in the organization. Training in job-related skills and personal continued learning and education add to what people bring to an organization.

There will be a need for investment in research and development of new products or services. Capital investment to keep the infrastructure in good order, to build new buildings, or to purchase major equipment is a part of the investment in improvement. Present accounting methods often seem to induce leaders to favor more tangible investments.

It seems obvious that investment is needed, but it takes leadership and good character for an organization to invest in a balanced way. Balanced investment usually takes years to have its full impact. It is tempting to delay some needed investments to make the organization look good in the short term.

Subject Matter Knowledge

Improvements in quality come from the application of knowledge. The higher the level of relevant knowledge in an organization, the more effective the improvements will be. Identifying what the im-

portant areas of knowledge are in a particular industry is an important function. In health care, the relevant subjects of knowledge are numerous, such as physiology, psychology, nutrition, pharmacology, and so on.

Health care organizations usually assess the types of subject knowledge available by examining the professional education, training, and certification of prospective staff. They have relied on academic programs and their certification standards to help in identifying and interpreting the qualifications of prospective employees and coworkers.

Identifying those internal or external to the organization who have or are developing discipline-specific knowledge is necessary. Tapping these sources of knowledge can be accomplished, for example, through seminars, informal exchanges in the organization, or joint ventures with other organizations.

It is often the case that personnel within the organization possess knowledge that, if shared, would improve the abilities of coworkers. Developing an atmosphere of cooperation to encourage the spread of knowledge enhances an organization's ability to improve the quality of its services. Fear thwarts cooperation. Whether the organization can identify the sources of fear and build cooperation depends on its policies, practices, habits, and traditions. Increasing cooperation is another leadership priority.

Improvement Knowledge

The fourth prerequisite, improvement knowledge, is at the heart of the new approach to continual improvement. Deming's system of "profound knowledge" is the core of improvement knowledge.[7] It consists of four elements that interact with one another, and together they can ground new types of efforts to improve health care. The four elements are

1. appreciation for a system
2. knowledge of variation
3. knowledge of psychology
4. theory of knowledge

Appreciation for a System

The first of these four elements builds on an awareness that the means of producing something, the means of improving it, and the aim of the production and improvement are connected in a system capable of continual improvement (see Figure 4-3).

The means of producing something involves knowledge of what is actually made or created, the customers or beneficiaries who receive it, the work processes used to produce it, the inputs to these processes, and the suppliers who provide the inputs.

The means of improving something involves knowledge of the plan for improvement and its relationship to the vision for the future, the specific design and redesign activities that flow from that plan, and the relationship of those improvement activities to the suppliers, inputs, and work processes used to produce the improved output.

The aim of the system is based on knowledge of the underlying social or community needs and of the customers and the integration of this knowledge into the vision for the future of the organization.

Understanding these interrelationships and interdependencies is central to understanding how to proceed with improvement (see Figure 4-4). Without this understanding, suboptimization of improvement will occur, adding cost and waste.

The arrows in Figure 4-4 help define the key relationships necessary to organize health care work as a system. They also indicate the work and responsibility of leadership and management. Connecting, establishing context, working on the whole system and its aim, and integrating the parts are things top leaders must do.

The arrows could be drawn in both directions. More arrows could be drawn. These directional arrows are intended to signal a pathway for planning, identifying, and guiding improvement work.

Understanding and clarifying the flows from one category to another is an exercise in integration that top leaders and managers must lead. The arrows in many ways signify their work. Optimization of a part of the system is not the primary job of leaders. Optimization of the system requires knowledge of the parts, their connections, and the environment of the entire system.

Creating measures of successful system performance becomes possible when the entire organization is viewed as a system. Selecting a balanced set of measures that will serve as the key success indicators requires knowing the core process and results as well as the important customers.

Figure 4-4 can be used by senior leaders to show workers their contribution to the organization's operations and to enroll the workers in the work of the system as a whole. Those who seek to improve the work of the system can also use this figure for sponsoring and relating new improvement efforts to the general work of the organization.

Knowledge of Variation

Walter Shewhart and his student W. Edwards Deming have suggested that by studying and understanding variation and its sources, managers can develop an understanding of how the processes that generate it work, improve them, and reduce variation.

Traditionally managers have thought of signals of variation as being good or bad. The admission numbers are up, the average length of stay is down, the pharmacy costs are down, the serum potassium is up. Such facts are usually thought of as either good or bad news, depending on one's perspective.

Walter Shewhart suggested that those who manage processes should think about variation differently. He suggested that they should divide varia-

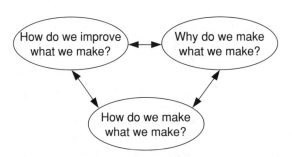

Figure 4-3 System capable of continual improvement

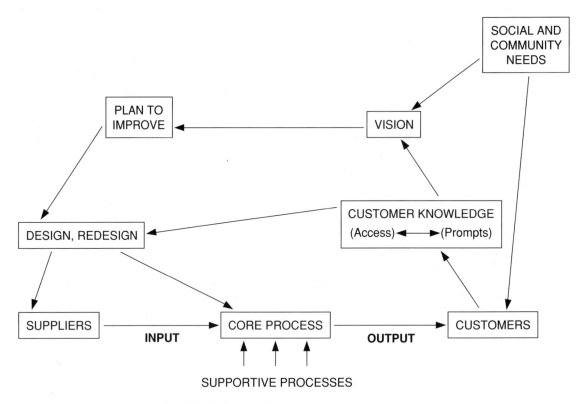

Figure 4-4 Organizing the Production of Health Care as a System

tion into two categories: (1) variation whose causes are found within the regular occurrences of a process and (2) variation that is unexpected or irregular. He called the first type "variation due to common causes," since it arises from causes found within the regular operation of the process. He labelled the second type of variation, "variation due to an assignable or special cause,"[8] since it arises from a specific circumstance that was not part of the regular operation of the process. Action on special causes often takes the form of solving problems.

This distinction between common and special cause variation is significant because the two different types of variation require different responses from leaders seeking to improve a process. Since it is usually possible to identify the special cause, the object is to understand the source of the variation and, if the effect is undesirable, prevent the cause

from recurring. If the special cause has produced a desirable effect, however, action should be taken to sustain it.[9] Once the special causes are acted upon, fundamental improvement can begin.

To improve a process that contains only common causes, a fundamental change usually will be necessary. This change can be developed by using current knowledge about the process or by first deepening the knowledge of the system of causes at work and using the new knowledge as a basis. The use of statistical methods to relate aspects of the process to measures of quality can increase the understanding of the system of causes at work.

Two types of errors sometimes occur when a response is made to variation in measurements. The first type of error is to react to variation due to common causes as if it were a result of special causes. The second type of error is to react to variation due to special causes as if it were a result of common causes. The use of statistical control charts to analyze measurements over time helps to minimize the net economic loss from the two types of errors.

Examples of the error of reacting to common causes as if they were special causes abound in health care. For instance, setting arbitrary thresholds for quality assurance measures and taking action when a threshold is exceeded gives rise to this kind of error. It is usually assumed that a measurement above the threshold is the result of a discoverable special cause. If the measurement exceeded the threshold because of common causes, taking action and changing the process based on the individual measurement has the potential of increasing variation and making the situation worse. This is not to say that exceeding the threshold because of common causes is a reason for feeling all is well. However, improvement will come from a fundamental change in the system, not from looking for and acting on nonexistent special causes.

Another example concerns the delivery of medications to hospital patients. Many sources contribute to the usual variation in medication delivery. In one hospital, however, a dose was delivered very late on a given occasion. The pharmacy was blamed, and almost immediately special systems were installed for notification of impending critical doses: critical medications lists were established; and special procedures were added, such as contacting newly designated, beeper-carrying "on-call pharmacy liaison representatives" in the event of a difficulty and maintaining additional stocks of critical medications on the units. When the pharmacist responsible was spoken with, however, he indicated that the pharmacy that day had had a sink overflow that resulted in a minor "flood." Since this was a special cause, no modification in the process of medication delivery was indicated. Instead, precautions to prevent sink flooding in the pharmacy were needed to avoid recurrence of the incident.

Reacting to the effect of common cause as if it were the effect of a special cause increases variation. Deming refers to this as "tampering."[10] It occurs when managers fail to study variation and simply respond to each point of variation as if it were the result of a single cause rather than many common causes working together.

Variation is linked to the decision to take action and the type of management action required. Variation is studied to understand and guide management action. Statistical thinking can assist in understanding special and common cause variation and clarifying cause and effect. This type of analytic thinking is further described by Deming and by Moen, Nolan, and Provost.[11]

Knowledge of Psychology

The third element of improvement knowledge is built on the belief that most workers are intrinsically motivated to improve and to do their best. This belief is at odds with the belief that seems to underlie most human resource development activities today. It seems to be assumed that ordinary workers are deficient in motivation and that part of the job of the human resource professional is to classify workers so that leaders can then provide the "right" type of motivation for each worker.

Deming suggests that, instead of wasting energy on classifying people, managers should try to better understand the sources of intrinsic motivation, joy, pride in work, and self-esteem that are to be found in every worker. Further, he suggests that managers who wish to increase motivation in the workplace should direct their attention to the factors that crush or form barriers to motivation.

For example, in health care organizations, the factors that serve as barriers to motivation are sometimes found in policies, practices, habits, and traditions. By directing the attention of human development personnel to these determinants of behavior, their unintended demotivating effects can be identified and eliminated.

Extrinsic motivators (e.g., pay incentives, employee of the month awards, etc.) impact the behavior of everyone in the workplace. However, designing extrinsic motivators so that they truly optimize a whole system of work is complex and is usually not attempted. More often, extrinsic motivators are used to encourage optimization of a part of the work of an organization or system. The call for a sharp focus on intrinsic motivation is not new; Herzberg suggested it many years ago.[12] Intrinsic motivation is the least likely to detract from the optimization of the system as a whole.[13]

Theory of Knowledge

C. I. Lewis asserts that a prime purpose of knowledge is to predict the future.[14] Leaders who aim to sustain their organizations must be able to predict trends. Prediction requires building knowledge by using accepted methodologies, such as scientific experimentation.

Knowledge for prediction can be garnered by an iteration of theorizing and observation. For an organization to be effective at increasing the rate and impact of improvements, it must be willing to experiment (preferably on a small scale) and learn from both successful and unsuccessful experiments. The building of knowledge is accelerated by the use of statistical methods to design tests, conduct surveys, and analyze data to confirm or dispel theories or hunches.

Unfortunately, scientific experimentation is not commonly or systematically used by leaders as a way of improving health care organizations. Making experimentation simpler may cause many more leaders to try it and gain the power that flows from using experimental methods.

One such simplification is the PDCA (Plan-Do-Check[study]-Act) cycle. In Japan, the PDCA cycle is often referred to as the Deming cycle. This cycle provides a method to systematically build knowledge by conducting small-scale studies. If accessible to all in the workplace, it "democratizes the scientific method" and spreads knowledge building and improvement throughout all levels of an organization. (A list of questions to help guide the use of the PDCA cycle is found in Exhibit 4-2.)

When the four elements described above are taken together as a system of knowledge and then combined with subject matter knowledge, they underpin a new type of improvement—continual im-

Exhibit 4-2 Questions Helpful for Building Improvement Knowledge

1. What are we trying to accomplish?
2. How will we know that a change is an improvement?
3. What changes *can* we make that we *predict* will lead to improvement?
4. How shall we *plan* the first pilot?
5. What are we learning as we *do* the pilot?
6. As we *check* and study what happened, what have we learned?
7. As we *act* to hold the gains or abandon our pilot efforts, what needs to be done?
8. Looking back over the whole pilot, what have we learned?

Source: Reprinted from *Building Knowledge for Improvement* by P.B. Batalden and T.W. Nolan with permission of HCA Quality Resource Group, © 1992.

provement. When top leaders accept that they are responsible for building this knowledge throughout the organization, they will aim to restructure the organization to make learning easier. (Those wishing further information on how to develop a learning organization should read *The Fifth Discipline* by P.M. Senge[15] and Chapter 5.)

ACTIVITIES FOR LEADERS

In many health care organizations, there is intense interest in establishing an initiative to improve quality. However, far too many organizations expect to "implement" a quality improvement program in the same way they would implement a new computer system. That is, they look for a formula or set of steps, and often they wind up bringing in outsiders to "install a system."

This view of quality improvement misses the point. Application and integration of improvement knowledge and subject matter knowledge is at the heart of improving quality. The interaction of the system of work, the variation within that system, the human resources available, and the traditions and practices of learning in any given organization all come together to make the appropriate initiation approach unique to that organization. This explains why line leaders who learn continual improvement are often best able to lead improvement in their organizations.

To be successful in making quality the core strategy in an organization, there must be some understanding of the components of improvement knowledge (outlined above) and a mechanism for learning from the activities that are undertaken to improve quality. Discussed below are some aspects of the learning process through which leaders can gain the necessary knowledge.

Initial Education

The leader and his or her management team should seek to educate themselves in the basic philosophy, principles, and methods of quality. A reading list for beginning this task is provided in the "Additional Resources" section at the end of this chapter.

Through this education, the team members should be able to reach a consensus on what the improvement of quality means to them and whether to move forward. To help in this discussion, the team might consider these questions:

- What are the needs in the society or marketplace that the organization is intending to meet by offering its services or products?

- Who has these needs? (That is, who are potential customers?)

- How do our customers (or potential customers) judge quality? (Consider the relation of their judgment to the quality characteristics in Exhibit 4-1.)

- From the viewpoint of the customers, what improvements have been made in the quality of our services or products in the last two years?

- What is the system by which opportunities for improvement are identified, priorities are set, and designs or redesigns of products, services, or processes are executed?

The answers to these questions will almost always uncover opportunities for changing some aspect of the organization. However, at this point management teams sometimes get frozen into inaction because they are not sure of the "right" thing to do. To prevent this from happening, the team should ground their activities in the PDCA cycle and initiate small-scale studies to learn what works.

Based on the knowledge that has been gained through the initial education, ideas may arise for activities such as conducting a customer survey, identifying and removing barriers to intrinsic motivation of employees, redesigning a particular service, or developing a training program. The best strategy is to use the PDCA cycle to plan the chosen activity (preferably kept to a small scale), do it, study the results, and learn from the experience. The increased knowledge can then be used to determine whether to expand the activity, modify it and try again, or abandon the activity.

It may not be easy for leaders and managers to admit that they do not have all the answers and that they are learning. Admitting this may itself be a source of learning for everyone in the organization. If quality is to be improved continually, the culture of the organization must allow new approaches to be tested. Failed tests should not be a cause of embarrassment but should be viewed as vital to learning.

When a trial fails to produce the desired outcome, it should be studied. Without studying the causes of failure, little will have been gained. Asking these questions might be helpful: What theory was used? What prediction did not materialize? Which collected data were anticipated and which were not? What ideas occurred that could be incorporated into subsequent trials? Answers to these questions will encourage people to apply what they have learned in the next improvement pilot.

Initial Improvement Activities

Groups of people working in teams to improve services or internal processes are certainly essential to making quality succeed as a strategy. However, the purpose of the initial improvement teams is not only to accomplish improvements but to serve as an opportunity for learning. The initial teams should be thought of as part of a PDCA cycle and be used to answer the following questions:

- Can improvements that impact our customers be made?
- What are the barriers to improvement that exist in our organization?
- What support will people in the organization need in order to make improvements?
- What is the relationship between improved quality and costs?

The learning will be more effective if top leaders from management as well as providers of care lead the initial teams and answer these questions using experience guided by theory. Based on the answers to these questions, they will identify aspects of the organization in need of fundamental change if quality is to become the key strategy. This will generate more PDCA cycles from the leadership and more opportunities to learn. Through this continued learning, top leaders, managers, and providers of care will be increasingly able to lead the organization in the direction of continual improvement.

It will be tempting to choose only support processes to improve rather than processes that have a direct impact on care. A balance of clinical care processes and support processes should be chosen for the initial improvements. At least some of the initial efforts should be aimed directly at measures of clinical outcomes.

Building the Infrastructure

Eventually the organization must be designed as a system that integrates day-to-day management and the efforts of the improvement program. The key components of the integrated system should include the following:

A Statement of Purpose. This statement should include the mission of the organization, the needs in society that the organization intends to meet by offering its products and services, the beliefs and values that will guide members of the organization in carrying out the mission, and a vision of how the organization will be structured to accomplish its mission in the future.

A Process for Gaining Knowledge about Customers. This process might include surveys of customers, but it also should include recording of observations of customers when services are provided. Similar efforts to find out about potential customers will provide additional insights. This knowledge should be gained on an ongoing basis with small samples obtained over short intervals of time rather than by large surveys done infrequently.

A Definition of the System. This should include a sketch of how the 40–50 major processes in the organization link together. This helps people see how they must interact to deliver the services.

A Set of Measures of Success for the System. The definition of the system makes possible the identification of overall measures of success for the system. These might include measures related to customers, employees, operations, finance, clinical results, and community needs.

A Process for Planning Improvements. This process should identify the opportunities to improve quality that would have the biggest impact on customers and that would best help achieve the aim of the system. The process for gaining knowledge about customers will undoubtedly provide important input for this planning process. The extent to which planning for quality and strategic planning are integrated is a good measure of the strategic importance of improved quality for the future of the organization.

A Process for Managing Improvements. The resources for improvement, just like any important resource, must be managed. This management process typically includes assessing the need for training and providing resources for it, allocating time to work on improvements, reviewing and monitoring the effectiveness of improvement work, providing recognition to teams and individuals who are working on improvement, and providing guidance to teams and individuals to ensure that the resources for improvement are used wisely.

The building of infrastructure should be thought of as another vehicle for learning. The PDCA cycle should be used as the framework for building this infrastructure.

A small start on each of the components to be continually improved is preferable to a major effort directed toward any one component alone. The reason for this is that the components work as a feedback system and thus fuel improvement more efficiently as a group. If one of the components is missing, the other components will not be as effective. Examining the barriers to progress will often yield valuable information about the toxicities of the prevailing organizational culture. These should not be overlooked when the construction of infrastructure is undertaken.

CONCLUSION

Improvement comes from the application of knowledge. New types of improvement (e.g., continual improvement) in health care comes from the application of new types of knowledge. Figure 4-5 shows the relationship of the new knowledge and traditional professional knowledge to continual improvement in health care. Leadership and investment are essential for building this new knowledge. Systematic application and learning is the most efficient means of introducing the necessary changes.

ADDITIONAL RESOURCES

Berwick, D.M. Sounding board: Continuous improvement as an ideal in healthcare. *New England Journal of Medicine* 320 (1989): 63–66.

Buchanan, E.D., and P.B. Batalden. Industrial Models of Quality Improvement. In *Providing quality care: The challenge to clinicians,* eds. N. Goldfield and D.B. Nash. Philadelphia: The American College of Physicians, 1989.

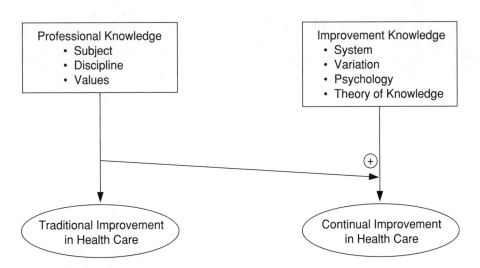

Figure 4-5 Traditional Improvement versus Continual Improvement

Deming, W.E. *Out of the crisis.* Cambridge, Mass.: Massachusetts Institute of Technology, Center for Advanced Engineering Study, 1986.

Moen, R.D., and T.W. Nolan. Process improvement: A step-by-step approach to analyzing and improving a process. *Quality Progress* 20, no. 9 (1987): 62–68.

Nolan T.W., and L.P. Provost. Understanding Variation. *Quality Progress* 24, no. 5 (1991): 70–78.

Scholtes, P.R., and H. Hacquebord. Beginning the quality transformation. *Quality Progress* 20, no. 7 (1988): 28–33.

Scholtes, P.R., and H. Hacquebord. Six strategies for beginning the quality transformation. *Quality Progress* 21, no. 8 (1988): 44–48.

Walton, M. *The Deming management method.* New York: Putnam, 1986.

NOTES

1. S.O. Foster, Smallpox Eradication: Lessons Learned in Bangladesh, *WHO Chronicle* 31 (1977): 245–247.

2. P.B. Batalden, Personal interview with smallpox eradication field personnel, Dacca, Bangladesh, January 1974.

3. GAO Report, NSIAD-91-190.

4. J.P. Womack et al., *The Machine That Changed the World* (New York: Rawson Associates, 1990).

5. Few data are available for evaluating organization-wide gains in health care at this time. Impressive examples of this new approach to improvement from the following institutions (offered by the CEOs) is indicative of a wider success. West Paces Ferry Hospital has saved more than $250,000 per year in staffing costs by careful examination of the process of staffing nursing units while simultaneously developing nurse extender programs offering upward mobility to hospital staff. By work on the process of planning C-section deliveries, they have also reduced the rates of C-section deliveries following prior C-section births from 21 percent to less than 15 percent, thus saving significant amounts of dollars and days of morbidity. Portsmouth Regional Hospital has saved several days per admission for joint replacement by examining the process of pain control and its relation to postoperative mobility training. West Florida Regional Hospital has saved in excess of $250,000 per year in antibiotic costs by modifying the process of physician notification of antibiotic sensitivities.

6. J.Q. Wilson, *On Character* (Washington, D.C.: AEI Press, 1991).

7. W.E. Deming, Profound Knowledge, in *The New Economics for Industry, Education and Government* (forthcoming).

8. Deming referred to "assignable" cause variation as "special" cause variation.

9. W.A. Shewhart, *Economic Control of Quality of Manufactured Product* (Washington, DC: D. Van Nostrand, 1931; reprint edition, American Society for Quality Control, 1980; reprinted by Ceepress, the George Washington University, 1986).

10. W.E. Deming, On the Distinction between Enumerative and Analytic Surveys, *Journal of the American Statistics Association* 48 (1953): 244–255.

11. W.E. Deming, "On Probability as a Basis for Action, *The American Statistician* 29, no. 4 (1975): 146–152; R.D. Moen et al., *Improving Quality through Planned Experimentation* (New York: McGraw-Hill, 1991).

12. F. Herzberg, One More Time: How Do You Motivate Employees? *Harvard Business Review* 65 no. 5 (1987): 109–120.

13. Deming, Profound Knowledge.

14. C.I. Lewis, *Mind and the World Order* (New York: Dover, 1956).

15. P.M. Senge, *The Fifth Discipline* (New York: Doubleday, 1990).

Barbara P. McCool

Organizational Learning

5

Purpose: This chapter discusses the learning organization that supports the individual, group, and organizational growth necessary to realize a health care institution's vision and goals. Human resource development occurs through incentives and structures that energize people to grow and develop and consistently provide clients with quality service. The department of education is the organizational unit that facilitates and coordinates learning programs for the health care organization.

INTRODUCTION

In today's environment, where consumers are greatly concerned about the cost and quality of health services, health care organizations must innovate or languish. Each organization must focus its energies on providing efficient, high-quality service. The human resource strategy should be to increase the use of effective work methods, increase productivity, and develop self-managed work teams. To meet the challenge, health care executives will be compelled to create a learning environment that encourages continuous learning and motivates personnel to develop new skills, adapt to

change, increase job competency, and deliver customer-driven service. Continuous learning must occur simultaneously at the individual, work group, and organizational levels.

Individual health care professionals must strive to improve their knowledge and skills and their ability to meet the needs and expectations of patients and the community. This means developing methods for determining the needs and wants of customers (including patients, physicians, community members, suppliers, employees, and government officials), delivering needed services efficiently, and defining clear outcomes that can be understood by those served. Individuals working in a high-performance health care organization are energized by the vision and values of the organization, are open to new and creative ways of thinking, and maintain a balance between work and outside interests to avoid burnout and other stress-related conditions.

Self-managed work teams that deliver a continuum of health services in multiple sites are needed to carry out the organization's mission and goals while responding quickly to demands of patients, physicians, and competitors. To accomplish goals, the work teams need to cut across the traditional departments and coalesce quickly to solve work process problems so that patient services meet defined standards.

A health care organization, through its leaders, needs to empower the staff by providing clear statements of its vision and its values. Mechanisms for communicating the strategic direction to all the stakeholders in the organization need to be put in place, and the strategic planning process must be used to help them learn and change their frame of reference.

Through the use of comprehensive information systems, progress on goal and quality attainment can be monitored so that corrective action can be taken. The culture of continuous quality improvement is a constant theme and creates an environment that encourages and supports individual and work team learning. Everyone in the organization is encouraged to ask questions and try new ways of providing services.

The continuous development of the work force is a major challenge for executives. As limits on available natural and financial resources are being encountered more frequently, health policy makers see more clearly that future growth has to focus on human capital. Therefore, the development of human potential becomes a key priority. Although physical assets can be better utilized, they cannot be increased; of all the resources available to society, people alone can grow and develop.

This chapter focuses on organizational learning and its role in employee and institutional adaptation to changing environmental forces. The health organization's learning system is discussed in relation to the learners, the processes followed, and the desired outcomes. The structure, staff, and resources needed for organizational training and education are defined. Finally, methods for maintaining quality in organizational training programs and the future challenges for organizational learning are discussed.

MANAGEMENT PRINCIPLES

There are several management principles that guide the development and nurturing of the learning organization.

1. Management should support an environment that facilitates individual, work team, and organizational vitality. A high-performance environment is characterized by the following:
   - a clear vision and a strategic direction that focuses on meeting customer needs
   - delegation of responsibility and authority to self-managed work teams
   - quick resolution of conflict to the satisfaction of all parties
   - honest and open communication up, down, and across organizational chains of command
   - individual and work team skill in using information for problem solving, decision making, and goal attainment
   - a culture and process that supports continuous quality improvement
   - rapid and creative adaptation to change

2. Guidelines for adult learning are used in the design and implementation of all training programs. These guidelines stress the following:
   - Adults have varying levels of knowledge and expertise because of different levels of experience. Each person should have an individualized assessment of his or her experience to determine the type and content of training.
   - Adults tend to be oriented to the concrete and useful. Therefore, instruction should include active participation of the learner and a focus on demonstrating skill in the workplace.
   - Adults learn best in environments that are physically comfortable and support trust, respect, freedom of expression, and diversity. Learning is also enhanced when supervisors find ways to reinforce newly learned behaviors of workers so that these behaviors will start to be used immediately on the job.
   - Adults are usually motivated to learn quickly when they recognize they suffer from a work skill deficiency that can be corrected through job training.

3. Training should be a means of improving the quality of services offered to patients and solving organizational problems. The content of training programs should flow from the needs of the organization and its clients and should stress competency development for meeting clearly stated standards of performance.

4. The human resource development function should be supported by management, adequately staffed and financed, and continually evaluated for effectiveness.

ORGANIZATIONAL ROLE AND FUNCTION

History

The history of training and development in health care organizations is summarized in Table 5-1. Health care organizations lagged behind industrial firms in maximizing the training function for

Table 5-1 History of Training in Health Care Organizations

Time Period	Educational Offerings*
1940–1950	Licensed practical nurse training
	Nurse's aide training
1950–1960	Nursing in-services
	Continuing education for physicians, nurses, and allied health professionals
1960–1970	Orientation programs
	Clinical ladder development
	Management development
	Technical skill training
1970–1980	Patient education programs
	Community health education programs
	Trustee education programs
1990	Quality improvement training
	Literacy training
	Life-style management programs

*The offerings are cumulative (i.e., the programs specified for a particular time period are offered in each successive period).

organizational renewal. One reason for this is the strong influence of physicians, nurses, and allied health professionals in determining the professional requirements for preservice and continuing education. As a result, until the 1980s hospital training was dominated by medical and nursing educators who focused mainly on the needs of their professional groups.

During World War II, when many health professionals served in the military, it became necessary to stratify the clinical care of patients in civilian settings and delegate functions reserved for professional clinicians to ancillary workers. Hence, the nurse's aide and licensed practical nurse roles evolved. Training ancillary workers was also stimulated by government initiatives that financially supported on-the-job training programs for nurse's aides and midlevel managers.

In the 1950s and 1960s, hospital training focused on the preparation of nurse's aides, in-service education, medical technology adaptation, and continuing education for physicians and nurses. There was some orientation for new employees carried out by the personnel department as well as broad-based management development programs for department heads. Training activities were housed in the department of nursing or the personnel department, and there was often very little coordination of educational functions by these two departments.

In the 1970s, as hospital cost controls became a major reality, administrators were forced to assess human resources in relation to their return on investment through increased competency and productivity. During this period, the Joint Commission on Accreditation of Hospitals reinforced the need to focus on the relationship between patient care audits and educational programming. As a result, deficiencies in patient care determined the content of learning programs for health care personnel.

The unions also stressed the need for orientation and career mobility for their members. One response was to create clinical ladders for nursing and the allied health professionals. Levels of competency became a dominant theme. Finally, increased malpractice activity contributed to the need to correct skill deficiencies and facilitate greater communication between physicians and nurses.

In the 1980s, the director of education emerged as the person responsible for planning, implementing, and evaluating a wide variety of educational programs for employees. The director was usually supported by a staff of educational specialists who worked with key managers in developing the programs.

In this same time period, it became apparent that elementary and secondary school systems were not providing the skills people needed to adequately function in a work setting. Many workers could not do simple calculations, write reports, or read instructions.

Departments of education began to assume responsibility for remedial programs in reading and writing to close the gap and to accommodate the increasingly varied backgrounds of employees in the health care labor market. Instituting such programs made good sense because 90 percent of the current workforce will still be employed in the year 2000.

Further demands were placed on the training staff to help health personnel retrain to keep up with the technological explosion and the generation of new knowledge about medical treatments. Also, with the advent of continuous quality improvement, bottom-line success became dependent on training people in process-improvement and facilitation skills to increase productivity, eliminate waste, and improve quality.

In the 1990s, as individuals commit themselves to lifelong learning, health care organizations must dedicate themselves to becoming learning institutions. A continuous learning philosophy encourages and nurtures the education of the work force. Through its policies and programs, such an organization can demonstrate each day that employee development is fundamental to its operations and key to employee adaptation.

As the problems of health care organizations grow in complexity and as hospitals merge to form larger systems of care, the necessity for interdisciplinary work team collaboration and problem solving will become the norm. The learning that takes place in the interdisciplinary work teams is essential for establishing new directions, more effective structures, and more relevant policies. The systematic solving of problems energizes everyone to adapt to new realities and shed old ways of thinking.

Learner Classification

A variety of learners develop new knowledge and skills within the educational system of a health care organization. These learners include health care personnel, managers, physicians, community groups, patients, and board members. Educational programs for clinicians, managers, and hospital employees include the following:

- Preparatory education programs that prepare persons for initial employment in medicine, nursing, health administration, social services, medical technology, occupational therapy, and other allied health professions.

- In-service education programs that assist employees to function effectively. In-service programs include orientation for new employees; skill training for adapting to new technology, updating computer and business systems, or upgrading clinical practice; continuing education for clinical personnel and midlevel and executive managers.

- Medical education programs that assist physicians in adapting to new advances in medical practice and technology.

- Career mobility programs that help a variety of workers move up in the organization.

- Continuous quality improvement programs that focus on the philosophy of quality service, team building, creative thinking, statistical process control techniques, benchmarking methods, and the total transformation of the organizational culture.

Patient education programs are offered to assist patients in understanding and taking responsibility for their disease process and healing protocols. Classes in diabetes, stroke rehabilitation, heart disease, and postoperative recovery and rehabilitation procedures are examples of such programs.

Community health education programs assist the well population to carry out life-style management and disease prevention practices more effectively. Examples include aerobic exercise, stress management, nutrition, and substance abuse programs.

Board of director programs assist policy makers in staying abreast of the latest developments in health care, such as the emergence of community-based networks of care, new financing and reimbursement mechanisms, and new health care reform proposals.

Learning Processes

The learning organization is responsible for assessing educational needs and designing, implementing, and evaluating educational programs. In fulfilling its responsibility, it must take into account the needs of patients; education and research advances; and the human, technological, and financial resources allocated for training. A diagram of the learning system is presented in Figure 5-1.

Assessing Needs

There is no more important element in the training function than the determination of learner

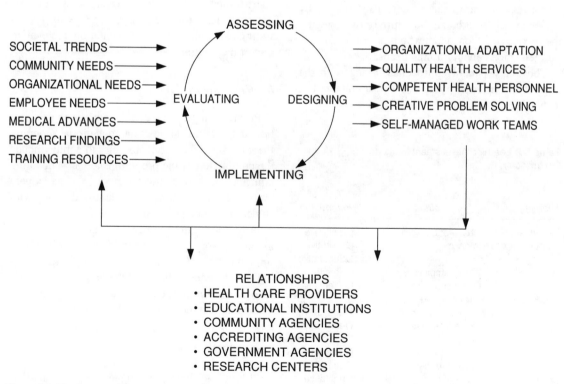

Figure 5-1 The Organizational Learning System

needs. An overarching principle of adult education is that a training activity that does not make sense to the adult learner will not succeed, for adults do not respond enthusiastically to education unless they see a relationship between the educational content and their deficiencies.

The purpose of the assessment process is to determine the training needs of employees, managers, physicians, patients, consumers, and board members as well as the organizational development needs of the institution.

Determining learning needs can be accomplished by examining learners directly through observation, interviews, skill inventories, work sampling, and surveys. Learning needs can also be assessed by analyzing turnover and absenteeism data, incident reports, equipment and supply purchases, and strategic planning and budgeting reports.

Finally, learning needs are influenced by trends in the delivery and financing of health care services. Assessment of these trends can be done by reviewing the health care literature or by engaging the services of a consultant who is able to make recommendations about training needs.

These assessment approaches, along with the type of information produced, are summarized in Table 5-2.

Table 5-2 Learning Assessment Methods and Information

Learning Level	Method	Type of Information
Individual or Work Group	Observation	Qualitative
	Interviews	Qualitative
	Tests	Quantitative
	Work sampling	Quantitative
	Questionnaires	Quantitative
Organization	Turnover and absenteeism records	Quantitative
	Incident reports	Quantitative
	Equipment purchases	Quantitative
	Questionnaires	Quantitative
	Focus groups	Qualitative
Society	Literature review	Qualitative
	Consultant assessment	Qualitative

Designing Programs

Designing learning programs involves defining learning objectives and developing educational activities that are based on adult learning principles and are relevant to job performance.

Clearly stated objectives are required for each learning program. These objectives define the desired outcomes of the educational sessions in terms of clearly defined learner competencies or additional knowledge, changed attitudes, and new skills. Well-defined objectives that clearly identify desired learner behavior are the basis for instructional strategies and program content. They also facilitate program evaluation and force the educational program to meet learner and organizational needs. (See Exhibit 5-1 for a sample learning objective taken from a course on the design of educational programs.)

The program design process defines the content, instructional methods, teaching aides, and evaluation procedures for an educational program. The resulting plan guides the implementation and evaluation of the program.

Implementing Programs

Program implementation comprises the institution and administration of an educational program. Prior to implementation, obstacles that may impede the completion of the program, such as scheduling conflicts, lack of faculty support, or inadequate training facilities, need to be identified, along with student reaction to the program.

In some situations, a panel of learners is formed as an advisory group to guide the development, implementation, and evaluation of a program. Using such a panel ensures that the program is responsive to the unique learning needs of the learner group and that the group will buy into the program.

Evaluating Programs

Program evaluation involves instructor, participant, supervisor, or patient assessment of the value

Exhibit 5-1 Sample Learning Objective

Student Outcome:	Demonstrate beginning skill in planning one instructional unit for a health-related program.
Measurement Criteria:	Submission of an individual lesson plan for one class session. The level of mastery should be at the 90th percentile, and the lesson should contain the following elements (the percentages indicate the weight to be given in determining the overall grade):

- session objectives   30%
- instructional strategies   20%
- teaching aides   15%
- audiovisual support   10%
- methods of evaluation   25%

of the educational activities. Evaluation is done to determine if the objectives were attained and if the program should be repeated, altered, or terminated. Evaluation should be seen as a continuing process that occurs immediately after the program and also later (e.g., at six-month or yearly intervals).

Training Outcomes

Outcomes of educational activities might include the acquirement of additional knowledge and skills by health professionals, a reduction in complaints from patients and visitors, innovations in the delivery of health care services, an increased ability on the part of the organization to adapt to change in a quick and orderly manner, and improvements in the quality of health care.

Through continuous improvement in skills needed on the job, individuals develop greater competency in carrying out their roles in the organization. At the same time, they become more aware of their feelings and reactions in work situations and their impact on others within their work groups.

The outcomes of work group training include shared accountability and responsibility for the work performed, a sense of a common purpose, trust and open communication between group members, and creativity in solving problems facing the organization and the group. There is a continuous evaluation of the effectiveness of the group and support for the team leaders.

Through relevant learner-based training programs, the organization strengthens its physical, financial, and human resources, improves communication between units, articulates and exemplifies its vision and values, and becomes more responsive to its clients.

Structure

Human resource development activities are carried out through a variety of organizational structures. Most large organizations have a centralized department of education responsible for all educational programming. The department is usually accountable to either the vice-president of human resources or an associate administrator for operations (or in some cases to the chief executive officer).

Within small organizations, the educational function is often assigned to a person with other responsibilities in the nursing or personnel department. In many cases, educational activities are developed and implemented in a consortium consisting of several small institutions. Economies of scale are realized through sharing a coordinator of educational programs; faculty members; educational equipment; and the development of in-service, continuing education, and management development programs.

Functions

The department of education is responsible for the following functions:

- Coordinating all educational programs.
- Planning and implementing educational programs that impact the productivity and profitability of the organization. A human resource development plan should be integrated into the

strategic plan of the organization so that strategic initiatives can be supported by qualified personnel when necessary.

- Consulting with department heads about educational programming for specialized learner needs.
- Maintaining appropriate records on employee learning needs and competency development programs.
- Orienting clinical learners and instructors who use the health care facility for clinical rotations.
- Working with executives, board members, physicians, and clinical work teams to determine training programs to assist in solving operational problems.
- Setting quality standards for all education programs and monitoring the effectiveness of educational programs.
- Formulating and implementing policies on reimbursement for continuing education programs.
- Collaborating with other educational institutions and hospitals to provide a full range of quality, cost-effective educational programs.
- Assessing the internal and external environment for trends and operational problems to be included in the content of educational programs so that the organization can respond to change more quickly.

RESOURCE REQUIREMENTS

The resources needed to run an effective training organization include competent staff and state-of-the-art instructional and audiovisual equipment.

Staff

The director of the department of education should have in-depth experience in health care administration, clinical practice, or organizational development and should have academic credentials in education. The department of education staff should consist of experts in education, organizational development, educational technology, and evaluation. The staff members typically function as resource consultants to the department directors in the health care organization as well as general coordinators for all educational activities.

Space and Equipment

The physical resources necessary for human resource development include space for learning and teaching. In particular, classrooms are needed that can accommodate a sizable number of people, as are small conference rooms for work teams to meet and solve operating problems.

Since educational space in health care institutions is heavily utilized, educational facilities should be aesthetically attractive and have ergonomically designed furniture. In the case of smaller organizations, which may not have educational space, arrangements can be made to rent space from hotels or other community centers.

Overhead and slide projectors, computers, learning resource centers, screens, chart pads, felt boards, writing boards, and rooms for viewing role-playing situations are among the necessities.

Quality Assurance

Quality standards for the educational programs offered by the department and for the other major departmental functions should be set and monitored.

For each educational program, a thorough needs assessment is done so that the objectives and program content reflect the needs of the learners and the organization.

A summary evaluation is done by the program participants and faculty. An assessment of each participant by his or her supervisor is also conducted to determine if the newly learned skills are impacting quality, productivity, profitability, or the ability of the organization to attain its goals.

Periodically the staff of the department of education evaluate the goals and major functions of the department in light of the organization's vision and strategic plan and the department's operational plan and budget.

THE FUTURE OF HUMAN RESOURCE DEVELOPMENT

The next decade will be taxing for everyone in health care and will continually reinforce the notion that an organization's human resources are its greatest strength. Without well-prepared, highly motivated personnel, health care organizations will not be able to deal with future challenges effectively.

Investment in the continuous training of the work force is simply a cost of doing business during times of rapid technological and societal change. The increasingly widespread use of information technologies will drive the need to re-educate a majority of the health care work force. Critical skills will include the ability to interpret and absorb information. Because office and medical system automation is thriving, the training needed by people to intersect with the developing technology is staggering. Health care personnel will require computer literacy, the capacity for complex thinking, and the ability to be flexible and to improvise.

The high illiteracy rate and the average performance of public school students on achievement tests raise questions about the future quality of the work force. Lack of basic reading and writing skills will cause health care employers to supply remedial education in basic skills to a substantial number of employees.

As a consequence, health care organizations and other businesses are taking the initiative by developing partnerships with local educational systems to influence the quality of the future labor pool. Health care administrators are giving time and energy to mentoring students, supporting school bond issues, and acting as resources for work study programs.

Within the health setting, consumers will demand more education on life-style management and more knowledge about health care reform so they can take more responsibility for their own health and make informed decisions about the future direction of health care delivery.

Other future health care organization trends will make demands on the department of education. These include the increased emphasis on continuous quality improvement, the expansion of leadership succession programs, and the growing need to foster creative approaches to delivering quality care in a constrained resource environment.

Continuous Quality Improvement

The management philosophy of continuous quality improvement is gaining momentum in health care. This new focus on the customer taxes the ingenuity of all health care professionals and executives, since it requires a change from telling patients what they need to trying to determine their needs and wants.

The department of education plays a key role in the implementation of this philosophy. The specialized education staff members can be invaluable in helping to assess the organization's major strengths and weaknesses. Their expertise is also needed to educate the managers, board members, and physicians about the characteristics and guiding principles of total quality management. In addition, they can help to strengthen work teams and give team members the necessary facilitation and statistical process control skills to solve operational problems related to improving customer service.

Continuous quality improvement training reinforces the idea of just-in-time training (i.e., that the skills needed by the staff will be supplied to them in training modules as they need them). This approach allows people to recognize the relevance of the training they are receiving and to apply the new skills immediately in problem solving. Just-in-time training places great demands on the education staff. Staff members must quickly uncover the needs of the quality teams and respond with clear, relevant learning materials that are user-friendly.

Training within the context of continuous quality improvement demands that each team member eventually master the range of technical and interpersonal skills necessary to competently perform his or her work responsibilities. Therefore, all training has to focus directly on the job at hand and the readiness of the learner to move to another level of proficiency.

The other challenge is to customize the training for the learner group. A board member does not need in-depth knowledge of statistical process control techniques as much as a working understanding of the process and culture of continuous quality improvement. However, nurses and physicians not only must be proficient at using statistical process control techniques in clinical areas but must also be able to motivate groups to develop creative solutions to operational problems.

Finally, education about continuous quality improvement should provide not only the technical tools for self-correction and self-monitoring but also the motivation for the work force to apply the concepts of continuous quality improvement to every aspect of customer service.

If delivering quality service is at the core of organizational processes, then organizational learning occurs naturally. As quality work teams solve problems, the organizational structures and procedures are altered to support these changes. In other words, "double loop learning" occurs as new ideas are supported by adaptation in the organizational structures and culture.

Leadership Succession

As discussed in Chapter 1, complex health care organizations need management stability so that system activities are orderly and executive transitions are not disruptive. Within the past several years, the importance of leadership succession planning has been stressed by boards of directors to ensure continuity of management talent.

Leadership succession planning entails many tasks:

- determining the competencies needed for key leadership positions
- assessing the knowledge and skills of each key manager against the stated competencies
- devising individualized development programs for the managers so that they are trained in all the functional areas of management
- assigning mentors who will coach young managers and be their advocates within the organization

Broadening the skills of physicians, nurses, and other health care professionals is also an important priority. In some health care organizations, year-long onsite management development programs are being offered for physicians. These programs, which cover accounting, finance, organizational behavior, marketing, and strategic planning, provide doctors with new knowledge and skills so that they can play a meaningful role in the governance and operational management of their health care organizations.

From the viewpoint of the manager, career counseling and developing a broad range of managerial skills are essential for career advancement. People who have financial expertise should learn more about marketing and strategic planning. Likewise, people with general management expertise should develop competence in computers, investment analysis, and organizational development.

The creation of an individualized learning plan will force an individual to examine his or her unique strengths and weaknesses and provide motivation to seek the courses and learning experiences that will maximize opportunities for professional development.

From the viewpoint of the organization, careful planning for future leaders ensures that there is an abundance of high-potential employees within the organization who can be promoted when the need for new leadership arises. Extolling mentoring as a development philosophy also encourages mature executives to give of themselves so that the younger managers can tap their experience and seasoned judgment and thus accelerate their own learning.

The department of education coordinates the leadership succession program. The staff members assist the managers in determining their strengths and weaknesses, consult with them as they develop their learning plans, and facilitate learning experiences when this is feasible. Learning laboratories and assessment centers are useful for this effort. Simulated experiences give the managers an opportunity to test their new skills in comfortable surroundings with a minimum amount of risk.

Creativity in Problem Solving

Because the health care system is so complex and many of the problems being faced today have no precedent, it is incumbent upon executives to welcome and support new ways of approaching problems and encourage continuous learning by everyone in the organization.

People in health care do not have time to rest on their laurels. The rate of change in how health care is delivered and financed is swift, technology becomes obsolete quickly, and new skills are needed to compete in regional, national, and international health care markets. An organization can no longer depend on the chief executive officer to do all the adaptation and forward thinking. This responsibility rests with all of the people in the organization.

New ways have to be found to solve operating problems. Using art, music, imagery, rituals, movement, and other forms of creative expression needs to be encouraged as a method of stimulating creativity and team building. An emphasis on systems thinking and on the interdependence of the parts of the organization is essential for creating an adaptive organization.

People at all levels of the organization must get excited about its vision and values and assume responsibility for making them come alive. They must completely redesign the organization around what the customer needs and wants and put their individual preferences in the background.

The ability to use data to describe and solve problems of variation should be part of everyone's repertoire. In addition, when the causes of a problem are made known, the reaction should not be finger pointing. Instead, a self-managed work team should attempt to make the situation better for the customer as quickly as possible.

The organization of the future will have to be open, adaptive, and focused on quality service. The executives will have to create a supportive environment that rewards the search for new ideas, the development of new skills, and the use of new ways of thinking about health care delivery.

CONCLUSION

This chapter has discussed the need for executives to develop health care organizations that encourage continuous learning by individual workers, work teams, and organizations as a whole. The mindset of continuous learning will be essential for ensuring that customers receive high-quality, efficient, and comprehensive health services.

The department of education is responsible for coordinating the activities of the learning organization. It serves a variety of learners and carries out an educational process that defines learner needs, plans and implements relevant programs, and evaluates the extent to which the programs contribute to organizational productivity and profitability.

In the coming decade, continuous quality improvement, leadership succession, and creative problem solving will present many challenges for the health care educational system. However, if organizations are to survive, they must renew and adapt, and focused learning in the workplace will be a key strategy.

ADDITIONAL RESOURCES

Argyris, C., and D.A. Schon. *Organizational learning: A theory of action perspective.* Menlo Park, Calif.: Addison-Wesley, 1978.

Joint Commission on Accreditation of Healthcare Organizations. *Striving toward improvement: Six hospitals in search of quality.* Oakbrook Terrace, Ill: Joint Commission on Accreditation of Healthcare Organizations, 1991.

McCool, B. *Organizational healing.* Master's thesis, Institute of Transpersonal Psychology, Menlo Park, Calif., 1991.

Orsburn, J., et al. *Self-directed work teams.* Homewood, Ill.: Business One Irwin, 1990.

Robson, G. *Continuous process improvement.* New York: The Free Press, 1991.

Rosen, R. *The healthy company.* Los Angeles: Jeremy P. Tarcher, Inc., 1991.

Senge, P.M. *The fifth discipline.* New York: Doubleday Currency, 1990.

Tracey, W. *Human resources management and development handbook.* New York: Amacom Publishing, 1985.

Part II

Organization and Management

Gerard F. Anderson
Stephanie L. Maxwell

6

The Organization and Financing of Health Care Services

Purpose: The organization and financing of a country's health care system are influenced and shaped by a variety of historical, social, economic, and political forces.

INTRODUCTION

Health care systems perform a variety of interrelated activities, including patient care, research, and education. How health care services are organized and delivered is influenced by a multitude of factors. This chapter begins with an exploration of how changes in medical practice in the late 1800s and early 1900s fundamentally altered the health care delivery and clinical educational system that had prevailed for centuries. As scientific advances led to more effective preventive and curative care, the role of health care organizations evolved. For example, the hospital shifted from being primarily a custodial care facility for the poor and insane to a modern medical center where patients from all socioeconomic backgrounds are treated for multifarious conditions and have a better opportunity for beneficial clinical outcomes.

During this same period a variety of political, economic, social, and regulatory forces were influencing the method of organizing and financing health care services. These forces, which are both internal and external to health care systems, have guided their evolution and are a major reason for the tremendous diversity in health care systems in the world today. Although access to clinical information is basically the same in every country, the degrees of emphasis placed on preventive versus curative care and on primary versus tertiary care, the access to care, the quality of care, and the provision of specific services vary substantially. This chapter provides a brief overview of the forces that have already had and will continue to have a major influence on the development of health care systems in various countries.

A critical determinant of the organization of any health care system is the corresponding financing system. Countries allocate different percentages of their gross domestic product to health care; spend different percentages of the health care dollar on hospital, physician, preventive, and other services; use a variety of mechanisms to generate health care funds; and employ a variety of methods to control health care spending. This chapter provides an overview of the financing and regulatory systems that are used in various industrialized countries.

As the twenty-first century approaches, managers of health care organizations will face a new set of challenges. They will be required to respond to constraints on health care spending, new methods of allocating health care resources to individual providers, a desire for increased allocative and technical efficiency, an increased level of concern for access and equity in the health care system, and a growing interest in identifying and paying for effective medical care. Managers will need to be aware of the changes in the health care environment and be prepared to take appropriate action.

MANAGEMENT PRINCIPLES

The following principles are intended to guide managers in monitoring and responding to the external environment.

1. Managers should continually monitor the external environment in order to be able to respond quickly to the changing economic, regulatory, and social conditions.

2. Managers should monitor broad social policy and not simply health policy, since health policy is influenced by the general social policies of the country.

3. Managers should understand the historical, social, economic, and political environment in which they operate. This environment determines the set of options they have available.

4. Managers have some degree of control over the external environment. They can, for example, exert some influence over the regulatory and financial environment by effective negotiation, lobbying, and other types of intervention.

5. Managers should develop a set of institutional objectives that are responsive to the external environment. These objectives should help guide their managerial decisions.

6. Managers in the twenty-first century must be aware of new management challenges, which will include an increased emphasis on medical effectiveness, technology assessment, technical efficiency, and allocative efficiency.

HEALTH SYSTEM ORGANIZATION

History and Background

Health care organizations and health care delivery systems are not preordained. They are forged by individuals and institutional objectives that are continuously influenced by a variety of internal and external forces. There is no predetermined role of any institution in a health care system and no fixed trajectory for institutional and health care system development. If there was a uniform evolutionary pattern, then all health care systems in the world would pass through the same phases and all organizations would be similar at some point during their development.

Between 1850 and 1920, most health care organizations were affected by the broad forces of urbanization, industrialization, and immigration. They were also affected by forces specific to health care systems, including changing perceptions of disease and science, an increased level of clinical professionalism, the development of health insurance in Western Europe, and a changing balance between philanthropists, administrators, and clinicians within institutions. These forces shaped the development of the health care system in each country and are partially responsible for the tremendous variation in the health care financing and delivery systems that exist today.

One of the major factors that shaped health care systems during this period was the increased effectiveness of curative and preventive care. Newfound medicines such as digitalis, quinine, and mercury gave promise of relief for certain conditions, while morphine reduced the manifestation of pain. The development of anesthesia vastly expanded the realm of surgery and allowed surgeons to perform such procedures as draining abscesses in the brain and removing benign and cancerous tumors from the body. Other physicians improved their diagnostic capabilities by using x-rays, laboratory tests, and other techniques. These advances helped make hospitals and other health care institutions become places where treatment and the alleviation of pain were possible for a wide variety of diseases.

Preventive care also became more effective. Public health efforts included draining marshes to control insectborne diseases such as malaria, developing sewage and clean water systems to control diarrheal diseases, and emphasizing personal hygiene and exercise as means of promoting health. Other public health and disease prevention developments included improved epidemiological techniques to help control disease, the discovery of vaccines for diseases such as polio, and the development of screening tests for diseases such as tuberculosis. The tuberculin test, introduced around 1890 and refined in 1907, disclosed that latent tuberculosis infection was widespread in the population. The discovery that many people could have the disease without exhibiting obvious symptoms prompted a variety of public health activities.

In general, the scientific advances of the era pushed health care systems to become more scientific, professional, clean, and organized. The roles of clinicians and the institutions where they worked changed dramatically during this era, and for the first time health care organizations started to resemble the entities of today.[1]

At the turn of the century, physicians, nurses, and other clinicians began to cultivate a new professionalism that was supported by the development of science-based expertise, the increased effectiveness of surgery, the evolution of new diagnostic techniques, and the growing strength of professional organizations. Working through professional organizations, providers were better able to shape public discussion and to have a major influence on issues such as licensing, fees, and practice arrangements.

The current roles of administrative actors in health care institutions emerged in this era as well. Inside the hospital, authority was being taken away from the lay trustees, who through philanthropy had exerted tremendous control over daily operations. Yet as the costs and sophistication of hospitals grew, the importance of employing business practices and principles in hospitals greatly increased. As the management needs of hospitals evolved, power shifted from lay trustees to professional managers, who incorporated business practices developed in other industries and who were trained in modern business techniques. Managers looked to management techniques employed outside the health care industry to improve their housekeeping, accounting, and public relations operations. Hospital administrators began to apply techniques of scientific management, such as those espoused by Frederich Taylor, in order to improve productivity. Hospital management became a balancing act that involved ensuring a steady flow of funds from patients, government, and philanthropy; maintaining the good will of the trustees; and retaining certain physicians, especially those with private pay patients. Physicians with private pay patients exercised much greater control over the care of patients, including almost complete control over admission, discharge, and treatment decisions.

As the importance and professionalism of the medical enterprise grew, there were calls for formal rules to guarantee that providers would meet specific clinical, safety, and operational standards. Two areas perceived to be especially in need of upgraded standards were medical education and clinical care.

In 1910, a critical report on American medical education was published by the Carnegie Foundation.[2] Commonly known as the Flexner report, it proposed that medical schools be linked with hospitals so that medical students could have clinical training as part of their medical education. The Flexner report identified the integration of the Johns Hopkins Hospital and Medical School as the type of organizational arrangement capable of producing the best-trained clinicians. The hospital was the site for clinical training of medical students, and the clinical departments in the hospital were under the direct control of the medical school professors.

The leadership at Johns Hopkins had been trained in the German system of scientific medicine, which stressed the value of incorporating scientific training and research into clinical training. Clinical training in other medical schools in Canada and the United States was soon patterned after the Hopkins example. The Flexner report also lambasted proprietary medical schools, and most of them closed soon after its publication.

Regulation of hospitals and clinical practice also developed around the turn of the century. Initially, physicians wanted licensure in order to protect themselves against competition from untrained professionals. In the United States, physicians began persuading states in the 1870s to license physicians. In 1901, the American Medical Association was recognized and began to argue for standards for physicians and physician training. In 1913, the American Hospital Association agreed in principle to the inspection, classification, and standardization of hospitals, leading to the accreditation bodies of today.

Other initiatives designed to improve quality of care were less successful. In the early twentieth century, Dr. E. A. Codman proposed to define quality in terms of the actual outcomes of care of the patient.[3] Codman argued, for example, that surgeons should be judged on the basis of their ability to treat patients and not on the basis of their prestige. After several years of intense debate within the clinical community, this standard of measuring quality was rejected. It is only recently that Codman's original idea of using outcome measures to gauge the effectiveness of medical treatment is being revived.

In Europe, an important factor in the evolution of health care systems was the adoption of universal health insurance by several countries. The resulting insurance systems provided a source of funding for health care providers. Additionally, each health insurance system gave the government a certain degree of power over the health care delivery system generally and health care institutions specifically. Governments have used this power to directly control aggregate spending, and in some cases they have dictated managerial policies and procedures for individual institutions.

In 1883, Germany became the first nation to institute some form of universal health insurance. Germany adopted an employer-based health insurance system that was soon copied by other European countries (Table 6-1). Over time, countries developed alternative health insurance models, including national health service, national health insurance, and variants of the German employer-based insurance system.

In North America, the evolution of health insurance developed much more slowly, but insurance has still had a major influence on how the Canadian and U.S. health care systems have evolved. In fact, health insurance is one of the major factors that explains the differences in these two health care delivery systems.

Although universal health insurance was proposed as early as 1919 in Canada, insurance through the 1920s and 1930s was provided through a variety of indemnity and prepaid plans. A British-style national health plan was proposed in 1945, but most Canadians considered the plan to be too centralized. By 1955, five provinces had developed their own single-payer hospital insurance systems, in large part to stabilize hospital finances. Pressure on the federal government for matching funds led to

---

Table 6-1 Development of Universal Health Insurance Systems in Selected Countries

Country	Date
Germany	1883
Austria	1888
United Kingdom	1911
France	1945
Sweden	1955
Japan	1961
South Korea	1989

Source: Information from *Health Affairs*, Vol. 8, No. 2, p. 25 and *Comparing Health Systems: Descriptive Analyses of Fourteen National Health Systems* by M.W. Raffel, ed., Pennsylvania State University Press, 1984.

a federal law that induced every province to have a hospital insurance system in place by 1961. Later legislation provided similar incentives for broader coverage, and provincial medical insurance plans were established in all provinces by 1971. As a result, Canada has a universal, single-payer system of health insurance that is run by the nation's ten provinces and two territories. This single-payer system gives provinces great authority to control certain aspects of health policy, such as setting hospital payment rates, directly controlling capital spending, and defining payment rates for clinical specialties.

Although the insurance system is publicly managed and financed, most Canadian health care facilities are operated privately. Canadian hospitals are mainly private, nonprofit facilities. The hospitals negotiate annually with each province to determine their operating budgets prospectively. Separate controls exist for capital spending, which is allocated by the provincial governments based on considerations of need, clinical expertise, and other factors. Canadian physicians have an all-or-nothing choice of operating or not operating within the Canadian health insurance system. If they elect to operate within the system, their fee schedule is fixed and they have no opportunity to bill for the unpaid balance. In addition, an expenditure target constrains growth in utilization.

Health insurance in the United States was first established in the nineteenth century, when insurers offered income protection insurance that compensated individuals for lost income due to unemployment caused by illness. In 1929, the first private health insurance plan was developed. In this plan, called the Baylor University Hospital Plan, the public school teachers of Dallas, Texas, were insured for 21 days of hospital care in return for a monthly fee of 50 cents.[4]

A second type of health insurance plan was developed in the United States by remotely located mining, lumber, and construction companies. These plans, in which the provider also played the role of insurer, spread to urban areas and were adopted by consumers and governments as an alternative to fee-for-service medicine. The plans, which became known as health maintenance organizations, offered comprehensive health care services for a set payment rate.

At about the same time that private health insurance was beginning to develop in the United States, progressive era social reforms, as well as rising medical costs, prompted an increased interest in national health insurance. The first national health insurance bill was drafted by a labor group in 1915. The bill, if passed, would have established compulsory, employer-based medical and income protection insurance for those under a set income level, similar to the German system developed by Bismarck in 1883. Various proposals for national health insurance have been put forth in almost every decade since the 1915 proposal.

The modern United States health insurance industry, which originated during the Depression with the creation of the Blue Cross hospital insurance plans, greatly expanded in the 1940s and 1950s as a result of the growth of commercial health insurance. Much of the growth in private health insurance has been traced to changes in federal tax laws during the 1940s, especially the creation of a tax deduction for employer-based health insurance. Tax deductibility encouraged corporations to offer private health insurance as an employee benefit. In 1965, Congress passed legislation establishing the Medicare and Medicaid programs, which provided insurance for the elderly and for certain categories of poor persons. When these programs were implemented in 1966, the number of Americans with health insurance coverage increased dramatically.

The focus of public policy at this time was on ensuring access to high quality care for the greatest number of Americans. However, the issue of cost containment would become a dominant issue after 1970, since health care costs continued to increase and insurers began looking for ways to improve allocative and technical efficiency in hospitals and among other health care providers.

The roots of inflationary health care costs largely lie in the method for paying hospitals developed by the Baylor University Hospital Plan in 1929 and used by other insurers. From the beginning, Blue Cross and the commercial insurers reimbursed either full allowable costs or full charges to institutional providers. These types of reimbursement did not give institutions any incentive to become more productive, since all allowable costs were paid under cost reimbursement and charges were fully paid under the other system. A similar system allowing the physicians immense flexibility in setting their own rates evolved for physicians as well.

When the Medicare and Medicaid programs were being designed, providers insisted that these programs adopt reimbursement systems similar to those used to pay Blue Cross, Blue Shield, and commercial insurance claims. Therefore, with the passage of Medicare and Medicaid and the expansion of private health insurance, hospitals, physicians, and other providers were assured full payment of their full costs or charges for treating most patients. These payment systems helped foster the rapid increase in health care spending in subsequent decades, which in turn has prompted recent health care reforms in provider reimbursement and cost containment.

Components of Health Care Delivery Systems

By the early 1920s, the various components of the typical modern health care system were in place. Table 6-2 compares the distribution of personal health care spending in the United States in 1929 and 1990 and shows how the distribution of health care spending changed during these 61 years. Institutional care (hospitals and nursing homes) grew dramatically in importance, while the proportion of health care spending on physician services, dental services, and drugs declined.

In the United States, Canada, and other industrialized countries, the majority of health care dollars are spent on acute care services. Hospitals and physician services typically account for 60 percent of health care spending. When drugs, dental care, and other acute care services are included, the percent-

Table 6-2 Personal Health Care Expenditures in the United States by Distribution Percentages, 1929 and 1990

	Percentage of Funds Spent	
Type of Expenditure	*1929*	*1990*
Hospital Care	17	43
Physician Services	32	22
Dental Services	16	6
Drugs	19	9
Nursing Home Care	—	9
Home Care and Other Professional Services	11	7
Other Personal Care Expenses	5	4
Total	100	100

Source: Information from *Medical Care and Costs in Relation to Family Income* by the U.S. Social Security Administration, 1947, and from K.R. Levit et al., National Health Expenditures, 1990, in *Health Care Financing Review*, Vol. 13, No. 1, pp. 1–15, Health Care Financing Administration, 1991.

age spent on acute care services approaches 80 to 90 percent in most industrialized countries. Where there is variation across countries, most of the variation occurs within the components of acute care spending and reflects different emphases placed on the provision of different services.

One area where the distribution of health care spending varies substantially is expenditures on drugs and devices. Japan, Korea, Taiwan, and other countries in East Asia have traditionally spent a much higher proportion of total health care expenditures on drugs and devices. This may be the result of the financing system in these countries where physicians derive most of their income from dispensing drugs and relatively little from providing diagnostic and therapeutic services.

A second area of variation is hospital expenditures. The United States and to a lesser extent Canada have developed health care delivery systems that place a great emphasis on hospital services. Other industrialized countries have placed a greater emphasis on primary care and therefore allocate a greater percentage of their health care dollar to ambulatory care services.

Given the resources devoted to delivering acute care services, it is not surprising that most policy development has centered on these services. Policy makers have placed great emphasis on achieving both allocative and technical efficiency in the provision of acute care services. Allocative efficiency results from creating an optimal mix of health care services so that cost can be minimized while access to appropriate high-quality medical services is ensured. Allocative efficiency is concerned with the appropriate mix of preventive care versus curative care and the appropriate balance between hospital care, long-term care, and home care. Technical efficiency results from ensuring that costs are minimized when a specific provider produces a certain bundle of goods and services. Health care systems often differ in the relative importance they place on cost containment, access to care, quality of care, and other factors that could influence their calculations of allocative and technical efficiency.

Within the acute care sector, most of the regulatory emphasis has been on monitoring either the quantity or the price of services. Given that price multiplied by quantity equals total expenditures, the division of policy options into controls on price and controls on quantity is not surprising. Countries have used a variety of ways to control the price of and the demand for health care services.

Most countries have utilized two general methods for controlling the prices and quantities of services that are delivered: competition and regulation. Exhibit 6-1 shows some of the specific policy initiatives that have been developed in various countries to influence the development of their health care delivery systems and to change the behavior of specific institutions.

Compared to acute care, preventive services and resource development account for a much smaller percentage of health care spending in all industrialized countries. Preventive services consist of clinical preventive services, patient education, and counseling. Clinical preventive services include primary preventive measures such as immunizations and dental fluoride treatments. Clinical prevention also involves secondary preventive mea-

Exhibit 6-1 Policy Alternatives To Influence Consumer and Provider Behavior

Controlling Prices through Competition
- Development of alternative delivery systems that will compete on the basis of price.
- Antitrust enforcement to encourage providers to compete against each other.
- Physician and patient education to make the provider and consumer more aware of their alternatives.
- Cost sharing to make the consumer more sensitive to the costs of health care.

Controlling Prices through Regulation
- Setting of payment rates for individual providers. For example, many systems use budget review to set hospital rates.
- Setting of payment rates for a class of providers, with specific adjustments for input and output differences. The Medicare prospective payment system is an example of this regulatory strategy.

Controlling Quantity through Competition
- Revision of the tax code to reduce or eliminate tax deductibility of health insurance. This will reduce the amount of health insurance that is purchased.
- Development of clinical practice guidelines so that physicians and patients can be more informed.
- Development of alternative delivery systems that use hospital services less intensively.

Controlling Quantity through Regulation
- Queues for elective services.
- Global budgets to control aggregate spending.
- Direct control over capital budgets to control the diffusion of unnecessary technology.
- Health planning to control the diffusion of unnecessary technology.
- Utilization review to reduce the number of inappropriate hospital admissions and hospital days and the use of unnecessary procedures.
- Coverage restrictions to prevent the use of unsafe, ineffective, unproven, or non-cost-effective medical treatments.
- Technology assessment to ensure that services are effective and perhaps cost-effective.

sures, such as screening for hypertension, cancer, and other diseases. Patient education and patient counseling are generally aimed at promoting healthy behavior and reducing risk factors for disease. Education and counseling activities include exercise, stress management, and smoking cessation programs as well as programs to reduce the consumption of alcohol and dietary fats.

Resource development includes research, education, and construction. Biomedical research is sponsored by government and private industry. In the United States, expenditures for biomedical research were an estimated 22.6 billion dollars in 1990, or less than 4 percent of the total amount spent on health care.[5] Biomedical research spending has remained a relatively stable proportion of total health care spending since the 1970s, although a greater proportion of the funds now are coming from private industry. The level of spending on biomedical research and the types of projects that are funded can have a major impact on health care systems in the future, since much of the growth in spending on new technology can be attributed to the creativity of scientists in government, universities, and private industry.

The education of medical students, residents, nurses, and allied health professionals is organized primarily through universities and hospitals and is financed through a variety of sources. Since the Flexner report in 1910, there has been a strong emphasis on combining scientific and clinical training. In general, this has meant involving students in the health care system relatively early in their training. As a result, institutions that include education as a part of their missions have an additional set of responsibilities. In most European countries, education is financed primarily by the government, and students pay a relatively small proportion of the cost of their education. Once students enter the clinical phase of their education, the health insurance system pays most of the cost of their training. In the United States, the scenario is quite different, and students pay a larger percentage of the cost of their undergraduate and medical school education. Because a greater proportion of educational costs is self-financed by American physicians, nurses, and allied health professionals, they have been given greater autonomy in their professional activities and greater remuneration for their services. This constrains the ability of regulators and managers to control the activities of health professionals.

Capital expenditures can indirectly affect the utilization of health care resources and thus the level of health care spending. Control over capital spending has much greater policy significance than the relatively small percentage of health care spending on construction, renovation, and medical equipment would suggest. This is because capital spending greatly influences what services are available, who has access to specific services, and how long patients have to wait to receive services. As a result, much of the discussion about health care rationing centers on the level and type of capital spending. Many countries have a surplus of competent physicians, nurses, and allied health professionals but still have queues for certain health services—a result of controlling the number of surgical suites and hospital beds and the specific technologies in use in their health care systems.

Policy makers, in trying to achieve the correct level and distribution of capital expenditures, have used three primary methods. The first is direct regulation of capital construction. In this method, used by most European countries and Canada, the government allocates capital directly. A second method involves private financing but public regulation. The United States followed this approach during the 1970s with the institution of certificate-of-need programs in all states. Many states continue to use health planning and certificate-of-need programs to control capital expenditures. A third approach is increased competition. In order to promote competition, the U.S. Department of Justice and the U.S. Federal Trade Commission have used antitrust enforcement. The objective of antitrust enforcement is to compel providers to compete against each other on the basis of price, quality of care, access to services, and other factors and to allow consumers to select the combinations that best fit their needs. The expectation is that by offering more choice, there will be greater efficiency and consumer satisfaction. The competitive strategy is in direct opposition to health planning, which uses planning and coordination of services to control costs.

Economic Factors

A number of economic factors influence the size and shape of any health care delivery system. As shown in Figure 6-1, there is a relationship between the gross domestic product (GDP) per capita and the level of health care spending in industrialized countries. As the GDP per capita rises, more dollars are spent on health care.

In addition to the macro issue of how much in aggregate is spent on health care, the economic issues of price and quantity have a major influence on health care delivery systems and health care organizations. In any health care system, it is necessary to control consumer demand. One option is to allow price to moderate consumer demand. In Canada, patients pay virtually nothing out of their own pocket for most covered health services, whereas in the United States a variety of coinsurance, deductibles, and other financial mechanisms have increased the sensitivity of consumers to health care costs. Studies such as the Rand Health Insurance Experiment have demonstrated that health care utilization is affected by the amount that consumers pay for health care services.[6] Queues and rationing are other available alternatives for controlling consumer demand. Many European countries and Canada use queues to manage consumer demand. Whether the dominant constraint on demand is based on money or waiting time has a major influence on any health care system.

Social and political factors also have a major impact on health care systems. One important factor is tolerance of inequalities in access to social services. Most European countries have a tradition of providing social services through an elaborate compulsory

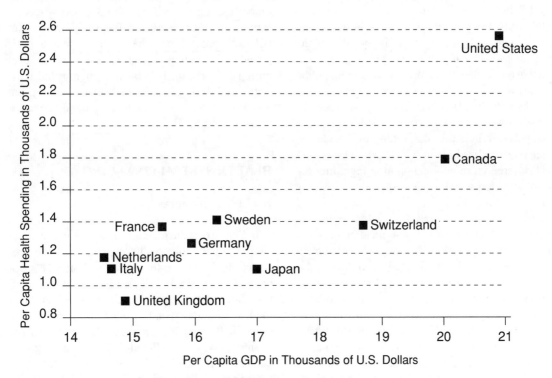

Figure 6-1 Per Capita Health Spending Related to Per Capita Gross Domestic Product, 1990. *Source:* Information from the Organization for Economic Cooperation and Development 1991 Health Data File.

social welfare system. Financed through payroll deductions and general tax revenues, such systems redistribute income across different income strata. Traditionally, welfare systems combine retirement, health care, income security, and other social programs into one funding mechanism.

The systems for financing health care services are a natural extension of the European social welfare philosophy. In most European countries and in Canada there is agreement that at least a minimum of health services should be accessible to everyone. At one level, this becomes the manifesto that health care is a right and that everyone is entitled to access to the health care system regardless of financial situation. The United States does not have this same social welfare tradition and historically has not endorsed the concept of income redistribution. As a result, the concept of health care as a right remains less acceptable to American policy makers and has not been incorporated into the U.S. health care system.

Probably the greatest difference between the U.S. system and other systems is the role of the government. Table 6-3 shows the percentage of national health care expenditures coming from public sources in selected industrialized countries. The data show that the U.S. health care system receives a much lower percentage of its health care dollar from public sources than the systems in Canada and other industrialized countries. These numbers reflect differences in political opinion regarding the extent to which social services should be privately or publicly funded.

There is significant variation across countries with respect to the degree of centralization in health care systems. In Canada, the national government provides some of the funding and coordinates national policy, but most of the detailed policy making is left to the provinces. Britain, Spain, and other European countries gradually are moving from centralized to decentralized health care systems where more of actual decision making is left to the regional governments. In the United States, virtually all of the models of centralization and decentralization have been used. The Medicare program is a

Table 6-3 Percentage of National Health Expenditures from Government Funds in Industrialized Countries, 1990

Country	Percentage of Expenditures from Government Sources
Norway	96
United Kingdom	85
Spain	78
Japan	75
France	74
Canada	74
Germany	73
United States	42

Source: Information from the Organization for Economic Cooperation and Development 1991 Health Data File.

highly centralized national program, whereas the Medicaid program gives much more authority to the states. Much of the regulation of private insurance occurs at the state level, but most major corporations are self-insured and are governed by federal Employee Retirement and Income Security Act (ERISA) provisions. The United States experimented with capital regulation at the federal level during the era of the Hill-Burton program and at the state level during the era of health planning, but now it has turned over the major capital allocation decisions to providers.

HEALTH SYSTEM FINANCING

Health Expenditures

In Figure 6-1, the relationship between per capita GDP and per capita health expenditures was presented. In Table 6-4, the percentage of GDP spent on health services in selected industrialized countries during 1990 is presented. The data suggest that the United States spends a much larger proportion of its GDP on health care than other industrialized countries. While the United States is spending 12.4 percent of its GDP on health care services, most other industrialized countries are spending in the 6–9 percent range.

Table 6-4 Percentage of Gross Domestic Product Spent on Health Care in Industrialized Countries, 1990

Country	Percentage of GDP Spent on Health Care
United States	12.4
Canada	9.0
France	8.9
Germany	8.1
Norway	7.2
Japan	6.5
United Kingdom	6.1

Source: Information from the Organization for Economic Cooperation and Development 1991 Health Data File.

Monitoring trends in health care spending suggests that health care policy makers, providers, and consumers can influence the rate of increase in health care spending. Figure 6-2 compares the percentage of the GDP spent on health care in Canada and the United States from 1970 to 1990. The data suggest that, in 1970, both countries were spending a little more than 7 percent of GDP on health care

services. Since 1970, Canada has experienced a relatively slow rate of growth, especially between 1970 and 1980 and between 1985 and 1990. The United States, on the other hand, has experienced an almost continual rise in expenditures since 1970.

Policy makers are concerned about the level and rate of growth in health care expenditures for several reasons, although most of these reasons are summarized by the economics term *opportunity costs*. Opportunity costs reflect the value of alternative uses of scarce resources. For example, more government spending on health care can reduce a government's ability to fund other social programs, fund national defense, reduce budget deficits, or lower taxes. Increases in health care spending by private industries can affect their profit margins, international competitiveness, or ability to increase wages and salaries for their employees. The issue of opportunity costs has prompted policy makers to give considerable attention to the level of health care spending in their country.

The 1990 distribution of health care spending in the United States is shown in Table 6-5. As noted earlier, expenditures for hospital and physician ser-

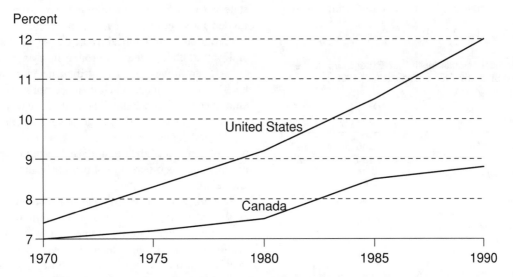

Figure 6-2 Health Expenditures as Percentage of GDP in Canada and the United States, 1970–1990. *Source:* Information from the Organization for Economic Cooperation and Development 1991 Health Data File.

vices represent the largest share of the health care dollar. More importantly, changes in the health care system are revealed by examining trends in the distribution of the health care dollar. Table 6-6 shows annualized increases by expenditure category since 1980. The areas showing the most rapid growth were nursing home care, home health care, and physician services, with hospital services showing much slower growth. Much of the change was in response to explicit policies designed to transfer inpatient services to less expensive outpatient and ambulatory care settings.

Sources of Health Care Resources

As noted in Table 6-3, governments play different roles in financing health care services. In Canada, for example, the government pays the full cost of all covered health services and does not permit balance billing and cost sharing. Most of the major health system decisions are made at the provincial level, with the national government having only a limited role in policy development. In Germany, the government plays a relatively small role, with private insurers developing their coverage policies and providing most of the insurance cover-

Table 6-6 Annualized Rate of Increase in U.S. Personal Health Care Expenditures, 1980–1990

| | Percentage Increase | |
Type of Expenditure	Nominal Dollars	1982 Dollars
Hospital Care	10%	3%
Physician Services	12	4
Dental Services	9	2
Drugs	10	2
Nursing Home Care	10	4
Home Care and Other Professional Services	14	7
Other Personal Health Care	10	3

Source: Information from K.R. Levit et al., National Health Expenditures, 1990, in *Health Care Financing Review,* Vol. 13, No. 1, pp. 1–15, Health Care Financing Administration, 1991.

age to the population. Recently the role of the German government increased when it established guidelines and limitations for the rate of growth in the nation's health care spending. In the United States, the Medicare, CHAMPUS, Department of Defense, and Veterans Administration programs are national, the Medicaid program is a federal-state partnership, and public health programs are funded and operated by a variety of mechanisms.

Private financing of health care can occur in several ways, although there are four primary systems.

First, employers may contribute to employee health insurance plans. In Germany, employers and employees each pay half of the cost of employees' health insurance. A variety of arrangements exist in the United States. For example, some employers pay 100 percent of their employees' insurance premiums whereas others do not pay for health insurance at all.

Second, individuals may pay for insurance directly out of their own pocket. In Germany the wealthiest citizens are not compelled to purchase health insurance through their employers, and they may buy insurance privately or choose to self-insure. Approximately 8 percent of Germans have private coverage or simply self-insure.[7] In the

Table 6-5 Personal Health Care Expenditures in the United States by Type of Expenditure, 1990

Type of Expenditure	Dollars (in billions)	Percentage
Hospital Care	256	43
Physician Services	126	22
Dental Services	34	6
Drugs	55	9
Nursing Home Care	53	9
Home Care and Other Professional Services	39	7
Other Personal Health Care	23	4
Total	586	100

Source: Information from K.R. Levit et al., National Health Expenditures, 1990, in *Health Care Financing Review,* Vol. 13, No. 1, pp. 1–15, Health Care Financing Administration, 1991.

United States, almost 15 million Americans purchase health insurance directly.[8] Individually purchased health insurance is typically much more expensive than group insurance and frequently has pre-existing exclusions, waiting periods, higher deductibles and coinsurance levels, and other limitations. As a result, persons with individual insurance policies pay more for coverage than individuals with group insurance. Legislation requiring open enrollment and health insurance reform in the United States is designed to respond to these problems.

Third, individuals may pay for health care through coinsurance and deductibles. Many countries ask patients to pay a portion of the cost of their health care visits. The purpose of per day or per visit fees is to discourage unnecessary utilization. For example, the United States, France, and Korea all place great importance on cost sharing. Of the three, Korea has the highest coinsurance rate—almost 50 percent. In the United States and France, the typical coinsurance rate is 20 percent, although considerable variation exists among insurance plans and among health care services. Canada and some European countries do not have any coinsurance.

Finally, individuals may pay for health care by paying for services directly out of pocket. Individuals who lack any insurance pay for their health services directly. In addition, all persons pay out of pocket for those services not covered by insurance at all. Drugs and dental services, for example, are frequently not covered by insurance.

Financial Constraints on Health Service Delivery

Governments and private insurers have developed a variety of mechanisms to control health care prices and utilization in order to promote allocative and technical efficiency. It has been recognized that without a constraint on health care prices, the income of health care providers will increase to a level that reduces the overall welfare of society. Without a constraint on health care utilization, the demand for

health care services will increase. Seven major control mechanisms are discussed below.

For many years, Europe and Canada have used expenditure targets to limit overall spending on health care. To employ expenditure targets, the government or some other entity defines an aggregate amount of spending for health care and frequently determines the total level of spending for specific types of providers or geographic regions. Providers are reimbursed according to a payment formula; if the aggregate level of spending exceeds the predetermined limit, however, the payment level declines. Both Germany and Canada have used expenditure targets to control expenditures for physician services, and the United States has recently adopted volume performance standards to control expenditures for physician services in the Medicare program.

Budgeting is a second method of controlling health care spending. Many countries, such as Canada, develop an annual budget for each institution in the country. The budget defines the total amount of resources the institution will receive during the year.

Capitation is a related cost-control method. In a capitation system, a provider or group of providers receive a fixed amount of money for treating patients for the year. Both budgeting and capitation shift the responsibility for controlling health care expenditures to providers and encourage them to become more productive. The impact of these cost-control methods on the quality of and access to care is uncertain and is highly dependent on the specifics of the system.

Prospective payment is a fourth method intended to improve the technical efficiency of providers. Prospective payment uses a formula approach to determine payments to individual providers for treatment of specific patient conditions. It is designed to encourage providers to produce services with enough efficiency that costs are lower than payment rates. The Medicare program began using a prospective payment system to pay hospitals in 1983. States such as Maryland, New Jersey, New York, and Massachusetts have used prospective payment systems for several years. All of the programs have shown some success in controlling the rate of increase in hospital expenditures.[9]

Other types of controls target utilization of health care services. One way of controlling utilization is to limit the services covered by insurance. Studies have shown a high correlation between utilization of health care services and insurance coverage.[10] As a result, medical care ostensibly covered by insurance policies is closely monitored to ensure that the services rendered are appropriate, medically necessary, and beneficial to patients. However, there is wide variation across countries and across insurance plans within the United States regarding what health care services are covered. Most of the recent debate over coverage decisions centers on services involving costly technologies, expensive new drugs or devices, or experimental procedures.

In addition to coverage restrictions, several other constraints on utilization of health care services have been adopted. Referral criteria, utilization review, second-opinion requirements, and managed care activities such as the use of a gatekeeper are all examples of attempts to monitor and control utilization. They are basically designed to allow review of physicians' decisions. Recent studies in the United States showing that a sizable (but unspecified) percentage of care may be unnecessary have stimulated insurers to become more aggressive in using utilization controls.[11]

Finally, the state of Oregon has proposed a new system that would allocate funds based on a set of priorities. The state proposes to rank all medical conditions from highest to lowest priority and fund programs and services in rank order until all available funds are exhausted. This system would have a major impact on Oregon's health care managers, as they would need to monitor the ranking of services and restructure their mix of services accordingly.

THE FUTURE OF HEALTH CARE ORGANIZATION AND FINANCING

The preceding sections suggest that a multitude of factors influence the behavior of health care managers and clinicians and that these factors explain the wide variety in organizational systems that exist today. In the next few decades, additional factors are likely to exist, including further constraints on health care spending, new ways to allocate resources to individual providers, an increased desire for more allocative and technical efficiency, and a growing interest in effective medical care.

In most industrialized countries, an increasing share of the gross national product (GNP) is spent on health care. Nowhere is that more true than in the United States, where health care costs are projected to be 18 percent of the GNP by the year 2000. It is common for politicians to state that health care costs are "out of control" and that some way to constrain cost increases must be found. Although there are many reasons for rising health care costs, one of the most frequently cited reasons is the use of expensive new technologies. Governments and health care institutions will need to develop technology assessment programs to evaluate new and established technologies. The choice of who will conduct technology assessments will probably depend on the financing system of each country. In the United States, the Medicare prospective payment system essentially turns over technology assessment responsibilities to hospitals, whereas cost- and charge-based insurers continue to conduct their own assessments. In most other countries, the government plays a major role in conducting technology assessments. Regardless of who has the responsibility for assessing technologies, managers and clinicians in the next century will need to become much more involved in the technology assessment process.

In Europe and North America, where there is a recognition that many health care institutions are inefficient, governments and insurers are looking for ways to encourage productivity gains. One method that is winning favor is to use formulas to set payment rates for providers and then allow the providers greater flexibility in working within the financial constraints. In the United States, Medicare's prospective payment system, physician payment reforms, and method for reimbursing health maintenance organizations are based on this principle. Other countries are employing similar strategies to allocate resources to individual providers, whether they use a fee-for-service, institutional budget, or other system. The basic process of developing a formula-based payment system is to identify the output of providers, determine why some providers are more expensive than others, make specific adjustments for differences in input costs and outputs, and then pay the providers based on the formula. As the use of this type of payment system increases, more managers will have to adjust to established payment rates. This will require managers and clinicians to work within stricter financial constraints than they have been accustomed to.

As governments and insurers search for ways to achieve greater allocative efficiency, health care systems will need to find less expensive ways to achieve similar outcomes. For example, Europe and Canada have not adopted outpatient surgery to the same extent as the United States. This difference in use is primarily due to the existence of financial incentives promoting inpatient care in most countries and to the fact that insurance policies in the United States usually do not pay for inpatient care for certain types of surgery. On the other hand, the U.S. system continues to encourage the use of high-technology services and specialty care and pays relatively little attention to disease prevention. In order to achieve allocative efficiency, this imbalance will need to be rectified.

Managers in the next century also will need to respond to research on effective medical care. Several research projects in the world are examining current medical practice and finding that some medical care is inappropriate, that a scientific basis does not exist for many procedures performed today, and that some commonly performed procedures actually may be harmful to patients. Managers and clinicians will need to be aware of this research in order to operate efficiently, since governments and insurers will begin using this type of research in making coverage decisions.

Finally, managers in the future will need to respond to the mandate to contain costs while im-proving quality. Managers will have to experiment with new management methods to increase operational efficiency and responsiveness and to develop a better understanding of community needs. As they have done in the past, health care managers will need to borrow strategies, such as total quality management and continuous quality improvement, from other industries and tailor them to the health sector in order to meet the management challenges of today and tomorrow.

ADDITIONAL RESOURCES

Anderson, G.F., et al. 1989. *Providing hospital services: The changing environment.* Baltimore: Johns Hopkins University Press.

Davis, K., et al. 1990. *Health care cost containment.* Baltimore: Johns Hopkins University Press.

Iglehart, J.K. 1990. Canada's health care system faces its problems. *New England Journal of Medicine* 322:562–568.

Iglehart, J.K. 1992. The American Health Care System: Introduction. *New England Journal of Medicine* 326:962–967.

International Health Care System Edition. 1991. *Health Affairs* 10, no. 3.

Levit, K.R., et al. 1991. National Health Expenditures, 1990. *Health Care Financing Review* 13, no. 1:29–54.

NOTES

1. For a discussion of the development of the modern U.S. health care system, see P. Starr, *The Social Transformation of American Medicine* (New York: Basic Books, 1982); or R. Stevens, *In Sickness and in Wealth: American Hospitals in the 20th Century* (New York: Basic Books, 1989).

2. A. Flexner, *Medical Education in the United States and Canada,* Bulletin no. 4 (New York: Carnegie Foundation for the Advancement of Teaching, 1910).

3. Stevens, *In Sickness and in Wealth,* 76–77.

4. Starr, *The Social Transformation of American Medicine,* 295.

5. Office of Program Planning and Evaluation and the Division of Research Grants, National Institutes of Health, *NIH Data Book 1991* (Bethesda, Md.: National Institutes of Health, 1991), 1.

6. J.P. Newhouse, Some Interim Results from a Controlled Trial of Cost-Sharing in Health Insurance, *New England Journal of Medicine* 305 (1981):1504.

7. B.L. Kirkman-Liff, Health Insurance Values and Implementation in the Netherlands and the Federal Republic of Germany: An Alternative Path to Universal Coverage, *JAMA* 265(1991):2500.

8. U.S. Congressional Budget Office, *Selected Options for Expanding Health Insurance Coverage* (Washington, D.C.: U.S. Government Printing Office, 1991), 4.

9. G.F. Anderson, All-Payor Ratesetting: Down But Not Out, *Health Care Financing Review,* 1991 Annual Supplement, 36.

10. J. Hadley et al., Comparison of Hospital Care of Privately Insured and Uninsured Patients: Condition on Admission, Resource Use, and Outcome, *JAMA* 265(1991):377.

11. For examples of studies examining the appropriateness of medical procedures, see M.R. Chassin et al., Does Appropriate Use Explain Geographic Variations in the Use of Health Care Services? *JAMA* 258(1987):2533–2537; or G.L. Goyert et al., The Physician Factor in Cesarean Birth Rates, *New England Journal of Medicine* 320(1989):706–709.

G. Ross Baker
Lutchmie Narine
Peggy Leatt

7

Organizational Designs for Health Care

Purpose: The purpose of an organizational design is to structure work relationships and decision making in the organization. Effective organization designs provide knowledge of the external environment, facilitate the management of work, and create a context for delivering high-quality care.

INTRODUCTION

Health care organizations have been described as among the most difficult of all organizations to manage. The internal challenges faced by health care managers include the technical complexity of the services provided by health care professionals, the need to control costs while assuring high-quality care, and the difficulties of managing professionals who value autonomy in carrying out their work. In the last 15 years, growing regulatory pressures, increasing competition from other provider organizations, and problems assessing the effectiveness of new ways of delivering health services have been among the major external challenges. Strategic vision and individual skill alone are insufficient to meet these challenges: Effective organizations require resilient organizational designs that

harness the productivity of the work force while permitting sufficient flexibility to empower workers and managers to respond to external demands and achieve internal coordination.

Organizational design refers to the arrangement and relationships of individuals, work groups, departments, and divisions within an organization.[1] Managers often identify the design of an organization with the reporting relationships arrayed on the organizational chart, although in fact the organizational design (or organizational structure) includes other elements, including job descriptions, committee structures, and information systems, that are more difficult to portray in a simple chart.

The organizational design determines how work is organized, how authority is exercised, and how information is transmitted within the organization. An effective organizational design can contribute to efficient communications, promote adaptive behavior in response to changing goals and external challenges, and ultimately help determine the success or failure of the organization in achieving its goals and surviving in a changing environment.

This chapter discusses the factors that need to be considered in designing organizational structures in health care and describes existing organizational designs used by health care organizations. Recently, an increasing number of organizations have adopted a "program management design" to implement their strategic vision and align their organizations with the rapid pace of external change. Given the interest in program designs, this chapter focuses heavily on their strengths and weaknesses and on their potential for supporting organizational efforts to decentralize managerial control and budgeting and to create an effective context for the development of effective quality improvement programs.

MANAGEMENT PRINCIPLES

- Which organizational designs are appropriate for an organization depends on the complexity and rate of change of the external environment as well as the range and difficulty of management reponsibilities.
- Organizational designs should clarify responsibilities for managers. Overly complex designs may create confusion and conflict rather than flexibility.
- For effective management, organizational designs must incorporate physicians and other professionals in decision making.
- Appropriate organizational designs must balance the information and coordination needs of the larger organization with the autonomy unit managers require for managing their resources.
- Organizational designs should be crafted to ensure effective use of the human resources within the organization. When replacing individuals, changes in structure need to be considered as well as changes in personnel.
- There is no one best organizational design, and many organizations will combine elements of several design types.
- Functional designs are best adapted to smaller organizations or larger organizations with few key stakeholder groups and slowly changing external environments.

- Divisional designs are most appropriate for larger organizations whose divisions have clearly differentiated missions.
- Program management and other designs that align organizational structures with clinical care processes offer major advantages when it comes to developing effective budgetary and quality management responsibilities.
- Managers in program management need to monitor professional issues to compensate for the de-emphasis on professional identification and discipline-based work groups within the organization.

MAJOR DETERMINANTS OF ORGANIZATIONAL DESIGN IN HEALTH CARE

Organizational theory suggests that effective organizational designs should fit the information and coordination needs that are created by the external environment and internal operations.[2] A number of environmental and operational issues influence the design requirements of health care organizations.

Professional Membership

Historically, the most important factor affecting the design of health care organizations has been the professional nature of the work force. As professional bureaucracies, health care organizations have traditionally grouped like professionals together, placing physicians, nurses, pharmacists, and other professionals into separate departments. Such functional designs derive their strength from the common training and similar attitudes of the individuals who make up each professional group. The concurrence of departmental and professional group membership has also supported peer review, continuing education, and other professional activities within departments.

Physician-Hospital Relationships

The traditional professional autonomy of physicians has had a critical impact on the structure of health care organizations. In many hospitals and some other health care organizations in North America, physicians are not employees but rather members of a medical staff organization who are given practice privileges. Decisions on granting these privileges are made by an organization's governing body, not by management, and the medical staff is considered to be self-governing. Indeed, there is usually a separate medical staff committee structure that is parallel to and independent of the hospital committee structure. The existence of these two separate decision-making hierarchies greatly complicates the relationship between physicians and hospital management and staff. Although physicians work both as members of the medical staff and as participants in the complex operations of the entire organization, having a separate medical staff structure creates managerial and psychological barriers to collaboration and hampers the coordination of work activities, the development of strategic plans, and the shared management of organizational resources.

The existence of this dual hierarchy is based on the assumption that administrative decision making can be separated from medical-clinical decision making, that is, that health care managers can effectively manage costs while clinicians control services and service quality. In practice, however, clinical decisions have administrative consequences, and administrative solutions reduce or increase the resources supporting physicians' practice. Management in such circumstances succeeded in the past largely because the economic environment favored the continuing expansion of health care institutions and papered over the inherent conflicts between managers and physicians. In the environment of the 1990s, new organizational designs are required that develop mechanisms providing a more direct and more effective coordination of physicians, other professionals, and managers and that integrate all professionals into decision-making structures.

Technology

Studies of organizations in the health care and other industries indicate that the nature of organizational technology influences effective organizational designs.[3] *Organizational technology,* in this context, refers to the knowledge, tools, techniques, and activities used to transform inputs into outputs.[4] The technology of health care organizations is complex, highly variable, dependent upon careful coordination of personnel, and heavily reliant on the use of sophisticated scientific analysis and expensive diagnostic and treatment machinery. Effective organizations must provide structures that allow a high degree of coordination between units and monitoring of units while at the same time enabling a high degree of decentralized decision making by individual professionals.

Ironically, despite the enormous resources devoted to new health care technology, efforts to evaluate the effectiveness of these technologies have been limited.[5] Recent initiatives to strengthen the assessment of medical technology and to develop treatment protocols or guidelines that standardize professional practice create new management challenges. Decisions about adopting new technologies, changing staffing and work patterns, or utilizing new approaches to care delivery require collaboration between health professionals and managers. Here too organizational structures may facilitate or hinder effective communication and decision making.

Corporatization and Integration

In the past ten years, there has been considerable consolidation of health care organizations into larger entities and the development of numerous multi-institutional networks. These new corporate forms include formal mergers, investor-owned chains, and partnerships as well as voluntary organizational networks and strategic alliances. Although these new forms may provide competitive advantages and economies of scale, the organizational structures and the responsibilities of management are substantially altered, particularly the balance between head office tasks and individual unit tasks. In voluntary networks, hospitals may benefit from economic efficiencies and strategic advantages without being required to meet the formal requirements that accompany new ownership.[6] But as the need for coordination and external communication increases, these hospitals may also alter their management structures and organizational processes to maintain awareness of strategic and operational issues affecting network hospitals and to participate in strategy formulation and shared services or joint ventures undertaken by such networks.

Competition and Cost Constraints

Unlike the era of cost reimbursement, when hospitals could expect to receive payment for the costs of service delivery, current reimbursement policies in both the United States and Canada are creating increasing incentives for ensuring efficient use of hospital resources. This crucial policy shift was exemplified by the development of a prospective payment system (PPS) for Medicare patients in the United States and by the incorporation of analogous case-costing methods in provincial grants to Canadian hospitals. As a result, health care organizations have faced spiralling pressures to evaluate the effectiveness of care, including the effectiveness of management structures and administrative expenditures. At the same time, the increasing pressure to control cost has altered the incentive structures facing hospitals and physicians. Prior to prospective payment systems, managers and physicians could commit, without concern for costs, to the provision of virtually any patient service that would be covered by third-party insurers. The development of PPS reimbursement, coupled with other programs such as preferred provider arrangements, has created incentives for hospitals to try to control costs. As a result, previous relationships between hospital managers and medical staff members based on the exchange of physician access to hospital facilities in return for patient referrals, and care provision

have become untenable.[7] Effective organizational structures must therefore enable health care organizations to identify and select cost-effective patient care programs and to integrate physicians in the management of those programs.[8]

CHOOSING ORGANIZATIONAL DESIGNS

In the relatively stable health care environment prior to the 1980s, structural changes were relatively infrequent, but in the last decade the pace of change has accelerated. To adapt to this change, each health care organization must initiate a strategic planning process to evaluate external pressures and examine the capabilities of the organization to meet these challenges. Review of the organizational design is a crucial element in the strategic planning process. This process should include the CEO and other senior managers, board members, and physician leaders. Input from the community is also essential. The effectiveness of such planning is increased when the strategic decisions, including the choice of an organizational design, are based on consultation with key members of the organization and important external stakeholders. Soliciting a variety of perspectives will help the organization develop a broader understanding of its mission in the community and its effectiveness in carrying out that mission. This understanding provides the basis for developing a strategic plan and the organizational design needed to implement it.

Although regular review of the organizational structure is appropriate, some circumstances require review, such as the following:

- *Changes in organizational mission.* The structure of an organization reflects the understanding managers have of the key needs that the organization meets, the key customers whom it serves, and the core processes that benefit external customers or support the activities of the organization. As these needs, customers, and processes change, the structure of the organization must be realigned to fit the new focus.

- *Evidence that organizational processes are inefficient or ineffective.* The recurrence of situations in which managers find it difficult to reach decisions or find that decisions are reversed or situations in which workflow suffers from bottlenecks and the productivity or quality of work is low is a sign that the organization may suffer from an inappropriate organizational design. Recognition of these problems often occurs only when competition or changes in reimbursement formulas emphasize prevailing difficulties.

- *Consistent conflicts between groups, departments, or divisions within the organization.* Conflicts over work responsibilities, ambiguities in reporting relationships, and battles over departmental roles are indications of an ineffective design.

- *Significant changes in the rate and areas of external change.* The organizational design not only structures the workflow and decision making within the organization but also configures the organization's relationships with external stakeholders. In cases where the pace of change increases and the change activities become more complex, organizations often need to reconfigure their operations to be able to react to change more quickly and more effectively.

Structure versus Individuals

When confronted with the problems listed above, managers often attempt to identify and replace the individuals responsible for the problems rather than change the structure or improve the work processes. Deming has argued that 85 percent of work problems are system problems and are not attributable to individual workers.[9] In such cases, blaming workers for inefficiencies or poor quality does not create a basis for improving operations. Similarly, ineffective management often results from defects in the structure of the organization rather than from a lack of motivation or skill. Therefore, replacing individuals is usually no solution, since the alignment

between the external environment and the information needs or decision-making processes of the organization has not been altered. Considerable costs and the loss of experience and knowledge are also incurred by replacing managers. Thus careful consideration must be given to the organizational design and its interaction with the skills and capabilities of individual managers when managerial changes are being contemplated.

At the same time, a carefully selected organizational design will not suffice when individuals are not provided with the skills to manage or where the relationship between medical staff and administration is contentious. Effective human resource strategies and training are as necessary for productive management as an appropriate organizational structure.

FUNCTIONAL AND DIVISIONAL ORGANIZATIONAL DESIGNS

The most common organizational designs in health care organizations have been functional designs and divisional designs. As noted above, a functional design divides the organization into departments on the basis of specialization (e.g., finance, nursing, and radiology) and separates the hospital support services from the clinical services.[10] This kind of design is most prevalent among relatively small acute care hospitals, chronic care facilities, and nursing homes (see Figure 7-1).

Besides the simplicity and logic of functional designs, they have several other advantages. In smaller organizations, the hierarchical reporting structure enables effective accountability and centralized decision making. Department heads, who are usually promoted from within the organization, have extensive knowledge in their functional areas of responsibility. Moreover, department managers usually serve dual roles as administrators and clinical leaders. These managers then are able to deal effectively with departmental issues (e.g., the staffing mix) that require knowledge of professional skills and patient needs as well as knowledge of budget implications and supervisory requirements.

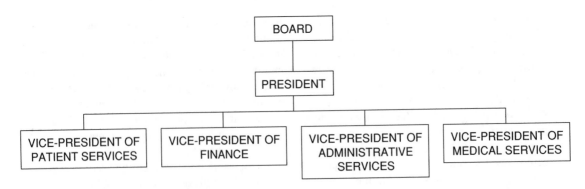

Figure 7-1 A Sample Functional Design

Larger health care organizations such as academic medical centers or large multispecialty group practices find simple functional designs inefficient. Management decisions on resource allocation or conflicts between professionals or departments are typically referred upward to department heads or vice-presidents. As the numbers of employees, the types of professionals and services, and the geographic spread of these organizations increase, the demands on management to solve problems become overwhelming. Senior managers find themselves in an endless cycle of firefighting and are unable to address broader policy issues. The information-processing capacity of functional designs also tends to be insufficient to ensure coordination between units or departments, since middle managers are heavily dependent on senior leaders for information. As a consequence, many large health care organizations have adopted divisional designs.

In a divisional design, the organization is subdivided into several smaller units on the basis of groups of services or markets.[11] For example, a hospital may create divisions providing inpatient acute care, ambulatory services, and rehabilitative services. Each division is a semiautonomous unit with the authority to make operational decisions and each takes responsibility for managing its own clinical and financial affairs. Accordingly, each unit has its own management team, which includes representatives from the administration, finance, nursing, and medicine. In effect, a divisional design creates an organization consisting of linked subunits that may each be viewed as a miniorganization (see Figure 7-2).

Functional and divisional designs have come under increasing criticism for being unresponsive and wasteful and for lacking accountability.[12] Functional managers are responsible for groups of professionals and other workers, not for work processes or patient groups, which typically require coordination across departments. Grouping similar professionals in departments, as occurs in functional organizations, encourages professional development, but the members of the departments can become insulated from the goals of the entire organization and fail to understand the perspectives of those with other functions. Nurses, pharmacists, social workers, and other types of professionals focus on optimizing the resources and activities of their departments, which frequently detracts from the outcomes of the organization as a whole. In addition, since departmental boundaries coincide with professional boundaries, functional design organizations institutionalize conflict, since each unit competes with others for scarce resources. In such circumstances, the mission of the health care organization, which is to serve the needs of its clients, can be displaced by the goal of serving the vested interests of the organization's constituent groups.

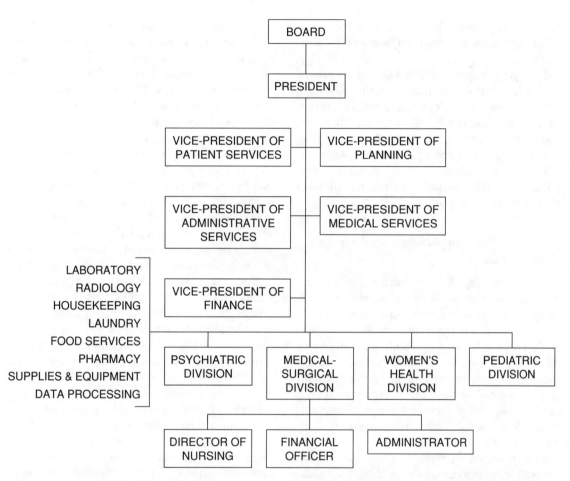

Figure 7-2 A Sample Divisional Design

As Mintzberg notes, in functional design organizations the patient "is treated not so much as one integrated system with interdependent parts, but as a collection of loosely coupled organs that correspond to the different specialties."[13]

The insularity of functional departments within large health care organizations can also reduce efficiency. For example, the divisional structure, with its autonomous units, can result in the duplication of activities and resources. Each division may have its own finance staff, although economies of scale require that financial planning and accounting be performed in a single centralized department.[14] De-

cisions about which functions to centralize and which to decentralize are political issues for divisional organizations. Also, the autonomy of work units in divisions may discourage collaboration that cuts across disciplinary, divisional, or functional lines. In fact, interunit conflicts might well cancel out efforts at achieving excellence. Finally, the control that professionals have over their practice makes it difficult to establish accountability. Claiming the right to exercise professional judgment, a physician can continue to provide inappropriate and expensive care virtually unchallenged. Since physicians are notoriously reluctant to act against one of their own, and because good measures of treatment outcome are difficult to obtain, such professional judgments are difficult to challenge.[15]

In response to these criticisms, attention has been focused on developing mechanisms to encourage greater professional accountability and increase coordination across functional groups and divisions. The object of developing such mechanisms is to counter the natural tendency of functional organizations to channel communications vertically and to solve problems by delegating them upward through the administrative hierarchy.

Improving Traditional Designs by Promoting Integration

Health care organizations use a variety of management techniques and mechanisms to promote integration across functional departments, including appropriate policies and procedures, interprofessional task forces and committees, and managerial and clinical information systems that link data from various departments and professional activities. Individuals also assume roles as integrators, whose duties include fostering horizontal (cross-departmental) communication and discouraging unproductive conflict.

One technique is to create managerial positions whose major responsibilities center on the coordination of activities across departments. A common example is a director of planning, whose job responsibilities often include organizing and planning tasks that involve all divisions of an organization. Quality management staff play a similar role in facilitating problem identification and problem solving among different groups. Integration results from coordinating similar processes within different departments, ensuring parallel methods and comparable results, and leading project groups with members from different departments. In cases where integrator positions are permanent, their incumbents serve as facilitators or liaisons, eliciting cooperation and commitment from other organizational members. Other integrator roles are assumed on a temporary basis when the needs of the organization require coordination between departments. In such cases, the integrators are often department managers or staff members who serve as project managers or task force chairs and have responsibility for planning, organizing, and coordinating task groups.

Integrators often must be able to influence the decisions of individuals without having direct authority over them. Successful integrators require excellent communication skills and a sound knowledge of group psychology as well as an appreciation for the history and culture of the organization in which they work. Since the chief purpose of integrators is to break down the barriers existing between groups, they must know individuals in all parts of the organization and be trusted by them. In addition, integrators must understand the group processes required to facilitate decision making and develop support for the decisions made by task groups. Building consensus often requires skilled negotiation and the effective use of group decision-making techniques, such as nominal group techniques and brainstorming.[16] Many hospitals and other health care organizations have educational staff or organization development professionals who provide training in these techniques. Other organizations send managers to seminars in group process skills.[17] More recently, many health care organizations have focused on teaching integrator and group process skills to the facilitators and team leaders of quality improvement projects.[18]

Task forces and project groups serve as "a temporary patchwork on the functional structure used to short-circuit communication lines in a time of high uncertainty."[19] They permit the organization to make more decisions and to process more information without overloading the vertical communication channels. By using such groups to address periodic crises or facilitate planning, organizations can retain the advantages of having a simple organizational design. Where line personnel are heavily taxed by direct managerial responsibilities or where the external environment is complex and unstable, such as the health care environment during the last decade, integrator roles and other integrative mechanisms may be insufficient.

MATRIX ORGANIZATIONS

A different approach to encouraging integration, decentralization of decision making, and lateral communications is to use a matrix design. This type of design is characterized by dual authority relationships through which project managers or program coordinators coordinate or supervise people and resources for major clinical areas. A matrix design basically superimposes a structure focused on clinical program components on top of a functional structure. It thus permits the organization to continue to reap the efficiency associated with functional specialization and a departmental structure but adds a cohort of managers responsible for coordinating programs across the departments (see Figure 7-3).

The major advantage of a matrix design is that there is a correspondence between the management of program resources and the structure of health care teams. Unlike managers in functional or divisional organizations, program managers in matrix organizations are responsible for the groups of patient care providers involved in such programs as long-term care, oncology, cardiac surgery, or women's health. Clinical management decisions are thus more clearly linked to resource decisions.

In a matrix design, each care provider has two supervisors: the director of the provider's functional department and the manager of the provider's project or program. This dual authority is the principal weakness of the design, since it frequently creates conflicting expectations and ambiguity in work assignments, which can lead to frustration for both employees and managers.[20] The larger management structure and the need to maintain dual accounting, budget, control, and reward systems, as well as the development of an additional layer of management, impose additional costs. A further limitation is the complexity associated with two reporting structures. This complexity makes a matrix organization difficult to manage, and considerable time and energy must be devoted to meetings between department and program managers in an attempt to keep everyone apprised of program activities and departmental goals.

The responsibilities and power of the department and program managers vary among organizations. In some cases, program managers are limited to coordination and planning activities, and these managers must negotiate with department managers to encourage them to meet the needs of the program. In other cases, program managers have the main responsibility for work assignments, and functional managers are limited to providing advice on recruitment, selection, and training.[21] Since program managers are typically added to an existing functional structure, department managers are likely to have greater powers unless the design specifically gives program managers authority over program staff. Successful implementation of matrix management requires continuing care to ensure that neither department managers nor program managers commandeer powers that unbalance the management of departmental resources or the direction of program activities.

PROGRAM MANAGEMENT

To achieve the benefits of a matrix structure while limiting the disadvantages, some organizations have adopted a program structure, eliminating or de-emphasizing departmental groupings and appointing managers responsible for specified clinical areas such as medicine, surgery, ophthalmology, and maternal health. Johns Hopkins Hospital in Baltimore is recognized as a pioneer in program management.[22] The hospital adopted a program structure that created departments under physician leadership, supported by nursing and administrative coordinators. Each program was given responsibility for budgets and staffing and contracted out for central services provided by the hospital. The decentralization of budgetary decision making increased clinicians' awareness of the costs of medical and nursing care. Program-by-program negotiating on the costs of support services created pressures to limit costs charged by service departments.[23] The change to program management at Johns Hopkins Hospital has been credited as a major factor in reviv-

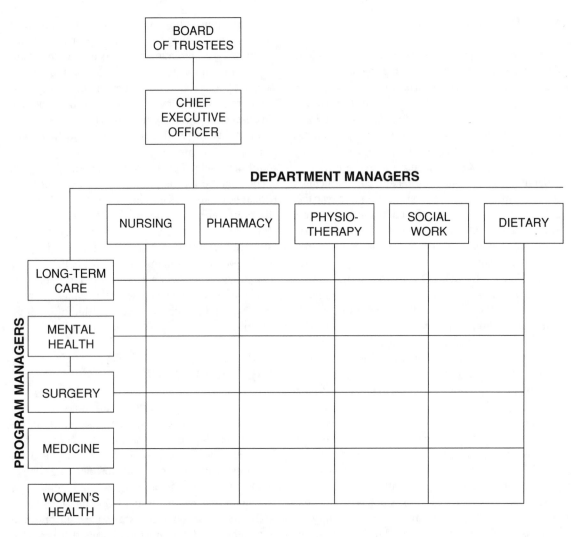

Figure 7-3 A Sample Matrix Design

ing the financial health of the hospital.[24] Although the hospital has become part of the much larger Johns Hopkins Health Care System, the program structure continues to be used for tertiary services within that system.

Program management realigns management activities and resources to focus on specific types of care or patient groups. For example, West Park Hospital, a 400-bed continuing care and rehabilitation facility in Toronto, Canada, has adopted a program model focused on six groups of patients: amputee rehabilitation, respiratory care, continuing care, geriatrics, transitional living, and neurological rehabilitation (see Figure 7-4). Each program is managed by a team consisting of a service director and a medical program director in concert with the

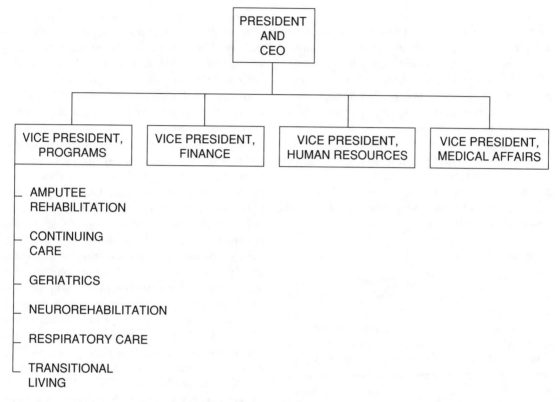

Figure 7-4 Program Design for West Park Hospital, Toronto, Ontario

vice president of programs. Traditional professional departments such as physiotherapy, nursing, occupational therapy, pharmacy, and social work have been disbanded, but West Park has created peer groups for each discipline to set and monitor standards, and has designated senior clinical positions for larger disciplines. To support the implementation of program management, West Park initiated a review of its hospital information resource strategy. Based on this review, the hospital is restructuring its information systems management to focus on program-specific information, and is developing program indicators of resource use, quality of care, and patient outcomes. One innovation developed at West Park is the creation of two new board committees focused on programs: one for continuing

care and geriatrics, the other for transitional living. These committees are charged with strategic planning and assessing quality and risk management reports for the programs. The existence of these board committees, along with the program management teams and new information strategy, has enabled the hospital to respond more quickly and effectively to recent budgetary restraints.[25]

The Impact of Program Management

In complex organizations such as large teaching hospitals, it may be difficult to assess the extent to which organizational changes lead to decentralization of decision making. A recent study of the clinical unit structure at Sunnybrook and its impact on the roles of managers found that physician and nurse managers did perceive an increase in their discretion on the job and a decrease in the influence of senior managers on the setting of unit goals and objectives and on the administration of their budgets.[26] At the same time, however, decentralization raised certain issues. At Sunnybrook, clinical managers found that their greater budgetary power caused concern about possible conflict between their roles as managers and as clinicians.[27] Ethical dilemmas may in fact increase as program management structures become more widespread among health care organizations.

Program Budgeting

The development of management information systems, particularly patient costing systems, in hospitals and other health care organizations has encouraged the adoption of program budgeting. In program budgeting, decisions and control over budgets are delegated to program directors. Program budgeting provides improved financial control since it resolves the main problem of department budgeting—that the linkage between department inputs and outputs (such as patient care) is unclear. By contrast, program budgeting offers managers set budgets based on patient revenues and patient volumes: Existing resources must be managed to meet workload requirements. This strategy has considerable appeal for hospital administrators, who have been continually squeezed between limited funding and clinician demands for greater resources. Put bluntly, program management permits senior health care executives to delegate the responsibility of managing services. Program budgeting creates incentives for cost savings and aids the development of effective utilization management techniques.

Quality Improvement

The increasing focus of health care organizations on organization-wide quality improvement also supports the development of program management approaches.[28] Current accreditation guidelines and quality assurance processes are largely departmental in focus, but administrators, quality professionals, and accrediting bodies are becoming increasingly aware of the structural inadequacies of current quality assurance systems. In its Agenda for Change, the Joint Commission on Accreditation of Healthcare Organizations supported the development of continuous quality improvement (CQI) approaches to address some of the deficiencies of current quality monitoring and evaluation. Accreditation requirements, both in the United States and Canada, are being changed to incorporate CQI components.[29] CQI (or total quality management) approaches focus on aligning the work of the organization with customer needs. Quality teams are formed that include individuals from all departments involved in specified work processes. (For example, a quality team focused on a discharge planning process might include representatives from admitting, social work, nursing, administration, medicine, and other disciplines.) These teams use a variety of sophisticated but easy-to-learn tools for analyzing work processes and improving the quality of care.

The development of quality improvement approaches to quality of care will encourage the establishment of quality review and improvement processes that parallel work processes rather than traditional departments. Program management, which focuses on clinical services and cross-functional activities and incorporates individuals from several different disciplines, provides a natural context for CQI.

Successful implementation of CQI requires considerable delegation to work groups of problem analysis and potential solution testing. Front-line staff must be empowered to address the problems of unnecessary complexity, rework, and waste found in existing work processes. Many hospitals that use a CQI approach have created quality councils to craft problem statements and support the work of CQI teams, by making decisions, for example, on the implementation of solutions developed by the teams. As these hospitals develop greater experience with CQI activities, and these activities expand to incorporate more and more areas of organizational decision making, existing management structures may meld with the quality councils and CQI teams. These hospitals may evolve structures much more decentralized and flattened than exist in current hospitals. Substantial changes in managerial roles and organizational culture will be required to make such an evolution possible. The hospitals will also have a critical need for information on program activities, costs, and outcomes so that managers and professionals can analyze and improve the key processes on which they work. Program management, because it encourages cross-functional thinking and decentralized decision making, provides a framework for the development of such organizational designs.

Professional Issues Raised by the Development of Program Management Models

Since program management provides an improved organizational context for dealing with the two most important policy issues facing health care organizations, financial control, and quality improvement, it is unlikely to be a passing phenomenon. Like most innovations, however, program management does have some negative consequences that need to be addressed. Some methods and mechanisms for addressing these consequences are discussed below.

Professional Reference Groups

Since program management can lead to the distribution of professionals across different programs, these professionals may feel cut off from their disciplinary colleagues. Although working with other types of professionals in a program can be rewarding, organizational mechanisms such as professional interest groups are also needed to foster professional identification and promote professional development.

Awareness and Adaptation of Professional Practice Standards

Practice standards are currently developed separately by each profession, and practitioners learn and adapt these standards to their work situations largely through professional interactions with disciplinary colleagues. Some professionals in organizations with program management may interact less frequently with disciplinary colleagues, limiting the diffusion of new practices or the improvement of care processes. However, the increasing emphasis on cross-disciplinary work processes and the development of "care maps" or practice guidelines that incorporate several professional groups provide a means to overcome this problem. To the extent that program management encourages the coordination of practice standards across disciplines, it may lead to the development of professional practices that support the effective use of all staff in the delivery of patient care.

Assessment and Improvement of Quality

The structures and processes of quality assessment and improvement are changing as health care organizations begin implementing CQI, but many professionals wish to maintain the use of discipline-based quality reviews. To some degree, this desire reflects an urge on their part to assert professional roles and responsibilities to counteract the diminishing visibility of professional groupings within the organization. It is unclear to what extent department- and discipline-based reviews of quality of care are necessary in the context of broader organizational quality activities such as CQI.

Discipline

A key concern professionals have about program management is that they will be supervised by managers who are not trained in their discipline. The worry is that the managers will be unable to identify inadequate or inappropriate care and they may also lack an understanding of the professional activities required to deliver services. How should professional care be reviewed in these circumstances? Who should have the responsibility for assessing actions and possible sanctions? One option is to develop professional councils composed of senior clinicians in each profession. These councils could advise managers on professional issues and provide guidance in developing practice standards.

Managerial Training and Career Advancement

Program management places a greater burden of responsibility on managers. Consequently it increases the range of knowledge and skills required for managerial positions. Many department managers have acquired their knowledge and skills on the job, but this method has obvious drawbacks when managerial promotion is based on proven skills and educational accomplishments, as increasingly it will be. Professionals who aspire to managerial positions need to be aware of the implications and plan accordingly. There should also be provisions made for those professionals who wish to advance their careers though clinical specialization and clinical career ladders (i.e., nonmanagerial promotion).

Recruitment and Retention of Professionals

Some observers believe that the de-emphasis in program management on professional identity will adversely affect the ability of an organization to attract professionals and hold on to those already employed. Other observers believe that the reactions of professionals vary: Some individuals may feel threatened by program management whereas others may find the interaction of different professionals to be more rewarding than traditional working arrangements.

These issues pose considerable challenges to managers of professional services. Managerial styles that have proven successful in traditional organizations will likely be dysfunctional in a program organization. Furthermore, while the need for managers to adopt new orientations in a program structure is acknowledged in the literature on program management, too often these managers are given only a general orientation to the goals of the new structure and little assistance in examining what their own needs are. Failure to address the educational and social needs of managers will increase the turmoil and extend the time necessary to implement a program design.

CONCLUSION

To be effective, organizations must adopt designs that will help in dealing with the external challenges they face and create a structure for managing the work they do. The professional work force, complex technology, and rapidly evolving health care environment make the selection of an appropriate design complicated and difficult. But not only must an organizational design be chosen, it must be adapted to fit the human resources and work flow of the organization, which means matching managerial talents with organizational responsibilities and balancing and developing the strengths of individuals to meet organizational needs. Indeed, most organizations find themselves incorporating components of several models.

Functional, divisional, matrix, and program designs exist in health care today. Although each is suitable to certain types of organizations, each also imparts particular strengths and brings particular problems. Program designs have drawn attention in recent years for several reasons. Many believe that decentralizing decision making is necessary to create more responsive organizations and to free senior managers to deal with strategic issues rather than engage in endless firefighting. Program budgeting has been heralded as a key managerial tool for creating more cost-conscious and more effective organizations. Perhaps most importantly, the growing interest in CQI has alerted managers to the importance of breaking down barriers between functional departments. Quality improvement teams are being created in many organizations and given mandates to develop knowledge of processes that stretch across the traditional units. These teams are currently uncovering evidence of unnecessary complexity, rework, and waste in activities throughout these organizations. Team members and managers recognize that much of this waste stems from departmental and disciplinary perspectives that focus on limited parts of health care work. As more and more evidence of waste is provided to senior managers, they will become increasingly committed to developing managerial structures that are better aligned with care processes. Here too program management will be seen as an effective response.

ADDITIONAL RESOURCES

Allcorn, S. Using matrix management to manage health care delivery organizations. *Hospital and Health Services Administration* 35 (1990): 575–590.

Daft, R.L. Organization structure and design. In *Organization theory and design.* 4th ed. St. Paul, Minn.: West, 1992.

Duncan, R. What is the right organizational structure? *Organizational Dynamics,* Winter 1979, pp. 59–80.

Leatt, P., et al. Organization design. In *Health care management: A text in organization theory and behavior.* 2d ed., eds. S.M. Shortell and A.D. Kaluzny. New York: Wiley, 1988.

Mintzberg, H. *Structuring in fives: Designing effective organizations.* Englewood Cliffs, N.J.: Prentice-Hall, 1983.

NOTES

1. Leatt et al., Organization Design, in *Health Care Management: A Text in Organization Theory and Behavior,* 2d ed., eds. S.M. Shortell and A.D. Kaluzny (New York: Wiley, 1988).

2. D.A. Nadler and M.L. Tushman, A Model for Diagnosing Organizational Behavior, *Organizational Dynamics* 8:35–51; W.A. Randolph and G.G. Dess, The Congruence Perspective of Organizational Design: A Conceptual Model and Multivariate Research Approach, *Academy of Management Review* 9, no. 1 (1985): 114–127.

3. J. Woodward, *Industrial Organization: Theory and Practice* (London: Oxford University Press, Argote, L. 1982); Input Uncertainty and Organizational Coordination in Hospital Emergency Units, *Administrative Science Quarterly* 27: 420–434.

4. C. Perrow, A Framework for the Comparative Analysis of Organizations, *American Sociological Review* 32 (1967): 194–208; D. Rousseau, Assessment of Technology in Organizations: Closed versus Open Systems Approaches, *Academy of Management Review* 4 (1979): 531–542.

5. P. Caper, Defining Quality in Medical Care, *Health Affairs* 7, no. 1 (1988): 49–61.

6. D. Pointer et al., Managing Interorganizational Dependencies in the New Health Care Marketplace, *Hospital and Health Services Administration* 33, no. 2 (1988): 167–177.

7. G.L. Glandon and M.A. Morrisey, Redefining the Hospital-Physician Relationship under Prospective Pricing, *Inquiry* 23 (1986): 166–175.

8. S. Shortell et al., *Strategic Choices for America's Hospitals* (San Francisco: Jossey-Bass, 1990).

9. W.E. Deming, *Out of the Crisis* (Cambridge, Mass.: Massachusetts Institute of Technology Center for Advanced Engineering Study, 1986).

10. A. Kaluzny et al., *Management of Health Services* (Englewood Cliffs, N.J.: Prentice-Hall, 1982); Leatt et al., Organization Design.

11. Leatt et al., Organization Design.

12. Kaluzny et al., *Management of Health Services;* F. Garner and L.P.F. Smith, *Strategic Nursing Management.* (Gaithersburg Md.: Aspen Publishers, 1990).

13. H. Mintzberg, *Structuring in Fives: Designing Effective Organizations* (Englewood Cliffs, N.J.: Prentice-Hall, 1983), 207.

14. P. Robbins, *Essentials of Organizational Behavior,* 2d ed. (Englewood Cliffs, N.J.: Prentice-Hall, 1988).

15. Mintzberg, *Structuring in Fives.*

16. J.R. Galbraith, *Designing Complex Organizations* (Reading, Mass.: Addison-Wesley, 1973).

17. S.L. Gill and S.S. Meighan, Five Roadblocks to Effective Partnerships in a Competitive Health Care Environment, *Hospital and Health Services Administration* 33 (1988): 505–520.

18. D. Berwick, *Curing Health Care* (San Francisco: Jossey-Bass, 1990); P.R. Scholtes, *The Team Handbook* (Madison, Wis.: Joiner Associates, 1988).

19. Galbraith, *Designing Complex Organizations,* 51.

20. Leatt et al., Organization Design; S. Allcorn, Using Matrix Management to Manage Health Care Delivery Organizations, *Hospital and Health Services Administration* 35 (1990): 575–590.

21. Allcorn, *Using Matrix Management.*

22. R. Heyssel et al., Decentralized Management in a Teaching Hospital, *New England Journal of Medicine* 310 (1984): 1477–1480.

23. R.N. Anthony and D.W. Young, Summary: The Well-Managed Organization, *Management Control in Non-Profit Organizations,* eds. R.N. Anthony and D.W. Young (Homewood, Ill.: Richard D. Irwin, 1984).

24. Heyssel et al., Decentralized Management in a Teaching Hospital.

25. B. Monahan et al., Transition to Program Management, *Leadership in Health Services* 1, no. 5 (1992): 33–37.

26. Hospital Management Research Unit, Department of Health Administration, University of Toronto, *Changing Times: About Your Job, about Your Work Unit* (mimeo, 1991).

27. L. Lemieux-Charles et al., Ethical Issues Faced by Clinical Managers in Resource Allocation Decisions, *Hospital and Health Services Administration* (in press).

28. D. Berwick et al., *Curing Health Care.*

29. Joint Commission on Accreditation of Healthcare Organizations, *An Introduction to Quality Improvement in Health Care* (Oakbrook Terrace, Ill.: Joint Commission, 1991).

Gordon D. Brown
Kenneth Bopp
Michael R. Soper

Managed Care's Evolving Role

8

Purpose: Managed care organizations assume direct financial risk for health services provided to a defined population. Because of this risk, managed care organizations must create structures and processes to influence the behavior of providers and consumers to function within the limits of the risk exposure as measured by a capitated fee.

INTRODUCTION

Managed care incorporates many transferable design features intended to aid in controlling unit costs, controlling utilization, and coordinating care across institutional boundaries. The term *managed care* does not refer to a single model of care provision but embraces a range of types of delivery sys-

The authors hold appointments in the National Center for Managed Health Care Administration, a cooperative center of the University of Missouri and Group Health Association of America.

Portions of this chapter are based on *Balancing the Triad: Cost Containment, Quality of Service, and Quality of Care in Managed Care Systems,* by M. Soper, J. Stallmeyer, K. Bopp, and M. Wood, National Center for Managed Health Care Administration, Kansas City, 1989.

tem. Some types are specifically based on managed care concepts, such as health maintenance organizations and preferred provider organizations. Other types, such as fee-for-service medicine and indemnity insurance plans, have incorporated some managed care concepts into more traditional designs.

Managed care is called coordinated care by most U.S. government agencies because of the implications of stating that a provider is "managing" health services for the public it serves. This demonstrates an appropriate sensitivity, but the concepts of managed care go beyond merely coordinating services and in fact require that the provision and utilization of services be managed.

Regardless of the differences in models of prepaid health care, there have emerged common elements that serve as the foundation of managed care as it exists today. These principles include the following:

1. an agreement by or on behalf of a specific set of health care providers to accept responsibility for the delivery of needed medical services *to*
2. a defined population of enrolled consumers, *in exchange for*
3. a specific, per-person sum of money agreed upon in advance and paid on a regular (typically monthly) basis.[1]

The first two elements differentiate managed care from traditional fee-for-service delivery models and indemnity insurance plans. In the case of the first element, we might add "as agreed to in a benefit package" to the phrase "needed medical services." The premise of managed care is that if providers assumed risk for a defined population, the costs of providing care would be low as a result of financial incentives. In addition, providers would be motivated to control costs due to excess utilization by keeping the enrolled population healthy and controlling access to high-cost services. Low-cost health care was thought to be a natural result of managed care plans, making them competitive in the market and popular with consumers. Cost containment thus became a policy expectation when HMOs were identified as an instrument of social policy.

The other side of the cost equation is the concern for quality. Although early models were supported because they offered a high-quality option, they were frequently developed in areas that had limited health services or none at all (e.g., the Kaiser Plan for workers at the Grand Coulee Dam). When managed care plans started to enter competitive markets, and once the federal and state governments became primary payers for health services, there developed a concern that quality of care might be sacrificed for low cost. The public sector has spent many decades putting into place what are hoped to be adequate measures and reporting systems to maintain the level of quality. The issue of quality versus cost continues to be a major social policy issue today.

HISTORY AND BACKGROUND

The prepaid health care movement in the United States evolved gradually during the last two centuries. Beginning with pristine models that met specific needs, the prepaid health movement acquired new dimensions as it adapted to such developments as medical group practice and group health insurance. As it evolved, prepaid health care assumed new forms, including, eventually, the health maintenance organization and subsequently managed health care systems.

Prepaid health care in the United States can be traced as far back as the eighteenth century when the Colonial Army was served by individual physicians under contract.[2] Prepaid group practices, however, have their roots in the transportation industry. One of the first prepaid medical group practices was the U.S. Marine Hospital Services, established in 1798. Merchant seamen received care in American ports by the local marine hospital, with payments for health care services made through nominal payroll deductions (20 cents per month).[3] In 1864, the railroads also began to finance health care services for employees through its railroad employees hospital association programs.[4]

Although there were isolated examples of prepaid health plans in the United States during the late nineteenth century and early twentieth century (e.g., the French Hospital Plan established in 1851 in San Francisco[5] and the Western Clinic established in 1906 in Tacoma, Washington),[6] one of the most noteworthy events during this period was the creation of the medical group practice. This occurred in the 1880s when William and Charles Mayo joined their father in building a large general practice with an emphasis on surgery. In following years, the father retired and the Mayo brothers recruited new members to the practice who would handle primary care, thus allowing the brothers to concentrate on surgery. During the next 20 years, other physicians joined the practice with expertise in diagnostic work and research. The practice became a prototype for prepaid group medical practices throughout the country.[7]

Another significant development was the advent of Blue Cross plans. Although health insurance began to provide accident protection for workers in the steamboat and railroad industries in the mid-1800s,[8] the Blue Cross Plan established in Dallas in the late 1920s was considered experimental. Beginning with an agreement by Baylor University Hospital to provide 21 days of hospital care per year to 1,500 school teachers for a rate of six dollars per person, the Plan was later extended to include other groups. The premise of the Plan, "to assume and redistribute the income from a group,"[9] laid the groundwork for hospital reimbursement on a retrospective, cost-plus basis; community-wide premium rating; and other features that shaped mainstream medicine for years to come.

During this period, prepaid plans began to emerge as alternatives to fee-for-service medicine and the new insurance arrangements. In fact, staff model HMOs often trace their history back to several large cooperatives established between 1920 and 1950. These cooperatives, many of which are in existence today, were among the best examples of coordinated prepaid systems.

Unlike their successors, the early cooperatives were not primarily motivated by cost containment. Rather, their founders "were often visionaries with strong beliefs concerning the superiority of prepayment and group practice"[10] and were driven by an altruistic desire to make positive reforms in health care delivery. Many focused on making specific health care reforms to help meet the immediate needs of employee groups and families within their communities.

Cooperatives established in Oklahoma and California are considered by many as the first major prepaid group practices. The Elk City, Oklahoma, Farmers' Cooperative Clinic was founded in 1927 by Dr. Michael Shadid as a consumer-sponsored cooperative.[11] When the cooperative began, Dr. Shadid sold consumers $50 shares in an association that would build a new community hospital and provide ownership of the health center; in exchange, shareholders would receive a discount for medical services.[12] This approach received widespread support by consumers, but a national controversy ensued because of tremendous opposition by the county medical society. After Dr. Shadid was ostracized by the medical community, he filed an antitrust suit against the county and state medical societies, which ultimately was settled out of court. As the cooperatives evolved into the Farmer's Union Cooperative Association, Dr. Shadid added comprehensive benefits and a prepayment plan for enrolled subscribers.

Around the same time that the Farmers' Cooperative Clinic was established by Dr. Shadid, others were engaged in similar activity in California. The Ross-Loos Medical Clinic was established in Los Angeles in 1929 by Drs. Donald Ross and H. Clifford Loos. Starting out as a fee-for-service partnership, the clinic soon contracted to provide prepaid medical care to employees of the Los Angeles Water and Power Department. The clinic later entered similar contracts with numerous other groups of municipal employees.[13]

In 1937, another important prepaid organization was created, the Group Health Association (GHA) of Washington, D.C. Established as a nonprofit staff model for federal employees from the Home Owners Loan Corporation, GHA eventually opened its membership to all federal employees, with the exception of those in the armed services.[14] Because government agencies were not allowed to sponsor health care organizations, GHA was consumer owned at its inception—and it remains consumer owned today.[15]

Perhaps the best known of the early prepaid prototypes, however, was the Kaiser-Permanente Medical Care Program, which was established in 1938. The plan began when the Kaiser construction company hired Dr. Sidney Garfield to develop a prepaid medical program (similar to one he had developed in the southern California desert) to provide medical care to Kaiser employees and their families at Washington State's Grand Coulee Dam. Based on the positive reception of that program, Kaiser next assigned Dr. Garfield to develop a similar program to provide comprehensive services for Kaiser shipyard and steel mill workers in three different areas. The new programs took a different form than other prepaid plans. Using its own complete facilities, which offered hospitals and clinics to its members, Kaiser-Permanente was able to produce even greater efficiencies than other models. Following several expansions, which included opening up membership to the public, Kaiser-Permanente became the nation's largest non-government prepaid program for hospital and medical care.

Another notable prepaid program was the Health Insurance Plan of Greater New York, which was established in 1947 to compensate for the inadequate care available to city public works employees. That same year, the Group Health Cooperative of Puget Sound was created through a merger of union groups and the Medical Securities Clinic to provide prepaid care to employees of the lumber industry in Washington and Oregon.[16]

Other prototypes, such as the San Joaquin Medical Foundation established in 1954 by the medical society in San Joaquin, California, were developed to incorporate physicians who were averse to staff or group model prepaid health plans. These medical care foundations, which were networks of independent physicians who contracted directly with a health plan and received payments on a fee basis, were forerunners of the current foundation health plans and individual practice associations.

MANAGED CARE ORGANIZATION MODELS

Although there are basic elements common to all managed care organizations, several general types of organization can be distinguished and each type has many variations.

Staff Models

In a staff model HMO, care is provided to subscribers through one or more multispecialty clinics owned and operated by the HMO. While most patient problems are handled by salaried primary care and selected specialty physicians within its own facility, the HMO arranges for more extensive care on an as-needed basis through contracts with hospitals and specialists.

Staff model HMOs developed in the mid-1970s organized their medical staffs by employing the physicians directly. The primary purpose of each HMO's medical staff was to serve the members, and there was little incentive, interest, or capacity for additional fee-for-service activities. Issues of accountability and autonomy of employed physi-

cians required constant management attention. Many of these staff model HMOs have since reorganized, and now physicians often form their own medical groups, which then contract with the HMOs. This does not alter the nature of the autonomy and accountability issues, but it does change the structure in which they are addressed.

Group Models

Created Medical Groups

In some cases, physicians form a medical group that is legally separate from the HMO. This arrangement may evolve from a staff model HMO, as noted above, or may be established from the onset. As with the staff model HMO, the primary purpose of the medical group is to serve the HMO's members according to an exclusive arrangement. There have been isolated instances in which a created medical group has pursued independence from its parent HMO (e.g., the Hawthorne Medical Group vis-à-vis Maxicare), established a separate identity through fee-for-service practice, and even contracted with other HMOs.

Typically, however, the created medical group maintains such a close relationship with the HMO that it is difficult to distinguish one from the other. Kaiser-Permanente's group model, for example, often has been mistaken for a staff model, because it is not immediately obvious to the public whether the physicians are hired by the HMO or the group and because the Permanente medical groups have no purpose or identity outside the context of their relationship with the Kaiser Health Plan. Such a high degree of mutual dependence requires a high degree of interaction. The entities have been described as Siamese twins joined at the heart. All conflicts must be resolved without threat of dissolution, since it is commonly known that separation would be fatal to both.

Pre-existing Medical Groups

This type of group model occurs when an HMO contracts with a pre-existing medical group to provide physician services to the HMO's members. The contract may or may not involve an exclusive arrangement between the medical group and the HMO. Regardless of whether the group contracts with other HMOs, however, the group keeps its HMO-related business separate from its fee-for-service business.

As an example of an exclusive arrangement, Maxicare Texas, Inc. (which was later purchased by Sanus HMO) entered a joint venture agreement with Kelsey-Seybold Clinics, a corporation of multispecialty medical groups in Houston and elsewhere, to provide care for Maxicare members. Although the physicians in Kelsey-Seybold clinics maintained their substantial fee-for-service practice, their exclusive contract with Maxicare prohibited them from entering into contracts with other HMOs.

In nonexclusive group model arrangements, the medical group contracts with several HMOs to provide physician services to each HMO's members. Given the independence of pre-existing medical groups and the proliferation of HMOs, nonexclusive arrangements are expected to increase. Thus, there is increasing interest by HMOs in securing exclusivity through the shared ownership of joint ventures. In some cases (e.g., the Ochsner Clinic in New Orleans), a medical group has created its own HMO.

Networks

In a third variation, an HMO may contract with multiple medical groups. These are usually pre-existing medical groups, although in some instances a created medical group also may be included in the network. An example of this model is HMO Colorado (sponsored by Blue Cross and Blue Shield), in which five medical groups located throughout Denver are affiliated with the HMO.[17]

Independent Practice Association Models

During the late 1970s and early 1980s, private practice physicians became more interested in HMOs primarily for defensive reasons (i.e., to pro-

tect themselves from the loss of patients). At the same time, federal funding was being phased out to free up market forces. Because high development costs and diminishing federal funds made it increasingly difficult to create staff model HMOs, independent practice associations (IPAs) became more attractive. The 1976 amendments to the HMO Act, which allowed IPA physicians to decrease the percentage of HMO patients from 51 to 35 percent, further opened the door to physicians who previously had been reticent to join a managed care plan. Even this minimum percentage did not need to be achieved during the early years of operation.

IPA model HMOs contracted with independent physicians who practiced from their own offices, thus avoiding the high building costs and fixed personnel fees, including the salaries of full-time physicians, inherent in other types of managed care systems. IPAs are currently responsible for much of the growth in managed care. According to InterStudy, more than half of today's HMOs are IPAs.[18]

The growth of IPAs made possible an infusion of new subscribers to managed care who otherwise were reluctant to join. Patients who desired greater convenience and a broader selection of facilities from which to choose (more like mainstream medicine) found it easier to adapt to prepaid health care through IPAs than through staff model HMOs. For one thing, they were still able to see their physicians of choice while obtaining the benefits of an HMO product.

In IPAs, physicians are employed neither by the HMO nor by a medical group contracted by the HMO. Rather, they provide services to members as part of their individual contracts with the HMO while still seeing their fee-for-service patients. According to 1983 statistics, prepaid patients in IPAs "typically account for under 15 percent of the physicians' caseload."[19] That percentage may be considerably higher today, particularly for primary care physicians who are active participants.

IPA physicians are paid individually for providing care to IPA members, mostly on a fee-for-service basis. Through this arrangement, the "HMO has much less influence over the organization and method of physician practice"[20] than under the group and staff model arrangements. Throughout the years, many types of IPAs evolved, but four types have been the most predominant: the created IPA entity, the individual direct contract, the independent practice organization (IPO), and a combination model. These four types are described below.

Created IPA Entities

Created IPA entities were the historical basis for other types of IPAs. In fact, the original HMO Act of 1973 allowed only for this type of IPA, since it required that the IPA be a separate legal entity and there existed few entities at the time with the appropriate legal status.

A created IPA entity is an IPA that an HMO constructs and contracts with for physician services. The IPA then contracts with individual physicians to provide services for the HMO's members. Because the HMO created the IPA, their relationship is exclusive. The created IPA entity model is similar to the created medical group model, but the individual physician's association with the IPA is much more tenuous than a physician–medical group relationship.

In effect, the early HMO-created IPAs were "pass-through" organizations established to meet the requirements of the initial HMO Act. In order for an HMO to remain in business, it had to ensure the financial viability of its IPA. Thus the HMO retained the financial risk, except to the extent that this risk was imposed directly on individual physicians by up-front membership fees or ongoing withholds of a portion of fee-for-service payments (these practices were constrained by physician resistance).

The IPAs required tight management by the HMOs that established them. Although the IPAs provided a structure for physician involvement, physicians, because of the closeness of the HMO-IPA relationship, often considered themselves to be dealing directly with the HMOs. In some cases, the medical director of an HMO even served as the president of the IPA. This kind of dual leadership role is also common in created medical groups, but the sense of the relationship is reversed; it is the president of the medical group who serves as medical director of the HMO.

Since physician behavior is more likely to be influenced by fellow physicians, it would seem that HMOs could have benefited from IPAs that accepted greater authority and accountability for medical management, even though this would require greater autonomy and an independent identity. Several factors inhibited such a development. First, for marketing reasons, an IPA model HMO tended to seek participation from a large number of physicians who had little reason to support their connection with the HMO. Second, since the HMO was not bound by exclusivity, neither were the individual physicians. The association was neither strong nor characterized by loyalty. Third, the physicians were not likely to provide the capital to establish the reserves needed for the IPA to bear meaningful financial risk. Thus, for all practical purposes, and the created IPA entity notwithstanding, the HMO was dealing directly with individual physicians.

Individual Direct Contracts

Some HMOs contract directly with individual physicians, which became permissible after amendment of the HMO Act. This arrangement better matches the function described above. It is somewhat similar to the structure of a staff model HMO, except that the physicians are independent contractors with much looser bonds to the HMO than employed physicians in a staff model. Although there is no formal IPA entity, participating physicians constitute an informal association, and their connections with each other are supported through peer review and medical advisory committees (similar to the practice of staff model HMOs).

An example of individual contracting is HMO of Pennsylvania, which is a subsidiary of U.S. Health Care Systems, Inc. Its IPA model HMOs were predominantly established by directly contracting with individual physicians.

Independent Practice Organizations

In contrast to a created IPA, an independent practice organization (IPO) establishes an independent identity and resists a pass-through role for the HMO. Generally, an IPO is an organized entity that independently establishes itself by contracting with individual physicians from a wide array of physician specialties. The IPO is thus the IPA analogue of the pre-existing medical group. Although it functions as a multispecialty group practice, it is not structured as one, since the contracted physicians practice from their own offices and do not share the facilities or medical records.

IPOs tend to be small and frequently are organized around a hospital. Many IPOs are very loose associations of all physicians on the medical staff and function primarily as collective bargaining units. Such IPOs refuse to accept meaningful financial risk but expect control of aspects of medical management, including physician selection, fee schedule setting, and utilization management. They urge their physician members to avoid directly contracting as individuals with HMOs, promoting a "we must all hang together or we will hang separately" mentality.

However, some IPOs with growing experience in prepaid practice have developed effective medical management systems and programs and also support goals (particularly cost-containment goals) that are congruent with the purposes of managed care. Such IPOs not only accept but vigorously seek meaningful financial risk. Their primary care physicians are exclusively associated with the IPO and typically provide the medical leadership and are the driving force of the organization. Since the medical management structure within an IPO is much closer to the physicians, it is easier to change physician behavior or recognize those physicians who are not supporting the goals of the organization. Thus, an IPO of this type provides considerable benefits to any HMO it is associated with.

An effective IPO can assume responsibility for managing the health care delivery system of an HMO, but it cannot by itself serve as a managed care organization. The IPO does not assume HMO responsibilities such as marketing, financing, or pricing. In addition, the IPO is not licensed as an HMO to sell directly to employers, and it usually covers a geographically limited portion of the market area. Therefore, the IPO must contract with an HMO. Their association is usually not an exclusive one unless the parties share ownership of a joint venture.

Combinations

Some IPAs are essentially combinations of one or more of the other types of IPAs. For example, an HMO may contract for physician services with several IPOs but also directly contract with individual physicians to cover a market area completely. Regardless of their differences, these models are all considered IPA-model HMOs, or simply IPAs. It is less certain how to categorize the mixed model that results when a staff model HMO also contracts directly with individual physicians to add an IPA element to its basic structure. This model, which is becoming increasingly common, allows HMO members to choose a primary care physician from the HMO's staff or from the list of independent physicians who have contracted with the HMO.

Other Managed Care Organizations

Preferred provider organizations (PPOs), exclusive provider organizations (EPOs), designated provider organizations (DPOs) and many other new terms recently have come into vogue. These are best understood through a discussion of the health benefit plans (or products) currently available. These differ in terms of benefit design and requirements.

Indemnity Plans

Indemnity plans offer traditional health insurance, and until recently were by far the most common product. Preventive health care is usually excluded from coverage, and out-of-pocket expenses are imposed through deductibles and co-insurance (a percentage of the medical service fee). Such cost sharing at the point of service has increased substantially since the early 1980s. An indemnity plan does not require a delivery system, and medical care may be obtained from any physician.

Managed Indemnity Plans

Managed indemnity plans are growing rapidly—at the expense of traditional indemnity plans. They require that a utilization management company be notified whenever hospitalization occurs or is recommended. Notification may also be required for certain outpatient procedures. Benefits are reduced for noncompliance with this provision. The utilization management company provides certification of hospital admissions, assigns expected lengths of stay, and performs continued review if a stay is extended. Second opinions may be required for certain procedures. No delivery system is required, and medical care may be obtained from any physician.

HMO Plans

All traditional HMO products are closed panel products, meaning that, except for emergencies or with prior approval of the HMO, benefits are available only from the HMO's established delivery system. The comprehensive nature of the benefits and the various delivery system models have been discussed previously.

Open HMO Plans

Also called a non-lock-in or open reservation plan, a leak product, or an HMO plan with an escape hatch, an open HMO plan is identical to a traditional HMO plan, except that certain benefits also may be received outside of the HMO's delivery system (i.e., from any physician), subject to an out-of-pocket fee typical of indemnity plans. Prior to the 1988 amendments to the HMO Act, an HMO could offer such a product only to a self-funded employer or in association with a licensed insurance company.

Preferred Provider Options

Preferred provider options, also called preferred provider arrangements or designated provider options (or arrangements), are second only to the managed indemnity plans in terms of growth. In 1983, there were only a scant number of these products throughout the country; by 1986, there were more than 400, with enrollments nearing 10 percent of the population.[21]

A preferred provider option is essentially an indemnity plan or a managed indemnity plan that offers an incentive, in the form of a reduced deductible or coinsurance fee, to receive care from designated preferred providers (physicians and hospitals). Any of the types of IPAs discussed above may serve as preferred provider organizations (as may some types of medical groups and a few types of staff model HMOs).

IPOs in particular, especially those that function more as collective bargaining units than as managed care providers, are likely to present themselves as PPOs to insurers and self-funded employers. Some may contract only with such entities to support a preferred provider option, eschewing contracts with HMOs, since HMO plans are viewed as contrary to a provider's interests.

Exclusive Provider Options

For all practical purposes, an exclusive provider option is a traditional, closed panel HMO plan but is constructed in a manner that escapes HMO regulations. Loosening of the regulations, as occurred as a result of the 1988 HMO Act amendments, may lessen the perceived need for this product. Any of the HMO delivery system types may serve as the exclusive provider organization.

HMOs for Special Populations

Aiming to save costs, the federal government is urging its 31 million Medicare beneficiaries to consider enrollment in HMOs.[22] Currently, 150 HMOs in 33 states are providing care to Medicare recipients who enroll by paying an additional premium along with their Part B fee for physician coverage.[23] And not only are existing HMOs providing care to special populations, such as the elderly, along with their usual mix of subscribers, but some HMOs are being established to provide care solely to special population groups. One example is the Social Health Maintenance Organization (S/HMO).

Although S/HMOs share many characteristics with HMOs, enrollment is limited to the elderly. S/HMOs are few in number, and most are demonstration projects created by HMOs, chronic care organizations, skilled nursing facilities, and case management agencies. Through funding from Medicare, Medicaid, subscriber premiums, and other sources, S/HMOs attempt "to control institutional care through increased availability of home and community based programs such as home health care, homemaker chore services, adult day care, and home delivered meals.[24]

Single-Specialty Managed Care Companies

Provider organizations have now emerged for specific specialties and services. For example, managed mental health organizations provide psychiatric care, substance abuse, and employee assistance programs for HMOs, insurers, and self-funded employers. Such organizations may be structured in a manner similar to any of the various HMO types discussed in this chapter.

ORGANIZATION AND MANAGEMENT STRUCTURE

Managed care organizations perform a number of basic functions in the health system that are intended to increase the effectiveness of health services. It is not the nature of the management tasks that is unique to managed care organizations, but the context in which they are carried out. Managers must not lose sight of these critical areas of organizational performance.

First, managed care organizations play a brokering role by assembling relevant information about buyers' needs and providers' competence and efficiency, thereby facilitating the task of market searching for buyers and sellers. In the brokering role, the managed care company also negotiates agreements with buyers and sellers, which allows the company to serve as their agent. As agent, the company gets buyers (employer groups and members) and sellers (physicians, hospitals, and other vendors) to commit to a benefit package. As the health system becomes more complex and segmented, the brokering role played by managed care companies becomes even more valuable to providers and consumers.

A second service offered by managed care companies is to provide information to buyers and sellers to improve their performance in the market exchange. A managed care company might inform employers about safety or preventive measures they might take to reduce work-related injury or illness. It might advise physicians on office management or management of patient participation in the medical encounter to increase practice effectiveness and efficiency.

A third service is managing resources through various types of structural arrangements for delivering health services. Managed care companies monitor and manage resource exchange through cost negotiation, utilization management or case management, and quality assurance. The systems and structures for managing resources depend on the type of managed care organization. Regardless of the type, however, the success of the organization will be primarily dependent on its ability to manage resource exchange.

Systems Differentiation and Integration in Managed Care: The Dynamic Network

The focus of systems differentiation and integration is on structuring work and coordinating and controlling the units in which work is distributed. To get work done, it is necessary to divide responsibilities across different individuals and organizational units or even entities outside the organization. The work of producing and delivering health services is highly differentiated, and much of a managed health care organization's work is assigned to specialized personnel and units, some inside the organization but many outside, including whole other organizations. This differentiation leads to interdependence. That is, the people and work units depend on one another to get the work done. Therefore, the personnel and work units need to be linked together and coordinated; otherwise, they may pursue their own goals while ignoring the larger mission of the organization. Without appropriate coordination and control, the managed care organization will become fragmented, fractious, and ineffective.

Because most managed care organizations rely on outside entities, they may be characterized as dynamic networks. Miles and Snow suggest that dynamic networks have the following characteristics and components[25]:

1. *Vertical disaggregation.* Functions such as product design and development (benefit packages), service delivery system design, marketing, service production, and service delivery, typically conducted by a single organization, are performed by independent organizations within a network.

2. *Brokering.* Because each function is not necessarily part of a single organization, the business partners are assembled through brokers. The managed care organization usually serves as the broker but may use other entities to accomplish the task of assembling the partners to carry out the managed care functions.

3. *Market mechanisms.* The major functions are held together primarily by market mechanisms rather than plans and controls. Contracts and payments for results are used more frequently than standard operating procedures and hierarchical supervision.

4. *Full-disclosure information systems.* Miles and Snow suggest that broad-access computerized information systems must be used as substitutes for lengthy trust-building processes based on experience if a dynamic network is to succeed.

Participants in the network first must agree on a general payment structure for value added and then must be linked together by means of a continuously updated information system so that contributions can be mutually and instantaneously verified.

This dynamic network framework can help provide further understanding of the four managed care models: staff, group, network, and independent practice association. First, the models vary in their degree of vertical disaggregation. In a fully integrated staff model, benefit package design and development, marketing (although some plans may use outside brokers), and all health care service production and delivery are done internally (see Figure 8-1). The more typical staff model will internally produce most health care services, with the exception of hospital and highly specialized services (see Figure 8-2). An IPA, which is at the other extreme, designs and develops the benefit package and markets the package and all the service production, but service delivery is done by outside entities. Furthermore, the IPA's disaggregation extends down to individual physicians. The degree of disaggregation in the group and network models falls between the staff model and the IPA model.

The magnitude of the brokering role is a function of the degree of disaggregation and the number of participating partners. In the staff model, the broker role—locating potential network participants, negotiating agreements, monitoring and maintaining relationships, and enforcing agreements—requires a smaller percentage of the organization's total management effort than is the case for an IPA. The IPA's high degree of disaggregation and large number of participating business partners make the brokering task substantial.

Organizational Effectiveness and the Dynamic Network

In the IPA form of organization, the disaggregated functions and participating partners are held

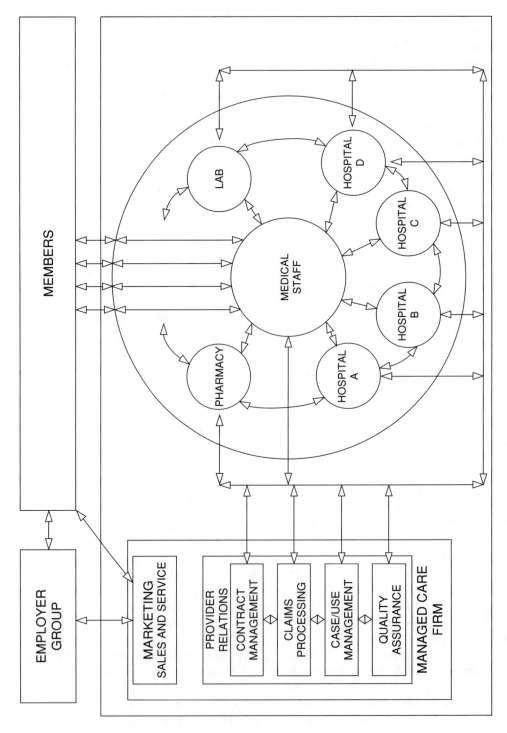

Figure 8-1 Operations Management: Fully Integrated Coordination Model

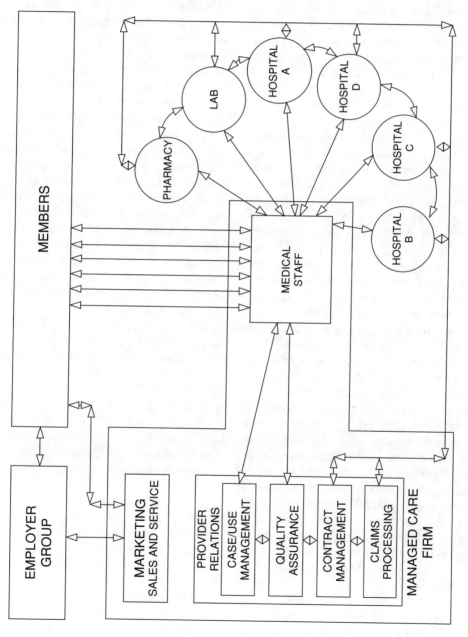

Figure 8-2 Operations Management: Staff Coordination Model

together primarily by market mechanisms. In a market relationship, the transactions between the parties are mediated by a price mechanism in which the perception of exchange equity for the involved parties is dependent on the existence of a competitive market. Market transactions are governed by contractual relationships with specified responsibilities (e.g., render services specified in benefit package to assigned members), terms and conditions for compensation (e.g., managed fee schedules, salary schedules, capitation rates, and productivity standards), regulatory and control processes (e.g., utilization management methods such as gatekeeper, prospective, concurrent, and retrospective reviews), and quality improvement processes. However, given the performance ambiguities associated with medical technology and member (patient) participation, together with the limited mental capacity of the individuals negotiating the contract, it is impossible to write complete contracts that specify what the future obligations of each party would be under every future eventuality.

Contracts will succeed only if each party can trust the other to not be opportunistic—to pursue their common interests rather than pursue their individual interests. Here lies the heart of the coordination problem in the IPA models. The individual providers and the managed care organization have only partially overlapping goals. Left to their own devices, individual physicians and medical groups loosely affiliated with a managed care organization will pursue their own goals, which are likely to be incongruent with the managed care organization's goals. To the degree that affiliated providers' goals are incongruent with those of the organization, their efforts will not be coordinated and organizational effectiveness will suffer. In order to maintain relationships with providers and protect itself from the potential opportunism, the managed care organization will have to go to considerable expense to negotiate safeguards and monitor and enforce the performance of the providers. Miles and Snow suggest that the monitoring and control system must be a full-disclosure information system that is continuously updated and allows the parties to continuously moni-

tor one another's contributions and mutually and instantaneously verify their performance.[26]

With such information systems, managed care organizations could tolerate relatively high levels of goal incongruence and opportunism in market relations if there is little ambiguity over performance.[27] However, the great ambiguity surrounding the medical tasks and the associated ambiguity in measuring performance does not bode well for the dynamic network organizational form, particularly the IPA model's effectiveness in terms of transaction costs.[28] Negotiating agreements, monitoring performance, and enforcing agreements with a multiplicity of autonomous providers pursuing independent practice ideologies and behaviors are formidable coordination and control tasks. If the transaction costs become too high, market relations will fail and a bureaucratic structure, despite its inefficiencies, may be relatively more efficient.

Although a group or network managed care organization relies on market relations between the organization and the medical group to mediate transactions, the relations are fewer and the potential for goal congruence is greater (see Figures 8-3 and 8-4). If the organization and the medical group can achieve a relatively high level of goal congruence, then the group's bureaucratic structure can be used to guide the performance of individual providers.

Organizational Effectiveness and the Bureaucratic Structure

A bureaucratic organization, such as a staff model HMO, has two principal advantages over use of market relations (see Figures 8-1 and 8-2). First, it is based on the employment relationship, which is an incomplete contract. In accepting employment, health care personnel agree to receive a salary in exchange for the legitimate right of the organization to appoint superior officers who can (1) direct the work activities of the employee from day to day (within some domain or zone of indifference), thus overcoming the problem of dealing with the future in advance and all at once, and (2) closely monitor

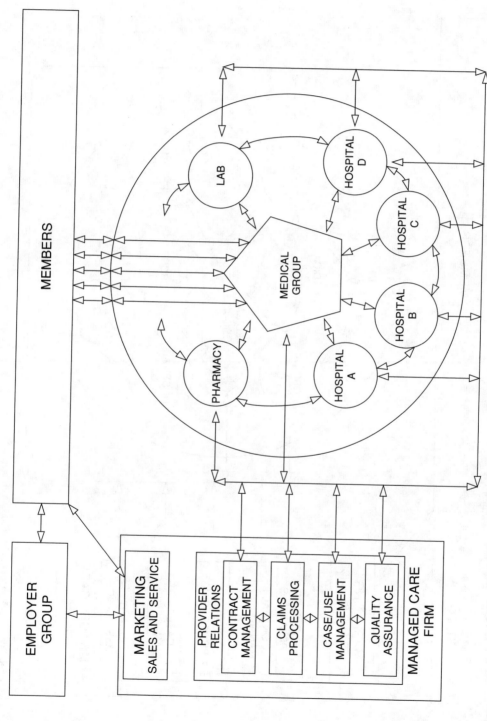

Figure 8-3 Operations Management: Group Coordination Model

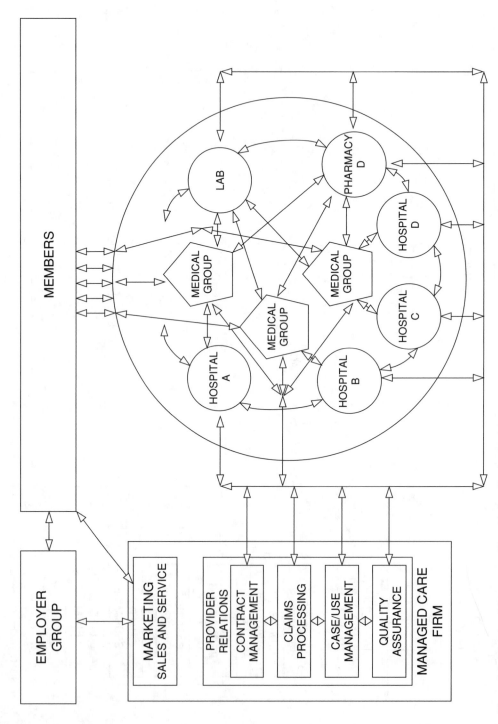

Figure 8-4 Operations Management: Network Coordination Model

the employee's performance, thus minimizing the problem of opportunism.

Second, the bureaucratic organization can create an atmosphere of trust among employees much more readily than a market can among parties of a market exchange. Because members of an organization assume some commonality of purpose and because they perceive that long-term relationships will reward good performance, they develop some goal congruence. This reduces their opportunistic tendencies and thus the need to monitor their performance.

However, bureaucratic relations are also limited in their capacity to efficiently deal with performance ambiguity and goal incongruity. Bureaucratic organizations operate according to a system of hierarchal surveillance, evaluation, and direction. In such a system, coordination and control are implemented by establishing roles, rules, and procedural specifications that guide service providers in the execution of their activities, and adherence to these prescribed roles, rules, and procedures is maintained through hierarchal supervision.

As illustrated in Figure 8-5, the direct interaction between the service provider and the patient is a transaction in which information is being exchanged; mutual adjustment is required of both parties, because the transaction involves the continuous transmission of new information or feedback. Health care personnel involved in such transactions are engaged in task activities that require the interpretation of information that is equivocal to varying degrees.[29] Not only does the information lend itself to various interpretations, but the interpretations often conflict with one another. Consequently, it is impossible to specify a priori the full range of idiosyncratic demands or the required conversion activities that could arise in a given transaction. If only formal structural or bureaucratic mechanisms (rigid rules and procedural specifications) surround the transaction, this suggests that there is only one decision that health care personnel can correctly make.[30] This is because the interpretation of the information provided in the transaction is limited by the perceived rules and regulations. Such bureau-

cratic constraints inhibit front-line personnel's responses to patient needs and diminish patient satisfaction and organizational effectiveness.

Furthermore, in provider-patient transactions, it is not appropriate or even possible for a supervisor to be present who can exercise ongoing, immediate quality control or utilization management. In these transactions, the individual providers are on their own. Their decisions and actions cannot be directly influenced at that "moment of truth." Additionally, the task complexity of medical technology—coupled with the high input uncertainty, the task interdependence stemming from the patients' involvement in the production process, and the difficulty of specifying outcomes in detail—makes it hard for supervisory personnel to evaluate the performance of front-line providers.

Although bureaucratic structures and governance mechanisms are appropriate for service production functions that can be standardized and do not directly involve patients, they are counterproductive in coordinating and controlling front-line patient-provider interactions. Yet coordination and control of these interactions is key to achieving organizational effectiveness, because they are the locus of decision making regarding quality (technical and service) and resource use.

Organizational Effectiveness: Augmenting Formal Structure with Value Structures

In provider-patient transactions where mutual adjustment is required and a multitude of decisions are possible, professional value structures (culture) traditionally have served as the means of deciding what decisions to make and determining the "correctness" of the decisions made.[31] However, for a value structure to be effective in coordinating and controlling front-line providers' decisions and behavior, it must create a harmony of interests within the organization, and thereby erase the possibility of opportunistic behavior.

In the managed care context, a value structure, including professional norms, is substituted for

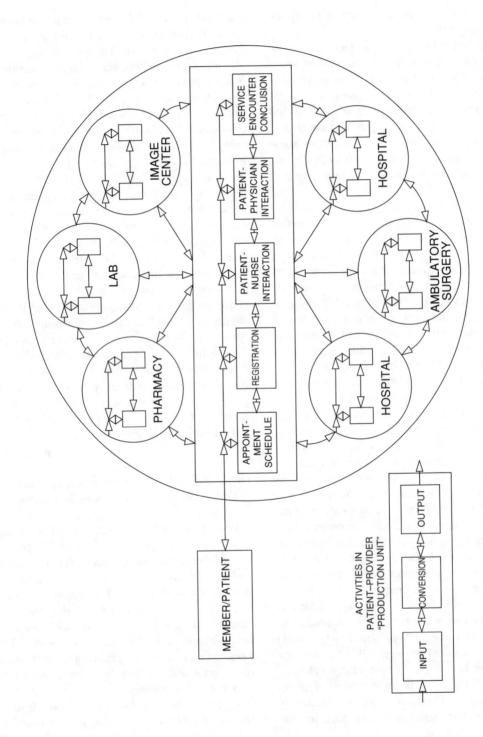

Figure 8-5 Member–Provider Transactions: The Heart of the System

leadership and supervision in provider-patient transactions. Within the broad boundaries of the practice ideologies and patterns of their various specialties, front-line health professionals exercise self-management. This means that these professionals take responsibility for the management of their own task-related activities rather than have their activities closely monitored by a supervisor. The decisions made in the provider-patient transactions are dependent on the types of individuals recruited to affiliate with the firm and on their values. These health care professionals, for the most part, are trained and socialized outside the organization.[32] They enter the organization with the values, ideologies, and skills they have acquired in medical school, nursing school, allied health school, residencies or internships, and past work and other experiences. Thus, the value structures employed to guide front-line provider decisions and actions are actually determined outside the managed care organization through accepted practices and procedures for patient care. Furthermore, changes in the technology usually occur as a result of external research that is imported by the affiliated providers.

Externally generated professional values typically do not provide the kind of harmony of interests that will erase opportunistic behavior and the need for explicit organizational guidelines and the auditing and evaluation of performance. As noted above, the medical professions do not share a unitary set of values but exhibit a variety of ideologies and practice patterns. The lack of a uniform value structure and the propensity of physicians to resolve uncertainty by committing more resources limits the effectiveness of professional norms as mechanisms for coordinating and controlling front-line provider actions.

For a value structure to be effective in coordinating and controlling provider behaviors to achieve the managed care organization's goals, all the members of the organization must undergo a socialization process that instills in individual providers and reinforces a set of shared goals that are compatible with the goals of the organization. If a congruence of goals occurs, auditing of performance is unnecessary except for educational purposes, since members will not attempt to depart from the organization's goals. Few medical organizations, with the exception of longstanding medical groups such as the Mayo Clinic, have a shared value structure that is truly effective in coordinating and controlling health professionals' decisions and actions. It appears that a value structure mechanism is easier to employ in staff and group model managed care organizations than it is in IPAs.

In summary, the different managed care organizational models and the associated governance mechanisms vary in the degree to which dependency relationships require regulation and also vary in their amenability to cybernetic regulation.[33] Staff and group model managed care organizations, which tend to develop a shared value structure, create dependence relationships that may not require performance auditing regulations except for quality improvement and educational purposes. Furthermore, their organizational structures may be more amenable to regulation through cybernetic control processes and may be less costly to regulate. On the other hand, IPAs, which are linked to autonomous practitioners via market mechanisms (competition and price) and lack bureaucratic and value structure mechanisms to facilitate coordination and control, appear to suffer from excessive transaction costs. An IPA's susceptibility to goal incongruence and opportunism, coupled with the performance ambiguity surrounding medical treatment, suggests that extensive negotiations, monitoring, and agreement enforcement will be required to achieve organizational effectiveness. Furthermore, the IPA dependence structure is less amenable to cybernetic regulation than those of the other models, further increasing its transaction costs.

Organizational Effectiveness: Managing Interdependence with Cybernetic Control

Although the effectiveness of a managed care organization is partially dependent on controlling the transaction costs associated with the coordination and integration of the "production units" that make up the health care production and delivery system, many market-driven organizations have given little attention to the transaction costs associated with the different organizational models. Theoretically, the staff and group models should be more efficient in terms of transaction costs than the IPA models. Organizational structure and associated coordination mechanisms are an important part of the comprehensive schemes that an organization uses to ensure the flow of resources from dependence relationships and are intimately tied to the process of control. Although different organizing schemes are more or less effective in regulating the activities of the production units and the work and information flow among the production units, regulation by means of organizational structure does not possess cybernetic validity and is not true control. To be effective, a managed care organization must control and constrain activities within and among production units to ensure that (1) information and resources flow in appropriate quantities; (2) resources, processes, and outcomes possess certain characteristics (quality); and (3) resources (information, personnel, facilities, and information) are available when needed (workflow scheduling). To the extent that the managed care organization's formal structure and associated coordination mechanisms (the market, the bureaucratic structure, and the value structure) are insufficient for coordinating production and workflow among the production units, cybernetic control mechanisms must be employed.

As indicated above, true control has cybernetic properties.[34] The control process thus has a feedback loop that uses standards of performance, measures the system's performance, compares that performance to standards, feeds back information about unwanted variances in the system, and modifies the system's comportment. The implementation of cybernetic control processes in managed care will require broad-access computerized information systems that link together the production units and allow the managed care organization to prospectively remind providers of organizational performance standards, to continuously monitor production unit performance, and verify that it conforms to resource use standards and technical and functional quality standards.

Organizational effectiveness is also diminished when a production unit has to wait on other units for inputs, inspect the inputs to ensure their quality, or rework the inputs because they are defective. Therefore, the cybernetic control process should monitor the effectiveness of system differentiation and integration technology (accuracy and timeliness of the flow of work and information between production units) as well as medical and customer relations technology. As indicated above, each interface transaction between a service provider and a patient is part of the process of producing and dispensing the service to the patient.

There is a great deal of uncertainty regarding the workflow, because the arrival, demands or needs, and behavior of patients generally cannot be anticipated. Since patients are involved in all stages of the service production process (input, conversion, and output), they may find, in interacting with any one of the many production units of the production and delivery system in defining outcomes and conforming to the mutually derived expectations of both provider and consumer. Furthermore, the transactional nature of the interaction within the conversion process invites recycling, skipping, and aborting. Thus, the conversion process may be composed of several information exchange subprocesses, but these constitute reciprocal rather than linear sequences. Consequently, service technologies are insufficient, because patient demands and behavior are never totally understandable.[35] The management of the linkages and exchanges between the production units relies on the system's structural configuration and the associated market, bureaucratic, and value structure mechanisms.

MANAGING UNIT COSTS

One of the major outcome considerations in managed care organizations is the control of costs.

This was one of the major social expectations of the managed care movement and continues to be a major social and political issue. This section examines processes to control unit costs, one of the key components of cost. There is no single managed care process for controlling unit costs, but instead, a range of controls and incentives, each related to the nature of the organization and management structure.

One of the key ways to control costs in managed care is by working to achieve a reasonable unit cost (price) for services at each stage of production so as to achieve a low overall unit cost. This effort requires "movement toward the least cost method of producing a given service."[36] Compensation, physician productivity, and the buying power of the managed care organization are three important factors that can be used to contain unit costs.

Compensation

Since their inception, managed care organizations have controlled unit costs by opting for salary, capitation, or a combination thereof. Although some managed care organizations have employed a modified fee-for-service schedule, pure fee-for-service reimbursement has no place in managed care. Because fee-for-service reimbursement tends to be inflationary, it is antithetical to managed care objectives.

Practice behaviors that result in excessive utilization were deeply ingrained in the costly fee-for-service system. Since most physicians received their experience in fee-for-service practice, they had become accustomed to receiving rewards for revenue-producing practice styles and behaviors. Inducements to increase costs occurred in several ways. First, because physicians in fee-for-service practice were paid a certain amount for each service, they were encouraged to increase costs by itemizing for each aspect of patient care. Second, indemnity insurers reacted passively to escalating health care costs by paying for equipment costs without requiring justification. Third, physicians historically have set their fees based on the ability of patients to pay.

Managed Fee Schedules

Desiring an alternative to fee-for-service practice, managed care organizations have established their own managed fee schedules for their physicians. These schedules are then used as the basis for salaries and capitation rates. Adjustments normally are made by specialty and locale so that managed care organizations can be competitive in the market and attract physicians.

Establishing a managed fee schedule saves costs in two ways. First, it is administratively more efficient to determine one fee schedule for all physicians than to negotiate a separate fee schedule for each physician.

Second, an established fee schedule for all physicians allows the managed care organization to realize tremendous savings on high-priced physician services. Generally, these savings occur because salaried specialists receive less than if they were paid fees for their services. Primary care physicians, on the other hand, are paid salaries commensurate with the amount they could make in fee-for-service practice, and thus the managed care organization does not realize great savings in this area.

The downside of managed fee schedules, however, is that they do not entirely remove the financial incentive to increase services. Even when fees are tightly restrained, providers find that they still can increase their income by increasing services or billings. The tendency of physicians to compensate for controls on the amount they are paid for services also has been evident in Medicare, which has experienced double-digit inflation due to increased utilization and billings. Other similar efforts to control fees have met with similar fates, such as the federal price controls on physician fees imposed in the 1970s. As each control was implemented, physicians reacted by increasing their services and billings,[37] thus demonstrating that even stringent efforts to reduce unit costs through fee schedules or other methods may not have a major effect on fee-for-service pricing patterns.

Why Physicians Accept Managed Care Fee Schedules

Although HMOs must try to offer primary care physicians roughly the equivalent of a typical fee-for-service income, they are rarely able to provide high-priced specialists and subspecialists with salaries that compare with their potential earnings in private practice. Nevertheless, there are several professional and philosophical reasons why lower fees do not always dissuade physicians from joining managed care organizations.

First, many physicians find that staff and group model HMOs enable them to focus on the practice of medicine rather than on the business side of medicine. They "may have no taste or gift for business and therefore for the incorporation strategies, tax deductions, stock options, dissolvings, corporation purchases, and the rest that medical partners and groups must work out collegially."[38]

Second, some physicians find that staff and group model HMOs are more suited to their individual practice styles. Because most patient problems and conditions are treated in-house, many physicians find that managed care affords them a greater opportunity to perform the specialized procedures they were trained in. Also, the patient volume that characterizes managed care organizations is an alluring feature for subspecialists who enjoy being busy and can see a large number of patients without depending on referral sources.

Third, some physicians are attracted to the quality-of-life aspects of group practice. Predictable schedules, possible opportunities to teach at nearby institutions, shorter hours, retirement, and other benefits are often preferable to the rigors of a private practice life style.

Fourth, some physicians prefer managed care organizations for economic reasons. They may be attracted to the idea of a guaranteed base salary that they receive without having to be involved in collections or to deal with bad debts. Likewise, recent residency graduates who join a managed care organization can acquire a full patient load from the out-set rather than having to face the huge debts required to start a new practice or the long wait before a full clientele is developed.

Another reason specialists accept managed care fee schedules is that working in managed care gives them a good opportunity to receive patient referrals from primary care physicians. Many physicians believe that, unless they sign on with a managed care organization, they may lose the chance of acquiring new patients within the managed care system and may also risk losing their non-managed-care patients as well.

Salaries

Salary compensation is the most prevalent means to contain unit costs in staff and group model HMOs. Based on physician contracts (a separate one for each physician), an HMO pays a predetermined amount for physician services regardless of the volume of patients.

Because salary compensation removes the financial incentive to increase services, staff and group model HMOs typically experience lower utilization rates than fee-for-service practices or HMOs with managed fee schedules. Although salary compensation removes the incentive to increase the volume of billable services, its drawback is that it also removes the incentive for productivity. This results in a need for managed interaction by providing financial incentives in the form of bonuses, profit sharing, and so on.

In some staff and group models, the incentives are fairly modest and mainly serve a symbolic function. When this is the case, incentives (bonuses and merit increases) are tied to a more comprehensive evaluation by rewarding cost-effective care, high-quality care, and high-quality service.

Some staff and group model HMOs have introduced profit-sharing programs in which physicians receive a portion of organizational savings when expenditures are not as great as projections. Typically, such profits are shared with the entire group, and various methods of dividing up the funds are used.

Capitation

Capitation, in which the HMO pays a predetermined per member fee, is another popular method of compensation in managed care organizations. IPAs generally use capitation as their method of compensation for primary care physicians. While early models paid a strict capitation rate, a more sophisticated system of capitation has developed throughout the years that makes adjustments for age, sex, and other characteristics of the patient population.

Regardless of these adjustments, however, capitation requires that each physician have a defined and captive HMO member panel. It is by means of these panels that the HMO is able to calculate the capitated amount that each physician is paid. Since a physician is paid a certain dollar amount for each member, the HMO must know the number of members for each physician so they can prepare the appropriate monthly check. Each monthly check is based only on the membership and the capitation formula; it does not vary on the basis of the number of services or procedures.

Making a panel captive is achieved by requiring that members select a primary care physician from whom they will receive all of their care. This allows the HMO to ensure that it is not paying more than one primary care physician for each patient's care.

Although capitation is a common method of compensating primary care physicians in IPAs, it is less common for specialists because of the difficulty in defining their patient population. Especially in the case of IPAs with large service areas, it is difficult to predict which specialists can best attend to a patient's future health care needs.

Because capitation is similar to the salary approach, capitation has a similar effect on unit costs by removing the fee-for-service incentive to increase utilization. However, capitation also removes the incentive to increase effort. To maintain this incentive, IPAs generally have relied on risk-sharing arrangements and physician incentive payments.

Risk Sharing

Historically, the first IPAs were required to enter into agreements with the HMOs that stipulated that the amount of payment to the IPAs would be based on a common fee schedule that would not exceed a certain amount per member per month. Problems arose, however, when payments were expected to exceed that set amount.

Since IPAs normally were not capitalized, they lacked the resources to compensate for shortfalls. Therefore, it became necessary to pass the risk on to IPA physicians through a fee schedule and capitation rates in which a modest amount was withheld (e.g., 10 or 20 percent).[39]

The withhold from physician fees enabled an IPA to create a reserve fund. The disposition of those funds was determined at the end of each fiscal year. For example, if the payments received by the IPA were not sufficient to cover their overruns in referral or service fees, the withhold would be used to cover the shortfall. On the other hand, if the total cost of the IPA was kept down, the physician would receive a portion of those funds on a pro rata basis. Because physicians were not at risk for an amount greater than their contribution to the reserve fund, they were afforded some degree of protection.

This risk sharing was clearly intended to provide IPA physicians with an incentive to avoid overutilization. Today, risk sharing exists in several different forms, with varying degrees of risk assumed by the physicians and by the managed care organization. Although many plans use withholds, some do not. Similarly, some plans tie their bonuses to the amount of risk assumed by physicians through their individual capitation pools.

Although risk sharing (through withholds) may play a nominal role in controlling utilization, it plays a greater role in lowering unit costs. When an IPA withholds an amount for the reserve fund, it reduces the amount the physician receives, which many consider tantamount to providing discounted services. Thus, services are provided to IPA members at a lower unit cost rate.

Physician Productivity

Increasing the level of productivity is another way of containing unit costs in managed care organizations. This is particularly important because, in many cases, the unit costs for primary care services in staff and group model HMOs are comparable to or even greater than the unit costs in other systems of care.

Productivity is measured differently in managed care than in a fee-for-service practice. In fee-for-service health care, productivity is measured primarily by revenue, that is, collections or billed charges. In managed care, however, productivity is measured by the number of members served. In addition to examining the number of visits, however, it is also necessary to examine the style and content of patient visits "to determine whether quantity is achieved at the expense of quality."[40]

In order to determine the unit costs for physician services in staff model HMOs, physician salaries are divided by the number of output units provided by each full-time physician per year. Since salaries are a fixed annual expense, unit costs (e.g., costs per visit) are affected by the number of each physician's total patient visits.

Because the salary schedule of most HMOs compensates each physician specialty the same amount, salary alone does not provide a financial incentive for maintaining productivity. Some physicians prefer spending a substantial amount of time with each patient, thus reducing the level of productivity and escalating the unit costs. For this reason, it is necessary to balance this effect by careful management of physician workloads. This can be accomplished by setting productivity standards for full-time salaried physicians in managed care. As in the case of any employer-employee relationship, it is incumbent upon the managed care organization to inform each physician about its expectations regarding work output.

Buying Power

Due to the buying power of groups, it is possible to purchase services and related items at reduced rates.

Most profitable HMOs have at least 25,000 members,[41] and hospitals, laboratories, and pharmaceutical companies are usually willing to provide discounted rates and package deals in exchange for substantially increased sales. Discounted rates and package deals are more easily attained by large closed panel plans, which can better restrict their purchases to a single supplier, such as one hospital, and thus deliver—or threaten to remove—a large volume of business. Large medical groups are also better able to consider producing (rather than buying) services (e.g., laboratory services) as a strategy for controlling unit costs, which further strengthens their bargaining position.

MANAGING UTILIZATION

The second component of controlling costs is the management of utilization. Although there is tremendous value in reducing unit costs, most managed care organizations have historically focused on utilization management, since "HMO cost advantages are almost entirely attributable to utilization patterns."[42] Utilization management consists of actions by payers or administrators intended to influence providers of health care services to increase the efficiency and effectiveness of services.[43] This is accomplished by conducting evaluations and reviews on ambulatory as well as hospital care.

It is helpful to distinguish utilization management from utilization review. Although *utilization review* was once synonymous with *utilization management,* the terms are now considered to have different meanings. *Utilization review* developed with the initiation of Medicare to describe the first type of utilization control: retrospective review of hospital medical charts. At the time, chart review was the predominant method of monitoring utilization. As additional mechanisms to assess and influence utilization came into being, however, the term *utilization management* began to be used to encompass the broader range of activities.

Most of the focus of utilization management is on physician behavior. This is logical, since more than "two-thirds of the HMO's budget is controlled directly by the individual physician."[44] Therefore, managed care organizations employ several incentives and control mechanisms that encourage physicians to utilize resources in the most cost-effective manner.

Utilization management is not geared only toward costs, however. It also must take into account quality of care and member satisfaction. In order to avoid deficiencies in either area, caution must be exercised to ensure utilization controls do not deny patients access to the system or to necessary medical care.

Staffing

Most HMOs have their own utilization management staff and rarely contract out for utilization management services. Companies that offer such services, some of which are owned by large commercial carriers, contract mainly with insurers and self-insured entities.

In most cases, utilization management staff members are nurses and other health professionals and are supervised by a utilization management coordinator, a medical advisory committee, and the medical director.

Functions

The utilization management staff are responsible for several specific functions. They determine whether care that is requested or provided is medically necessary, if it is being provided in an appropriate setting and in a timely manner, and if the resources are being utilized appropriately.

Utilization management efforts are directed at care in both inpatient and outpatient settings. Because most managed care organizations have been successful in generating savings through controlling inpatient care utilization, much of the recent focus has been on controlling the costly overutilization of outpatient facilities.

Utilization Management Methods

The first HMOs mirrored the approach to utilization used in traditional care; that is, utilization was based on each individual physician's professional judgment. Utilization was not perceived as a problem at that time, except as being too low. Thus, public policy was directed at increasing access rather than reducing it.

This meant that controls on utilization were not developed for the purpose of cost containment or to modify inappropriate behaviors. HMOs were established to improve access to health care by better coordinating and arranging for services. The effectiveness of HMOs in controlling utilization was essentially a byproduct. When cost control became a pervasive issue, however, the effectiveness of HMOs in this regard was noted, and this gave rise to the HMO movement.

Utilization management was achieved in the first HMOs in several ways—primarily through structure, reviews, programs, and culture.

Structure

Earlier in the chapter, the organizational structure was stated to have a tremendous bearing on the ability of managed care organizations to control costs. To be efficient, HMOs require a structure in which allied health care providers and primary care physicians contain costs by decreasing the utilization of specialty services. The primary care physician is in the best position to assess the patient and provide treatment, usually without the need for specialty referral. When such referral is necessary, the primary care physician can direct the patient to the best source for care. By expecting specialists to document their consultations, the primary care physician is able to maintain control of the patient's continuing and comprehensive care.

By routing patients first to primary care physicians, who, as gatekeepers, can navigate patients through the intricacies of the health care delivery system, many inappropriate treatments, unnecessary diagnostic tests, and other wasteful practices can be avoided. Since primary care physicians can treat the vast majority of patient problems and conditions, ambulatory care is emphasized and costly specialty care is utilized only when appropriate and necessary.

Although gatekeeping is an integral function in group and staff model HMOs, it has also become standard in the IPA model. Through arrangements made at the time of member enrollment, IPA model HMOs require each member to select a participating primary care physician and seek all care from or through this physician. The member's primary care physician must refer the member to any needed specialist in order for the services to be covered under the plan. This requirement prevents the member from self-referring to specialists and "discourages the member from shopping for care at several sites, such as specialists' offices, hospital outpatient departments, and emergency rooms."[45]

Prospective, Concurrent, and Retrospective Review

Utilization reviews are aimed at controlling utilization before a patient is hospitalized (prospective review), while a patient is hospitalized (concurrent review), and after the patient is discharged (retrospective review).

Prospective Review. When utilization within the hospital was first assessed, it was normally through utilization review studies conducted after the fact. Also, reviews were based on "diagnosis independent criteria"[46] (i.e., the same criteria were applied to all patients regardless of diagnosis). The single intent of such reviews was to assess whether hospitalization had been justified.

As other types of utilization management evolved, hospitals began using prospective reviews that were based on criteria related to diagnoses and other factors and that weighed admission decisions against benefits, risks, and costs.

Prospective review is now popularly known as preadmission certification. In classical preadmis-

sion certification, physicians are required to contact the HMO before admitting any IPA patient to the hospital except in case of emergency. The HMO (usually a preadmission certification nurse who bases admission decisions on predetermined standards) confirms the patient's membership in the managed care organization, the medical necessity and appropriateness of the admission, and the appropriateness of the facility and the providers.

Next the nurse discusses the case with the admitting physician, and they decide whether to approve hospitalization or recommend an acceptable alternative. In the event of a disagreement, the HMO's medical director intervenes to render a final decision. The physician will generally comply with preadmission certification decisions. Without approval for the patient's hospitalization, the physician either would not be paid or would face some form of penalty (e.g., a reprimand, corrective action, suspension, or even termination).

Once the patient admission is deemed necessary, the preadmission workup is evaluated to make certain that necessary diagnostic testing is completed prior to hospitalization whenever possible, that results have been reviewed, and that arrangements for necessary hospital services have been made.[47] Based on predetermined criteria, a length of stay is assigned. When a treatment plan has been devised, the preadmission certification checks whether planned procedures are covered.

Since preadmission certification is aimed at ensuring appropriate and efficient utilization of hospital services, less costly outpatient services are recommended for minor or elective procedures whenever possible. The timing of hospital admissions is also considered (e.g., patients are admitted the day of the surgery rather than three days before). Preadmission testing is conducted either in the hospital on the day of admission or in the managed care organization prior to admission. In many instances, the managed care organization contracts with laboratories and other facilities to conduct preadmission testing at discounted rates.[48]

By limiting or avoiding expensive hospital stays through the provision of services and treatments in less costly settings, preadmission certification has had a tremendous impact on utilization. In fact, it is known to have an even greater impact on utilization than concurrent review.[49]

Concurrent Review. Concurrent reviews are conducted to assess inpatient care at the time it is provided. Although concurrent reviews originally focused on the length of time a patient stayed in the hospital, they were later expanded to include other aspects of a patient's ongoing hospitalization. Today, concurrent reviews assess "the use of resources, the timeliness with which treatment is provided, and the adequacy and timeliness of discharge planning."[50]

In a large plan, one or more nurses are stationed in an office at each of the plan's major hospitals to assess patient status on a regular basis. In other types of organizations, staff who conduct concurrent review are based in offices at organization headquarters and make frequent visits to the hospitals.

In either case, concurrent review begins on the day of the patient's admission, and the first task is to validate the appropriateness of the admission. The status of each patient is documented in a daily census report, and the medical charts of each managed care patient are assessed through a comprehensive review or by spot-checking. The concurrent care coordinator uses the information to monitor all aspects of the patient's ongoing care, with a special focus on medical necessity and risk management.

In order to evaluate the continued appropriateness of the setting and health care resources as well as the medical necessity of the prescribed treatment, several criterion lists are used. These instruments include the Intensity of Service, Severity of Illness, and Discharge Screens, developed by InterQual; the Appropriateness Evaluation Protocol, originally developed at Boston University; and the Standardized Medreview Instrument, developed by Systemetrics. The increased knowledge of the efficacy of alternative treatment patterns, the related development of treatment protocols and clinical practice guidelines, and the development of advanced information systems is giving rise to a new generation of concurrent review processes

conducted by the attending physician or care giver. In some organizations, these clinical practice guidelines take the form of monitored institutional standards, while in others they are presented as practice norms that remind physicians of the efficacy of alternative treatment patterns.

As clinical practice guidelines are subjected to increased specific scientific testing and as information is disseminated to practice settings and used to guide care giving, information will be increasingly accepted as a clinical intervention that influences patient as well as provider behavior. There is potential to decrease health care costs by decreasing utilization through the use of advanced information systems. The Columbia registry of Controlled Clinical Information Service Trials provides the first systematic collection of scientific evidence on the efficacy of information as a clinical intervention.[51]

One of the major elements of concurrent review is continued stay review. Continued stay review programs control hospital costs by curtailing unnecessary days of hospitalization. This is a significant method of utilization management, since "one extra day in the hospital costs as much as 15 or 20 additional office visits."[52]

Another aspect of concurrent review is discharge planning. Discharge planning begins on the first day of a patient's hospitalization and involves conducting a discharge planning needs assessment (determining the patient's special needs based on the anticipated outcome), working with the patient to arrange an early morning discharge, and assisting hospital discharge planning staff to expedite the discharge process. When continued care is required, the managed care organization's coordinator also arranges for a transfer from the hospital to a residential, rehabilitation, long-term care, or other facility as appropriate.

Retrospective Review. Retrospective utilization review originally assessed whether care could have been provided in a more appropriate setting than the hospital. The value of this type of review was basically as a guide for future admissions. Utilization review now encompasses a much broader range of care. A review is conducted following a patient's discharge from the hospital and also for any patient who has received ambulatory treatment. In addition to assessing whether the level of care was appropriate, utilization review evaluates whether the resources were used appropriately by each provider and identifies problem areas and inefficiencies. It also examines whether the care provided matched the type and severity of the patient's illness.

In many cases, several types of data are assessed in utilization review. For example, hospital activities and inpatient procedures are tracked weekly or monthly, and any deviant patterns are reported. Reports also are made on inpatient consultations and referrals; laboratory, radiology, and ancillary services; physician productivity; and any out-of-area services. Similar reports are made on ambulatory services. Because of the detail required in the compilation of these reports, most reviews are computerized.

Through use of such reports, the managed care organization develops several types of profiles, including profiles of the providers, the facility, diagnoses and procedures, and the subscribers. These profiles make it possible to compare trends as well as to conduct financial audits on the care provided.

Programs

Educational programs aimed at individuals and groups are offered as a part of the typical members' benefits package. These programs cover a broad array of topics, such as nutrition, weight control, substance abuse, exercise, stress reduction, prenatal care, and childbirth. Although expensive to institute, programs can save cost in the long term by educating members about the proper utilization of the system and about the care and treatment provided to them. Such programs enable members to develop more realistic expectations and place fewer unreasonable demands upon the providers and the system. Also, proper education often makes patients less dependent upon or less expectant of protracted hospital stays. In addition to these cost-and-quality benefits, educational programs have marketing value because of their appeal to potential and current subscribers.

HMOs have developed special services (after-hours care, home health care, home health education, and pre- and postoperative education) to provide less costly alternatives to hospitalization.

Although collaboration among all types of health professionals is essential, nurses play a particularly active role in the development and implementation of programs and services. Many physicians initially resisted nurses' involvement, which they perceived as an intrusion into the doctor-patient relationship. Today, however, physicians recognize the benefits of such collaboration, and many consider it a vital adjunct of their practices. In fact, many physicians have found that it is easier to care for patients who are educated about procedures or conditions beforehand. As an example, most obstetricians today would prefer to provide care for first-time mothers who have received education regarding labor.

Because staff model HMOs function through a centralized facility, it is much easier for these HMOs to establish programs and services than it is for IPAs. In staff model HMOs, there is greater opportunity for collaboration on program development and implementation, and it is also easier to obtain higher levels of member participation because programs can be more easily publicized among the membership.

Physicians in IPAs may find it more difficult to establish programs, because interprofessional collaboration and management control of programs and services are not as easy to accomplish in decentralized settings. In addition, these physicians may not be able to attract as many program participants, since IPA members may only constitute a small percentage of the patients they see. Nevertheless, many IPAs are finding ways to build such programs into their delivery systems. For some, their future success may depend on it.

Culture

Costs can be contained by influencing physician behavior through the organizational value structure or culture. The organizational culture includes the standards of practice (community standards) used by the organization and the peer influence exerted by colleagues.

When physicians become a part of an HMO and receive feedback from colleagues who are accustomed to a certain style of practice, they normally conform to the practice standards of that group. This feedback affects physician behavior, since physicians are often strongly influenced by comparisons with their peers. For example, physicians who receive feedback that the rate of tonsillectomy in their county is five times the rate in other areas in the state are likely to change their practice behavior. Their motivation would be to avoid appearing as outliers who engage in a deviant practice style. Thus, by sharing peer review data, physicians are likely to change their practice style in ways that may reduce utilization and costs.

Affecting utilization through the organizational culture is more feasible in group and staff model HMOs than in IPAs. IPA physicians do not have the same opportunity for acquiring a common culture, since the physicians often practice in a variety of settings. Many observers believe staff model HMOs always will have an edge over IPAs in management effectiveness for this reason.

THE MANAGEMENT OF QUALITY

The management of quality encompasses the quality of care (or technical quality) and the quality of service (as perceived by the patient and family). The management of quality is important to managed care organizations because of the increased interest by the public in quality and the increased accountability of health providers for providing quality. These reasons are not unique to the managed care industry. What is unique is the structure of managed care organizations within which quality of care is provided, assessed, and assured. This creates special management requirements and challenges.

Quality of Care

The quality of care in a managed care organization is partially determined by the measurement and

management of processes and structures to improve quality. The issues of measurement are not unique to managed care, but it is likely that managed care and traditional care organizations differ as regards process and outcome indicators of quality. Quality of care is an area of current research and much is yet to be learned. Interestingly, much of the research is focused on hospitals and will likely result in measures and systems that might not, and probably will not, be transferable to managed care organizations, particularly HMOs. There is a need to increase the research on the measurement of outcomes and processes of managed care organizations, first, because these organizations have been neglected, and, second, because they probably will resemble health care organizations of the future in the United States and other countries. The management of processes and structures to improve the quality of care involves the same design issues addressed in the previous sections. The tasks include working across organizational units to develop a shared perspective and commitment to quality, to develop an information system that measures and monitors performance, and to design management systems and structures that actually improve quality. Management challenges include getting institutional commitment to standards and protocols to be used to manage care and changing the performance of individual units so that they contribute more toward achieving the broader institutional goals and mission. Managing an organization so it is able to accomplish a broad mission requires new approaches that will require the traditional new structures, management systems, and management skills.

Quality of Services

Services provided by health organizations are not objects—they are processes or sets of interrelated processes. Although members may have no idea of the process underlying a medical service, the quality they perceive is a function of the design of the process. This design facilitates and constrains provider-patient interactions and influences members' perceptions of the quality of the service. Although a process is intangible, its design serves to structure members' exposures to the facilities, equipment, and people involved in providing the service. Therefore, a critical factor in the management of the quality of a service is the design of the process.

The management of the quality of a service includes managing (1) the service process that prescribes the provider-member contact points and establishes the boundaries of the interactions, (2) the role of the member in the interactions, (3) the attitudes and behaviors of the providers, and (4) the physical environment surrounding the interactions. The necessary management activities cross intrainstitutional and often interinstitutional boundaries, which makes the management process complex and far reaching. Its importance in managed care organizations is probably greater than in more traditional delivery systems, because managed care organizations raise expectations among members that services will be available, coordinated, and oriented primarily to their welfare.

The actual management process consists of (1) determining member expectations, (2) evaluating the service concept and system, (3) redesigning the service concept and system, (4) developing a system to monitor performance, and (5) developing an internal marketing system. Each of these steps is more difficult if multiple organizational units or multiple organizations are involved. Determining member expectations requires use of patient satisfaction questionnaires, focus groups, and other techniques typical of health care settings. In a managed care organization, however, the concern is to ensure that members are satisfied with the entire system, including service access and provision, referrals and transfers, insurance benefits, and overall cost.

In like manner, other steps in the management of quality process must be considered from a systems perspective. Evaluating and redesigning the service concept and system involves assessing performance across a wide range of services and organizations. Carrying out this assessment requires managing across organizational unit and multiple organization boundaries and integrating a range of service types. Service evaluation in managed care organizations focuses on the transfer points between organizations and between units within organizations. Although this makes the evaluation process exceedingly difficult, the focus of attention is important, because it is at these transfer points that the delivery of health services most frequently breaks down. While the process is challenging, managed care organizations at least have the organizational framework and the incentive to make it a focal point of concern and attention.

The final steps in the process of managing service quality are to develop a system for monitoring performance and to develop a system for internal marketing. The necessary tasks include creating an integrated information system to support the monitoring of operations and to provide information needed to make decisions on system management and redesign. This task also requires crossing the boundaries of organizations and units.

The process of managing service quality is more difficult in IPAs or PPOs, because they are made up of multiple organizations and delivery units. In contrast, staff model HMOs have more traditional organizational structures, and the services are provided within a single organizational framework. However, it is advisable not to prejudge the ability of different structures, including multiple organizational structures, to manage complex processes. U.S. Health Care, an IPA model organization, has developed a strong concept and created expectations shared by its participating members, and its feedback and control system for measuring quality and making corrections is impressive.

THE FUTURE OF MANAGED CARE

Much can be learned from the history and development of various types of managed care organizations. They have focused on, but not resolved, the most publicized health care issues: cost, access, and quality. Many of their techniques and structures will be incorporated into the design of future health systems, which will be characterized by more organizational control over the provision of services, more integration of services, greater rationing of technology, and more orientation toward primary care.

The various models of managed care, which were once clearly differentiated, now are often blended together. As a result, there are many new options to go with the more common benefits and services. Managed care has taken what has worked and incorporated it into its organizational models. The fee-for-service system has also adopted many of the utilization review and cost-control mechanisms developed by managed care organizations.

Managed care organizations have not been successful in meeting the goals of the social agenda, which served as the rationale for their development in the past two decades. They have demonstrated some effectiveness in controlling costs but have not resolved the social issues of high-cost care and the rationing of technology. One expectation was that they would provide increased access, but they have had little success in bringing health care to the poor. There is nothing in the design of managed care organizations that guarantees resolution of these issues, but they have joined the debate and must continue to contribute approaches to solutions.

Managed health care organizations can aid in the development of new system structures and management techniques that will be increasingly incorporated into new system designs. They should not be viewed as static models or as alternatives to more traditional and individual-oriented systems. Managed care systems have demonstrated their effectiveness in addressing some of the major health issues facing the country, and for this reason they can be instructive to policy makers, managers, and educators and provide a fruitful area for research.

The existing types of managed care organizations cannot be considered as fully mature, even though they have been around for a number of years. They will continue to evolve and assume forms that have not yet been envisioned. Managers must not lock into existing designs and patterns and defend the status quo. The challenge to management is to create new organizational forms, some that might challenge assumptions long held by the industry. Managers must create better functioning and more effective health systems, not to enter into the ideological debates frequently fostered by professionals and professional societies. The goal is to provide high-quality, low-cost health services that are accessible to all.

ADDITIONAL RESOURCES

Organizations and Agencies

American Association of Preferred Provider Organizations, 401 N. Michigan Avenue, Chicago, IL 60611-4267; 312/644-6610. Professional association of preferred provider organizations.

American Managed Care and Review Association, 1227 25th Street, N.W., Suite 610, Washington, DC 20038; 202/728-0506. Quality assurance and accrediting agency for managed care organizations.

Group Health Association of America, 1129 Twentieth Street, NW, Suite 600, Washington, DC 20036; 202/778-3200. Professional association of managed care organizations.

National Center for Managed Health Care Administration, University of Missouri, 5100 Rockhill Road, Kansas City, MO 64110-2499; 816/235-1478. Reference center; provides executive course in managed care administration.

Books and Periodicals

Berkowitz, E.D., and W. Wolff. *Group Health Association: A portrait of a health maintenance organization.* Philadelphia: Temple University Press, 1988.

Boles, K.E. *Strategic financial management in managed care: A primer.* Kansas City, Mo.: National Center for Managed Health Care Administration, 1989.

Bopp, K.D. *Marketing managed care: Getting and keeping members.* Kansas City, Mo.: National Center for Managed Health Care Administration, 1989.

Brown, G.D. *Strategic management in managed health care organizations.* Kansas City, Mo.: National Center for Managed Health Care Administration, 1990.

Cowan, D.H. *Preferred provider organizations: Planning, structure, and operation.* Gaithersburg, Md.: Aspen Publishers, 1984.

DeMarco, W.J., and T.J. Garvey. *Going prepaid: A strategic planning decision.* Denver: Center for Research in Ambulatory Health Care Administration and Medical Group Management Association, 1986.

Edgdahl, R.H., and D.C. Walsh. *Industry and HMOs: A natural alliance.* New York: Springer-Verlag, 1978.

Flautt, S.M., and T.G. Kirschbraun. The social health maintenance organization: New boundaries for the HMO. In *Proceedings of the 1986 Annual Meeting of the Group Health Association of America.* Washington, DC: Group Health Association of America, 1986.

Hale, J.A., and M.M. Hunter. *From HMO movement to managed care industry: The future of HMOs in a volatile healthcare market.* Minneapolis: Inter-Study Center for Managed Care Research, 1988.

Hicks, L.L. *Role of economics in managed health care systems.* Kansas City, Mo.: National Center for Managed Health Care Administration, 1990.

Kongstvedt, P.R. *The managed health care handbook.* Gaithersburg, Md.: Aspen Publishers, 1989.

Luft, H.S. Health maintenance organizations and the rationing of medical care. In *Securing access to health care.* Vol. 3. Washington, D.C.: U.S. Government Printing Office, 1983.

Luft, H.S. *Health maintenance organizations: Dimensions of performance.* New York: Wiley, 1981.

Mackie, D.L., and D.K. Decker. *Group and IPA HMOs.* Gaithersburg, Md.: Aspen Publishers, 1981.

Mayer, T.R., and G.G. Mayer. HMOs: Origins and developments. *New England Journal of Medicine* 312 (1985):590–594.

Mayer, T.R., and G.G. Mayer. *The health insurance alternative: A complete guide to health maintenance organizations.* New York: Perigee Books, 1984.

Nelson, J.A. The history and spirit of the HMO movement. *HMO Practice* 1 (1987): 75–82.

Shouldice, R.G. *Introduction to managed care.* Washington, D.C.: Information Resource Press, 1991.

Soper, M., et al. *Balancing the triad: Cost containment, quality of service, and quality of care in managed care systems.* Kansas City, Mo.: National Center for Managed Health Care Administration, 1989.

Stack, R.H. *HMOs from the management perspective.* New York: American Management Association, 1979.

Welch, W.P., et al. Toward new typologies for HMOS. *The Milbank Quarterly* 68 (1990): 221–243.

NOTES

1. J.A. Hale and M.M. Hunter, *From HMO Movement to Managed Care Industry: The Future of HMOs in a Volatile Healthcare Market* (Minneapolis: Inter-Study Center for Managed Care Research, 1988), 2.

2. J.A. Nelson, The History and Spirit of the HMO Movement, *HMO Practice* 1 (1987): 75–80.

3. Ibid.

4. Ibid.

5. R.H. Stack, *HMOs from the Management Perspective* (New York: American Management Association, 1979).

6. R.G. Shouldice and K.H. Shouldice, *Medical Group Practice and Health Maintenance Organizations* (Washington, D.C.: Information Resource Press, 1978), 22.

7. P. Starr, *The Social Transformation of American Medicine* (New York: Basic Books, 1982), 210–211.

8. T.R. Mayer and G.G. Mayer, *The Health Insurance Alternative: A Complete Guide to Health Maintenance Organizations* (New York: Perigee Books, 1984), 31.

9. Ibid.

10. H.S. Luft, Health Maintenance Organizations and the Rationing of Medical Care, in *Securing Access to Health Care,* vol. 3 (Washington, D.C.: U.S. Government Printing Office, 1983), 331.

11. T.R. Mayer and G.G. Mayer, HMOs: Origins and Developments, *New England Journal of Medicine,* 312: 9 (1985): 590–594.

12. Nelson, History and Spirit of the HMO Movement, 78.

13. Mayer and Mayer, HMOs.

14. D.L. Mackie and D.K. Decker, *Group and IPA HMOs* (Gaithersburg, Md.: Aspen Publishers, 1981), 21.

15. E.D. Berkowitz and W. Wolff, *Group Health Association: A Portrait of a Health Maintenance Organization* (Philadelphia: Temple University Press, 1988), 9.

16. Shouldice and Shouldice, *Medical Group Practice,* 22, 27.

17. W.J. DeMarco and T.J. Garvey, *Going Prepaid: A Strategic Planning Decision* (Denver: Center for Research in Ambulatory Health Care Administration and Medical Group Management Association, 1986), v.

18. C. Shaeffer, Second Thoughts on HMOs, *Changing Times* 34 (1987).

19. Luft, Health Maintenance Organizations, 315.

20. S.J. Williams and P.R. Torrens, *Introduction to Health Services* (New York: Wiley, 1980), 313.

21. D.R. Cohodes, The Loss of Innocence: Health Care under Siege, in *Health Care and Its Costs,* ed. C.J. Schramm (New York: W.W. Norton, 1987), 75–76.

22. HMO: The Three Letters That Are Revolutionizing Health Care, *Business Week,* March 1987.

23. Shaeffer, Seconds Thoughts on HMOs.

24. S.M. Flautt and T.G. Kirschbraun, The Social Health Maintenance Organization: New Boundaries for the HMO, in *Proceedings of the 1986 Annual Meeting of the Group Health Association of America,* 1986.

25. R.E. Miles and C.C. Snow, Organizations: New Concepts for New Forms, *California Management Review* 28, no. 3 (1986).

26. Ibid.

27. D.E. Bowen and G.R. Jones, Transaction Cost Analysis of Service Organization–Customer Exchange, *Academy of Management Review* 11 (1986):428–441.

28. Transaction costs are the costs of negotiating, monitoring, and enforcing the exchanges between parties to a transaction. The sources of transaction costs are goal incongruence and performance ambiguity. The greater these are, the higher the transaction costs will be. See Bowen and Jones, Transaction Cost Analysis of Service Organization–Customer Exchange.

29. P.K. Mills and T. Turk, A Preliminary Investigation into the Influence of Customer-Firm Interface on Information Processing and Task Activities in Service Organizations. *Journal of Management* 12, no. 1 (1986): 91–104.

30. H.A. Simon, *Administrative Behavior,* 2d ed. (New York: Macmillan, 1957).

31. Ibid.

32. S.R. Hernandez et al., The Relationship between Technology and Task Design in Hospital Nursing Units, *Health Services Management Research* 3, no. 2 (1990): 137–148.

33. Cybernetic regulation is a control process that comprises the establishment of performance standards, the ongoing measurement of system performance, the comparison of performance and standards, the feeding back of information about unwanted variances in the system, and the modification of system comportment.

34. S.G. Green and M.A. Welsh, Cybernetics and Dependence: Reframing the Control Concept, *Academy of Management Review* 13 (1988): 287–301.

35. P.K. Mills and D.J. Moberg, Strategic Implications of Service Technologies, in *Service Management Effectiveness,* ed. D.E. Bowen et al. (San Francisco: Jossey-Bass, 1990).

36. H.S. Luft, *Health Maintenance Organizations: Dimensions of Performance* (New York: Wiley, 1981), 25.

37. R.G. Evans et al., Controlling Health Expenditures—The Canadian Reality, *New England Journal of Medicine* 320 (1989): 575.

38. L.D. Brown, *Politics and Health Care Organizations: HMOs as Federal Policy* (Washington, D.C.: Brookings Institution, 1983), 56.

39. R.H. Edgdahl and D.C. Walsh, *Industry and HMOs: A Natural Alliance* (New York: Springer-Verlag, 1978), 44.

40. Luft, *Health Maintenance Organizations,* 158.

41. S. Gannes, Strong Medicine for Health Bills, *Fortune* 71 (1987).

42. Luft, *Health Maintenance Organizations,* 165.

43. S.M.C. Payne, Identifying and Managing Inappropriate Hospital Utilization: A Policy Synthesis, *HSR: Health Service Research* 22 (1987): 712, 733.

44. Mackie and Decker, *Group and IPA HMOs,* 112; Mayer and Mayer, *Health Insurance Alternative,* 40.

45. Edgdahl and Walsh, *Industry and HMOs,* 41.

46. Payne, Identifying and Managing Inappropriate Hospital Utilization.

47. D.H. Cowan, *Preferred Provider Organizations: Planning, Structure, and Operation* (Gaithersburg, Md.: Aspen Publishers, 1984), 171.

48. P.R. Kongstvedt, *The Managed Health Care Handbook* (Gaithersburg, Md.: Aspen Publishers, 1989), 87.

49. Luft, *Health Maintenance Organizations,* 98.

50. Cowan, *Preferred Provider Organizations,* 172.

51. Columbia Registry of Controlled Clinical Information Service Trials. Health Services Management, University of Missouri, Columbia, Mo.

52. Mackie and Decker, *Group and IPA HMOs,* 181.

Steven R. Orr

Multiunit Systems

9

Purpose: By combining hospitals, multispecialty clinics, nursing homes, home health care agencies, and a variety of other health care facilities and organizations, multiunit health systems are able to leverage their collective resources, provide a common focus and directed momentum, and maximize the use of assets to achieve more in improving health services delivery than could be accomplished by a mere collection or alliance of autonomous facilities.

INTRODUCTION

The evolution of multiunit systems seems at odds with the old saying that "form follows function." Their creation was in many cases stimulated by political, social, or organizational considerations. Sometimes the explicit goal of efficient and effective delivery of health care services was only tangential. These systems now have a pragmatic need to provide services in a way that capitalizes on their unique characteristics. Their growth and development served as a catalyst for the creation of operating principles that are fundamental to the way they are now managed. This chapter will

briefly describe some of the ways in which multiunit systems were created, outline underlying organizational principles that have evolved, and explore their implications for the management of these organizations.

ORGANIZATIONAL ROLE AND FUNCTION

According to American Hospital Association data, multiunit health care systems now own, lease, or manage over 53 percent of the acute care hospitals in the United States. Besides adding free-standing hospitals, systems are also adding and integrating primary care clinics, nursing homes, home health agencies, multispecialty clinics, rehabilitation centers, and other types of facilities. In effect, multiunit systems are becoming the core of the nation's health care delivery system.

Although these organizations currently exhibit remarkably similar characteristics, their historical formation was stimulated by a wide range of factors. In the 1960s, as urban dwellers accelerated their migration to the suburbs, increasing numbers of physicians established or moved their practices to locations close to their patients. Combined with the desire of suburbs to develop their own municipal identities, the establishment of a critical mass of practitioners led to the creation of hospitals located in these centers of growth. The departure of the medical staffs, together with the creation of new free-standing hospitals, exerted pressure on existing inner-city institutions. It resulted in lost prestige, leveled off growth, severed some of their historical ties to constituent groups, and, most important, reduced their financial capabilities. All of these factors served as stimuli to prompt these organizations to devise a response—the creation of satellite facilities.

In most cases, the embryonic multiunit systems replicated history by placing the constituent institutions within organizational structures that reinforced their independence and individual development. Generally they were geographically separated hospitals that functioned independently except for ownership. The most common form of structure was adapted from "holding company" models. The underlying operating principle was to reserve as little control as possible at the parent level.

During this early period, two other developments were occurring that encouraged the growth of multiunit systems: the establishment of a market presence by investor-owned hospital chains and the development of a philosophy of collective health delivery by religious groups. Although historically there had been many privately owned, taxable hospitals, it was not until the 1960s that privately held multihospital corporations began to grow and gain national visibility. This visibility was particularly enhanced when these organizations began to access a different capital market by being publicly traded. This created a need to define characteristics that would distinguish their approach to providing hospital services from those in the tax-exempt or public hospital sectors. The main distinguishing feature was their emphasis on their ability to adapt management techniques that had been successfully developed and used in other industries for use in a multihospital setting. They particularly underscored the value of creating a critical mass that would permit

economies of scale. The approach was to leave the clinical areas to the discretion of each hospital and focus on areas in which larger-scale operations would make a difference (e.g., group purchasing and centralized reimbursement).

There is another essential characteristic of these organizations that distinguishes them from the original holding companies. Given their patterning on other industries and the fact that they were not based on existing older organizations, both governance and management control were created as corporate or central responsibilities. Management control might, in turn, be delegated, but the power to decide to do this was retained by the corporation. This is in contrast to the holding company approach, which, by convention, allowed considerable autonomy to remain at the individual unit. The units chose which activities and decisions to refer to the corporation.

The second stimulus to the development of multiunit systems came from religious groups that owned multiple hospitals (particularly the Catholic religious communities). These groups historically had operated individual hospitals within an organization that made collective decisions. Implicitly, the emphasis was not on how to manage the institutions collectively as a hospital system but how to manage the individual hospitals within a system that had other responsibilities (i.e., to the church or the religious community). During the late 1960s and early 1970s, many of these groups began to move their health care activities, particularly their hospitals and nursing homes, into newly created and separate legal entities. While in most cases the groups retained ownership, these new multiunit corporations had their own governing and management structures. Because of the collective memory and experience of individuals within each new corporation, they retained the historical decision-making approach and philosophy of their founding group. In many cases, this was constantly reinforced because of the interaction of individuals in the group and the corporation. The corporation's mission and management philosophy and the balance of authority between individual units and the corporation were formed and reformed based on the prevailing approach of the sponsoring group.

Over time, two other trends affected the development of the early systems. Multihospital structures allowed smaller or weaker hospitals to join a system and yet continue to exist and retain a certain amount of independence. The addition of these hospitals created a higher degree of dissimilarity within the system. Initially, the less the amount of control exerted by the parent, the easier the assimilation and the less impact the new facility had on the overall organization. As more varied institutions were added, the cumulative impact began to create pressures—only because of the increased complexity. Organizations that were based on the holding company approach lacked internal experience that would help reduce these pressures. They needed to create new responses. The only sources of experience were to be found in other industries or other systems confronting similar issues.

The investor-owned chains had to take into account two additional considerations. First, a greater portion of their growth occurred by building new facilities. Second, because of greater central control, the systems tended to use a similar approach to each new facility, which created great conformity. It also made assimilation of free-standing facilities difficult. Greater change was required of the additions for them to successfully make the transition into the systems. As a result, resources had to be continually balanced. All of this occurred in a public arena that was still adjusting to the concept of a publicly held company providing health care.

The nonsecular multiunits faced a different set of pressures as new facilities were added. The interaction between the sponsoring groups and the systems became increasingly complicated. The demands of running a health care system competed with non-health-care demands. For the Catholic religious communities that had fewer and fewer individuals participating in health care delivery, this competition was especially acute. There were not enough individuals available to maintain the historical relationship between the sponsoring community and the new facilities.

The other major trend affecting multiunit systems was the merger and acquisition of systems by systems. Not only did organizations with a similar historical development merge, but so did systems with dissimilar backgrounds. All of the possible combinations of these historical disparate groups occurred. For example, investor-owned systems not only acquired and merged with other investor-owned systems, but they acquired both holding company and nonsecular systems.

Several factors influencing these mergers have become clear. Many of the systems, prior to the mergers, were still in a developmental stage. Individually they were composed of institutions, boards, medical staffs, and communities that were still uncertain about how a system operated. Numerous issues such as governance relationships, capital formation and disbursement, corporate cost allocation, and the role of the medical staffs had not been adequately addressed and resolved. The merger of even similar systems involved these issues. However, the merging of the organizations now placed them in a context of greater uncertainty.

The vehicle driving the growth of tax-exempt systems was merger, not acquisition. With acquisition there was a clear indication of the direction the new system would take. However, with most mergers of tax-exempts, there was a great deal of uncertainty as to who would take the lead. Mergers occurred that combined organizations with unequal assets, equal representation on the governing board, a mixture of the management groups, and historically competing hospitals and medical staffs. This all occurred at a time when there were few system mergers that had existed long enough to serve as examples. Nor, because of the uniqueness of the tax-exempt status, could the organizations look to other industries for similar experiences. For example, there was no stock to be valued and exchanged.

The varied historical paths that led to the development of multiunit systems, combined with other factors, created considerable heterogeneity across systems. Although the legal structures and generic organizational issues were similar, the operational specifics and the complexities of interaction were not. It is only recently that these organizations have had the time and collective experience to sort out what it is they have and how might they be managed. As this has occurred, certain underlying principles have begun to emerge.

LEVERAGING THE MULTIUNIT SYSTEM

Periodically a debate surfaces in the literature as to whether or not participation in a system adds value to the individual hospital. The increasing reliance the nation's health delivery system has on multiunit systems had altered the focus of this discussion from "if" to "how best?" For multiunit systems, the question is how to make the whole greater than the sum of the parts (or, from a slightly different perspective, how to make the part stronger because it is a part of the whole). Systems must use their existing capabilities or create capabilities to leverage their activities to accomplish more than would have been possible if each unit had remained free-standing. It is also critical at this stage in multiunit systems' development that this leveraging occur in such a way that they achieve more than they would as mere collections or alliances of autonomous facilities.

This leveraging appears to have gone through three phases. Initially, the effort was to combine those activities that used economies of scale to achieve specific benefits but did not require a high degree of interaction with the internal operations of the organization. Secondly, the focus targeted specific functions having high potential to achieve the benefits of economies of scale but required interactions with the operations of the organization. Finally, this has brought organizations to the point where leveraging is occurring through the integration of operations among the operating units and between the corporation and these units.

One of the early recognized benefits of creating a system was the potential to combine specific activities to achieve something that could not be accomplished when hospitals were free-standing. One ex-

ample of this was the use of a master indenture as a debt instrument. Nonprofit private hospitals historically accessed the tax-exempt bond market. They secured their debt with the buildings and equipment they purchased with the proceeds. The combined debt for these early systems was the accumulation of each of the issues for each of the facilities. The formation of the systems and the increasing number of facilities within these systems created a need to go back into the capital market more frequently. Where a single facility might access the market every ten years, systems were going to the market for their individual facilities much more frequently. This pressure caused the systems to behave initially as collections of facilities. A system would typically bundle its individual needs into a single issue, refinance old debt, and achieve savings by reducing the costs of processing. This leveraging was then extended with the use of a master indenture. This instrument took advantage of the single ownership to secure the debt, not through the identification of specific assets, but by "pledging" the assets of the whole system. It streamlined the system's ability to access the market by establishing debt covenants that, in turn, helped identify the debt capacity of the system. It also provided greater security to bondholders by establishing specific financial ratios that benchmarked the financial stability of the system. The financial health of a specific facility at a particular point in time became less important than financial strength of the multiunit system as a whole.

This example demonstrates several of the important and developing characteristics of these systems as they learned how to leverage their activity. They achieved benefits that could not have been realized by free-standing institutions or by a collection of facilities. They also were able to articulate to a new and external audience in an understandable and tangible way that they were really new kinds of organizations. Finally, specific opportunities existed in these organizations that did not depend on their being operationally mature, and there were several areas in which their experiences were similar (the formation of captive insurance companies is one other example).

As multiunit systems began to understand their capacities and as their internal operations stabilized, they were able to initiate a different phase of leverage. They focused their growing critical mass in functional areas that were, to some degree, internally insulated but where economies of scale could be attained. These areas included information systems, financial areas like accounting and reimbursement, public relations, and the human resources functions. The greatest impact was in those areas where there was a linkage between external suppliers and internal activity, such as purchasing and materials management. The most difficult were those areas that impinged on the individual institution's historical autonomy. Particularly sensitive were any changes that affected the clinical departments.

Experience with purchasing, and later materials management, illustrates some of the ways that multiunit systems were able to increase cost-efficiency. Initially, purchasing resembled the kinds of activities that did not require interaction with internal operations for the achievement of economies of scale. The system accumulated information describing what supplies individual facilities were purchasing, bundled it together so that suppliers might anticipate specific volumes, and negotiated prices based on those volumes. Purchasers quickly realized that they could gain additional savings if the volume of a specific item being purchased was increased and if they could assure the supplier that the estimated amount would actually be bought. This required active internal intervention. Increased committed volume could only be achieved by establishing internal processes that controlled the volume and purchase of specific items for the total system. Purchasing, because of the benefits that the leverage could produce, was usually the first intervention into clinical areas by a support department.

This second phase was important to the concept of leveraging for a couple of reasons. First, it continued to build on a principle that had been implicitly accepted earlier: that the systems could continue to provide benefits to their individual units that the units could not acquire individually. Second, it established the concept of system discipline, which would serve as a foundation for other future activities. In other words, it operationalized the idea that if a change would benefit the whole system and not negatively affect any individual institution, then it should be implemented. For example, if committing to volumes could achieve lower glove costs without lowering the quality, then the system had the right to choose the specific manufacturer and supplier. The concept of the system discipline also embodies another element. To achieve systemwide consistency within an appropriate time frame and to replicate this process in subsequent iterations, it required the system to confront who and which part of the system had specific responsibilities. It served as the test for resolving issues between the corporation and individual facilities, between individual facilities and other individual facilities, and between the clinical services and the support services.

Many multiunit systems have entered a third phase in the development of their leveraging ability. Their entry into this phase has been stimulated by a series of external pressures and is possible because of their increasing maturity as systems. The demands created by innovations such as DRGs, the necessity to respond to the requirements of managed care, and the continued increase in the use of ambulatory care services have pushed systems toward greater integration on multiple levels. This process is driven by an underlying premise that recombination and redesign can create organizational improvement. Fundamental to approaches such as total quality management is the ability of an entire system to leverage itself through collective learning and shared experience. This phase concentrates investments of time, people, and other resources in processes that, in turn, can be leveraged throughout the system.

Multiunit systems are creating internal educational and training programs that tailor external programs to fit unique system needs. They are establishing benchmarks in order to compare activity between the units. This is being done with the explicit intent of adapting similar approaches systemwide. Changes are being made to benefit programs, name recognition is being transferred from facilities to the corporations, and internal and external communications are emphasizing the interaction between units.

The most dramatic shift is occurring in the clinical areas. Case management, built around specific episodes of care, is being constructed by each system as a whole and then adapted to specific settings. The term *full service,* which often meant just *up-to-date,* is now used to refer to systems that really offer complete services. This capitalizes on the ability of systems to leverage the extent of its activity by having the discipline to implement differentiation.

It is important to note that, along with each of these emerging principles, there are key dimensions that allow them to be operationalized in a current time frame. Each has an essential core element. For example, leveraging depends on the ability to apply the assets of a greater whole in order to achieve a capability that is beyond what an individual unit of that whole could achieve. It is equally critical to recognize another dimension. For each principle, there needs to be an understanding of the evolution and maturing that occurs in the application of the principle. Each requires certain building blocks. Finally, it is important to recognize that the application of each principle is dependent on how it fits with each multiunit system's own history and maturing process. Again, using the example of leveraging, the second and third leveraging phases were dependent on explicit and implicit foundations laid by the preceding phase. The ability to move successfully from one phase to the next tests how firmly the base is in place within the overall organizational context.

COMMON FOCUS AND DIRECTED MOMENTUM

The history of multiunit systems demonstrates that these organizations were created for many reasons other than a common explicit organizational mission. As they mature, their discipline permits them to maintain sharp and consistent focus. They are evolving ways to concentrate their attention on specific activities and ignore or discard those that are distracting. Critical to each system's focus is its ability to achieve directed momentum as a single entity—its ability to take the critical mass that has been built up over time, consciously determine its direction, and create movement toward the future.

The development of the ability to have a common focus and directed momentum parallels the development of the ability to leverage. The initial systems were based on the premise that the purpose of the corporations was to support and supplement the individual facilities. The systems were seen as collections of hospitals with a common bond, and the corporations were mainly responsible for those activities that would permit the individual units to better carry out their roles. The focus was at the operating entities, not each system as a whole.

The holding company systems emphasized their ability to respond to a facility while letting it maintain its historical role and identity. It was this feature that attracted free-standing hospitals and nursing homes into these systems. The nonsecular systems did have a common focus derived from their founding groups, but this focus had historically been expressed through single facilities and was not necessarily limited to health care. The formation of a legal separate health care structure did not disturb this connection. This was particularly evident in cases where individuals in a health care organization retained active involvement in the religious community, many times assuming greater personal responsibilities there than they had in the organization.

The investor-owned systems did maintain a common focus to a greater extent. Stimulated by their need to demonstrate their ability to transfer management techniques from other industries, they concentrated on those functions that appeared to be similar, such as financial services. This left the clinical areas to develop independently (similar to clinical services in independent hospitals).

As multiunit systems continued to develop and to realize their potential as single entities, they began to develop similar ideas. The concept of a single corporate management that would be responsible for diverse activities took hold, as did the idea of maintaining a portfolio of activities and subsidiaries.

The historical independence of individual units made internal change difficult. This pushed attention outward. Systems acquired a wide range of enterprises. They acquired laundries, restaurants, and medical device companies. They constructed medical offices and formed land development companies. They moved into services traditionally provided by outside organizations. Architectural, computer, and supply distribution services are all examples of acquisitions or start-up operations developed by systems. Ironically, in many cases the services had markets that were external to the system's market. If a system provided services to its own facilities, it was common for it to compete with outside organizations for the business. The individual units retained the prerogative to choose who they felt would best meet their needs. Although there were different nuances caused by dissimilar backgrounds, all of the historically different systems engaged in this type of diversification.

Although diversification did not create a common focus or achieve directed momentum, it did serve to bring the systems closer to these outcomes. It taught the senior management collectively how to create focus and achieve momentum for individual subsidiaries, and it reinforced the notion that, despite the barriers, the most important markets were internal. The lack of management experience with integrating start-ups and acquisitions resulted in a high percentage of failures. These in turn fostered a better understanding of how to select and manage new companies. They also stimulated the development of capabilities to recognize failure and then successfully exit.

Multiunit systems are now beginning to acquire the capability to construct an organizational focus and are using it to produce directed momentum. In part this focus is being fostered by the health care delivery system itself. As pressures increase for more integration and less fragmentation, the lines between professional and institutional territories blur, and the payers seek entities to hold responsible for defined population segments, it becomes more evident what direction the systems need to take. Effective organizational integration can only

occur if redesign and reallocation also occur. The underlying dilemma is how to create something new while maintaining and transforming what exists. To some degree, the general characteristics to aim for are known, but how to get from point A to point B is not.

In a sense, multiunit systems are now faced with the same situation that architects confront and deal with by using modified fast-track construction. Architects are able to conceptually outline the way they want the building to look based on certain need parameters. However, because they face certain constraints, particularly lack of time, they begin the construction of the foundation before there is a complete plan and use the same period to further detail what will be built on top of it. However, this approach is particularly difficult for multisystems to use in that there is no historical experience base to rely on.

This dilemma suggests that systems are going to need to rethink the way they approach their organizational future. Thinking strategically and then determining tactics is difficult given the uncertainty about what the systems are capable of within a given time frame. Much of the existing health care delivery system (including the multiunit systems) is based on historical modifications of older delivery forms. The situation the systems now face is like a jigsaw puzzle where the picture on the box can be briefly seen. However, when the box is open, it is discovered not all the pieces are there. New pieces will need to be created, others will need to be reformed, and putting the pieces together will take a new set of strategies and tactics. During this process, some of the newly created pieces will need to be rebuilt and some discarded.

One of the key characteristics that make multiunit systems capable of completing this new puzzle is their maturing ability to construct a common focus and direct their momentum. The adoption of total quality management by some of the systems demonstrates this. When a system adopts this management philosophy, all components become involved in improvement efforts that force restructuring and reintegration of existing services. Activities are continually evaluated based on objective criteria. Those that cannot pass this evaluation are either redesigned or discarded. There is an understanding that the multiunit system as a whole has to have this focus. Finally, there is a clear realization that a major effort involving many years is required. Subsequently, management will have to create ways to maintain momentum in an organized and committed fashion. It is difficult to predict whether total quality management will be the vehicle to transform multiunit systems. It is clear that the experience gained by being involved in the process will create an additional foundation for making improvements in the future.

Multiunit systems started their existence with little or no common focus. They developed the ability to focus by concentrating on diversification and acquisition. To achieve a systemwide focus, they need to integrate individual perspectives into a single organizational whole. At least implicitly, there is starting to be a recognition of the need for directed momentum. It will take an application of system discipline for a system to use its critical mass to establish systemwide integration.

ASSET MAXIMIZATION

The health care system is different from other service industries. The particular nature of the services it provides has created social institutions with special status and societal obligations. This is particularly true for the tax-exempt organizations; their release from tax obligations is increasingly being weighed against their ability to demonstrate benefits to the community. The uniqueness of health care presents multiunit systems with special problems. As health care continues to increase its consumption of the nation's gross national product and multiunits accelerate their consolidation of the delivery system, the burden of redesigning the national health care system is going to fall on these organizations. Their existing role and image competes with their future responsibilities. For example, they are currently held accountable by their

constituencies for providing technological enhancements. There is a growing recognition that burdening the existing delivery system with these continuing additions will not be an accepted or viable option in the future. Multiunit systems are faced with having made tremendous capital investments in existing delivery vehicles without having a clear policy mandate as to how to change or access sufficient new capital to develop a new delivery model even if the direction was clear.

This challenge underscores the importance of the third principle—asset maximization. The cost of change is high. It is the capability of multiunit systems to take tangible and intangible assets, focus on what makes a difference, and institute changes that transform the delivery system. Critical to this transformation is the existence of a continuing balance between maintaining the old while substituting the new. The object is to use assets not just to institute change but to manage it in such a way that the stress of the change does not prevent the achievement of broad goals.

Asset maximization is probably most evident in the utilization of human resources. The greatest asset that multiunit systems possess is people. When the multiunits were created, individuals working in the component institutions suddenly had a better chance of being able to stay within the same organizational environment but still achieve personal growth. To some degree this was a function of the number of opportunities that were available because of the size of the systems. When individuals transferred from institution to institution in a given system, it created stability and continuity in the system as a whole. It also taught the individuals that they could rely on a single organization to provide them with room to develop professionally. This was essentially a new concept for the health care industry. For the systems, it began to lay the groundwork for career tracking.

As systems diversified, much of the growth was internally driven. Previously, people had accepted the idea of moving within the system but still thought in terms of moving upward in the traditional sequence. For example, an assistant administrator would become an associate administrator, then an administrator, and finally assume corporate officer responsibility. Now there were new positions in new institutions that were internally grown or acquired. An individual could become involved in a start-up venture or move to a newly purchased subsidiary. New careers were created in areas such as sales. People could choose these career alternatives while remaining in the same organization. The focus of career development shifted from taking positions in the right sequence to doing the right things. Opportunities for upward mobility expanded to allow several different approaches to the next position. For example, an assistant administrator could become a director of marketing in a subsidiary, then move to the presidency of a new acquisition, return to a line administrator position, and end up as a senior vice-president for affiliated services. Simultaneously the systems began to value the divergent experiences of their staff.

These changes created a new relationship between the systems and the individuals. Individuals moved from gaining experience within their functional areas to being encouraged to try new areas or at least apply old functions to new activities. They were given new measures of success and failure. Individuals began to distinguish careers in systems as opposed to single institutions. They began to view career commitment to a system as longer term than commitment to single hospitals, and they expected to gain access to a variety of roles and responsibilities in exchange for such a commitment.

The systems continue to evolve. They began to lay the groundwork to establish long-term agreements with current employees. The systems' unique needs (caused by the changes they were undergoing) and the lack of outside pools of individuals with compatible experience directed them internally. They learned to articulate their needs in an organized fashion and to value the new positions while maintaining a balance with the traditional hierarchy. As an example, compensation no longer was always based on position but tended to be based on whether an individual possessed the knowledge and skills to perform groups of activi-

ties. This permitted both the old and the new positions to achieve parity. Multiunits have learned ways of stimulating some people to seek new roles while retaining others to continue the traditional activities that are critical for their future success.

As multiunits move to become integrated delivery organizations, they will need to capitalize on what they have in order to create what they will become. Their ability to maximize their assets will be based on capabilities created during their development. They balanced the provision of existing services with the creation and addition of new ones and simultaneously created new delivery mechanisms. Existing assets were rearranged in organizational structures that mirrored and supported these new mechanisms. New assets were created by maximizing what existed.

The greatest organizational changes occurred in nonclinical areas. The clinical services were moved and shifted as the systems changed. Vertical integration was described as the organizational linking of subsidiaries such as hospitals, nursing homes, home health agencies, and outpatient clinics. It is only recently that clinical services have begun to be explicitly integrated based on episodes of care. The emphasis of shifting from mere working together to designing a seamless sequence of services intended to meet each individual's specific health care needs.

There are several catalysts accelerating this change in delivery design. The first is managed care, with its emphasis on providing total care for enrolled individuals. The second is the shift in payment mechanisms that now prospectively set reimbursement limits per case. Even competition has played a role, as the financial need to retain patients, residents, or clients becomes more evident. Whatever the particular history of a specific multiunit, most are going to again undergo major redesign. Given the inability of the U.S. economy to contribute more resources to support the conversion, their success will depend on their ability to capitalize on existing assets to effect the transition.

Using human resources again as an example, there are already indications that this transition is occurring. As case management envelops care outside an institution, clinical training is expanding to allow professionals other than physicians to accept greater responsibilities. This is particularly true in the supportive services (e.g., home therapy) or where the health condition lends itself to predetermined and prospectively agreed treatment (e.g., rehabilitation following hip replacement). This development has encouraged many multiunits to create their own internal education and training programs or to seek special relationships with educational institutions that will tailor curricula to meet their specific needs. The size of a particular system and numbers of individuals who enroll provide a basis for long-term programs. It is important to recognize that multiunits are again tapping internal pools. They have enough individuals with the specific organizational knowledge who, when trained properly, can facilitate the transitions they are pursuing. Also, by matching the size and scope of educational programs with the rate of organizational change, they can maintain the balance between redesign and the short-term financial viability. It is the size of the multiunits' assets,

coupled with their historical understanding of how to differentially maximize these assets, that makes them uniquely able to achieve this balance.

This maximization of human resources is evident in the changing relationships between physicians and multiunits. In most systems, the traditional interaction between medical staff members and their hospitals still exists. The difference is that there are also new and developing ties. Some multiunits are merging with physician group practices. Others are forming their own group practices and employing physicians. Systems are employing physicians in specific functions (e.g., as emergency room physicians or as locum tenentes). What is important to note is that many of these new arrangements are at the system level. It is at this level that the medical staff can best be directed and that knowledge has accumulated about how to manage professionals who do not fit traditional institutional positions. Many of the organizational human resource processes developed in early stages, such as compensation programs, are now being applied to physicians.

James E. Orlikoff

Governance

10

Purpose: The governing board is the ultimate authority of the hospital or system and provides oversight and direction for the planning, operation, and evaluation of all programs, services, and activities. It also hires and monitors the chief executive officer.

GOVERNANCE PRINCIPLES AND FUNCTIONS

The board is the ultimate authority of the hospital or health care organization and as such bears the final responsibility for everything the organization is, does, and becomes. Governance has been succinctly defined as "the fulfillment of the function of responsible ownership."[1] A more expansive description of hospital and health care organization governance is as follows: The responsible stewardship and allocation of health resources to produce a sustained benefit to the community and, in the for-profit sector, the shareholder.

Houle defines a board as "an organized group of people with the authority collectively to control and foster an institution that is usually administered by a qualified executive and staff."[2] Thus, a crucial point about governance is that the authority of the board rests with the board as a whole and not with any of its individual members.

The board has the fundamental responsibility for leadership but must employ negotiation and delegation to share this responsibility with the executive management and the medical staff. There are several broad categories of basic governing board functions, including mission stewardship and organizational oversight and evaluation, board organization and self-evaluation, management oversight and relations, planning oversight, quality oversight, medical staff oversight and relations, and financial oversight.

ROLE OF GOVERNANCE IN THE HEALTH SYSTEM

The Evolution of Hospital Governance

Benjamin Franklin became the nation's first hospital trustee when he founded the nation's first hospital, Pennsylvania Hospital, in Philadelphia in 1752. Franklin organized other local citizens into a board of trustees whose primary function was to donate and raise money for the construction and continued operation of the hospital. By doing this, Franklin ushered in the first, and longest-lasting, developmental stage of hospital governance: the board as philanthropic fund-raiser.

From these origins, hospital governance evolved in three stages (see also Figure 10-1)[3]:

1. the honorific-philanthropic stage (the emphasis is on fund raising)
2. the transition stage (the emphasis is on education)
3. the active-effective stage (the emphasis is on board effectiveness and self-evaluation)

The first stage of hospital governance, the honorific-philanthropic stage, lasted for over two hundred years, until the mid-1960s. During this stage, trustees on the hospital board were chosen primarily for their wealth, fund-raising ability, and stature as business or community leaders. The honorific-philanthropic board had very little responsibility for the oversight or strategic direction of the organization and practically no responsibility for the quality of care or the oversight of the medical staff. During this stage, hospital boards were largely fund-raising figure heads.

In the honorific-philanthropic stage, the effectiveness of the hospital was largely independent of the functioning of the board. Boards were insulated from the hospitals they supposedly governed and,

other than raising funds, had minimal impact. Over time, the mission, structure, function, and complexity of the hospital dramatically changed and the honorific-philanthropic model of hospital governance became increasingly inappropriate. In 1965, as a result of the advent of government payment for health care (with the inception of the Medicare program) and the landmark malpractice case *Darling v. Charleston Community Memorial Hospital,* the honorific-philanthropic stage of hospital governance in the United States ended and the transition stage began.

The transition stage saw the expansion of the legal basis of the board's responsibilities and functions as well as a significant increase in the board's legal duties. In particular, the board's legal duties of care, loyalty, and obedience were expanded or reframed during this period. The transition stage led, in the early 1980s, to the third and current stage of health care organization governance: the active-effective stage.

In the active-effective stage of governance, board members are selected who recognize and accept their ultimate legal and ethical responsibility for the governance of the health care organization. The active-effective model board defines its roles and responsibilities in relation to those of management and the medical staff, sets goals and objectives for itself, and evaluates its own performance relative to those goals and objectives. A key characteristic of an active-effective model board is that it

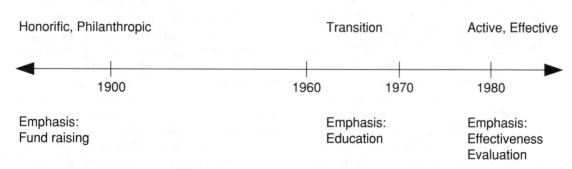

Figure 10-1 Evolution of the Governing Board's Role

recognizes the critical importance of collaboration between management, the medical staff, and the board for the development of an effective and viable hospital or health care organization.

In examining the transition of governance from the honorific-philanthropic stage to the active-effective stage, it is useful to look at the issue of responsibility for quality of care and oversight of the medical staff. From Franklin's first hospital in 1752 until the mid-1960s, the responsibility for quality rested primarily with individual physicians or groups of physicians. The putative ultimate authority of the hospital, the board, had no real responsibility for the quality of care provided by or within the hospital. Furthermore, the board had no real responsibility for meaningful oversight of the medical staff.

This is evident in the 1902 Michigan Supreme Court ruling in the case of *Pepke v. Grace*. Here the board of a Michigan hospital sought to be more active in overseeing the activities of the medical staff via more rigorous board involvement in the medical staff credentialing process. The medical staff took great umbrage at the board's actions and sued the board. The case went to the Michigan Supreme Court, which ruled as follows:

> The trustees of a hospital are laymen. The rules of the hospital provide for a medical board . . . who have charge of all surgical matters in the hospital. They examine applicants . . . and recommend such appointments to the trustees. . . . The trustees, who are laymen, must naturally leave the competency of the physician . . . to the judgement of those competent to determine such matters, since they are not qualified to make the determinations themselves. [The board] performed their full duty . . . in appointing a [medical] board to examine applicants.[4]

This ruling reinforced the prevalent and persistent view that the board's role in determining which physicians could be members of the medical staff and which clinical privileges they could have was basically to rubber-stamp the decisions of the medical staff. Similarly, the board during this period was also regarded as having no responsibility for oversight of the quality of care.

In 1965, the famous *Darling* malpractice case significantly altered the concept of the board's responsibility for quality and medical staff oversight. In this case, a malpractice suit was filed by Mr. Darling and his family against a physician and the Charleston Community Memorial Hospital. The suit alleged that the physician provided negligent care and the hospital was negligent in its failure to supervise the physician's treatment of Darling's fractured leg, which resulted in gangrene and the subsequent amputation of the leg.

The physician settled out of court and the case proceeded against the hospital, which became the sole defendant. In court, the hospital defended itself with the argument that the physician, not the hospital, was responsible for the practice and quality of medicine. Thus, it was the physician who should be held liable for the bad outcome, not the hospital.

In its ruling the court rejected the hospital's argument and ruled against the hospital. According to the court,

> Present day hospitals, as their manner of operation plainly demonstrates, do far more than furnish facilities for treatment. . . . Certainly the person who avails himself of hospital facilities expects that the hospital will attempt to cure him, not that its nurses or other employees will act on their own responsibility. . . . Licensing, per se, furnished no continuing control with respect to a physician's competence, and, therefore, does not assure the public of quality patient care. *The protection of the public must come from some other authority, and that, in this case, is the hospital board of trustees.*[5] (Emphasis added)

The court ruled that the hospital board had the ultimate responsibility for the quality of patient care and for the oversight and control of the medical staff and employees. This notion was a significant, if not revolutionary, development in the history of hospital and health care organization boards.

The far-reaching changes in governance that the *Darling* decision initiated are evident in the comparison of two simple graphs. Figure 10-2 shows the legal and conceptual relationship between the hospital governing board, the administration, and the medical staff as it existed prior to 1965 and the

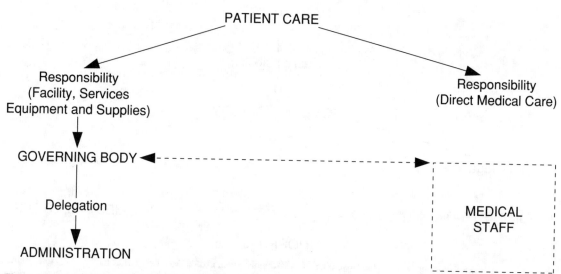

Figure 10-2 Legal Relationship between the Governing Body, Administration, and Medical Staff Prior to 1965. *Source:* Reprinted from *The Guide to Governance: A Manual for Hospital Trustees* by M.K. Totten, J.E. Orlikoff, and C.M. Ewell, p. 1, with permission of American Hospital Association, © 1990.

Darling decision. The responsibilities of the hospital board were limited to the facility itself and its equipment, nonmedical services, finances, and supplies. The board delegated these responsibilities to the hospital administration, although it maintained some responsibility for overseeing the administration.

Figure 10-2 also portrays the pre-*Darling* relationship between the board and the medical staff. The hospital board during the honorific-philanthropic period did not have organizational authority over the medical staff, and the board and medical staff are seen as coequal organizational bodies with authority over very different areas.

The impact of the *Darling* decision can be seen in Figure 10-3. The results of the decision and the changes in state laws and regulatory requirements it stimulated strikingly altered the organizational, legal, and conceptual relationship between the health care organization governing board, medical staff, and management. The ultimate responsibility for quality patient care, and indeed everything within the organization, is plainly seen as resting on the shoulders of the board.

The Changing Relationship of the Board to the Health Care Organization

As the health care environment changes, so does the character and function of health care organization governance. When hospitals were in a relatively unchallenged environment characterized by predictability and stability, the contributions of and the very need for a board (other than for fund raising) were questionable. However, since hospitals and other health care organizations now exist in an increasingly changing, challenging, and turbulent environment, it is almost universally recognized that the board and the way it functions inexorably influences the functioning and viability of the organization it governs. Kovner expresses this view by stating that "effective hospitals require effective boards. Hospitals cannot be effective, particularly when the environments they face are changing in important and often threatening ways unless they can make timely and appropriate decisions with due process for those affected by the decisions."[6]

If the board can indeed affect the health care organization, then it has the potential to be either an

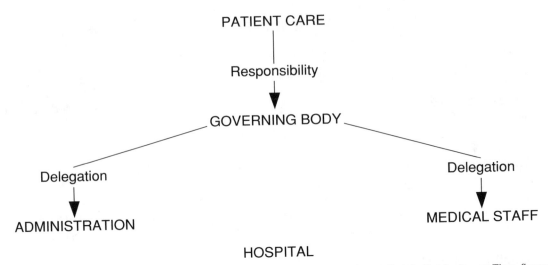

Figure 10-3 Legal Relationship between the Governing Body, Administration, and the Medical Staff at the Present Time. *Source:* Reprinted from Caniff, C.E., "Responsibilities and Relationships of the Medical Staff Administration, and Governing Body," Presentation at the American Medical Association seminar, Medical Staff: Physician Friend or Foe, April, 1980.

asset or a liability to the organization. This is in marked contrast to earlier days, when the board could be safely assumed to have no substantial effect on how the organization operated.

Furthermore, just as the changing environment requires constant adjustment in the planning, structure, and operation of the health care organization, it also requires change in the structure and operation of the governing board. Thus, the definition of good governance will evolve depending upon the circumstances confronting the health care organization and board. What was effective governance this year, what contributed to the success of the organization, may be ineffective governance next year and result in damage to the organization.

This indicates one of the key characteristics of an effective board—that it is a dynamic, evolving group. An effective board "must be elastic, able to stretch and adapt as circumstances warrant. Yet at the same time, it must be sufficiently resilient, disciplined, and self-aware to"[7] change shape and function when conditions change.

The dynamic and changing role of the nonprofit hospital board can be better understood by considering the relationship between hospitals and the community. This relationship is threatened by challenges to the tax-exempt status of nonprofit hospitals, the demand on hospitals to operate as efficient businesses and to provide charitable services to the community, and the erosion of traditional geographic competitive boundaries between hospitals, among other things.

As the important relationship between a hospital and its community is strained by such issues, a new role for the board emerges (or that role, if existing, becomes emphasized). To put it briefly, the board must act as a link between the community and the hospital. This role is reflected by the increasing consideration given by boards to the health status of the community as a whole, not just the patients being treated.

PROFILE OF HOSPITAL GOVERNING BOARDS

Just as board functions have changed since the inception of the hospital, so have board structure and composition changed. There have been changes, for example, in the method of selecting board members, in board size and composition, and in reporting relationships among multiple boards. Many of these changes have been stimulated by the profound changes in the health care field.

Board Size

The first hospital boards tended to be rather large (many had 75 members or more). Having a board with numerous members makes sense if the board's primary purpose is philanthropic: The more members on the board, the more money that can be donated or raised by the board members. Since the 1960s, however, boards have generally been decreasing in size.

Board size is often regarded as a significant structural characteristic that critically affects board functioning. Larger boards are often viewed as more likely to be ineffective because of their more cumbersome decision-making processes and the diffusion of board member commitment and involvement. Thus many governance consultants advocate smaller boards.

It is important to remember, however, that a board's structure and size do not inherently determine how the board functions; they can at most facilitate or inhibit the board's effectiveness. Thus the decision as to the size of a hospital board should be based on the individually defined roles and responsibilities of the board. Houle makes this point by saying that the board "should be small enough to act as a deliberative body . . . [and] it should be large enough to carry out the necessary responsibilities."[8]

Nevertheless, the trend toward streamlined boards is evidence of the emerging view that smaller boards tend to be better boards. In 1985, the average size of the board of all types of American hospitals was 14.64 members; by 1989, the average size of the board of all hospitals had decreased slightly to 13.86 members.[9]

Board Composition

The age distribution of board members has shown little change in recent years. For example, in 1985, 58 percent of all hospital board members were over 51 years of age, and in 1989 this figure had declined slightly to 57 percent. In 1989, the age of board members of all hospitals was distributed as follows: 1 percent were younger than 31 years, 42 percent were between the ages of 31 and 50, 52 percent were between 51 and 70, and, 5 percent were 71 or older.[10]

Board composition can also be examined in terms of the occupational background of board members. The current turmoil and change in health care calls for different expertise than in the past. This is reflected in a slight increase, during the years 1985–1989, in the proportion of board members with a health care background and a corresponding decrease in the proportion of those with a general business or financial background.[11]

Another aspect of board composition is the relative number of men and women. Research has shown that the overall number of women on hospital boards has not increased significantly from 1940 to 1980.[12] Unfortunately, national data on female membership on hospital boards past 1980 are unavailable. In 1940, approximately 17 percent of hospital trustees were women; in 1979, this figure had decreased slightly to 16.7 percent.[13]

Terms of Office

There has been a long-lasting debate regarding whether there should be a limit on the number of years or consecutive terms a trustee should be allowed to serve on a board. The proponents of unrestricted trustee tenure argue that an arbitrary limit would expose the board to the risk of losing talented and valuable trustees.

The argument for setting a limit on length of tenure or number of terms rests on the premise that boards that do not have regular trustee turnover become stale and complacent. Currently, most argue that the days of the "lifetime" trustee are gone forever, as "it is unreasonable to expect a volunteer trustee to devote substantial time and energy in these challenging and demanding times for indefinite or interminable periods of time."[14]

As this view gains currency, there is a moderate trend toward instituting maximum limits on the number of consecutive years that a board member may serve on the board. In 1985, 43 percent of all hospitals placed maximum limits on board member service and terms, and in 1989 that figure had risen to 48 percent.[15]

The Relationship between the Board and the CEO

One of the relationships most important for the smooth functioning of the board and the effective governance of the hospital is the board-CEO relationship. Effective governance and effective management require an effective and integrated working relationship between the board and the CEO.

The most basic perspective from which to examine the board-CEO relationship is the actual involvement of the CEO with the board. The number of CEOs who were board members with full voting privileges increased from 38 percent in 1985 (for all types of hospitals) to 42 percent in 1989.[16]

Another measurable factor relevant to the board-CEO relationship is whether a written employment contract exists. A written employment contract holds out the promise of a more structured and therefore more stable relationship between the CEO and the board. A contract can provide advantages such as clear expectations regarding the performance and the evaluation of the CEO, clear distinctions between the role of the CEO and the role of the board, and a level of protection to the CEO from capricious or inappropriate board actions. The proportion of hospitals that offered CEO employment contracts increased, during the period 1985–1989, from 39 percent to 44 percent.[17]

Another method of strengthening the board-CEO relationship and improving governance and management is to institute a standardized CEO performance evaluation process based on pre-established performance criteria or standards. Recently there has been significant increase in the number of hospitals using a formal CEO evaluation process: In 1985, 39 percent

of hospitals used a formal process, and in 1989 that figure had grown to 66 percent.[18]

The Relationship between the Board and the Medical Staff

Just as the board-CEO relationship is crucial to the functions of governance and management, so too is the relationship of the medical staff to the board crucial to the functions performed by the board and the medical staff. The involvement of the medical staff in the governance of the institution and in activities such as policy development is almost universally viewed as essential for the effective operation of the modern hospital. One measure of the relationship between the board and the medical staff is the extent of physician involvement in the governance decision-making process via board membership. In 1989, 88 percent of hospitals had at least one physician on the governing board.[19] Among those hospitals, there was an average of 2.24 physicians on the board, and the mean percentage of board members who were physicians was 16 percent.[20]

Another way of strengthening the relationship between the medical staff and the board is to have nonphysician board members participate as members of committees of the medical staff (often minus voting privileges). Hospitals showed an increase in nonphysician board members serving on medical staff committees from 1985 to 1989. Nonphysician board member participation was most common in the following medical staff committees: quality assurance committee, medical staff executive committee, utilization review committee, and credentials committee.[21]

Corporate Boards and Interboard Relationships

The roles and relationships of the board of a single health care entity are complicated enough, but the challenges of governance become even more daunting in the case of multiorganizational enterprises. The evolution of multihospital systems and vertically integrated hospital organizations, for example, has brought with it changes in the structure and function of governance. Frequently, one result of these changes is the emergence of multiple boards with different but related responsibilities and authority.

Clearly, multiple boards within a health care organization create issues that must be addressed to ensure effective governance and smooth functioning. These issues include the following:

> How will the organization integrate the efforts of these multiple levels of governance? What should be the respective roles and relationships of these various levels of governance? How should key policy formulation and decision-making functions be allocated among the multiple levels of governance? What levels of governance are best suited to address the key strategic decisions demanded of our organizations? How effective will policy-making and decision making be, given these multiple layers of governance? To what extent will multiunit organizations be able to strike an effective balance of integration and differentiation with regard to governance activities?[22]

Although these issues are of key importance, no universally accepted approach to resolving them has been developed. It is essential that they be considered and resolved, since in 1989 one of every three U.S. hospitals belonged to a multihospital system (defined as two or more hospitals owned or sponsored by a single administrative entity).[23] Further, 61 percent of hospitals in 1989 reported that the hospital board was accountable to a higher authority or board.[24] Following are the higher authorities to which the boards reported and the percentage of boards accountable to them[25]:

- parent holding company (53%)
- unit of government (23%)
- religious order (13%)
- other (5%)
- for-profit corporation (4%)
- university or college (2%)

As a multihospital system exercises greater control to achieve operating economies and efficiencies, the relationship between the system board and the local

hospital board changes. Frequently, the local board becomes more advisory in nature. Such a change carries with it the potential for friction and conflict between the local hospital board and the system board. A survey of 29 multihospital systems found that 19 reported at least one dispute between the system board and a local hospital board.[26] The disputes were in the following areas: local board authority, hiring or firing the hospital CEO, transfer of assets from the hospital to the system, allocation of capital, closing of a hospital, and local board member selection.[27]

A system board usually has reserved powers that give it ultimate authority on certain issues. Different system board–local board relationships have different allocations of final authority. Frequently, when a system board has final authority, the local board will make recommendations to it for approval or will make a decision that is subject to reversal by the system board if it exercises its reserved powers. In the survey of 29 systems, 58 percent of the systems reported that the system board had exercised its reserved powers and reversed a decision made by a hospital board.[28]

Multigovernance arrangements affect not only the relationships and relative authority of the different boards but also other relationships, such as those with the local health care organization CEO and medical staff. Clearly, one key to effective governance in organizations with multiple boards is to clarify and communicate roles, responsibilities, accountabilities, and authority. Likewise, the implications for other key relationships must be identified and addressed. The less clear these distinctions in authority, role, and relationships are, the more ineffective the governance of the organization will be.

GOVERNANCE ROLES, RESPONSIBILITIES, AND FUNCTIONS

The Legal Responsibilities and Accountabilities of the Board

The legal responsibilities of health care organization boards are simply stated, less easily understood, and often improperly discharged. Each board has important legal duties, including its fiduciary duty to act as financial overseer of the organization. The fiduciary duty also involves the two more specific duties of loyalty and responsible action.[29]

The duty of loyalty requires the individual board members to place the interests of the organization above their own interests. More specifically, it entails that "no trustee is permitted to gain any secret profits personally, to accept bribes, or to compete with the corporation."[30]

The second duty is the duty of responsible action. This duty requires board members to exercise "reasonable care, skill, and diligence proportionate to the circumstances in every activity of the board."[31] This means that the governing board must actually govern and direct, that the board members are not simply caretakers. The board must exercise reasonable care in governing the health care organization.

Distinct from its legal duties, the functions that a board is legally required to perform can be summarized as follows. First, the board is required

> to develop policy and articulate plans for both short- and long-range institutional goals. Second, the board is directly responsible for the appointment of staff, including . . . senior administrative officers and medical staff members and the delineation of clinical privileges. Third, the board has ultimate responsibility for reviewing and evaluating the professional performance of both lay administrators and the medical staff.[32]

Although a board performs many more functions, most of them fall into one of the three categories stated above. Still, the above perspective is legalistic and is a fairly limited and limiting view of the full scope of governance. The following section reviews the many roles, responsibilities, and functions of the board in greater detail.

Overview of the Roles and Responsibilities of the Board

Governance and Management: CEO Relations, Selection, and Evaluation

The relationship between the board and the CEO is key to every aspect of the ongoing operation of the health care organization. This crucial relationship is, unfortunately, often built upon implicit assumptions about relative roles, expectations, and performance objectives instead of routine communication and explicit objectives and expectations. Consequently, the board-CEO relationship is frequently not as stable or as effective as it should be.

The practical relationship between the board and the CEO has as its foundation a conceptual distinction between governance and management. Unfortunately, this distinction is often not understood well enough to form a solid basis for constructing a stable board-CEO relationship.

For example, governance is frequently equated with policy development, and management is equated with the implementation of policy. Put another way, the board decides *if* a health care organization will do something, and management decides *how* it will be done.[33] Does this mean that management does not participate in policy development or that the board does not monitor the implementation of the policy or occasionally fine-tune it? No, there is rarely an absolute division of these two intertwined functions.

Although many boards and CEOs seek, and many governance consultants proffer, a fixed universal definition of the relationship between governance and management, it is important to recognize that such a universal definition does not exist. Umbdenstock and Hageman speak to the issue by describing governance and management as

> related functions at either end of the same line, namely, the continuum of corporate leadership. On one end is governance or the creation of policy, and on the other end is management or the implementation of policy. Neither function can be complete when held in isolation from the other. "Who is responsible for doing what?" will be answered as the parties together move up and down the continuum, taking on the most appropriate roles and responsibilities depending on the issue and circumstances at hand.[34]

Thus, the practical distinction between governance and management must be tailored to fit each individual organization, and it must be revisited and revised as new circumstances and issues arise.

The relationship between the board and the CEO begins with the selection hiring process. The selection of a CEO is frequently cited as the most important decision that a board makes.[35] In fact, the selection process constructed by the board will often reflect its view of the governance-management continuum and will establish the context of the board-CEO relationship once a new CEO is chosen.

Although many CEO selection processes exist, they all share certain characteristics. In each type of process, for example, the board establishes criteria for the new CEO; decides on a search method, such as the use of outside executive search consultants; decides on a mechanism for reviewing candidates, such as a board selection committee; decides how the board will make the final selection; and defines the relationship using mechanisms such as an employment contract. Finally, the board establishes CEO performance expectations and objectives (i.e., develops a CEO job description). The last two tasks—the development of a CEO contract and the establishment of performance expectations and objectives—form the basis for a function that is crucial to maintaining a positive board-CEO relationship: the evaluation of the CEO's performance.

This evaluation is not a simple task and should not be approached lightly, since it will typically involve a reaffirmation or revision of the board-CEO relationship—of the distinction between governance and management. Yet, as critical as the board evaluation of the CEO is, many boards are uncomfortable with this responsibility, and there is a surprising degree of variability in the care and consideration devoted to carrying it out.

An effective CEO evaluation process is planned, deliberate, objective, and fair. Moses states that "the key to any evaluation process is its fairness. If either party is not completely satisfied with the process that is to be used, the evaluation is almost doomed from the start. Also, criteria that are going to be the basis for the evaluation must be agreed on. This of course requires input from the CEO as well as the board."[36] Thus, while the CEO evaluation is a governance function, interaction between the board and CEO is required in all phases of the process.

Evaluation is a key component of effective leadership. Thus, it is incumbent upon both the board and the CEO to participate in the evaluation of the CEO and also the evaluation of the board (discussed in a later section). The two evaluation processes contribute to the establishment and maintenance of an effective and productive relationship between the board and the CEO and to the effectiveness of the leadership of the hospital or health care organization.

Mission Development and Evaluation

A key responsibility of the board is the establishment, monitoring, evaluation, and articulation of the mission of the organization. McMillan defines the mission statement as

> the job description of your hospital stated in community terms, and it considers the community's needs, the hospital's medical capabilities, and the hospital's financial ability to serve. The statement is a tool designed to communicate what the hospital stands for. It is the beginning point of discipline that will allow [the board] to sensibly appraise requests for money, new equipment, new staff, and new facilities. The mission statement is the beginning of [the strategic] plan.[37]

Unfortunately, most hospital mission statements are so general as to be useless; they provide no definition of the hospital and outline no direction for it. In failing to define a mission adequately, a board abdicates an important responsibility. As a practical matter, it will also find itself without a guiding light during times of crisis and at critical decision points.

The mission is the rudder of the hospital and the board. It is therefore essential for the board to develop a meaningful mission, evaluate the mission routinely to verify that it is still valid, modify it when appropriate, and ensure that the plans and practices of the hospital are consistent with it.

Strategic Planning

The mission provides a basis for the development of the strategic plan. Once the board has overseen the development or refinement of a meaningful mission, its next responsibility is to make certain that strategic planning occurs—that a strategic plan is developed and is implemented on a schedule.

It is common for a board to assign the responsibility for strategic planning to a standing planning committee. The committee will often perform all the tasks of the planning process, including gathering background information on the hospital, identifying key environmental trends, reviewing the hospital's mission, identifying the strengths and weaknesses of the hospital, identifying the opportunities and threats, developing goals and objectives, examining alternate approaches and solutions, and recommending a course of action.[38] The board then considers the work and recommendations of the committee and makes the final decision on the strategic plan.

Strategic plans, however, are not static, and thus planning involves evaluating and modifying existing plans and continually developing new ones. Due to the accelerating pace of change in health care, the time horizons of detailed strategic plans have generally been shortened to one to three years.

Since the planning process is fluid and ongoing, the board or its planning committee will have to constantly monitor changes in the environment and in the needs of the community and the hospital. A key responsibility of the board, a responsibility usually delegated to the planning committee, is to evaluate the relevance and currency of the strategic plan regularly.

Medical Staff Relations

The rapidly changing health care environment confronts organizations with severe pressures and challenges that require closer, more effective working relationships between boards and medical staffs. Paradoxically, these pressures often polarize boards and medical staffs rather than unite them.[39]

The increasing stress is straining many board–medical staff relationships to the breaking point. Current pressures include increasing organization and board scrutiny of physician performance and utilization patterns, National Practitioner Data Bank reporting requirements for actions adversely affecting physician privileges, economic competition, conflicts over the allocation of resources, and reductions in physician income and changes in physician behavior due to fundamental changes in reimbursement under the Medicare Resource-Based Relative Value Scales (RBRVS) system.

Profound adverse effects on the relationships among boards and medical staffs and between physicians are predicted to result from these pressures.[40] These relationships will be stressed because of increasing competition between physicians and hospitals; increasing physician reluctance to serve in medical staff leadership positions, at least not without compensation; the desire of many hospital-based physicians to renegotiate their compensation arrangements with their hospitals; increasing conflicts among physicians over who can perform which procedures and services, and conflicts for which hospital boards will be the ultimate referees.

Although the governing board and the medical staff both have a duty to try to maintain a good working relationship, the ultimate responsibility for preventing and managing conflict and for building and nourishing the relationship rests with the board. To develop an effective relationship, the board might consider the following strategies:

- conduct a structured assessment of the current relationship to identify strengths and weaknesses

- conduct activities that strengthen the medical staff as an organization, such as medical staff self-evaluation and role clarification

- improve the structure and flow of communication between the board and medical staff

- clearly define the roles and responsibilities of the board, management, and medical staff

- conduct regular leadership retreats to which the board, medical staff leadership, and senior management are invited

- look for opportunities to enhance the practice of physicians and to make the hospital more efficient from their perspective

- provide compensation for the elected leaders of the medical staff

- create the position of medical director or vice-president of medical affairs

Maintaining a healthy and productive relationship between the medical staff and the health care organization is critical to achieving the organization's mission, providing quality care, and ensuring continued financial viability. A healthy and productive relationship does not occur as a result of luck or benign neglect. It is achieved only through planning, managing change, monitoring, and revising, and these actions should be initiated and overseen by the board.

Financial Oversight

Most board members are familiar with the board's responsibility for financial oversight of the institution. The role of the board, however, has changed because of a number of factors, such as new payment mechanisms that threaten financial viability, increasing competition from alternative delivery systems, conflicting mandates from the government, and the rapid development of high-cost technologies.

Nevertheless, the board is ultimately responsible for maintaining the financial viability of the organization it governs. The board fulfills this responsibility by "approving financial goals and monitoring management's progress toward achieving those goals; establishing financial policies and monitoring adherence to those policies; monitoring the hospital's system of control to safeguard its financial resources and to ensure compliance with government regulations."[41]

Many people join a health care organization board with a basic understanding of finance acquired from running their own business or being on boards of other organizations. Nevertheless, it is critically important for all members of a hospital board to understand the unique characteristics of hospital finance.

First, a board must develop an understanding of the different revenue sources of the organization, including their unique characteristics and requirements. Next, it should develop an understanding of the cost of the care that the organization provides.

The board can then perform the important function of monitoring the cost of the hospital's care in relation to reimbursement rates.

In performing this function, the board should consider an important issue that relates to finance: the impact of finance and cost control on the quality of care provided. It is this issue that contributes most to the uniqueness of health care organization finance from the board's perspective. Bradford and Tiscornia point out that for a board to exercise meaningful financial oversight, "trustees of for-profit and not-for-profit hospitals alike must be able to make decisions that help their hospitals maintain patient care at a high level of quality while generating more money than [they spend]—and to understand how the difference can be allocated most effectively."[42]

Hospital and Community Advocacy

A hospital is a crucial resource for the community it serves, and many different groups in the community have a stake in the hospital. These groups also have power over the hospital—power to influence the hospital's reputation, stature, and viability positively or negatively. Thus, it is essential that the hospital communicate with the various groups and stakeholders to maintain good relations and to identify and respond to their concerns.

The board and its members are in a unique position to communicate the hospital's message to the community and to find out about community interests and concerns and communicate these back to the hospital. Many hospital boards are identified as "community representative boards," which emphasizes their role in community and hospital advocacy. There are many advocacy activities that a board or its members can perform. These include explaining the organization's position on issues to legislators; educating the public via the media and personal appearances about organizational issues and health issues; acting as a spokesperson for the organization; acting as an ambassador of the organization at important community gatherings; and serving as a host and guide when community, media, or legislative groups visit the organization.

Board Development

The board also has the responsibility to make certain that it develops as a deliberative and decision-making body. This function, broadly referred to as board development, encompasses such activities as new trustee recruitment and orientation, board continuing education, and board self-evaluation.

Trustee recruitment involves identifying prospective board members and persuading them to join the board. Typically this process is overseen by a committee of the board, such as the nominating committee. New trustee selection is not a function performed by the board if board members are politically appointed or are elected by the community or shareholders.

Once selected, each new board member should undergo orientation. The orientation should provide the board member with information about the unique nature of the health care organization and about the health care field in general. It should also focus on the roles and responsibilities of the board and the board members. The orientation should be regarded as an ongoing process lasting several months. The better the orientation, the more prepared the new board member will be to contribute effectively.

The end of the orientation process should not, however, mark the completion of the education of the board member. Ongoing education is a cornerstone of board development and effective governance, especially in turbulent and rapidly changing times. Thus, arranging regular board retreats and education programs, sending members to external educational events, and subscribing to publications and videotape series designed especially for health care organization board members are all part of a necessary continuing education process that can help a board improve the way it functions.

Board Structure and Organization

The board also has a responsibility to organize itself. For example, it must address such issues as board size, board committee structure, and meeting frequency. Decisions regarding board size and committee type and number should be based on the stated functions of the board.

Perhaps because of their larger size, hospital boards have traditionally had more committees than corporate boards.[43] The tendency toward smaller hospital boards, however, may lead to a decrease in the average number of committees. Most hospital boards conduct much of their work through their committees. A board's committees may perform detailed reviews, pursue agendas and objectives approved by the board, and make recommendations to the board for action.

The committee structure should reflect the board's method of functioning and its goals and objectives and should contribute to the board's effectiveness. For example, if a board is charged with the responsibility of electing its members and officers, one structural way of supporting this function is to establish a nominating committee. Executive, finance, nominating, planning, quality improvement, and joint conference committees are common standing committees. The joint conference committee is often a forum for communication and resolution of conflicts between the board and the medical staff.

Regardless of the number and type of board committees, committee performance can be improved and maintained at a high level through effective board oversight. The board oversees its committees by establishing a charge for each committee and approving an annual work plan and objectives. The board then can monitor the progress of each committee in relation to its stated charge, objectives, and work plan. The committee structure should not be static but should change as the issues confronting the organization and board and the set of priorities change.

QUALITY MANAGEMENT

Since 1965 and the *Darling* decision, boards have been held increasingly responsible for the quality of care provided by the health care organizations they govern. The responsibility of the board for quality stems from four broad and often overlapping factors: the ethical obligations of the board, the legal accountability of the board, the legislative and regulatory requirements that pertain to the board's activities, and the fiduciary responsibility of the board.[44]

Yet many boards and board members are uncomfortable with and uncertain as to how to discharge their responsibility for quality. This is because, among other reasons, the board responsibility for quality is of relatively recent origin; the majority of board members are not physicians or health care professionals and consequently are unfamiliar with hospital practices and medical terminology; quality is an elusive concept and is difficult to define practically; and the fact that board quality oversight requires board members to oversee medical staff personnel, whom many boards are intimidated by.

To oversee quality of care effectively and to contribute to its continuous improvement, the board should recognize that it has three related responsibilities. First, the board must monitor the organization's quality improvement program. Second, it must determine what the actual level of quality of care provided by the hospital is and where quality is in most need of improvement. Third, it must oversee the medical staff credentialing process.

Medical Staff Credentialing

Perhaps the most important quality assurance responsibility of the board is the credentialing of the physicians on the organization's medical staff. For many hospital boards, this governance function is the least understood and the most difficult to perform effectively.

The purpose of a hospital's medical staff credentialing system is to ensure that only qualified physicians are granted practice privileges and that the physicians practice within the scope of their capabilities and expertise. The phrase *medical staff credentialing* encompasses the establishment and implementation of policies and procedures for the initial appointment and reappointment of physicians to the medical staff and the granting and renewal of clinical privileges.

Although much of the work in the credentialing process is performed by the medical staff, the governing board must make certain that appropriate credentialing procedures exist. The medical staff assesses each physician applicant and makes a recommendation regarding admission or readmission to the medical staff and delineation of specific clinical privileges, but it is the board that makes the final decision.

Unfortunately, many boards are unfamiliar with their responsibilities and requirements regarding credentialing. Other boards, although perhaps familiar with their responsibilities, are uncertain as to how to discharge them effectively.

In either case, the result is likely to be a board that routinely rubber stamps the credentialing recommendations of the medical staff. Rubber stamping is an improper approach to this key governance responsibility and results in ineffective credentialing. An inadequately credentialed medical staff in turn can compromise the organization's quality of care, expose the organization to malpractice liability, and also expose the board to liability.

The key to meaningful and effective credentialing is to develop a clear distinction between the roles and responsibilities of the board and those of the medical staff and to use clear and objective decision criteria that allow the board to oversee the medical staff's credentialing process and to verify that the credentialing recommendations are consistent with those criteria.[45] Such criteria will meaningfully integrate the results of the quality review of physician performance into the reappointment and privilege renewal process.

Board Self-Evaluation

On January 1, 1986, a requirement of the Joint Commission on Accreditation of Hospitals became effective; it stated that "the governing body evaluates its own performance."[46] Beyond this simple requirement, there are other reasons for a health care organization board to perform periodic self-evaluations. The unforgiving health care environment demands nothing less than excellence in governance, and a well-constructed self-evaluation process can help a board improve its performance. Self-evaluation can also facilitate quick and appropriate board responses to rapidly changing external and internal pressures and can help the board recognize, accept, and more effectively discharge its many responsibilities.[47]

Board self-evaluation has been defined as "an organized process by which the board regularly examines its goals and objectives, structure, processes, and collective and individual performance, and then reaffirms its commitment by adopting new goals and improved methods of operation."[48] Self-evaluation provides a board with a structured opportunity to both look back and plan ahead. The process allows the board members to ask themselves such questions as these: What are we doing well? What could we be doing better? What are our objectives? How well did we achieve our objectives? Why did we fail to achieve certain objectives? The board then uses the answers to develop and implement an action plan to improve its performance and establish new goals.

Typically, the board self-evaluation session consists largely of a facilitated discussion about the compiled anonymous responses of board members to a detailed questionnaire. This discussion is the real meat of the self-evaluation process.

During the discussion, a number of issues, questions, and concerns will arise. These will then form the basis for an action plan. The action plan lists areas to be addressed by the board, establishes the priority of the issues, establishes deadlines, and assigns responsibility for action.

Self-evaluation is an integral component of effective leadership. Boards that recognize this tend to integrate self-evaluation into their routine activities.

Indicators of Quality in Governance

Much of the focus on hospital governance concerns structure, process, function, roles, responsibilities, and the like. Ewell points out that there has been very little effort devoted to measuring the out-comes of board activities and suggests that this will soon become a focus of investigation.[49]

Ewell proposes the development of "governance indicators" that would measure the structure and process of governance and also the outcomes. He suggests that these indicators be developed for the key areas of responsibility, such as financial oversight, planning oversight, quality oversight, and management oversight. Measurement of outcomes of board activities in these areas could be achieved through comparative assessments of financial status, market position, and quality improvement over time and continuity of management and other personnel.[50]

Whatever governance outcome indicators are developed, a focus on outcomes will yield critical information. This information can then be used by the board to strengthen its performance and improve its outcomes, which will in turn improve the organization that it governs.

ISSUES IN GOVERNANCE

Board Member Selection

For boards that elect, appoint, or recommend their own members, a crucial question routinely faced is, Who should be on the board? Obviously, the members of the board will affect how the board operates and so should be chosen based on their likely contribution to the stated board functions.

The problem is that many boards do not have clearly stated or accepted functions. If this is the case, asking who should be on the board is putting the cart before the horse. The questions should flow in this order: What is the board supposed to do? What board members will contribute most to the board's effectiveness in doing what it is supposed to do? Although this is a logical progression, it is seldom simple to arrange for the issues to be dealt with in this straightforward way.

This is because most hospital boards have many functions, some explicit, some implicit. Each function places different, and frequently contradictory demands on the board. For example, if the board is supposed to "represent the community," that suggests the membership should represent a cross-section of the community. If the board is supposed to exercise business acumen, that points toward selecting trustees with business expertise. Individuals with professional backgrounds in health care may contribute to the board's effectiveness, so might individuals with legal or accounting or social service backgrounds, and so on. Clearly, the members of the board should be chosen based upon the purposes and functions of the board. Hageman states that "a board interested in improving its performance will recognize the need to develop an organized approach to recruiting and selecting trustees. It simply makes good sense to link the selection of individuals who meet specific criteria with the performance goals of the board."[51]

The problem of choosing board members is compounded by the current tendency toward smaller boards. Smaller boards may have advantages, but they make the process for selecting board members all the more important by eliminating the margin for error in selection allowed by larger boards. How then should a board select its members?

Board member selection can be made more effective by two strategies: determining the goals and objectives of the board and developing a profile of who is currently on the board to discover what strengths exist and what needs should be met.[52] In this way, each board can develop evolving and meaningful criteria for new board member selection and can build and maintain board effectiveness through focused board composition.

Board Member Compensation

The issue of board composition leads to other questions: Is a volunteer board appropriate given today's competitive environment? Should board members, especially of nonprofit community hospital boards, be paid?

The general trend is away from board member compensation. In 1985, 36 percent of hospitals provided some type of compensation to their board members; in 1989, that figure had significantly decreased to 23 percent.[53] Compensation, however, can take many forms, such as annual or per meeting fees or free or reduced medical services. When examined by type of compensation, the incidence of board compensation becomes clearer. In 1985, 21 percent of hospitals provided board members with a per meeting fee only, and this sharply decreased to 7 percent in 1989; the drop in this category accounted for almost all the decline in overall board compensation from 1985 to 1989. Interestingly, the incidence of annual fees only increased from 1 percent of all hospitals in 1985 to 2 percent in 1989.

Some argue for the use of professional board members who are paid to bring specific professional talents and services to the board. For example, Kovner states,

> Paying board members will ease the reticence of holding board members accountable and expecting them to give more time to board activities.... Paying board members does not necessarily diminish the community-oriented and charitable mission of the hospital. Paying board members can increase board diversity as lower-income members of the community may now be more willing to give of their time to the hospital. Perception of the benefits of this recommendation may depend upon the amount of compensation.[54]

Many others, however, reject the idea that board compensation is a valid approach to attracting and retaining better board members. For example, one observer states that "in developing a list of pros and cons, it quickly appears that the list of cons is lengthier than the potential advantages of paying hospital board members."[55] Among the cons are the following:

- It is inconsistent with the idea of trusteeship as a civic responsibility.
- It may offend the volunteer trustee's sense of engaging in a community service.
- It may generate conflicts of interest.
- It may change the loyalty of the board away from the mission and toward the short-term financial success of the institution.

- It may decrease routine turnover among board members.

Proponents of both sides of this issue are equally adamant. Although the trend from 1985 to 1989 was away from board member compensation, this issue is at a crossroads. It arises in most board rooms today and will likely continue to do so for quite some time.

The Role of the Board Chairperson

The effectiveness of a governing board is largely determined by its leadership. For most boards, the dominant leader is the chairperson, although leadership authority is shared to varying degrees with the officers of the board, the executive committee, and the chairs of the board committees.

The role of the board chair is to oversee or direct almost all board activities. Duties include devising meeting schedules and setting agendas, presiding at board meetings, planning for leadership succession, and initiating and overseeing the CEO evaluation and board self-evaluation processes, among many others.

Effective board leaders usually have a mixture of professional and personal characteristics. For example, they usually have tenure on the board; maintain good relations with management, medical staff leaders, and other board members; participate in the organization's strategic planning activities; are able to make a significant commitment of time and energy; and possess integrity, independence, and a balanced perspective.

Just as the selection of board members is an essential task, so is the selection of the board chair. Some boards take a successional approach to selection of the chair, requiring the chair to have served for several years in a series of lesser board leadership positions. The benefit of this approach is that each chair is fully oriented to the organization and the board. The main drawback is its inflexibility: Almost any individual on the leadership track will become chair regardless of his or her past performance in the lesser positions.

Other boards elect their chairs, using selection criteria or not. Whatever method is used, the approach to selecting the board chair should share many characteristics with the approach discussed earlier for selecting board members. The strategy is to determine the functions of the board, determine the kind of individual who would most effectively lead the board, and select the individual who displays most of the relevant characteristics.

Effective governing boards require strong, capable leaders. Unfortunately, many board leaders are chosen for reasons of political convenience, availability, tenure, or rotation or on the basis of other criteria unrelated to leadership ability. If a good leader emerges from such a selection process, it is often due more to luck than to planning.

A board leader can either help or hurt the board that he or she leads. The selection of a chair should be a planned, deliberate process. The final decision should be based on the stated functions, goals, and objectives of the board and on a clear job description of the position.

Ethics in Governance

Health care organization boards are increasingly called upon to make difficult decisions on issues that arouse extreme feelings among people in any way associated with or affected by the organization. Such issues might include policies on AIDS testing for patients and health professionals, abortion, termination or withholding of treatment, providing care for the medically indigent, allocation of health resources that denies certain populations access to care, and acquisition of new technologies. Decisions on such issues all have an ethical dimension.

Traditionally, ethics in governance was considered to be restricted to such issues as conflict of interest, self-dealing, and confidentiality. However, now ethics in governance is usually assumed to encompass the process of the entire board.

Essentially, ethical decision making involves establishing conceptual foundations that support enduring principles, and use of these principles in turn enables consistent choices and decisions to be made. In a health care organization, the conceptual foundations are usually to be found in the mission statement, and the enduring principles are usually to be found in those documents that codify the mission, such as the bylaws, strategic plans, and policies and procedures. Finally, the choices and decisions made by the board should flow from, reflect, and support the conceptual foundations and enduring principles.[56] The object is for the board to establish a common basis for decision making—a shared sense of purpose and shared values.

Ethical decision making is a necessity if a board is to function effectively in the current schizophrenic and volatile health care environment, which pressures hospitals to act simultaneously as businesses and charities. Boards require an ethical foundation to guide their decisions so they can avoid becoming paralyzed by attempting to respond to multiple, frequently contradictory demands. Ethically based decisions have a consistency, predictability, and focus that engenders trust and respect among the leaders and stakeholders of a health care organization.[57]

Directors' and Officers' Liability

Increased board responsibility and accountability brings increased board exposure to liability. The liability of the governing board is called directors' and officers' liability, and there are two separate categories: the organization's liability for the actions of its governing board and the personal liability of individual board members.

Historically, three types of lawsuits have most frequently been brought against hospital boards: injunctive relief suits, breach of contract suits, and damage suits.[58] There are four types of protection from directors' and officers' liability: indemnification provisions in hospital bylaws, liability insurance, state statutory "immunity," and board risk management.[59]

An indemnification provision in the health care organization's bylaws ensures that board members will be compensated by the organization for losses that board members are legally obligated to pay and that are related to their being members of the board. An indemnification provision, however, is only as good as the organization's financial ability to back it up.

The next level of liability protection is insurance. No insurance policy provides complete liability protection to board members and the hospital, as all policies contain coverage limitations and exclusions. Typically, insurance coverage limitations and exclusions are in the exact areas of a board's greatest liability exposure.

Many states have passed legislation to provide immunity from liability for directors of nonprofit organizations, and such state statutory immunity is the third level of protection from liability. However, each statute contains limitations and exclusions, vague language, and loopholes.

The exceptions and exclusions are quite broad and considerably limit the immunity granted by the statute.

Thus, it is quite possible for a board to be covered by an indemnification provision, a directors' and officers' liability insurance policy, and state statutory immunity and still have significant liability exposure. The foregoing approaches are not complete solutions to the problem of liability because, in addition to their significant individual weaknesses, they place no emphasis on preventing liability. That is the purpose of the fourth method of protecting boards and trustees from liability: governing board risk management.

Governing board risk management consists of a series of activities designed to minimize the board's liability exposure and reduce the risks of lawsuits while enabling the board to govern the health care organization effectively. A board risk management program usually has three main steps: (1) Determine potential areas of board liability exposure, (2) assess the degree of liability exposure in each area, and (3) implement actions to minimize liability exposure in high-risk areas.[60]

By instituting a systematic governing board risk management program, a board can prevent liability claims, significantly reduce its exposure to liability, and lessen its dependence on the frequently volatile directors' and officers' insurance market. In a demanding and competitive health care environment, no boards can afford to be timid or hesitant in its decision making. By knowing the strengths and weaknesses of their indemnification provision, directors' and officers' insurance, and state statutory immunity, trustees will have a clear picture of their liability exposure. Sound board risk management practices will then enable board members to govern and make difficult decisions without the paralyzing fear of liability.

THE FUTURE OF GOVERNANCE

The ability of a board to anticipate and respond to environmental change, along with its ability and willingness to change itself and the health care organization it governs, will partly determine whether the organization is successful or is even able to survive. Yet there are some who question the necessity of having an "effective" health care organization governing board. (In fact, some ask, why have a board at all?)

Why is having an effective board essential for a vital health care organization? Empirical answers to this deceptively simple question will soon emerge from recently initiated research into the relationship between the degree of success of health care organizations and the degree of effectiveness of the boards that govern them. Although the results of this research are not yet available, compelling empirical evidence on the necessity of boards and board effectiveness has been gathered in a similar sector.

Specifically, an investigation into the relationship between board effectiveness and institutional performance has been conducted in the area of higher learning. Chait and others studied 21 independent liberal arts and comprehensive colleges over three years. They found that "there is a positive and systematic association between the board's performance . . . and the college's performance, as measured against some conventional financial indi-

cators."[61] Why should not the same be true for health care organizations, especially in the current environment of constrained resources and tough choices?

Why is a board necessary at all? The answer is that it provides consistent direction and critical oversight, keeps a focus on the mission, and helps to manage the incredibly complex relationships that form the health care organization. These relationships are as critical to the success of an organization as they are complex and unstable, and they must be carefully nurtured.

Why is an effective board necessary? In other words, why is it necessary to have a board that does more than act as a figurehead, does more than rubber-stamp the decisions of others? The answer is that an ineffective board will contribute to organizational decline—financial instability, regulatory compliance problems, challenges to tax-exempt status (for nonprofit organizations), deteriorating relationships with the medical staff, poor relations with the community, and on and on.

What, then, defines governing board effectiveness? One persuasive view holds that an effective board has the following five critical components:

1. A common working definition as to *"What is governance?"* and what it means for the leadership roles, responsibilities and relationships within the particular organization;

2. A clearly defined mission with specific *goals* and *objectives* for the organization that drive virtually *everything* the board does;

3. A well planned *decision-making* process based on the specified priorities and ongoing responsibilities of the board, and supported by a continuing education process that prepares the board for critical decisions it knows it must make in the future;

4. A *board structure* that is tailored to the priorities at hand and which enables the efficient accomplishment of the board's work; and,

5. An *information, reporting and communication system* that keeps the priorities clearly in focus and that utilizes formats to help the board ascertain progress toward the accomplishment of its goals.[62]

To expand on this, Chait found that there are specific characteristics and behaviors that distinguish strong boards from weak boards. Although the research was restricted to college governing boards, it seems reasonable to suggest that the results of the research apply to the boards of health care organizations as well. The characteristics of strong boards are divided into six distinct dimensions:

I. *Contextual Dimension.* The board understands and takes into account the culture and norms of the organization it governs.

II. *Educational Dimension.* The board takes the necessary steps to ensure that trustees are well-informed about the institution, the profession, and the board's roles, responsibilities, and performance.

III. *Interpersonal Dimension.* The board nurtures the development of trustees *as a group,* attends to the board's collective welfare, and fosters a sense of cohesiveness.

IV. *Analytical Dimension.* The board recognizes complexities and subtleties in the issues it faces and draws upon multiple perspectives to dissect complex problems and to synthesize appropriate responses.

V. *Political Dimension.* The board accepts as one of its primary responsibilities the need to develop and maintain healthy relationships among key constituencies.

VI. *Strategic Dimension.* The board helps envision and shape institutional direction and helps ensure a strategic approach to the organization's future.[63]

Boards in the future will embody the above characteristics of effectiveness. Board members will recognize that they can be an asset or a liability to the health care organization they govern. They will accept that the organization's need for an effective board is a normal state of affairs rather than the result of a crisis. Senior management will also accept this and will embrace the notion that strong, capable managers require an effective board to complete the necessary strategic partnership required to lead any health care organization today and in the future.

It is important to note, however, that the characteristics of board effectiveness will not be static and will change as the environment changes. What will the characteristics of effective boards in the future likely be? Although no one can answer this question with any certainty, a reasonable prediction is that governing boards will be changemasters. Their main role will be to help their organizations embrace change and even create it—view it as an opportunity for organizational development. Further, future boards are likely to focus much of their attention on systems as opposed to a few component parts. They will strive to see the big picture, identify the patterns that combine to create it, and act to influence them.

Future boards will facilitate the development of a collective organizational vision among key stakeholders and then will actively attempt to articulate it. Finally, each board will probably go beyond focusing on its own organization to involve itself in the continuing reformation of the health care system.

As the health care environment changes, the character and functions of health care organization governance will also change. The current environment confronts organizations with constrained resources, increasing competition and regulation, and demands for the demonstrated provision of high-quality, cost-effective care, among many other daunting challenges. Clearly, in such a demanding and unforgiving environment, any health care organization needs effective leadership, and such leadership must be provided by the governing board.

ADDITIONAL RESOURCES

General Governance

Carver, J. *Boards that make a difference.* San Francisco: Jossey-Bass, 1990.

Chait, R.P., et al. *The effective board of trustees.* New York: American Council on Education and MacMillan, 1991.

Duca, D.J. *Nonprofit boards: A practical guide to roles, responsibilities, and performance.* Phoenix: Oryz Press, 1986.

Houle, C.O. *Governing boards.* San Francisco: Jossey-Bass, 1989.

Mattar, E.P., and M. Ball, eds. *Handbook for corporate directors.* New York: McGraw-Hill, 1985.

O'Connell, B. *The board members book: Making a difference in voluntary organizations.* New York: The Foundation Center, 1985.

Health Care Governance

Alexander, J.A. *The changing character of hospital governance.* Chicago: Hospital Research and Educational Trust, 1990.

Bader, B.S. *Three waves of change: Hospital board responsibilities in the new health care environment.* Rockville, MD: Bader & Associates, 1986.

Health Administration Press. *Frontiers of Health Services Management* 6, no. 3 (Spring 1990). (*Note:* This entire issue is devoted to commentaries on health care governance effectiveness.)

Mott, B.J.F. *Trusteeship and the future of community hospitals.* Chicago: American Hospital Publishing, 1984.

Rindler, M.E. *The challenge of hospital governance: How to become an exemplary board.* Chicago: American Hospital Publishing, 1992.

Totten, M.T., et al. *The guide to governance: For hospital trustees.* Chicago: Hospital Research and Educational Trust, 1990.

Umbdenstock, R. J., and W. M. Hageman, eds. *Critical readings for hospital trustees.* Chicago: American Hospital Publishing, 1991.

Periodicals

Action Kit for Hospital Trustees. Pittsburgh: Horty, Springer & Mattern, P.C.

Health Governance Digest. Chicago: Orlikoff & Associates.

Trustee Briefing. Chicago: Modern Healthcare.

Trustee: The Magazine for Hospital Governing Boards. Chicago: American Hospital Publishing.

NOTES

1. R.J. Umbdenstock, The Role of the Board and Its Trustees, in *Health Care Administration: Principles and Practices,* eds. L. F. Wolper and J. J. Pena (Gaithersburg, Md.: Aspen Publishers, 1987), 51–52.

2. C.O. Houle, *Governing Boards* (Washington, D.C.: National Center for Nonprofit Boards, 1989), 6.

3. M.K. Totten et al., *The Guide to Governance: A Manual for Hospital Trustees* (Chicago: American Hospital Association, 1990), 1.

4. *Pepke v. Grace,* 130 Mich. 493 (1902).

5. *Darling v. Charleston Community Memorial Hospital,* 33 Ill2nd, 326, 211 NE 2d 253 (1965).

6. A.R. Kovner, Improving Hospital Board Effectiveness: An Update, *Frontiers of Health Services Management* 6, no. 3 (1990): 15.

7. R.P. Chait and B.E. Taylor, Charting the Territory of Nonprofit Boards, *Havard Business Review,* January-February 1989, 54.

8. Houle, *Governing Boards,* 66–67.

9. J. Alexander, *The Changing Character of Hospital Governance* (Chicago: Hospital Research and Educational Trust, 1990), 4.

10. Ibid., 5.

11. Ibid., 6.

12. *Focus on Women on Health Care Boards: Their Changing Role* (Chicago: Hospital Research and Educational Trust, 1987), 12.

13. Ibid.

14. J.E. Orlikoff, Burnout in the Boardroom: Recognizing and Preventing a Growing Problem, *Trustee* 43, no. 6 (1990): 11.

15. Alexander, *Changing Character of Hospital Governance,* 8.

16. Ibid., 13.

17. Ibid.

18. Ibid., 15.

19. Ibid., 17.

20. Ibid.

21. Ibid., 19.

22. H.S. Zuckerman, New Issues and Expectations for Governance, *Frontiers of Health Services Management* 6, no. 3 (1990): 44.

23. Alexander, *Changing Character of Hospital Governance,* 11.

24. Ibid., 12.

25. Ibid.

26. J. Greene, Hospital, System Boards Adjust to Changing Role, *Modern Healthcare,* September 2, 1991, p. 22.

27. Ibid.

28. Ibid.

29. A.F. Southwick, *The Law of Hospital and Health Care Administration,* 2d ed. (Ann Arbor, Mich.: Health Administration Press, 1988), 114–115.

30. Ibid., 124.

31. Ibid., 126.

32. Ibid., 122–123.

33. R.J. Umbdenstock, *So You're on the Hospital Board!* 2d ed. (Chicago: American Hospital Publishing, 1983), 12.

34. R.J. Umbdenstock and W.M. Hageman, *Hospital Corporate Leadership: The Board and Chief Executive Officer Relationship* (Chicago: American Hospital Publishing, 1984), 6.

35. B. O'Connell, *The Board Member's Book: Making A Difference in Voluntary Organizations* (New York: The Foundation Center, 1985), 67.

36. R.P. Moses, *Evaluation of the Hospital Board and the Chief Executive Officer* (Chicago: American Hospital Publishing, 1986), 57.

37. N.H. McMillan, *Planning for Survival: A Handbook for Hospital Trustees* (Chicago: American Hospital Publishing, 1985), 40.

38. Ibid., 112.

39. J.E. Orlikoff, Brave New World: RBRVS and the Importance of Effective Relationships between the Hospital and the Medical Staff, *Health Governance Digest* 1, no. 6 (1991): 3.

40. *The Future of Healthcare: Physician and Hospital Relationships* (Chicago: Arthur Anderson and the American College of Healthcare Executives, 1991).

41. C.M. Bley and C.T. Shimko, *A Guide to the Board's Role in Hospital Finance* (Chicago: American Hospital Publishing, 1987), 3.

42. C.K. Bradford and J.F. Tiscornia, *Monitoring the Hospital's Financial Health: A Guide for Trustees* (Chicago: American Hospital Publishing, 1987), xiii.

43. Totten et al., *Guide to Governance,* 13–14.

44. J.E. Orlikoff and M.K. Totten, *The Board's Role in Quality: A Practical Guide for Hospital Trustees* (Chicago: American Hospital Publishing, 1991), 21–22.

45. J.E. Orlikoff and M.K. Totten, Medical Staff Appointments and Privileges: Key Role of the Governing Board, *Trustee* 41, no. 4 (1988): 14–15.

46. Joint Commission on Accreditation of Hospitals, *Accreditation Manual for Hospitals 1986* (Chicago: Joint Commission, 1985).

47. J.E. Orlikoff, Taking the Mystery out of Board Evaluation, *Trustee* 39, no. 1(1986): 24.

48. B.S. Bader et al., *Board Self-Evaluation Manual* (Rockville, Md.: Bader & Associates, 1986), 15.

49. C.M. Ewell, Measuring the Performance of Hospital Governing Boards, *Modern Healthcare,* February 19, 1990, p. 48.

50. Ibid.

51. W.M. Hageman, Targeting the Board's Strengths and Weaknesses, *Trustee* 40, no. 10 (1987): 28.

52. Ibid.

53. Alexander, *Changing Character of Hospital Governance,* 25.

54. Kovner, Improving Hospital Board Effectiveness, 18.

55. C.M. Ewell, Should We Pay Hospital Boards? *Trustee* 42, no. 7 (1989): 21.

56. J.E. Orlikoff, Ethics in Hospital Governance: A Decisionmaking Framework, *Trustee* 42, no. 7 (1989): 28.

57. Ibid.

58. J.E. Orlikoff and A.M. Vanagunas, *Malpractice Prevention and Liability Control for Hospitals,* 2d ed. (Chicago: American Hospital Publishing, 1988), 102.

59. J.E. Orlikoff, What Every Trustee Should Know about D & O Liability, *Trustee* 43, no. 1 (1990): 8.

60. J.E. Orlikoff, Preventing Directors' and Officers' Liability Exposure, *Trustee* 40, no. 6 (1987): 13.

61. R.P. Chait et al., *The Effective Board of Trustees* (New York: Macmillan Publishing and the American Council on Education, 1991), 2.

62. R.J. Umbdenstock et al, The Five Critical Areas for Effective Governance of Not-for-Profit Hospitals, *Hospitals and Health Services Administration* 35 (1990): 485–486.

63. Chait et al., 2–3.

Rockwell Schulz
Donald E. Detmer

Physician Organization and Management

11

Purpose: The main responsibilities of a medical staff organization are to develop effective working relationships among physicians so that patients receive optimal service; to help physicians apply advancing medical knowledge and technology in the treatment of their patients; and to establish management structures and processes that assure patients, other physicians, and payers that such treatment is provided appropriately, effectively, efficiently, and humanely.

INTRODUCTION

The role of physicians vis-à-vis organizations has changed dramatically in the last 50 years. Before World War II, most physicians were in solo general practice. Their organizational exposure was with hospitals that served as their workshops. Hospital management's role was to obtain nursing and facility resources to serve each individual doctor. The hospital roles of physicians increased after World War II. Increasing physician and other health worker specialization necessitated coordination of physician hospital practices through the medical staff organization. Even more important,

expectations for quality as defined by the Joint Commission on Accreditation of Hospitals imposed increasing organizational constraints on physicians to ensure high-quality care. While the medical staff was a self-governing organization, the *Darling* case (*Darling v. Charleston Community Memorial Hospital* 33 Ill. 2nd 325, 211 N.E. 2nd 253, 1965) made it clear that hospitals themselves, not just the doctors, have responsibility for quality of care. Hospital management was expected to make certain that the medical staff fulfilled its obligations for managing quality assurance. In the 1970s and 1980s, Medicare requirements for utilization and quality controls and especially diagnosis-related groups (DRGs) imposed hospital management on clinical practice. Not only did physician–hospital management relationships become closely intertwined, but increasing competition for patients forced many physicians into managed care organizations such as health maintenance organizations (HMOs) and preferred provider organizations (PPOs).

As physician practice moved from the office and bedside to complex organizational settings, physicians, organizations, and their managers have become increasingly interdependent. Physicians can no longer practice effectively outside an organizational setting. By the same token, health service organizations cannot survive and serve without effective physician services and leadership. It is the thesis of this chapter that management and all key participants, including physicians, share the responsibility for developing effective relationships to achieve organization goals.

Managing for Effective Organization-Physician Relationships

This chapter begins by proposing certain principles managers should consider in their relationships with physicians. Next it describes the organization of physician services in solo and organized settings.

Physicians are a select group of individuals who undergo long and rigorous training and who are essential resources for hospitals and other health service organizations. The supply of physicians is growing, but problems of distribution remain. Within the hospital or other health service organization, management has a responsibility for ensuring that physician services are efficient and of high quality. Quality management in hospitals is accomplished by establishing medical staff bylaws, credentialing physicians, and monitoring and evaluating physician services. Forces such as increasing competition, revenue constraints, government and corporate intrusions, malpractice litigation, and ethical issues strain the relationship between managers and physicians but underscore their interdependence. There are both organization structure and management process opportunities for integrating physicians and hospitals. The importance of a team approach to the challenges of the 1990s and beyond is emphasized.

Management Principles in Physician Organization and Management

The following principles are useful for developing an effective physician-organization relationship:

1. Physicians have primary legal responsibility for patient diagnosis and treatment and as such should serve as patient advocates. Managers too should serve as patient advocates, since the primary purpose of the organization is to meet health care needs of the local community.

2. There should be adequate staff, facilities, systems, and procedures for physicians and other caregivers to serve patients and their loved ones effectively and efficiently.

3. The organization structure, systems, and procedures should ensure high-quality care by physicians and other caregivers. They should also promote patient satisfaction.

4. There should be a culture that emphasizes working collaboratively in pursuing the organization's mission and objectives. The culture should foster early and ongoing physician involvement in strategic planning and implementation; respect for physicians; open, honest, and persistent communication; development of strong physician leadership; willingness to explore alternative organizational forms; willingness to collaborate; and a knack for managing the pace of change.[1]

THE ROLE OF THE PHYSICIAN

The physician's historic leadership role in diagnosis and treatment has not changed substantively in recent years, but patterns of medical practice and the role of the physician in hospitals have changed dramatically.

Mission

The mission of physician services has remained essentially unchanged over the years. It is best described by the oath most physicians take upon graduation from medical school. In the past, this was the Hippocratic oath, but because of changes in positions on abortion, the Declaration of Geneva adopted by the General Assembly of the World Medical Association in September 1948 is now more frequently used. This pledge is as follows:

> At the time of being admitted as a member of the Medical Profession:
> —I solemnly pledge myself to consecrate my life to the service of humanity;
> —I will give to my teachers the respect and gratitude which is their due;
> —I will practice my profession with conscience and dignity;
> —The health of my patient will be my first consideration;
> —I will respect the secrets which are confided in me;
> —I will maintain by all the means in my power the honor and the noble traditions of the medical profession;
> —My colleagues will be my brothers [and sisters];
> —I will not permit considerations of religion, nationality, race, party politics or social standing to intervene between my duty and my patient;
> —I will maintain the utmost respect for human life, from the time of conception;
> —Even under threat, I will not use my medical knowledge contrary to the laws of humanity;
> —I make these promises solemnly, freely and upon my honor.

While the mission of medicine may have changed little, the organizational role of physicians has changed a great deal over time, especially in the last decade. In the early part of this century, the physician could carry most of the standard medical equipment in a leather bag and apply the accepted technologies at the patient's bedside. As medical technology advanced, medical practice moved into the hospital and increasingly into organized practice settings. Competition for patients has been another stimulant to physicians moving their practices into settings such as HMOs and PPOs.

The practice of medicine has historically been accorded professional status. A profession has been generally defined as "an occupation that regulates itself through systematic, required training and collegial discipline; that has a base in technical, spe-

cialized knowledge, and has a service rather than profit orientation enshrined in a code of ethics."[2]

In his classic book *The Social Transformation of American Medicine,* Paul Starr described the profession's gaining control over technology in the early 1900s, which was legitimized by the Flexner Report.[3] The medical profession was successful in obtaining practical autonomy from governments, corporations, and other payers. Physicians had not only clinical autonomy but organizational and economic autonomy. In recent decades, such autonomy has been eroded considerably by federal and state government and by corporations. It has also been diminished by the citizens, who have sought legal recourse in cases of malpractice in ever-greater numbers. Moreover, as knowledge and technology increased and funding and markets became more competitive, managers of health services organizations gained much greater authority over and control of the resources needed by physicians. Nevertheless, physicians are accorded legal authority for the care of individual patients and are thus considered to be clinical leaders.

Patterns of Physician Practice and Reimbursement

Although there are many different models for delivering physician services, they fall into four basic categories: (1) independent solo practice, (2) single-specialty group, (3) multispecialty group, and (4) hospital-based practice.

Independent Solo Practices

Although increasing numbers of physicians are joining group practices, independent solo practices (i.e., physicians who practice alone or practice with others but without pooling income or expenses) still dominate in some communities. In many respects, *independent solo practice* is a misnomer. Much of a physician's practice centers around the hospital he or she is associated with, involves other health professionals, and is subject to peer review by hospital colleagues. Moreover, increasing numbers of solo practitioners provide care to HMO and PPO patients in managed care settings.

Solo practice has certain theoretical advantages for both the physician and patient. The physician has more independence than in other models of care. The solo practitioner also has more flexibility in referring fee-for-service patients. This may be an advantage to the patient, since referral can be to the most competent physician instead of being limited to the physician's group. By dealing with one physician in the practice, patients are likely to have more continuity in their relationship with their doctor. Disadvantages of solo practice include less coverage for both the doctor (call and insurance coverage) and the patient and less professional interaction and quality review. With the growing supply of doctors and the greater prevalence of managed care, it is becoming increasingly difficult for physicians to enter solo practice because of the high cost of purchasing a practice or establishing a new one (unless in a rural area where the community provides assistance). Practitioners are also joining groups to avoid the administrative burdens of trying to manage complicated insurance, fiscal, and regulatory matters and to be more price competitive.

Single-Specialty Groups

In a single-specialty group practice, physicians in the same specialty (e.g., pediatrics or orthopedic surgery) pool their expenses, income, and offices. A group practice with three or more physicians is usually sufficiently large to employ some sort of business manager. The single-specialty group model resembles the solo practice model more than the multispecialty group model, except that the physicians can take emergency calls for each other and at least have informal quality reviews and interaction.

Multispecialty Group Practices

A group practice encompassing different medical specialties would be considered a multispecialty group. The Mayo Clinic in Rochester, Minnesota, was one of the pioneers of multispecialty practice. This model provides for more professional interaction (which can support quality assurance) and has the potential for skilled management. On the other hand, physicians are less independent, they have less freedom to refer to physicians outside the group, and costs and revenues are frequently higher because of greater use of ancillary services. Dividing incomes between procedure-based specialties, such as surgery, and cognitive-based specialties, such as pediatrics, is a frequent source of tension in multispecialty groups.

Many of the larger multispecialty groups have added a group model HMO to their fee-for-service practice. The experience of practicing together and pooling income and expenses has facilitated adoption of a managed care HMO practice. Some group practices have also vertically integrated their group with hospital services. Examples include the Cleveland Clinic and Hospital and the Mayo organization and the Methodist and St. Mary's Hospitals in Rochester, Minnesota. The Permanente Group of the Kaiser Health Plan is an example of a large multispecialty group organized as a staff model HMO.

Hospital-Based Practices

Increasing numbers of physicians are basing their practices in hospitals, especially tertiary care centers. Traditionally this has been true of pathologists, radiologists, and anesthesiologists. Physicians employed by the Veterans Administration, mental health institutions, medical schools, and some large public hospitals have also been hospital based. More recently, hospitals have contracted or employed full-time emergency room physicians. Larger hospitals have also employed physicians as medical directors and full-time department chiefs (frequently minus clinical duties). Moreover, as described later, increasing numbers of physicians are selling their practices to hospitals.

Physician reimbursement within group practice models varies widely. Expenses are usually taken off the top, and the balance of revenue is distributed on the basis of fees for service or some formula that takes into account a combination of factors. Physicians in staff model HMOs are usually on salary, as are those in the VA system, many large public hospitals, and medical school settings. Except for the VA and staff model HMOs, some sort of incentive might be incorporated, with the base salary determined by physician billings for services. Pathologists, radiologists, anesthesiologists, and emergency room physicians frequently have contract, rental, or percentage arrangements with hospitals. Physician reimbursement practices have been a source of controversy among physicians, the institutions in which they practice, managed care payers such as HMOs and PPOs, and third-party payers such as Medicare, Medicaid, and commercial carriers. The growth of contracts for care is creating new pressure for larger systems, especially in cities, and the current environment is quite dynamic and likely to remain so as managed care becomes one of the organizing principles of American health care reform. Table 11-1 summarizes the strengths and weaknesses of alternative bases for physician compensation.

Medical Staff Organizations in Hospitals

The Joint Commission on Accreditation of Healthcare Organizations states,

> There [should be] a single organized medical staff that has overall responsibility for the quality of the professional services provided by individuals with clinical privileges as well as the responsibility of accounting therefore to the governing body. There [should be] a mechanism to assure that all individuals with clinical privileges provide services within the scope of individual clinical privileges granted.[4]

The Joint Commission defines clinical privileges as "permission to provide medical or other patient care services in the granting institution, within well-defined limits, based on the individual's professional license and his experience, competence, ability, and judgment."[5]

Traditionally, the medical staff has been considered a self-governing body responsible to the organization's governing board for the quality of care provided by individual physicians. An example of the relationships of a traditional hospital medical staff organization is shown in Figure 11-1. In this model, the medical staff is self-governing but accountable to the board for quality of care. A joint conference committee composed of board and medical staff officers, the CEO, and the medical director is commonly used as a liaison committee for formal communications between the governing board, medical staff, and hospital management.

Except where the medical staff is small, there is often an executive committee of the medical staff on which the hospital CEO or his or her designate serves with or without vote. Each clinical department or major clinical service monitors and evaluates the quality and appropriateness of care provided by member physicians and meets monthly to consider its findings. Chairpersons of the clinical departments are accountable or responsible for

- all professional and administrative activities within the department
- continuing surveillance of the professional performance of all individuals who have delineated clinical privileges in the department
- recommending to the medical staff the criteria for clinical privileges in the department
- recommending clinical privileges for each member of the department
- ensuring that the quality and appropriateness of patient care provided within the department are monitored and evaluated[6]

Because of the effort and time required to fulfill these responsibilities, many larger hospitals employ full-time medical directors and department chairs. In 1985, nearly half of the hospitals over 200 beds reported having paid medical directors.[7] The use of paid medical directors and department chairs is just one indication of the increasing integration of physicians and hospitals.

Table 11-1 Strengths and Weaknesses of Alternative Bases for Physician Compensation

Base	Advantages	Disadvantages
Fee-for-Service (individual procedure)	Automatic adjustment for case complexity	Provides incentive for overservicing per case treated
	Provider's reward is closely linked to his/her output of services	If fees for particular services do not stand in constant proportion to the cost of these services, fee-for-service compensation may tilt the treatment modality toward more profitable procedures
	Patients have economic clout over physician	
	Provides transparency of the physician's profile of practice	Inflationary tendency through ever finer decomposition of treatments into distinct, billable tasks
	Widely used throughout the world and typically preferred by physicians	
		Difficult to budget *ex ante*
Diagnostic-Related Groups (DRGs) (the medical case)	Logically the most compelling definition of the physician's "output"	It is technically difficult to force all cases into a finite list of DRGs
	Fairly good adjustment for variation in case mix (albeit not a perfect adjustment)	There may be a substantial variation of case complexity within a defined case category (DRG)
	Provider's reward is fairly closely linked to his/her output of services	To the extent that case complexity varies significantly within DRGs, physicians may engage in adverse risk selection of patients
	Provider has economic incentive to minimize the resource cost per medical case treated	Physicians may underservice their patients for the sake of economic gain
	Patients retain economic clout over physicians	Physicians may misrepresent diagnoses (DRG creep)
	Fairly good transparency of the physician's practice profile	The method is relatively untried here or elsewhere in the world
		Difficult to budget *ex ante*
Capitation (number of patients under continuing care)	No need to decompose physician's work into procedures or cases; therefore, administratively simple	Physicians have incentive for adverse risk selection and may dump patients with complex, costly conditions onto other providers
	Facilitates budgeting for health care *ex ante*	Physicians have incentive to underserve patients they do accept (to the extent that patients remain unaware of it)
	Provider's effort still somewhat linked to his/her effort	If average case mix varies greatly among physicians under one capitation system, capitation may be viewed as unfair
	Medical treatments are not influenced by the relative profitability of individual procedures	There is little transparency of the physician's practice profile
	Physicians have incentive to minimize the cost of medical treatments	
	Patients still have some economic clout over physicians if patients can change physicians from time to time	

continues

Table 11-1 Continued

Base	Advantages	Disadvantages
Salaried Practice (month or year)	Administratively simple	Unless salary can be linked somehow to output and patient satisfaction (as it is in group practices), patients lose economic clout over the physician who renders care as an act of noblesse oblige
	Medical treatments are not influenced by the relative profitability of individual procedures	
	Facilitates cooperation among physicians in treating complex cases	Physicians may underserve patients
	Facilitates budgeting for health care expenditures *ex ante*	There is little transparency of the physician's practice profile

Source: Reprinted from *Journal of Medical Practice Management,* Vol. 3, No. 2, pp. 85–95, with permission of Williams & Wilkins, © 1987.

In the 1980s, some physicians and hospitals jointly developed HMOs and PPOs to compete with other managed care organizations. Other types of joint ventures included ambulatory surgery centers, diagnostic testing centers, sports medicine centers, and primary care satellite clinics. According to Shortell, a hospital and a group of physicians might start a joint venture in order to increase patient referrals and revenue sources, extend the continuum of care by being able to move patients out of the hospital to less costly sites, bond the physicians to the hospital, and prevent the physicians from doing things exclusively on their own that would compete with the hospital's best interests.[8]

Organization of the Medical Profession

The American Medical Association (AMA) has long been the political voice of American physicians. It has worked to improve the quality of physician services and to protect physicians' clinical and economic independence. Over the years the power of the AMA has waned as more physicians have become specialists and have directed more of their attention to their own specialty societies. In 1975 a little more than half of all physicians were members of the AMA; by 1991 only 41 percent were members.[9]

Perhaps the main criticism of the organization among doctors is that the AMA does not represent the physicians' interests vigorously enough. There

are liberal groups in medicine, such as the Medical Committee for Human Rights and the Physicians for Social Responsibility; however, their membership is small. Much faster growing are conservative groups such as the Association of American Physicians and Surgeons and the Congress of County Medical Societies. In the view of these and other physician groups who are unhappy with the control of nonprofessionals over medicine, one answer is to unionize. Although AMA leadership remains opposed to true unionization (seeing it as a sellout of professional integrity), the physician union movement could gain support.

Specialty boards, (e.g., the American Board of Surgery) and specialty associations (e.g., the American College of Surgeons) have considerable influence on physicians and on the type of medical care received by consumers. The principal stated objective of specialty boards and associations has been to upgrade the qualifications of specialists. Over the years this has meant increasing training time, setting standards for specialty and subspecialty certification and recertification, developing subspecialties, and sponsoring numerous continuing education programs and professional journals.

RESOURCE REQUIREMENTS

In almost all health services organizations, physicians, who are the leaders of the clinical team, are

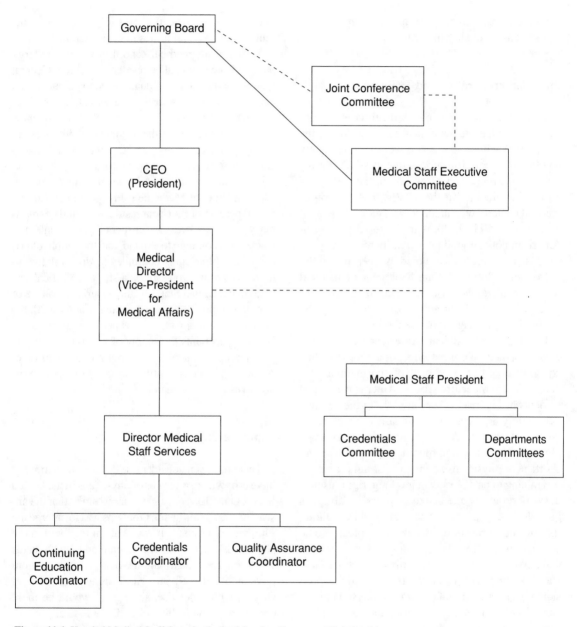

Figure 11-1 Hospital Medical Staff Organization and Services Department Relationships

essential resources. Physicians are a select group who undergo an especially long and rigorous period of formal training and continuing education. Because physicians order the technologies to be ap-

plied to patient care, most health care costs are attributed to physicians. A potential surplus of physicians has important implications for costs. In addition to providing technological staff and facility resources, hospitals need to provide support services to ensure quality of medical care.

Physician Preparation and Training

Competition for entry into medical school is substantial. For the medical class entering during the 1991–1992 school year, there were approximately 33,000 applicants for approximately 17,000 positions.[10] This represents a reversal of the steady decline of applicants in the 1980s. The "average" medical student, with an undergraduate grade point average of 3.40 in 1990, is in the top 5 percent of American college graduates. An increase in applications of 14 percent was noted in 1991 over 1990.

In 1968–1969, less than 8 percent of medical school graduates were women. This increased to 23 percent by 1978–1979 and to over 40 percent by 1990. The percentage continues to increase.

In 1990–1991, African Americans constituted over 12 percent of our nation's population, but they constituted only 6.5 percent of the medical students. The number of African American medical students has increased very slightly in the last few years. Only 3 percent of physicians in practice are African American. Although there is a surplus of physicians in many communities, there is a severe shortage of physicians serving racial minorities.

Training to be a physician is a long, rigorous process. It typically means four years to obtain a bachelor's degree, four years of medical school, three to eight years of residency, and typically some practice time before becoming certified as a specialist. Most graduates of U.S. medical schools pass state licensing exams on their first try, and few physician licenses are revoked. Once a physician is licensed, he or she, depending upon the state of practice, may or may not have to submit evidence of continuing education. Because of the rapid advances in medical knowledge, there have been attempts to make continued medical education mandatory. The American Academy of Family Practice requires it for continued certification, and a number of states require it for registration or continued

licensure. Recertification and relicensure are currently controversial issues in organized medicine.

Virtually all medical school graduates undergo postgraduate or so-called residency training. General practice, which most graduates used to go into after a one-year rotating internship, has essentially been replaced by family practice, which requires a residency. Less than 9 percent of the residents in 1988 were in family practice, but another 30 percent were in general internal medicine and pediatrics, also considered primary care specialties. A National Academy of Sciences Institute of Medicine study recommended that 60–70 percent of first-year residents should be in primary care.[11] However, subspecialty residents and residencies continue to expand, and the supply of primary care physicians continues to drop relative to need.[12] As long ago as 1975, a study of surgical services in the United States by the American College of Surgeons reported there were already at least 20,000 to 34,000 too many physicians performing surgery.[13] By many accounts the supply of general surgeons is nearly proportionate to need, but a number of other surgical specialties continue to grow out of proportion to estimated demand.

Supply of Physicians

There has been considerable debate whether or not there is or will be a surplus of physicians in the United States. Only 30 years ago it was assumed that the answer to America's health problems was to enlarge the supply of physicians. It was thought that, with more physicians, access to medical care and health status would improve; distribution would improve as more physicians filtered into rural areas; and medical charges would not rise, since there would be more competition. With this in mind, the federal government poured billions of dollars into increasing the number of medical schools by over 60 percent, expanding medical school class sizes, and developing physician extenders such as physician's assistants and nurse practitioners.

However, by the 1970s it became evident that medical care alone does not improve the health status of a population and that increasing the supply of physicians increases health care costs. Furthermore, as the number of physicians increased and the number of patients per physician declined, physicians performed more services and increased fees per patient. Even though each added physician has tended to increase aggregate health costs, it has been difficult to slow the production of physicians, nurse practitioners, and physician's assistants. In responding to national needs and incentives, medical and other health profession schools must find ways to increase the numbers of primary care physicians and stem the tide of subspecialists.

A 1980 report of the graduate Medical Education National Advisory Committee to the Secretary of the Department of Health and Human Services suggested that there will be 150,000 too many physicians in 20 years unless steps are taken to reduce the production and importation of physicians and extenders.[14] Since 1980, higher standards for admission of foreign-trained physicians has reduced the flow of physicians from abroad. However, medical school enrollments and the number of physicians in specialty and subspecialty training only declined slightly in the past few years. Ginzberg notes that, on the assumption that physicians are responsible for the decisions that govern about three-quarters of all health expenditures, an excess supply of physicians in 1990 of 25 percent "translates into a questionable outlay of $123 billion."[15]

Some speculate that there will be an even larger surplus because competitive medical plans (e.g., prepaid group practices and other managed care plans) will suppress the demand for services. However, another view proposes there will be no physician surplus by the year 2000.[16] Projections of no surplus are supported by estimates of increased demand from technological advances, an aging population, the need to serve those who are currently un- and underinsured, the desire for more leisure time by practitioners, and the move by more physicians into nonpatient care activities such as management. Whether or not a nationwide surplus will exist in the next century, shortages will probably remain in poor inner-city and sparsely populated rural areas, while surpluses will remain in many urban and suburban areas. Further, a maldistribution of generalist versus subspecialist physicians is also likely to persist despite efforts to balance the scales.

Support Services for Physicians

In addition to physicians, there are nearly 5 million other health workers, for a ratio of nearly 10 health workers per physician. Table 11-2 contains the ratio per physician for the more prominent health occupations. As might be expected, it shows that nursing is the largest group of health workers. In addition to these health workers and managers of health services, there are many administrative support staff in hospitals, doctor's offices, insurance companies, and other settings.

The number of physicians per organization vairies widely depending upon the type of institution; the services provided; the number of hospitals with which the physicians are associated; and the number of medical staff members in various categories, such as active, courtesy, associate, consulting, or honorary. Even a small hospital can have over 100 physicians on its medical staff.

The medical staff organization is considered to be self-governing under authority delegated by the hospital governing board.[17] (For more on medical staff/board relations see Chapter 10 on governance.) To fulfill its obligations, it should be given nine specific responsibilities, according to Thompson.[18] In particular, it should:

Table 11-2 Support Workers per Physician

Registered Nurses	2.94
Aides	2.50
Licensed Practical Nurses	.82
Clinical Laboratory Staff	.60
Therapists	.52
Pharmacists	.35
Radiology Staff	.25
Managers	.21
Dietitians	.16
Physician's Assistants	.10
Other	1.2

1. recommend to the governing board action on new medical staff applications
2. evaluate practitioner performance based on comprehensive data
3. recommend to the governing board action on applications for renewal or expansion of clinical privileges
4. provide continuing medical education
5. recommend to the governing body corrective action
6. provide corrective action for potential behavioral or practice problems that can be handled before they require governing board action
7. provide coordinated input to the CEO and the governing board regarding individual practitioners' concerns
8. submit regular and special reports to the governing body, including evaluation of practitioner performance, activities and recommendations of the medical executive committee, key features to support applications and renewals for individual staff appointments and privileges, and recommendations for corrective action
9. update medical staff bylaws and related documents

To meet these responsibilities, the medical staff organization must be provided with support services by the hospital.

QUALITY MANAGEMENT

Ensuring quality of care is a primary responsibility of management. The medical staff is delegated accountability for quality by the governing board. Management and physician leaders must be diligent in their efforts to make sure that the medical staff organization fulfills its responsibilities regarding quality assurance. The quality assurance system for physician services typically includes the establishment and enforcement of medical staff bylaws, rules, and regulations; credentialing and granting matching clinical privileges; and monitoring and evaluating the quality of care provided by the physicians.

Medical Staff Bylaws, Rules, and Regulations

Medical staff bylaws are the ground rules for the provision of services in the hospital. The hospital governing board approves and adopts the medical staff bylaws, and all members of the medical staff must sign an agreement to abide by them. Physicians have a responsibility to be familiar with the bylaws, rules, and regulations, and the hospital management and physician leadership serve as referees to ensure that they are followed and as scorekeepers and team managers to help the medical staff inform the governing board how the medical staff as a whole and individual physicians are performing. To help individual physicians be aware of the contents of the bylaws, rules, and regulations, they should be written as clearly and simply as is practical. Exhibit 11-1 presents an outline of typical components of medical staff bylaws.

Medical staff rule and procedure manuals are likely to contain rules such as those related to timeliness and completion of medical records and dictation of surgical reports. Other items might include specified meeting times, nominating procedures, and standard procedures for general staff meetings.

Credentialing

Quality assurance begins with credentialing of physicians to ensure they are qualified and competent to provide patient care services in the hospital. Indeed, court cases such as *Darling, Purcell v. Zimbelman* (Court of Appeals of Arizona; 500P. 2d 335 [1972]), *Johnson v. Misericordia Community Hospital* (301 NW 2d 156 [Wisc.1980]), and *Elam v. College Park Hospital* (132 Cal. App. 3d 332 [Ca 4th Cir, May 27, 1982]) attest to the legal responsibility hospitals have for the qualifications and competence of medical staff members. Credentialing is a process to help ensure qualifications and competence.

Exhibit 11-1 Components of Medical Staff Bylaws

Medical staff bylaws might include the following:
- A preamble describing the purpose and content of the document
- Definitions of terms to avoid misunderstandings and disagreements over meanings
- A description of what the medical staff is supposed to do and why
- Appointment provisions describing who is eligible and specific appointment procedures
- Categories of medical staff membership (e.g., active, provisional, courtesy, consulting, and honorary) and prerogatives and responsibilities of each
- A statement to the effect that staff members may exercise only those clinical privileges that they apply for and are granted
- Rules and procedures for considering membership for and requests to use hospital services by individuals who are not licensed physicians (e.g., psychologists, dentists, certified nurse anesthetists, podiatrists, and chiropractors)
- A description of the medical staff organization
- A description of the process by which the medical staff and governing board will institute corrective action for unacceptable physician behavior or practices
- A brief statement referring to bylaws-related documents (e.g., rules and procedures)
- Rules for adopting amendments to the bylaws
- Miscellaneous provisions (e.g., a statement about the position of medical director and its range of authority)

Medical staff bylaws will usually state criteria for membership as a first screen for applicants. For example, they usually include such items as type of practitioner (e.g., physician, podiatrist, dentist), appropriate professional license, appropriate educational and training credentials, professional liability coverage, and in many hospitals, board certification or eligibility.

The typical application form for medical staff membership and privileges requires considerable information, such as education and training, past and present professional service and society affiliations, licenses and certificates, litigation and liability history, references, and clinical privileges requested. It also usually contains a list of questions to help detect previous professional problems as well as a series of pledges, to which the applicant must agree, regarding professional and ethical conduct.

It is incumbent upon the hospital (e.g., the medical staff services department) to validate the information and investigate past performance for the medical staff credentials committee and the department to which the applicant is requesting privileges. Although reference and past performance investigations are usually informative, the hospital might also require a personal interview with the applicant. The hospital must query the National Practitioner Data Bank in the U.S. Department of Health and Human Resources. This databank stores information on actions related to professional conduct and competence, licensing status, and malpractice payments. In addition to the requirements for obtaining information about applicants, hospitals must query the databank every two years to check on the status of current medical staff members and privilege holders.[19]

Delineation of clinical privileges properly performed and monitored is the most important function of the medical staff and governing board. Each medical staff member must have specified clinical privileges based precisely on his or her training, experience, and proven clinical competence. The limits of the clinical privileges must be clear.

The credentialing process is also important for the reappointment of medical staff members. Using information furnished by the monitoring process, the clinical privileges of current medical staff members are reassessed at regular intervals. If a physician infrequently performs certain procedures in the hospital and elsewhere, continuation of the relevant privileges needs to be justified.

Monitoring and Evaluating Medical Staff Members

Traditional approaches to evaluating quality of care usually consider structure, process, and outcomes. Appraisal of structure involves evaluation of the personnel, equipment, and supplies that are needed and available. While structural properties may facilitate the provision of quality care, by themselves they do not ensure quality. Evaluating the process of care through peer review involves using implicit or explicit criteria to assess conformity to current professional standards. Process, however, does not necessarily relate to outcomes of care. Assessment of outcomes—the end results in terms of health and satisfaction—provides the final evidence of whether care has been good, bad, or indifferent.

In a classic study of five methods of process and outcome evaluation, Brook and Apple found the evaluation of care depended on the method used.[20] For the 296 patients reviewed, from 1.4 to 63.2 percent of the patients were judged to have received adequate care, depending on the evaluation method used. Judgment of process using explicit criteria yielded the fewest acceptable cases. The Joint Commission has focused on an organization's quality assurance system, physical facilities, and quality-monitoring processes. However, in the 1990s the Joint Commission is developing outcome measures and focusing on continuous quality improvement. Further, clinical guidelines for common conditions are also being widely developed.

Quality of care can be reviewed prospectively, concurrently, and retrospectively. A prospective review is a preadmission screen or second opinion that is intended to confirm or question the necessity and appropriateness of care plans. A concurrent review involves monitoring care while the patient is under treatment. A retrospective review evaluates quality through an examination of medical records. The growth of computer-based record systems holds the promise of far more useful screening in the years ahead. (For more on these subjects see Chapter 3, Managing Quality.)

THE FUTURE OF PHYSICIAN ORGANIZATION AND MANAGEMENT

There will be many pressures on physicians and managers in the next decade, and only by functioning as team members will they be able to adjust to their changing environments successfully. This section suggests ways that management can structure the organization to integrate physicians into the organization, and ways that management can encourage physicians to use a team approach in attaining common goals.

It is difficult today for physicians to make patient care decisions based solely on their perceptions of clinical criteria and patient needs. Pressures from others, such as patients (who have rising expectations and greater knowledge), payers, legal systems, competitors, and colleagues, diminish the clinical autonomy of physicians. For example, payers are rationing costly technologies, and many physicians are expected to ration services as well. A growing number of payers (e.g., managed care plans) require physicians to obtain approval prior to costly treatments. Payers such as Medicaid in Oregon and elsewhere are setting explicit rationing rules that directly affect clinical decisions. Physicians who are in capitated managed care plans are expected to be gatekeepers to ensure that costly procedures are only performed when necessary. Medicare reimbursement using DRGs and concerns over malpractice litigation are also influencing clinical decisions.

Advancing technology has raised many new bioethical issues that in turn tend to restrict physician autonomy further. These issues include abortion, passive euthanasia, prolongation of life, physician-assisted suicide, therapeutic use of fetal tissue, behavioral control through psychosurgery and involuntary commitment, and use of genetic interventions and reproductive technologies. Other ethical problems arise in the hospital setting as a result of greater empowerment of patients, institutional resource constraints, disputed hospital priorities (e.g., should the organization commit dollars to high-tech tertiary care programs over primary and preventive care?), and various factors that limit patient access to care. Decisions in which such issues are involved may be facilitated via organizational mechanisms such as hospital ethics committees and related consultation services.

Increasing competition is another factor that makes organizational integration and a team approach to physician and hospital services sensible strategies. The potential surplus of physicians and the growth in HMOs, PPOs, and multispecialty groups suggest that competition between physician groups will only become more fierce. Physician groups are also competing with hospitals for outpatients, who are a growing source of revenue. Indeed, competition for outpatients and manged care headed the list of causes for conflict between hospitals and physicians in a 1987 survey.[21] Hospital-physician competition is wasteful and perhaps debilitating. Until the federal antitrust statutes for health care are reversed, however little real progress in dealing with costly system redundancies will occur.

Structural Integration of Physicians and Hospitals

Physicians and hospitals can be integrated by appointing physicians to hospital governing boards, appointing physicians to hospital management committees, appointing a medical director and salaried chiefs of services, and by instituting a number of formal structural changes.

Although physician membership on hospital governing boards was a controversial issue just a few years ago, it is now an accepted means of integration. Management-oriented medical staff committees, such as for planning or cost containment, are another mechanism for formally involving physicians in hospital decisions. Participation can be fostered by the appointment of physicians to management positions such as medical director or department chiefs. Figure 11-2 shows one way of structuring medical staff and joint hospital–medical staff committees to involve physicians in hospital decisions that directly affect patient care.

Shortell conceptualized three medical staff–hospital integration models as alternatives to the traditional departmental model (Figure 11-1): the divisional model, the independent-corporate model, and the parallel model.[22] The divisional model is characterized by the placement of functional support services within medical divisions such as medicine or surgery, which are organized along de-

partmental lines (Figure 11-3). Each medical division leader is responsible for management, including financial management. It is a physician-dominated model, with each division headed by a physician. There is no separate medical staff in this model, and physicians are totally integrated into the organization. The Johns Hopkins Hospital in Baltimore and Rush-Presbyterian-St. Luke's in Chicago are organized along these lines.

In the independent-corporate model, which is at the opposite end of the continuum from the divisional model, the medical staff becomes a separate legal entity that negotiates with the hospital for its services in return for receiving support services (Figure 11-4). The Kaiser-Permanente HMO system is an example of this model. The Permanente group practice and the Kaiser Hospital system have sole source contracts under the Kaiser Health Plan.

Shortell's parallel model (Figure 11-5) involves the creation of a separate organization in order to conduct certain activities that are not handled well by the formal hospital organization. The parallel model has been adopted by many community hospitals in recent years as a way to retain the traditional departmental structure (Figure 11-1) and medical staff independence. It allows hospitals and physicians to collaborate as management partners while still competing in certain situations. Examples include hospitals that have joined with physicians to establish an HMO or PPO, an ambulatory surgery center, a diagnostic testing center, a sports medicine center, or primary care satellites. In his case studies of 10 hospitals with effective medical staff relationships, Shortell found that most had established parallel models.[23]

A team model (Figure 11-6) in which the medical director, administrator, and nursing director function by consensus as a team of equals, is used in many European hospitals. Local health services in the British National Health Service, for example, used a team management model that required consensus among six managers representing administration, nursing, finance, community medicine, general practitioners, and specialists.[24] Although the decision process was slower, it resulted in

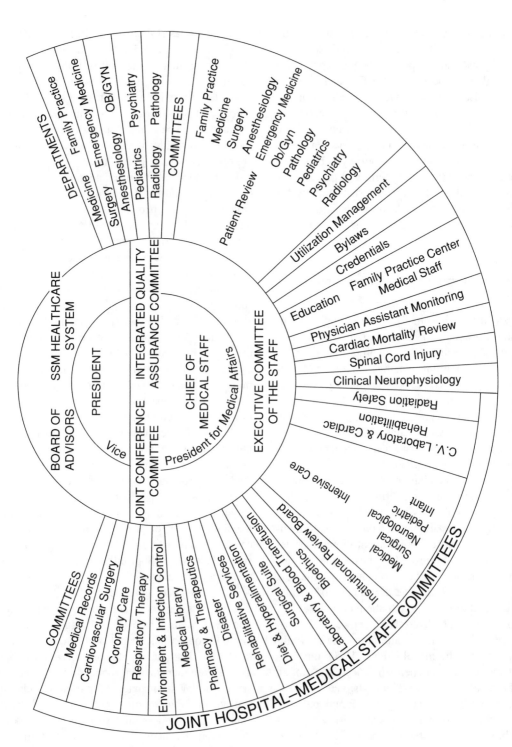

Figure 11-2 Integrative Medical Staff Organization Structure. *Source:* Courtesy of St. Marys Hospital Medical Center, Madison, Wisconsin.

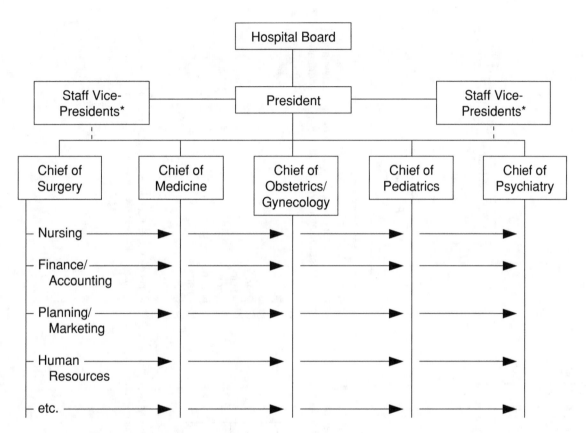

*Hospital or corporate-wide vice-presidents for nursing, finance, planning and marketing, human resources, etc. They are staff positions reporting directly to the president. They serve in a consultative or advisory position to the division chiefs, as indicated by the dotted lines.

Figure 11-3 The Divisional Model. *Source:* Reprinted from S.M. Shortell, The Medical Staff of the Future: Replanting the Garden, in *Frontiers of Health Services Management,* Vol. 1, pp. 3–48, with permission of Health Administration Press, Ann Arbor, Michigan, © 1985, Foundation of the American College of Healthcare Executives.

agreement among parties responsible for implementing top management decisions. The team model was also used in the United States in the 1960s—at Evanston Hospital in Illinois.[25]

As external pressures continue to mount in the future, there will be more hospital-physician consolidations and mergers. Mergers can be created by hospitals purchasing medical practices, by physician organizations taking control of hospitals, or by consolidating on equal terms. For example, in 1987

over 23 percent of hospitals said that they had purchased physician practices.[26] While employed physicians report average earnings that are $38,000 a year less than those of self-employed physicians, they work fewer hours; consequently, the hourly pay is not that much less.[27] The prestigious Cleveland Clinics Hospital is an example of a salaried physician–hospital arrangement. On the other side is the takeover of hospital operations by physicians. The Mayo Clinic, for example, has taken

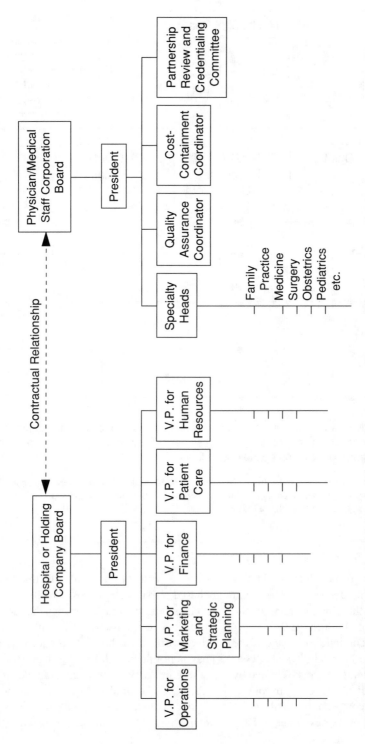

Figure 11-4 The Independent-Corporate Model. *Source:* Reprinted from S.M. Shortell, The Medical Staff of the Future: Replanting the Garden, in *Frontiers of Health Services Management,* Vol. 1, pp. 3–48, with permission of Health Administration Press, Ann Arbor, Michigan, © 1985, Foundation of the American College of Healthcare Executives.

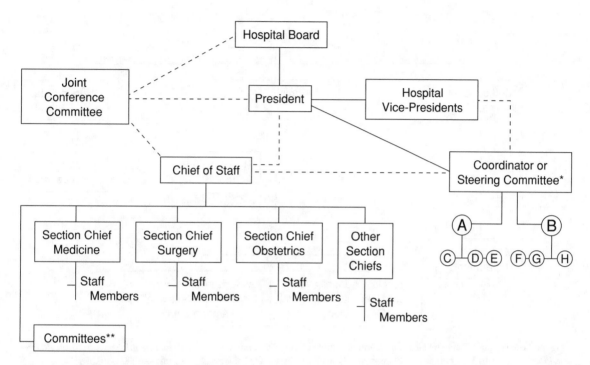

*The coordinator or steering committee of the parallel organization and the individuals involved are carefully selected from the formal medical staff organization structure shown on the left. Relevant criteria for selection include: maturity, expertise relevant to the mission of the parallel organization, credibility to both administration and medical staff, communication and listening skills, creative abilities, and representation from different specialties, committees, and age groups. In the example shown, individuals A and B serve as co-coordinators for two subgroups made up of individuals C, D, and E and F, G, and H. It should be noted that members from nursing, other health professions, and administration may also be members of the parallel organization. The parallel organization may have as its major charge the development of a strategic plan for providing more cost-effective health care to current and future markets in ways that are consistent with the hospital's mission and medical staff interests.
**Executive Committee, Credentialing Committee, Quality Assurance Committee (Utilization Review, Medical Audit, Tissue), Medical Records, Pharmacy and Therapeutics Committee, Infections Committee, etc.

Figure 11-5 The Parallel Model. *Source:* Reprinted from S.M. Shortell, The Medical Staff of the Future: Replanting the Garden, in *Frontiers of Health Services Management,* Vol. 1, pp. 3–48, with permission of Health Administration Press, Ann Arbor, Michigan, © 1985, Foundation of the American College of Healthcare Executives.

ownership of its primary hospitals—St. Marys and Methodist. Other group practices could well attempt to acquire ownership of their primary hospitals in order to compete more efficiently with other providers and to help reduce the adversariness of their relationships.

Building Physician-Hospital Teams

Goldstein and McKell propose a process for building successful hospital–medical staff partnerships.[28] This process includes steps to analyze competitors, the hospital's medical staff, and possible alli-

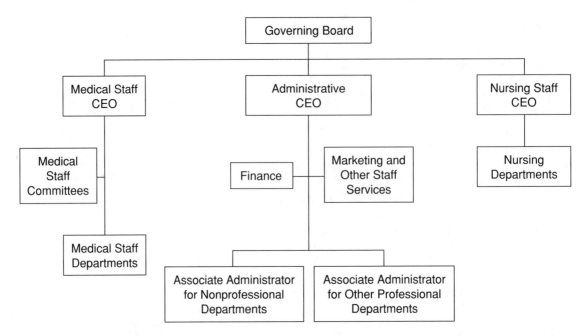

Figure 11-6 Hospital Team Organization. *Source:* Reprinted from *Management of Hospitals and Health Services: Strategic Issues and Performance,* by R. Schulz and A. Johnson, p. 139, with permission of C.V. Mosby Company, © 1990.

ance strategies. It also includes the development of a mission, goals and objectives, a budget, a cost-benefit analysis, an alliance program description, an implementation timetable, and evaluation procedures.

A joint American Medical Association and American Hospital Association task force on hospital–medical staff relationships proposed an analytical framework for avoiding, minimizing, or resolving differences.[29] It suggested a continuum for analyzing the allocation of decision-making responsibility between the hospital governing board or administration and the organized medical staff. Some decisions require the hospital or the medical staff to be singly responsible. Some require consultation, with either the hospital or the medical staff having final responsibility. Some decisions should be made using a formal process for sharing information (although the final decision still rests with only one party). Finally, some decisions require joint responsibility and the concurrence of both parties.

Building physician-management teams is not merely a matter of appointing physicians to managerial positions. Specific steps that management might consider to achieve an effective hospital-physician culture include the following[30]:

Clarify goals. Agreement may exist on general goals, such as quality of care and efficiency of service, but specific goals and priorities are seldom agreed on or even understood. Goal setting is an essential component of strategic planning. Formal definition of hospital objectives and goals, including an outline of priorities, can provide a foundation for joint efforts by the board, medical staff, and administration. Clarification takes time. Furthermore, it can occur only if it is accorded ongoing attention and everyone involved has realistic expectations. Researchers have found that goal congruence among physicians is an important predictor of perceived autonomy and work satisfaction.[31]

Specify responsibilities in formal terms. Cooperation and support will increase to the extent to which responsibilities can be identified. One reason teams fall apart is a lack of clear understanding of the role of the CEO vis-à-vis the medical or nursing staff. Role ambiguity and conflict invariably follow. Many crises in hospitals and much work dissatisfaction actually are manifestations of goal and role ambiguities.[32]

Encourage physician participation in strategic planning task forces, project groups, and coordinating committees. Joint planning and problem solving can be achieved through project groups created to devise strategies for achieving mutual goals. Other opportunities for collaboration are provided by search and screen committees for key positions such as the medical director and the vice-president of nursing. If the staff is sufficiently interested in a proposal or venture, they will devote time and energy to putting it in motion—with the end result that teamwork becomes the natural way to achieve goals. Shortell found strong physician involvement in strategic planning to be a "best practice."[33] Other researchers found that physician participation in management decisions helped to predict perceptions of autonomy and work satisfaction.[34]

Utilize liaison personnel. In addition to assuming certain executive responsibilities, the medical director should serve as a liaison between the medical staff, the administration, and the board. Opportunities for persons who have had training in liaison boundary-spanning work are beginning to develop.

Improve communication skills. Some pointers for improvement are as follows:

- Spring no surprises. It is natural for people to be resentful when they are not consulted about decisions that affect them. If, for example, the medical staff is allowed to collaborate in identifying a problem and alternatives for solving it, it is more likely to help develop a good working solution. On the other hand, if the CEO or the board decides on a course of action and simply announces it, the chosen solution may never be accepted and implemented. Shortell reports that holding discussions with physicians before meetings is a "best practice."[35]
- Encourage closeness. Common meeting areas and mutual involvement can help to break down the distinctions that create conflict and mistrust. Group meals and social events can help promote understanding among managers, physicians, nurses, and fiscal officers.
- Focus on problems, not personalities. It is critical to face the issues at hand rather than to point fingers of blame at individuals. Threatening language, aggressive postures, and certain physical gestures are manifestations of conflict and will quickly cease when people sit down and talk rationally about the problems that need to be addressed.
- Minimize power and status. Cooperation among factions in hospitals will grow when it is recognized that each person or group has equal power. It also should be recognized that cooperation instead of competition should be the standard approach. Having the power to compete, coupled with the good sense not to use it, encourages joint efforts and accomplishments. Examples of best practices paraphrased from Shortell's survey include
    - returning phone calls promptly (within at least two hours)
    - indicating the number of days to solve routine problems
    - providing feedback to physicians on difficult issues
    - immediately telephoning physicians when changes occur that affect them

Make dissension work for, not against you. Research shows that cooperation is increased when persons who are on the same side are not afraid to disagree out in the open—in one another's presence. Cooperation and the resulting benefits are maximized when everyone agrees to talk out any differences, focusing on problem solving and not just on maintaining preconceived positions.

Work toward personal and group goals simultaneously. It is unrealistic and perhaps immoral to assume that people will compromise their own values and goals for the good of the organization. To encourage joint effort, methods must be devised to help each person obtain what he or she personally wants from a given situation while contributing toward the achievement of the organization's goals.

Share information. Suspicion and mistrust tend to arise whenever important information is withheld. On the other hand, when physicians, for example, are kept fully informed, they perceive themselves as more autonomous and experience increased work satisfaction.[36]

Send signals that say, "You're okay." It is only natural to be cautious about expressing approval of others, particularly in an institutional setting, but it is important to do so nonetheless. Taking time to demonstrate a sincere interest in others gets the message across that one honestly cares about them (e.g., a manager who joins a group of physicians or nurses at lunch rather than eating with other managers). A caring attitude opens the way to honest and healthy communication.

To be sure, the strategies cited here are only a few of many ways in which joint efforts can be encouraged within hospitals. Too frequently, the tie that binds the board, medical staff, and managers is avid competition with another hospital or conflict with regulatory bodies. These negative unifying forces can cloud the commitment to the hospital's goals and can act as obstacles to meeting community needs.

One technique that helps solidify cooperation is to arrange for an educational session in a team setting that includes management, medical, and nursing personnel. Getting away from the routine work environment can facilitate objective thinking and open the doors to constructive change.

A discussion of the art of joint effort would not be complete without acknowledging that some hospitals appear to have more success at nurturing cooperation than others. The reason: Inevitably there is at least one individual on the staff who has a knack for bringing diverse groups together. It makes sense, therefore, to look around and pinpoint individuals with this talent—to exploit their ability to everyone's benefit.

ADDITIONAL RESOURCES

Organizations

American Hospital Association, 840 N. Lake Shore, Chicago, IL 60611, 312/280-6000.

American Medical Association, 515 N. State Street, Chicago, IL 60610, 312/464-5000.

Books and Articles

Gassiot, C.A., and W. Lindsey. *Handbook of medical staff management.* Gaithersburg, Md.: Aspen Publishers, 1990.

Goldstein, D.E., and D.C. McKell. *Medical staff alliances: How to build successful partnerships with your physicians.* Chicago: American Hospital Association, 1990.

Griffiths, J.R. *The well-managed community hospital.* Chap. 10. Ann Arbor, Mich.: Health Administration Press, 1987.

Physician Executive. Journal of the American College of Physician Executives, Tampa, Fla.

Shortell, S.M. *Effective hospital-physician relationships.* Ann Arbor, Mich.: Health Administration Press, 1990.

Shortell, S.M. Revisiting the garden: Medicine and management in the 1990's. *Frontiers of Health Services Management* 7, no. 1 (1990): 3–33.

NOTES

1. S.M. Shortell, *Effective Hospital-Physician Relationships* (Ann Arbor, Mich.: Health Administration Press, 1990).

2. P. Starr, *The Social Transformation of American Medicine* (New York: Basic Books, 1982).

3. Ibid.

4. Joint Commission on Accreditation of Healthcare Organizations, *1991 Accreditation Manual for Hospitals* (Oakbrook Terrace, Ill.: Joint Commission, 1990), 99.

5. Ibid.

6. Ibid., p. 107.

7. Physicians Grapple with Changing Health Care Delivery, *Hospitals,* December 20, 1986, p. 56.

8. S.M. Shortell, Revisiting the Garden: Medicine and Management in the 1990's, *Frontiers of Health Services Management* 7, no. 1 (1990): 3–33.

9. Personal communication with AMA Research Department, 1992.

10. Medical Education in the United States 1990–1991, *JAMA* 266 (1991): 873–1036.

11. National Academy of Sciences, Institute of Medicine, *A Manpower Policy for Primary Health Care* (Washington, D.C.: National Academy of Sciences, 1978).

12. C.E. Lewis et al., How Satisfying Is the Practice of Internal Medicine? *Annals of Internal Medicine* 114, no. 1 (1991): 1–5.

13. American College of Surgeons and American Surgical Association, *Surgery in the United States: A Summary Report of the Study on Surgical Services for the United States* (Chicago: American College of Surgeons, 1975), 21–90.

14. Department of Health and Human Services, *Report of the Graduate Medical Education National Advisory Committee to the Secretary,* vol. 1, GMENAC Summary Report, KGPO #1980-0-721-748/266 (Washington, D.C.: U.S. Government Printing Office, 1981).

15. E. Ginzberg, Personnel: Challenges Ahead, *Frontiers of Health Services Management* 7, no. 2 (1990): 7.

16. W.B. Schwartz et al., Why There Will Be Little or No Physician Surplus between Now and the Year 2000, *New England Journal of Medicine* 318 (1988): 892.

17. AMA Addresses Medical Staff Self-Governance, *Hospitals,* June 20, 1988, p. 54; H.L. Lang, The Independent Self-Governing Medical Staff, in *Handbook of Medical Staff Management,* ed. C.A. Gassiot and S. Lindsey (Gaithersburg, Md.: Aspen Publishers, 1990), 71–74.

18. R.E. Thompson, The Medical Staff Organization, in *Handbook of Medical Staff Management,* ed. C.A. Gassiot and S. Lindsey (Gaithersburg, Md.: Aspen Publishers, 1990), 39–69.

19. Practitioner Data Bank Begins September 1: Confidentiality Remains Key Concern, *American Medical News,* July 27, 1990, p. 1.

20. R.H. Brook and F.A. Apple, Quality of Care Assessment: Choosing a Method for Peer Review, *New England Journal of Medicine* 288 (1973): 1323.

21. Survery Spots Tight Turns in MD-CEO Relations, *Hospitals,* February 5, 1988, p. 48.

22. S.M. Shortell, The Medical Staff of the Future: Replanting the Garden, *Frontiers of Health Services Management* 1, no. 3 (1985): 3.

23. Shortell, *Effective Hospital-Physician Relationships;* Shortell, Revisiting the Garden.

24. R. Schulz and S. Harrison, *Teams and Top Managers in the National Health Service* (London: King's Fund Centre, 1983).

25. J.M. Danielson, Organized Action: Management Advisory Councils, *JAMA* 196 (1966): 1062–1063.

26. Survey Spots Tight Turns in MD-CEO Relations.

27. SMS Survey: MDs Earning More but Working More Hours Too, *American Medical News,* November 20, 1987, p. 13.

28. D.E. Goldstein and D.C. McKell, *Medical Staff Alliances: How To Build Successful Partnerships with Your Physicians* (Chicago: American Hospital Association, 1990).

29. American Hospital Association and American Medical Association, *Report on the Joint Task Force on Hospital Medical Staff Relationships* (Chicago: American Hospital Association and American Medical Association, 1985).

30. R. Schulz and D. Detmer, How To Get Doctors Involved in Governance and Management, in *The Hospital Medical Staff: Selected Readings 1972–1976* (Chicago: American Hospital Association, 1977), 1–7; Shortell, Revisiting the Garden.

31. R. Schulz and C. Schulz, Management Practices, Physician Autonomy and Satisfaction: Evidence from Mental Health Institutions in the Federal Republic of Germany, *Medical Care* (1988): 750; R. Schulz et al., Perceived Autonomy and Work Satisfaction Amongst Psychiatrists in the NHS, *Journal of Management in Medicine* 5, no. 2 (1991): 53–64.

32. S. Jackson and R.S. Schuler, A Meta Analysis and Conceptual Critique of Research on Role Ambiguity and Role Conflict in Work Settings, *Organization Behavior and Human Decision Processes* 36 (1985): 17–78.

33. Shortell, Revisiting the Garden.

34. Schulz and Schulz, Management Practices, Physician Autonomy and Satisfaction; Schulz et al., Perceived Autonomy and Work Satisfaction.

35. Shortell, Revisiting the Garden.

36. Schulz and Schulz, Management Practices, Physician Autonomy and Satisfaction; Schulz et al., Perceived Autonomy and Work Satisfaction.

Joan Gygax Spicer
Diane E. Nitta

Nursing Organization and Management

12

Purpose: The purpose of nursing management is to optimize the application of available nursing resources in the diagnosis and treatment of human responses to actual or potential health problems, such as self-care limitations, pain and discomfort, emotional problems related to illness and treatment, or strain related to life processes, including birth and death.

INTRODUCTION

This chapter discusses the management of nursing resources. When appropriately managed, nurses, in addition to providing nursing care, emerge as integrators of patient care services and facilitators of the efforts of members of the multidisciplinary team. The chapter starts with a list of relevant management principles. There is then a review of the historical origins of modern-day nursing, including an account of the evolution of the nurse's role.

Following this is a discussion of standards for organized nursing services and decision making, nursing education and nursing research, the role of nursing within the organization, collaboration in

practice, and interdepartmental relationships. Allocation of nursing resources is quantified into dollar expenditures, and a review of the budget process is provided. Quality assurance is discussed next, and the chapter concludes with a summary of the worldwide challenges facing nursing leaders.

FUNCTIONS, ACTIVITIES, AND PROCESSES

The functions or activities that must be performed and the processes that must occur in the management of nursing resources include the following:

- *Nursing process.* The nursing process includes assessment, diagnosis, planning, intervention, and evaluation.
- *Planning.* Nurses must try to determine what combination of skilled personnel, including registered nurses, licensed vocational/practical nurses, and unlicensed assistive personnel, will best meet patient care needs while contributing to the achievement of the organization's mission.

- *Collaboration.* Collaboration is essential for integrating the resources and expertise of clinical disciplines and ancillary and support departments in the decision-making and care-providing processes.
- *Allocation of financial resources.* Allocation of resources supports the actual delivery of nursing services and the monitoring and evaluating of nursing care.
- *Management of human resources.* The object of human resources management is to meet the demand for highly specialized nursing care while simultaneously giving clinical nurses as much control over nursing practice as possible.
- *Quality management.* In order to maintain quality, clinical nurses must monitor and evaluate the quality and appropriateness of nursing care based on the standards of clinical nursing practice.

MANAGEMENT PRINCIPLES

1. Each member of the nursing staff is assigned clinical or managerial responsibilities based on educational preparation, clinical or managerial competence, and applicable licensing laws and regulations.
2. The nursing staff adopts standards of clinical nursing practice that guide policy and procedure development, resource allocation, and quality assurance activities.
3. Patients receive nursing care based on the nursing process, and the nursing process is documented.
4. Nursing staff members collaborate with physicians, other clinical disciplines, ancillary departments, and support services to provide each patient with the nursing care he or she needs.
5. The nursing department's organization chart and program plan encourage innovation in nursing practice, meet the needs of the patients, and support the organization's mission.

6. A budget plan exists to allocate nursing resources.
7. Appropriate and sufficient support services are available to allow nursing staff members to meet the nursing care needs of patients.
8. As part of the organization's quality improvement program, the quality and appropriateness of the nursing care provided is monitored and evaluated by clinical nurses.

Nursing management includes structuring the work setting to support the clinical practice of nursing, allocating and using resources efficiently and effectively, and ensuring that the standards of clinical nursing practice are met.

THE ORGANIZATIONAL ROLE AND FUNCTION OF NURSING

Historical Origins

In the middle of the nineteenth century, the eminent social reformer and humanitarian Florence Nightingale believed that nursing should be established as an independent profession. This energetic and committed woman established nursing principles and practices that became the foundation of the nursing process as it is known today. Her systematic evaluation of the effectiveness of the health care services during the Crimean War brought about substantial reform in the way such services were delivered. Not only did Nightingale change the outcomes of care, but her work during the Crimean War resulted in the emergence of nursing as a profession.

During the U.S. Civil War, the necessity of educating women to become nurses was recognized, and after the war schools of nursing began to evolve. Throughout this period, nurses typically worked in their patients' homes. During World War I, there was an acute need for nurses near the battlefield caring for wounded soldiers and in the hospitals caring for returning soldiers. Military and Red Cross hospitals were the first organizations to utilize nursing school graduates. During the Depression, nurses seeking economic security shifted from delivering nursing care in patients' homes to working as staff in hospitals. As technology advanced and treatment modalities became more sophisticated, it became more efficient to deliver care in hospitals than in homes.

The Nursing Process

Nursing functions can be categorized as dependent, interdependent, and independent. Dependent functions are the activities mandated by physician's orders, such as administering medications and initiating intravenous therapy. Interdependent functions are carried out in conjunction with other health team members, such as active or passive range of motion exercises, which will typically be decided upon by the physical therapist. Independent functions are activities considered to be within the scope of nursing diagnosis and treatment. These actions do not require a physician's order. Examples include increasing the frequency of vital sign measurements, initiating intake and output measurements, assessing skin condition and implementing skin protection measures, and initiating a social services consult.

The nursing process is the theoretical framework for the independent functions of nursing. It is a deliberate problem-solving approach that requires cognitive, technical, and interpersonal skills and is directed to meeting the needs of patients and families.[1]

By the 1960s, nurses were utilizing the nursing process as a framework to provide nursing care. Evidence of the use of the nursing process is one of the criteria used by accrediting and licensing bodies to ensure that appropriate nursing care is being delivered. The nursing process steps must be documented in the patient medical record. The steps include these:

- *Assessment.* This first step involves the systematic collection of information about the health status of the patient for purposes of identifying the patient's needs, problems, concerns, and basic responses.

- *Diagnosis.* The nursing diagnosis is derived from the health status data and provides the basis for conclusions regarding the patient's needs, problems, concerns, and human responses. The nursing diagnosis provides an efficient way to communicate the patient's problems.

- *Planning.* The nursing care plan is based on the nursing diagnosis. The plan includes priorities, nursing interventions, and desired outcomes.

- *Implementation.* Interventions by the health care team, the patient, or family help the patient to achieve the desired outcomes.

- *Evaluation.* Whether the patient has achieved the desired outcomes is determined by the patient and nurse. The patient's progress toward goal achievement directs further assessment, diagnosis, planning, and treatment.

Practice Settings

Hospitals remain the largest employer of registered nurses. In the United States, there are 2.1 million RNs, approximately 80 percent (1.68 million) are employed in nursing, and about two-thirds (1.1 million) of these are employed by hospitals.[2] Nurses have also traditionally worked in community or public health programs and long-term care facilities, including residential and skilled nursing facilities.

The goal of community health nursing is to enable people to cope with threats to health. The roles nurses play in the community include provider of primary health care, provider of personal care to unhospitalized patients, patient advocate, patient advisor, and change agent influencing public policy.

In skilled nursing facilities, nurses deal with patients who need nursing care or assistance with activities of daily living. The skill mix of nursing personnel usually includes a high proportion of unlicensed assistive personnel and a low proportion of licensed nurses. Nurses in this setting oversee other personnel, who provide the direct physical care. One of the goals of nursing in this type of setting is to create a wellness (rather than illness), recreational, and social milieu.

By the 1990s, societal influences, new technology, and changes in the reimbursement system had brought about a restructuring of the health care delivery system, a new emphasis on wellness and preventive care, and a broader range of treatments and surgical operations. For example, more care is being provided in ambulatory settings and the homes of patients. More emphasis is put on preventive care, which creates avenues for teaching and coaching roles in preventive care programs (e.g., smoking cessation, sexually transmitted disease awareness, nutrition, and exercise programs). Finally, owing to the application of more sophisticated knowledge and of advanced technology, members of society are living at home with health conditions that would have required more intensive management or even been fatal previously, creating additional areas for nursing specialization. Today it is estimated that there are well over 100 combinations of clinical settings and specialties in which nurses practice.

Nurse Practice Acts

Article X of the United States Constitution delegates police power to each state to protect the health and welfare of its citizens. Nurse licensing thus falls within the purview of each state and has led to the development of nurse practice acts. State nurse practice acts are diverse but share these elements:

- identification of a regulatory agency
- identification of components of nursing practice
- prohibition of medical diagnosis and treatment
- regulation of advanced practice[3]

A Social Policy Statement

The challenge of defining nursing was undertaken by the American Nurses' Association (ANA),

the dominant professional organization for nursing in the United States. The ANA's effort resulted in the publishing of *Nursing: A Social Policy Statement* in 1980. This document is recognized by nursing leaders as a significant guide to the practice and management of nursing. It addresses the social context of nursing, the nature and scope of nursing practice, and specialization in nursing practice. Nurses have an informal contract with society that gives them the right to practice. In return, nurses must meet needs and demands of society. Each professional nurse remains individually responsible for his or her clinical practice regardless of position in an organizational structure. The contract with society is individual as well as collective, and thus individual accountability cannot be denied or disclaimed.

Nursing: A Social Policy Statement delineates the nursing process, establishes the standards of nursing practice, and sets forth the professionally accepted definition of nursing as "the diagnosis and treatment of human responses to actual or potential health problems."[4] This definition reflects the historical evolution of the independent function of nursing.

Levels of Skilled Nursing Personnel

There are three levels of skilled nursing personnel recognized uniformly in the United States:

1. *Unlicensed Assistive Personnel.* These are unlicensed individuals who work as assistants to licensed nurses.
2. *Licensed Vocational/Practical Nurses (LVN/ LPNs).* These nurses perform technical and manual tasks under the direction of a registered professional nurse or licensed physician. The range of tasks allowed varies from state to state.
3. *Registered Nurses (RNs).* RNs are licensed to practice those nursing functions, including direct and indirect patient care, described in the relevant state nurse practice act.

Extended or Expanded Registered Nurse Roles

An RN may function in an extended or expanded role in the clinical setting, for example, as a clinical nurse specialist, nurse practitioner, nurse midwife, or certified nurse anesthetist.

Clinical Nurse Specialists. A clinical nurse specialist is an RN who, through study and supervised practice at the graduate level, has become expert in a defined area of knowledge and practice in a selected area of nursing.[5] The components of the role are: clinician, educator, consultant, and clinical leader.

Nurse Practitioners. A nurse practitioner is an RN who, through advanced study and supervised practice at the post basic or graduate level, functions in a role that includes elements of medical practice. In accordance with standardized procedures and under the supervision of the licensed physician, the nurse practitioner performs physical examinations, treats common illnesses, and promotes health maintenance through education and counseling.

Nurse Midwives. A nurse midwife is an RN who, through advanced study and supervised practice at the post basic or graduate level, functions in a role that includes elements of obstetrical medical practice. In accordance with standardized procedures and under the supervision of an obstetrician, the nurse midwife manages normal obstetrical patients through pregnancy, labor, delivery, and the postpartum course.

Certified Nurse Anesthetists. A Certified Registered Nurse Anesthetist (CRNA) is an RN who, through advanced study and supervised practice at either the post baccalaureate or graduate level, functions in a role that includes elements of medical practice. Nurse anesthesia is the oldest nursing specialty, and in fact, precedes the field of medical anesthesiology. In accordance with standardized procedures, the CRNA is trained and legally able to perform the same duties as an anesthesiologist.

Hospitals determine the limit of privileges granted, which may include regional and general anesthesia.

ORGANIZATIONAL STRUCTURE

The nurse executive must organize the nursing department so that members within the department can be responsive to patients, nursing personnel, physicians, and other members of the organization. An organizational structure is designed to ensure decision making occurs at the appropriate level; eliminates redundancy; establishes accountability; and defines administrative, educational, and research support for clinical nursing functions. Within the nursing department, any combination of organizational structures (e.g., centralized, decentralized, matrix, and committee structures) might be used. The nurse executive more often than not utilizes and changes combinations of structures within the department in order to respond to the growing complexity of health care and its challenging and sometimes turbulent environment.

The organization chart, which depicts relationships using boxes and lines, is accompanied by a program plan that describes how the organizational structure functions. The program plan delineates clinical authority and accountability, communication processes and communication structure, interdepartmental relationships, and management methodology.

Standards of Organized Nursing Services

The ANA published standards for organized nursing services that were put forth as guidelines to establish effective nursing organizations. These standards include the following:

Standard I. Philosophy and Structure: Organized nursing services have a philosophy and structure that ensure the delivery of effective nursing care.

Standard II. Nurse Administrator: Organized nursing services are administered by qualified and competent nurse administrators.

Standard III. Fiscal Resource Management: The nurse executive determines and administers the fiscal resources of organized nursing services. The nurse executive has an interactive role in the determination of the organizations's fiscal resource requirements and their acquisition, allocation and utilization.

Standard IV. Nursing Process: Within organized nursing services, the nursing process is used as the framework for providing nursing care to recipients.

Standard V. Environment for Practice: An environment is created within organized nursing services that enhances nursing practice and facilitates the delivery of care by all nursing staff.

Standard VI. Quality Assurance: Organized nursing services have a quality assurance program.

Standard VII. Ethics: Organized nursing services have policies to guide ethical decision making based on the code for nurses.

Standard VIII. Research: Within organized nursing services, research in nursing, health, and nursing systems are facilitated; research findings are disseminated; and support is provided for integration of these findings into the delivery of nursing care and nursing administration.

Standard IX. Cultural, Economic, and Social Differences: Organized nursing services provide policies and practices that address equality and continuity of nursing services and recognize cultural, economic, and social differences among recipients served by the health care organization.[6]

Decision Making

There are three types of decision making involved in managing nursing resources: centralized, participatory, and shared decision making. Different types are appropriate for different aspects of managing nursing resources. Centralized decision making, where decisions are made by a few, is appropriate for determining wage and benefit structures and how a labor contract is going to be admin-istered, for example. It may be exercised in relationship to the dependent functions of nursing, but it would not be appropriate for decisions impacting the independent functions of nursing.

In participatory decision making, there are parameters established that determine who will make or control the final decision. Participants in the process may act as advisors or have final decision-making authority, and they may include both administrators and clinicians. The peer review process, which involves evaluating professional performance and administering awards, may use participatory decision making. The interdependent functions of nursing would also be appropriate for participatory decision-making processes.

Shared decision making evolved when it was realized that decisions regarding the clinical practice of nursing (the independent functions of nursing) needed to be made by the nursing staff involved in delivering the care. In shared decision making, the nursing staff uses an organized and systematic process to establish standards of professional performance and standards of care, ensure achievement of desired patient care outcomes, and resolve practice problems.

New skills are required of nurse managers involved in shared decision making. They must release the latent abilities of employees so that the employees can develop to their full potential. They must have skills in coaching and counseling and exhibit supportive behavior. They must encourage thinking, learning, and creativity. In a shared decision-making process, nurse managers have the responsibility for ensuring that clinical nurses receive and understand available information, and the nurses have the responsibility to access established communication channels to obtain information, ask questions, and supply information to the nurse managers.

Shared decision making requires an environment in which clinical nurses are acknowledged as essential participants in decision making that could have an impact on the practice of nursing. It should also be recognized that autonomy in the practice of nursing directly correlates with clinical nurse job satisfaction.

Organizational Support Functions

Clinical Nurse Education

The following essential functions of nursing education are usually centralized in a staff support area within the nursing organizational structure:

- *Orientation.* Orientation is a mechanism for introducing new nursing service personnel to the organization's philosophy, goals, policies, procedures, and physical facilities.
- *In-service education.* In-service activities are designed to augment nursing staff members' knowledge of pertinent new developments in patient care and to maintain their clinical competence.
- *Cross-training.* Cross-training is an educational technique for preparing staff members to work in areas where overlapping skills and knowledge are required.[7]

The goal of nursing education is to ensure that the nursing staff members have the skills required for performance of designated roles in specific clinical settings. The educational activities are typically competency based. Competency statements describe the general types of behaviors that are essential for a specific skill (or activity or role). Then observable and measurable characteristics of these behaviors are identified. Alternative methods of learning the skill are outlined for the nurse. When the essential characteristics are evaluated as present in the nurse's performance of the skill, the performance is evaluated as being competent. (See Exhibit 12-1 for an example of competency-based training. Also see Chapter 5 for more on educational programs.)

Clinical Nursing Research

The nurse executive must help establish standards of clinical nursing practice and then must test, through research, whether these standards achieve the desired patient care outcomes. The goal of nursing research in the practice setting is to determine the relationship between nursing interventions and quality patient care outcomes.

Available resources within the organization will dictate the level of involvement nurses will have in research. Journal clubs, nursing grand rounds, and research utilization require the least amount of resources. Journal clubs encourage participants to review and critique existing research reports. Participants identify the applicability of the research to their practice setting or generate discussion on other questions that might be investigated. During nursing grand rounds, case studies are presented. The emphasis is on (1) which interventions had a basis in research and which did not and (2) what were the outcomes compared to the predicted outcomes. The participants explore similarities from their own cases, both in outcomes and unanswered questions.

The next levels of research, replication and generation of research projects, involve more time and require nurses prepared to do such research. *Guidelines for the Investigative Function of Nurses,* published by the ANA, recommends that the principal investigator be prepared at the doctoral level.[8] The guidelines contained in the publication can be used to assist nurse executives and clinical nurses in defining the responsibility for nursing research.

Key Management Positions within the Organizational Structure

Nurse Executive

The nurse executive (also sometimes called the director of nursing, chief nursing officer, or vice-president of nursing services) plays a critical role in determining the vision for nursing within the organization and setting the climate for professional practice. The nurse executive also serves as a role model and mentor in order to help prepare the next generation of nurses. The primary focus of the nurse executive is strategic. The nurse executive

- participates in the administration of the organization through membership on the executive policy-making committee

Exhibit 12-1 Competency-Based Training in Chesttube Drainage

Competency statement: Performs critical care procedures and patient care safely and according to quality assurance standards as articulated in the nursing policy and procedure manual.

CHESTTUBE DRAINAGE SYSTEM

Goal: Orientee will demonstrate competency in setting up and maintaining a chest drainage system.

Competency Criteria Statement	*Learning Options*	*Target Date*	*Method of Evaluation*
1. Lists or assembles equipment for chest tube insertion	1. Reads policy (M)* 2. Practice demonstration on unit (M)	1. Week 5	1. Demonstration 2. Verbal description
2. Sets up chest tube drainage system	1. Practice demonstration on unit (O)* 2. Simulation in lab (O)		1. Demonstration
3. Describes the difference between pleural and mediastinal chest tube	1. Reads nursing policy and procedure		1. Verbal description
4. States nursing responsibilities of maintaining a pleural and mediastinal chest drainage system	1. Reads nursing policy and procedure (M) 2. Nursing article (O) 3. Film (O)		1. Verbal description to include: a) chest x-ray once tube has been placed b) document amount, color, and consistency of chest drainage c) check patency of tube d) maintain water seal at 2 cm, suction control at 20 cm unless otherwise ordered e) assess water level in suction control chamber; maintain water bubbling unless at water seal f) prepare chest drainage system for transport g) describe the procedure for changing chest drainage system h) keep chest drainage system lower than pt. chest
5. States the reason and/or demonstrates procedure for correction of: a) tidaling b) air leaks c) addition of mercury to suction control chamber d) abrupt decrease or increase in chest drainage e) dislodged or disconnected chesttube	1. Reads nursing policy and procedure (M) 2. Nursing article (O) 3. Film (O)		1. Return demonstration

continues

Exhibit 12-1 Continued

Competency Criteria Statement	Learning Options	Target Date	Method of Evaluation
6. Describes the nursing responsibilities during chesttube removal	1. Reads nursing policy and procedure (M) 2. Nursing article (O)		1. Return demonstration or verbal description to include: a) equipment b) valsalva maneuver c) dressing d) assessment e) disposal of chest drainage system

*Learning Options: M = Mandatory, O = Optional.

Source: Courtesy of the Department of Nursing Education and Research, University of California, San Francisco, California.

- determines the goals and direction of the nursing department and devises an organizational structure to achieve the goals
- acquires and allocates appropriate resources (money, capital, equipment, and materiel)
- evaluates the efficiency and effectiveness of services
- provides leadership in human resource development
- provides channels for consumer input in policy development
- participates in developing and implementing mechanisms for collaboration between nurses, physicians, and other clinical practitioners[9]

Nurse Manager

The nurse manager (also sometimes called the head nurse, clinical coordinator, or assistant director of nursing) helps coordinate the clinical nursing staff. The nurse manager's primary focus is operations. The nurse manager

- plans, prepares, and demonstrates accountability for the budget
- supervises the delivery of nursing care
- collaborates with ancillary, support, and interdisciplinary team members
- recruits, selects, and trains personnel

- schedules resources
- evaluates staff members for promotion, transfer, disciplinary action, and separation of service
- serves as role model[10]

Clinical Nurse as Patient Care Manager

The clinical nurse coordinates and prioritizes the elements of treatment (i.e., procedures, medications, education, therapies, etc.). The primary focus of the clinical nurse is patient care. The clinical nurse

- coordinates and delivers nursing care
- collaborates with interdisciplinary team members
- serves as patient advocate
- contributes to the professional development of other staff members
- participates in monitoring and evaluating care

Collaboration in Practice

Collaboration in health care involves integrating the care practices of different members of the health care team into a comprehensive approach to meet the needs of the patient and family.[11] The impact of an integrated care approach is greater than if each discipline's regime was implemented in isolation. If collaboration is to occur and be effective, there must be a forum for the discussion of patient care and the evaluation of patient care outcomes by multiple disciplines; standards of practice for each discipline; integration of the patient record, with one progress note; and joint patient care record reviews. One documented benefit of collaboration is the enhancement of quality patient care outcomes.

Relationships with Ancillary and Support Departments

The nursing department's program plan, which accompanies the organization chart, should define and describe its relationship to the ancillary and support departments. In particular, the plan should include the following:

- *Consultation guidelines.* Guidelines for when the resources and expertise of the ancillary or support department should be utilized for consultation and treatment interventions.
- *Formal and informal communication mechanisms.* Formal communication mechanisms include standing meetings, committees, and ad hoc task forces. Informal communication mechanisms, such as walking rounds and discussion of incidents, provide for flexibility, speed, and more personal interaction.
- *A mechanism to establish acceptable standards for service.* Standards for service are negotiated between nursing representatives and ancillary or support department representatives. Quality assurance activities should be delineated to ensure that standards of service will be met.

Members of the nursing department work with personnel from the ancillary and support departments to achieve patient care outcomes. The nurse becomes the integrator of services, facilitating collaboration.

RESOURCE REQUIREMENTS

Budgeting for Human Resources*

Nursing is labor intensive, and in most organizations 50 percent or more of the total budgeted dollars for salary and benefits are allocated to the nursing department. The allocation is determined by the skill mix of personnel, by the position of patients on the illness-wellness continuum, by economies of scale that can be actualized, and by the labor market. Salary varies depending on the area and the labor market supply and demand. The percentages of type of personnel also vary (RNs usually represent 50 to 90 percent of the staff, with LVN/LPN or assistive personnel constituting the remaining percentage).

Labor Standards

Budgeting for human resources is based on forecasted units of service (UOS) and a predetermined labor standard. A labor standard is the amount of time it takes nurses to deliver care to a patient during a procedure, visit, or patient stay. Each of these may be called a UOS. The labor standard is expressed in time (e.g., hours per UOS or, for an inpatient unit, hours per patient day). Information useful for determining the labor standard is derived from several data sources: patient demographics, the patient classification system, unit activity, national standards, and laws.

Patient Demographics. Patient demographics (i.e., a statistical representation of the patient population) helps to establish a standard. Certain patient characteristics indicate the intensity of nursing time required to care for that patient:

- *Diagnosis.* Patient diagnoses indicate the complexity of the required care.

---

*The material in this section is adapted from J.G. Spicer, *Workbook for Nursing Managers Developing a Salary Budget* (Santa Clara, Calif.: Spicer and Spicer Associates, 1989).

- *Origin.* A patient's origin gives some indication of nursing time. The patient admitted through a trauma service has different needs than the patient admitted from home (who usually has had time to prepare for the hospitalization).
- *Age.* Patients on either end of the age continuum require increased time. Younger patients require time for parenting, and elderly patients require more time because providing safety for them requires greater care and because they have slower cognitive responses.
- *Procedures.* Types of procedures vary in the amount of nursing time required.
- *Length of stay.* The length of stay, including time spent transferring from unit to unit in the organization, is another factor. Shorter lengths of stay mean that more time per patient day is spent on admission and discharge procedures.
- *Discharge destination.* The destination indicates how much time will be involved in preparing the patient for discharge. If the patient is going home, there may be increased time spent on coordinating equipment and family education. If the patient is being transferred to another facility, there may be increased time spent on communication with the receiving staff.

The Patient Classification System. The purpose of patient classification systems, sometimes called acuity systems, is to group patients and to quantify the patient care requirements by increments of time. Patient classification systems provide indices of activities that nurses perform for patients, such as feeding, ambulation, treatment, medication, and education. The outcome is a quantity of time required to care for a patient. Patient classification systems provide adjunct information needed to make decisions regarding resource allocation. This information does not determine the quantity of resources but instead affects the allocation of available resources.

Patient Care Unit Activity. Each patient care unit has specific characteristics. For example, the per-

centage of occupancy may indicate that total workload is in inverse proportion to the census (i.e., when the census decreases, the percentage of acutely ill patients increases). Unit data to consider include the average daily census, the percentage of occupancy, designations of special services, and the unit's space and physical layout. Each system has a saturation point beyond which it fails. This saturation point is usually linked to the percentage of occupancy. Resources are usually allocated on the basis of a specified projected percentage of occupancy. Once that percentage is reached, the system begins to be stressed. For example, imagine a unit that is at 100 percent occupancy. The emergency department (ED) has a patient to be admitted to the unit, which is the only place the patient can be given the specialized care needed. The nurse on the receiving patient care unit must now obtain transfer or discharge orders for a patient in order to accommodate the new admission. The patient, who no longer requires emergency care, is occupying an ED bed and consuming the time of the ED nurse, who is not necessarily efficient at delivering nonemergency care. Also, the ED may not have the necessary physical resources to support care during this next phase. These are the kinds of problems caused by being pushed beyond the saturation point.

National Standards and State Laws. National standards are the standards used by most hospitals that are the same size and that offer the same services. At one time, standards were viewed only from a local perspective, but because of the advent of mass communications, the standards of similar hospitals across the nation are now considered. There are a few states with laws that regulate staffing levels or the qualifications of personnel.

Direct Productive Full-Time Equivalent

The first part of the salary budget to be developed concerns direct productive full-time equivalents (FTEs). A productive FTE, in accounting terms, is defined as 2,080 hours in a year. In the simplest terms, assuming an FTE employee works 40 hours a week and 8 hours a day, the following formula can be used throughout the development of the salary budget:

Projected Annual UOSs ×
Budgeted Labor Standard
$$\frac{\text{per UOS}}{2{,}080 \text{ hours per FTE}} = \text{Total Productive FTEs}$$

Example:

5,824 Projected UOSs ×
$$\frac{5.0 \text{ hours per UOS}}{2{,}080 \text{ hours per FTE}} = 14 \text{ Productive FTEs}$$

The projected annual UOSs are multiplied by the budgeted labor standard per UOS. This number then gives the total number of hours that have to be budgeted to deliver the amount of hours of care for each UOS. If the total hours are divided by the FTE hours (2,080), the resulting number is the number of productive FTEs required.

Skill Mix

The skill mix is the mix of personnel with different skill levels. The skill mix might include licensed, unlicensed, and clerical staff. The mix is determined by the financial resources available and the location of patients on the illness-wellness continuum. Exhibit 12-2 shows a staffing pattern using 10 FTEs. In this example, 60 percent of staff are licensed personnel (either registered nurses or licensed vocational/practical nurses), 30 percent are nonlicensed personnel, and the remaining position is a clerical one.

Contribution to Standard

The contribution to standard for a given skill mix category is determined by dividing the number of FTEs in the staffing pattern for that category by the total number of FTEs and then multiplying the resulting figure by the labor standard per UOS.

Number of FTEs per
Skill Mix Category ×
Labor Standard
$$\frac{\text{per UOS}}{\text{Total Number of FTEs}} = \frac{\text{Hours Contributed to}}{\text{Standard per Category}}$$

The contribution to standard is the number of hours a given skill mix category contributes to patient care (see Exhibit 12-3). Contribution to standard has an impact on the level of care delivered and the salary expense per UOS. The labor standard might be five hours, but only three of the five hours might be worked by licensed nursing personnel.

Indirect Productive Full-Time Equivalents

Indirect productive time might include the activities of the nurse manager, and some organizations classify the clerical activities of employees in the patient care areas as indirect. It is important to know which categories are included in direct and indirect when making comparisons, since this varies by organization.

Nonproductive Full-Time Equivalents

In addition to productive time, there is nonproductive time, or time the employee is paid for but during which the employee is not providing patient care (e.g., vacation, education, or sick time). Nonproductive time is estimated to range from 15–20% of the employee's time. This varies depending on the benefit package, the culture of the work group, and the practice of the personnel administration. If the total productive FTEs per skill mix category is multiplied by the percentage of nonproductive time, the total additional FTEs that are required to replace employees at the bedside when they are using nonproductive time can be determined.

Total Productive FTEs
per Skill Mix Category
$\times$ Percentage of $=$ Total Nonproductive
Nonproductive Time   FTEs per Category

See Exhibit 12-4 for a sample calculation of nonproductive FTEs.

Salary Expense per Unit of Service

Managing by salary expense per UOS is the current challenge for nurse managers. Although labor

Exhibit 12-2 Sample Staffing Pattern

| | Shift | | | | Percentage |
Category	0700–1530	1500–2330	2300–0730	Total	of Total
Licensed	2.0	2.0	2.0	6.0	60%
Nonlicensed patient care	1.0	1.0	1.0	3.0	30%
Nonlicensed clerical	1.0	0.0	0.0	1.0	10%

standard per UOS has been the focus in the past, salary expense per UOS is now the "bottom line" the nurse manager must meet. The salary expense per UOS is calculated by multiplying projected annual census by hours contributed per skill mix category and then multiplying that by the hourly salary rate per category (the result is called the productive salary). To this is added the nonproductive hours multiplied by the hourly salary rate per category (the nonproductive salary), and to this sum is added the indirect salary, which total is then divided by the annual census. The result is the salary expense per UOS.

$$\frac{\text{Productive Salary +}}{\text{Nonproductive Salary +}} = \text{Salary Expense per UOS}$$
$$\frac{\text{Indirect Salary}}{\text{Projected Annual UOSs}} = \text{Salary Expense per UOS}$$

See Exhibit 12-5 for a sample calculation of salary expense per UOS. To reduce the salary expense per UOS, the labor standard can be reduced, which in return reduces the number of FTEs. The skill mix

of personnel can be changed to use lower-paid personnel. There can be a reduction in the amount of overtime or premium time paid. The use of nonproductive time can be decreased. Figure 12-1 indicates how changes in budget components affect salary expense per UOS.

Delivery Systems

Possible delivery systems include the following.

Case Method. The nurse interfaces with and coordinates members of a multidisciplinary health care team, third-party payers, and patients and families. The nurse may or may not provide direct care, but he or she definitely does provide direction, review, and evaluation of care. A critical path is determined for each patient to follow in the health care system, and the nurse, as case manager, facilitates movement along that path. The method of assigning patients varies (e.g., they can be assigned by diagnosis, medical service, or geographical area).

Exhibit 12-3 Sample Calculation of Contributions to Standard

Average Daily UOS   = 16
Labor Standard per UOS   = 5
Total Productive FTEs   = 10

Number of FTEs per Skill Mix Category	÷	Total Number of FTEs	=	Percentage for Category × Labor Standard	=	Hours Contributed to Standard per Category
6 RN FTEs	÷	10 Total FTEs	= .60	× 5.0	= 3.0	
2 LVN/LPN FTEs	÷	10 Total FTEs	= .20	× 5.0	= 1.0	
2 Clerical FTEs	÷	10 Total FTEs	= .20	× 5.0	= 1.0	

Exhibit 12-4 Sample Calculation of Nonproductive FTEs

Nonproductive Time = 18 percent		

8.4	RN FTEs	× .18 Nonproductive Time =	1.51 RN Nonproductive FTEs
2.8	LVN/LPN FTEs	× .18 Nonproductive Time =	.50 LVN/LPN Nonproductive FTEs
2.8	Clerical FTEs	× .18 Nonproductive Time =	.50 Clerical Nonproductive FTEs
		Total Nonproductive FTEs =	2.51

Primary Nursing. The decision about which nursing care should be delivered is made by the primary nurse. The primary nurse, who has 24-hour responsibility, delivers direct patient care when on duty. In the primary nurse's absence, the plan of care is implemented by other personnel, sometimes called associate nurses.

Team Nursing. One nurse has the management role of overseeing all other members of the team. Integral to this delivery method is the care conference, where a goal-oriented plan is created for the patient.

Functional Nursing. Tasks for a group of patients are assigned to nursing personnel based on the complexity of the tasks. Unlicensed assistive personnel may be assigned to bathe and ambulate patients. A licensed nurse may be assigned to give all medications. One nurse is responsible for ensuring that all tasks are completed.

Table 12-1 compares the delivery systems described above. Which delivery system should be selected depends on the established standards, the degree of cost-effectiveness of each, patient satisfaction, nursing personnel satisfaction, the nursing process, and the physical layout of patient care areas.

Data Management

Data management and retrieval of data are important for supporting timely decision making and reducing risks in decision making. Automated sys-

Exhibit 12-5 Sample Calculation of Salary Expense per UOS

PRODUCTIVE SALARY			
Projected 5,824 Annual UOSs	× 3.0 RN Hours	× $15.66 Salary per Hour	= $273,612
Projected 5,824 Annual UOSs	× 1.0 LVN/LPN Hours	× $10.88 Salary per Hour	= $ 63,365
Projected 5,824 Annual UOSs	× 1.0 Clerical Hours	× $ 8.50 Salary per Hour	= $ 49,504
NONPRODUCTIVE SALARY			
1.51 RN FTEs	× 2,080 Hours per FTE	× $15.66 Salary per Hour	= $ 49,185
0.50 LVN/LPN FTEs	× 2,080 Hours per FTE	× $10.88 Salary per Hour	= $ 11,315
0.50 Clerical FTEs	× 2,080 Hours per FTE	× $ 8.50 Salary per Hour	= $ 8,840
INDIRECT SALARY			
1.0 Manager FTEs	× 2,080 Hours per FTE	× $21.60 Salary per Hour	= $ 44,928

$$\frac{\$386,481\ \text{Productive} + \$69,340\ \text{Nonproductive} + \$44,928\ \text{Indirect}}{5,824\ \text{Annual Projected UOSs}} = \$85.98\ \text{Salary Expense per UOS}$$

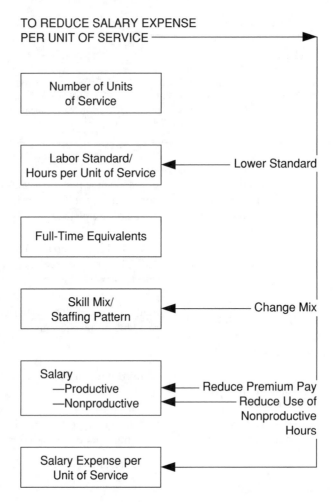

Figure 12-1 Ways to Reduce Salary Expense per Unit of Service. *Source:* Copyright 1986, 1989, 1991 Spicer and Spicer Associates, Santa Clara, California.

tems increase the nurse manager's ability to be responsive in a changing environment with diminishing resources. Key areas in need of computer-assisted management of data include nursing management and patient care.

Nursing management information systems provide managers with information for decision making and assist in communicating that information. Key components of a nursing management information system include the following:

- *Recruitment.* The recruitment component tracks the demographics of the applicant pool and the percentages of the pool being offered positions and accepting positions.
- *Position control.* The position control component tabulates budgeted versus actual positions by cost center.
- *Patient classification.* The patient classification component monitors and tabulates the acuity of patients and the use of nursing resources.

Table 12-1 Comparison of Delivery Systems

	Case Method	Primary Nursing	Team Nursing	Functional Nursing
RN Decision Making	24-hour responsibility	24-hour responsibility	8- to 12-hour shift responsibility	8- to 12-hour shift responsibility
RN Scope of Responsibility	Small groups of patients assigned by various designations	Small groups of patients from same geographical area	Large groups of patients from same geographical area	Large groups of patients from same geographical area
RN Focus	Managing critical pathways	Providing total patient care	Coordinating and planning care	Supervising delegated tasks

- *Staffing and scheduling.* This component formulates the need for nursing resources based upon indicators and also schedules employees based upon preset criteria.
- *Productivity.* This component compares resources used with target levels and provides variance analyses.
- *Quality assurance.* The quality assurance component tracks and trends critical indicators.

In the area of patient care, computer systems are most often part of a large organization-wide system. Typical components of a patient care system include the following:

- *Order entry.* The order entry component stores and communicates orders to departments responsible for carrying them out.
- *Vital signs.* This component tracks and analyzes vital signs, either directly from physiologic monitoring equipment or from data entry.
- *Care planning.* This component stores and updates patient care plans.
- *Nurses' notes.* Nursing progress notes are stored either in open format or in a predesigned "trigger" format, or both.

MANAGING QUALITY

Quality in the Context of Nursing

Quality in the context of nursing means ensuring accountability to the public for meeting the standards of clinical nursing practice. Nursing authority is based on a social contract between society and the profession. Society grants considerable professional autonomy and in turn expects nurses to act responsibly and be mindful of the public trust. The heart of this relationship is self-regulation to ensure competent performance. Quality assurance is a fundamental responsibility and is an integral part of clinical nursing practice. Participation in quality assurance activities should be expected of every nurse.

Indicators of Quality Performance

The standards of nursing practice were set forth by the ANA in 1973 and revised as standards of clinical nursing practice encompassing both standards of care and standards of professional performance in 1991.[12] The standards provide a broad basis for evaluation of performance and care and reflect recognition of the rights of those receiving nursing care. Because these standards have been accepted by leaders in the profession, quality can be defined in terms of the standards of care and professional performance. The standards of care include the following:

Standard I. Assessment: The nurse collects client health data.

Standard II. Diagnosis: The nurse analyzes the assessment data in determining diagnosis.

Standard III. Outcome Identification: The nurse identifies expected outcomes individualized to the client.

Standard IV. Planning: The nurse develops a plan of care that prescribes interventions to attain expected outcomes.

Standard V. Implementation: The nurse implements the interventions identified in the plan of care.

Standard VI. Evaluation: The nurse evaluates the client's progress toward attainment of outcomes.[13]

The standards of professional performance include the following:

Standard I. Quality of Care: The nurse systematically evaluates the quality and effectiveness of nursing practice.

Standard II. Performance Appraisal: The nurse evaluates his/her own nursing practice in relation to professional practice standards and relevant statutes and regulations.

Standard III. Education: The nurse acquires and maintains current knowledge in nursing practice.

Standard IV. Collegiality: The nurse contributes to the professional development of peers, colleagues, and others.

Standard V. Ethics: The nurse's decisions and actions on behalf of clients are determined in an ethical manner.

Standard VI. Collaboration: The nurse collaborates with the client, significant others, and health care providers in providing client care.

Standard VII. Research: The nurse uses research findings in practice.

Standard VIII. Resource Utilization: The nurse considers factors related to safety, effectiveness, and cost in planning and delivering client care.[14]

Additional standards may be derived from sources such as institutional policies, procedures, and practices or professional, licensing, or accreditation organizations.

Standards come in three types: structure, process, and outcome standards. Structure standards define the conditions and mechanisms needed to operate and control the nursing organization and are written in a policy format. They are generally viewed as governing the practice of nursing management. Process standards define the actions and behaviors of nurses giving care and the nature of that care. They are generally viewed as governing what clinical nurses do. Outcome standards define the end results of patient care.

A Ten-Step Monitoring and Evaluation Model

The Joint Commission on Accreditation of Healthcare Organizations has created a ten-step model (Figure 12-2) for monitoring and evaluation of nursing care.[15] The ten steps are as follows:

1. Assign responsibility. The overall responsibility for the monitoring and evaluation must be assigned (e.g., to the nurse executive, to a nurse manager, or to a staff support person). Ultimately the governing board has the authority and responsibility for quality patient care, and the quality assurance monitoring process must include a reporting line to the governing board.

2. Delineate the scope of care and service. A description of the scope of service should be developed. It should include types of patients served, conditions and diagnoses treated, treatments and activities performed, types of nursing staff providing care and service, all existing standards of care, sites where care is provided, and times when care is provided.

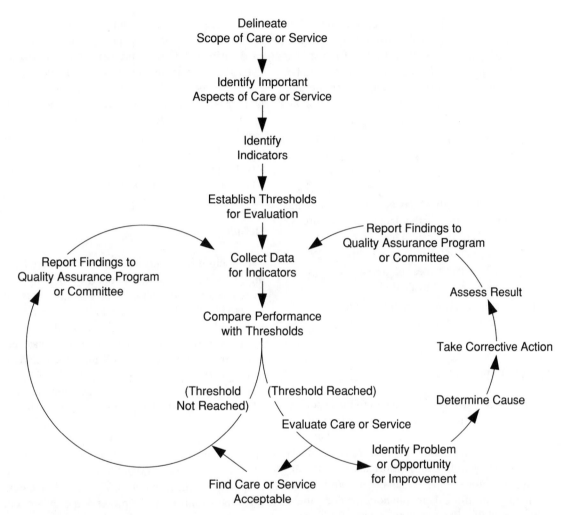

Figure 12-2 Monitoring and Evaluation Process Model. *Source:* Copyright 1988 by the Joint Commission on Accreditation of Healthcare Organizations, Oakbrook Terrace, Illinois. Reprinted from *Examples of Monitoring and Evaluation* series with permission.

3. Identify important aspects of care and service. Identify those aspects of care and service that occur frequently or affect large numbers of patients, that place patients at serious risk if not provided correctly, or that have tended in the past to produce problems for staff or patients. Important aspects of care may include skin integrity, patient safety, and medication administration.

4. Identify indicators related to the important aspects of care. Indicators are measurable variables that are related to the structure, process, or outcome of care and that provide information about the quality of particular aspects of care.

5. Establish thresholds for evaluation. Thresholds are the levels of compliance below which intense evaluation should occur.

6. Collect and organize data. This step includes identification of the study population, the study purpose, the time frame of the study, the manner in which the study is going to be conducted, and the individuals who are going to conduct the study.

7. Evaluate the care. In this step, the data collected in the previous step are interpreted.

8. Take action when appropriate for improvement if problems are identified. Responses include instituting continuing or in-service education, utilizing peer pressure, making administrative or environmental changes, and rewarding desired behavior.

9. Assess the effectiveness of actions. To assess the effectiveness of actions, data have to be collected and evaluated.

10. Communicate relevant information to the organization-wide quality assurance program.

Quality Improvement

Besides the quality assurance activities specific to nursing, there must be a focus on the flow of patient care and the processes and systems that support that flow throughout hospitalization. Nurses have a responsibility to support the quality improvement efforts of the overall organization and to bring to these efforts their collaboration and patient advocacy skills. By assuming a patient advocacy role, nurses can help maintain a focus on patient needs. Nurses can also, when working with other departments, use their collaboration skills to help look beyond specific problems and work toward a quality improvement orientation.

WORLDWIDE CHALLENGES FOR NURSING LEADERS

Nursing leaders worldwide are facing common challenges in managing nursing resources. These challenges include defining nursing, regulating nursing practice, restructuring human resource delivery systems, managing quality, supporting ethical decision making, and preparing nurse managers.

Partly responsible for these challenges is the rapid expansion in knowledge and technology that is increasing the range of available services. With this increase in range has come a growing disparity between the availability of services and the availability of economic resources to pay for them. Restructuring health care organizations and systems is an essential step to mitigate this disparity.

Defining Nursing

Nursing has no universal definition internationally, and even within most countries there appears to be no single definition. For example, it is not easy to identify the services nurses provide that can be provided by no other health care worker.

The scientific basis for nursing practice has been evolving, but that basis is still not as strong as in other professions such as medicine. Nursing research, which is essential for establishing a scientific basis for practice, is given a low priority during this period of diminishing resources. The outcomes of nursing services are also not well defined. Research is needed to document the specific outcomes of specific nursing interventions.

Ultimately the question is, Who will define nursing—the members of the profession or others outside of the profession driven by the economics of the health care industry? The challenge is to facilitate a process through which clinical nurses and nursing leaders define nursing.

Regulating Nursing Practice

Regulation of nursing has not kept abreast with the complexity and expansion of nursing roles as the nursing profession responds to the evolving health care needs of society. There are a number of groups with a special interest in the regulation of nursing practice. Specifically, these include the public, which needs affordable and accessible services from the profession; the nurses, who depend on the profession for social and economic benefits; and the employers, who are the intermediaries and are accountable to the public, through licensing and regulatory bodies, for the outcomes of care provided. Mediating the multiple interests of these groups and influencing which group will have the strongest impact in the regulatory process is a challenge for nursing leaders.

Restructuring Human Resource Delivery Systems

Nursing leaders have been prompted by the external environment to re-evaluate the current utilization of human resources. The economics of utilizing lower skilled and lower paid personnel is dictating the integration of increasing numbers of unlicensed assistive personnel into the nursing services delivery system. In some geographic locales, this same type of integration is driven by supply and demand or by a shortage of licensed practitioners.

This integration means that nursing leaders need to sort out those functions that must be done by registered nurses and those functions that can be done by unlicensed assistive personnel. It is desirable to have the legal system support registered nurses to perform all functions of nursing care that require a substantial amount of scientific knowledge and technical skill. For example, the assessing, diagnosing, planning, and evaluating elements of the nursing process should remain in the realm of the registered nurse.

Managing Quality

People are better educated today about health care and more likely to be involved in health care decisions. They are also more interested in prevention and self-care.

Managing quality as perceived by consumers, patients, and third-party payers, including insurance companies and the government, is a challenge. Quality in health care services exists in two spheres: the outcome sphere and the interactive sphere. The outcome sphere encompasses the measurable results of interventions, and the interactive sphere encompasses the interpersonal interactions between patients and providers of care. For nursing leaders, it is easier to manage the interactive sphere than the outcome sphere. Third-party payers, however, are beginning to link reimbursement to the achievement of outcomes, and nursing is not currently able to predict the outcomes of specific nursing interventions with a high degree of certainty.

Supporting Ethical Decision Making

The practice of nursing requires new levels of ethical awareness and sensitivity. An increasingly informed and assertive public is looking to nurses for information, guidance, and support concerning the ethical quandaries permeating health care. Unresolved issues range from the appropriateness of allocating limited health care resources to the right of individuals to deny extraordinary efforts to prolong life. An ethical decision-making structure must be developed and implemented. Establishing an ethics committee with interdisciplinary membership is one means of providing a support system for ethical decision making. The committee's functions could include consultation, counseling, prospective review, retrospective review, and making policy recommendations.

Preparing Nurse Managers

The era when nurse managers managed in traditional and stable organizations is gone. The restructuring of health care systems is now rapidly occurring, and the systems may never fully stabilize. Nurse managers must now be prepared to manage—to establish standards of clinical practice and to structure an environment in which the nursing process can be actualized—in a context of continuous change. Taking the two constants, standards of clinical practice and the nursing process, and using their knowledge and experience in the science of organizational development and administration, nurse managers must integrate nursing into organizations or health care systems as a whole to help achieve high-quality patient care and strong economic performance.

The challenge is preparing nurse managers of the future. Where will these nurse managers be educated and by whom? Will it be within schools of nursing and business administration? Given current economic constraints, how will nursing leaders be able to integrate and advance the science of nursing while acquiring the in-depth knowledge of organizational development and administration they will need?

If nursing leaders do not meet the challenges successfully, nursing will risk losing the identity it is struggling to maintain and strengthen, and the restructuring process will occur without strong input from the profession.

CONCLUSION

Historical developments dating back to the middle of the nineteenth century have influenced modern-day nursing. The dependent, interdependent, and independent functions of nursing evolved gradually, and by the 1960s the independent functions had been placed within the theoretical framework of the nursing process.

Organizational structures and roles vary, but the standards for organized nursing put forth by the ANA act as guidelines for establishing effective nursing departments. Shared decision making needs to prevail in the independent functions of nursing. This kind of decision making relies on the expertise of the clinical nurse.

Quality in the context of nursing means ensuring accountability to the public for meeting the standards of clinical nursing practice. Managing quality is the responsibility of every nurse and is an integral part of clinical nursing practice. Nurses must be involved in the overall organization's quality im-

provement efforts and contribute their skills in patient advocacy and collaboration.

Managing nursing resources in the future will present challenges for nursing leaders worldwide. These challenges include defining nursing, regulating nursing practice, restructuring human resource delivery systems, managing quality, supporting ethical decision making, and preparing nurse managers. These challenges must be met in order for nursing to maintain a strong presence in health care delivery.

ADDITIONAL RESOURCES

Organizations

American Nurses' Association, 2420 Pershing Road, Kansas City, MO 64108, 816/474-5720

American Organization of Nurse Executives, 840 North Lakeshore Drive, Chicago, IL 60611, 312/280-4190

International Council of Nurses, 3, place Jean-Marteau, 1201 Geneva, Switzerland, 011-41-22-731-2960

Joint Commission on Accreditation of Healthcare Organizations, One Renaissance Boulevard, Oakbrook Terrace, IL 60181, 708/916-5600

National League for Nursing, 10 Columbus Circle, New York, New York 10019, 212/989-9393

Periodicals

Journal of Nursing Administration, J.B. Lippincott Co., E. Washington Square, Philadelphia, PA 19105, 215/238-4200

Nursing Administration Quarterly, Aspen Publishers, Inc., 200 Orchard Ridge Drive, Gaithersburg, MD 20878, 301/417-7617

Nursing Management, 103 N. Second Street, Suite 200, West Dundee, IL 60118, 708/426-6100

Newsletter

Aspen's Advisor for Nurse Executives, Aspen Publishers, Inc., 200 Orchard Ridge Drive, Gaithersburg, MD 20878, 301/417-7500

Books and Articles

Carpenito, L. *Nursing diagnosis: Application to clinical practice.* Philadelphia: J.B. Lippincott, 1991.

Finkler, S.A. *Budget concepts for nurse managers.* 2d ed. San Francisco: Grune & Stratton, 1992.

Joint Commission on Accreditation of Healthcare Organizations. *Update on nursing services monitoring and evaluation.* Oakbrook Terrace, Ill.: Joint Commission, 1989.

Levine, J., and D. Groh. *Nursing manager bookshelf: Creating an ethical environment.* Baltimore: Williams & Wilkins, 1990.

Lewis, E.M., and J.G. Spicer. *Human resource management handbook: Contemporary strategies for nursing managers.* Gaithersburg, Md.: Aspen Publishers, 1987.

Lieske, A.M. *Clinical nursing research: A guide to undertaking and using research in nursing practice.* Gaithersburg, Md.: Aspen Publishers, 1986.

Mikulsky, M.P., and C. Ledford. *Computers in nursing: Hospital and clinical applications.* Menlo Park, Calif.: Addison-Wesley, 1990.

Osguthorp, S. Ancillary and support services. In *Managing the environment in critical care nursing,* ed. J.G. Spicer and M.A. Robinson. Baltimore: Williams & Wilkins, 1990.

Pinkerton, S., and P. Schroader. *Commitment to excellence.* Gaithersburg, Md.: Aspen Publishers, 1988.

Stevens, B.J. *The nurse as executive.* 3d ed. Gaithersburg, Md.: Aspen Publishers, 1985.

Strasen, L. *Key business skills for nurse managers.* Philadelphia: J.B. Lippincott, 1987.

U.S. Department of Health and Human Services. *Secretary's Commission on Nursing.* Vols. 1 and 2. Washington, D.C.: U.S. Department of Health and Human Services, 1988.

NOTES

1. P.W. Iyer, B.J. Taptich and I. Bernocchi-Lesey, *Nursing Process and Nursing Diagnosis,* 2d ed. (Philadelphia: W.B. Saunders, 1991).

2. K.H. Fenner and P. Fenner, *Manual of Nurse Recruitment and Retention* (Gaithersburg, Md.: Aspen Publishers, 1989).

3. American Nurses' Association, *The Nurse Practice Act: Suggested State Legislation* (Kansas City, Mo.: American Nurses' Association, 1981).

4. American Nurses' Association, *Nursing: A Social Policy Statement* (Kansas City, Mo.: American Nurses' Association, 1980), 9.

5. American Nurses' Association, *The Role of the Clinical Nurse Specialist* (Kansas City, Mo.: American Nurses' Association, 1986).

6. American Nurses' Association, *Standards for Organized Nursing Services and Responsibilities of Nurse Administrators across All Settings* (Kansas City, Mo.: American Nurses' Association, 1991), 3–8.

7. E.J. Serra, Orienting and Developing Professional Nurses in the Practice Setting, in *Human Resource Management Handbook,* ed. E.M. Lewis and J.G. Spicer (Gaithersburg, Md.: Aspen Publishers, 1987).

8. American Nurses' Association, *Guidelines for the Investigation Function of Nurses* (Kansas City, Mo.: American Nurses' Association, 1981).

9. American Nurses' Association, *Roles, Responsibilities, and Qualifications for Nurse Administrators* (Kansas City, Mo.: American Nurses' Association, 1978); Joint Commission on Accreditation of Healthcare Organizations, *The 1991 Joint Commission Accreditation Manual for Hospitals,* vol. 1 (Oakbrook Terrace, Ill.: Joint Commission, 1990).

10. American Nurses' Association, *Roles, Responsibilities, and Qualifications for Nurse Administrators;* Organization of Nurse Executives, *ONE-C Middle Manager Job Description* (Sacramento, Calif.: Organization of Nurse Executives, n.d.).

11. D.A. England, *Collaboration in Nursing* (Gaithersburg, Md.: Aspen Publishers, 1986).

12. American Nurses' Association, *Standards of Clinical Nursing Practice* (Kansas City, Mo.: American Nurses' Association, 1991).

13. Ibid., pp. 9–17.

14. Ibid., pp. 9–17.

15. Joint Commission on Accreditation of Healthcare Organizations, *Update on Nursing Service Monitoring and Evaluation* (Oakbrook Terrace, Ill.: Joint Commission, 1989), 5–37.

Part III

Information Management and Planning

Charles J. Austin
Richard C. Howe

Information Systems Management

13

Purpose: Information systems management provides a foundation upon which a hospital can develop and manage its information resources. The resultant computerized information systems can provide timely, accurate, and relevant information to hospital managers and clinical personnel for improving managerial decision making, promoting quality patient care, improving the efficiency of operations, controlling the use of institutional resources, and supporting service delivery throughout the organization.

INTRODUCTION

Carefully planned information systems are important assets for hospital management. Although computers are only incidental to the processing of information, they provide a powerful tool to improve the speed, accuracy, and communication of information throughout the organization. Advances in computer technology have brought the costs of these systems within the financial capability of even very small hospitals. However, computers are only tools to assist in accomplishing a broader set of goals. Careful analysis and planning of informa-

tion requirements in light of institutional priorities should always precede decisions on acquisition of computer hardware and software.

Computer systems should be planned to support the following management functions in the hospital.

Strategic Planning. Hospital computer systems can provide information to assist management in mission development, goal setting, program planning, and evaluation.

Quality Assessment and Improvement. Hospital computer systems can provide clinical information extracted from medical records for quality assessment purposes and can be used to process information obtained from surveys of patient satisfaction and employee attitudes within the organization.

Financial Analysis and Cost Containment and Avoidance. Hospital computer systems can provide assistance in financial analysis and forecasting.

Productivity Improvement. Computer systems can provide cost and productivity information on specific services and compare the organization's productivity with the productivity of other hospitals providing similar services in the community.

Performance Assessment and Service Evaluation. Hospital computer systems can provide periodic service statistics on inpatient occupancy, ambulatory patient visits, diagnostic tests performed in the clinical laboratory, and other quantitative measures of organizational activity.

Reporting to Government Agencies and Other External Organizations. Hospital computer systems can assist in generating the reports required by external organizations, including government agencies, accrediting bodies, third-party financing agencies, and major employers who provide health insurance for their workers.

Research and Education. Many larger hospitals, particularly those affiliated with educational institutions, use computer systems to support clinical research and to assist in the education and training of clinical personnel.

MANAGEMENT PRINCIPLES

The following management principles should guide the planning, design, and implementation of computer-based hospital information systems:

1. Treat information as an institutional resource. Hospitals are information-intensive organizations, and information must be treated as a major resource of an organization, on a par with its human, financial, and capital resources.

2. Obtain top executive support for information systems planning. Support for information systems development from the hospital's chief executive officer (CEO) and chief operating officer (COO) is essential for success. The planning and development of systems should be coordinated by a corporate-level executive, the chief information officer (CIO).

3. Employ a user-driven focus in the information systems planning process. Active involvement of personnel from all segments of the hospital organization (management, operating departments, and medical staff) is essential. This participation should start with the definition of information requirements and continue through all phases of analysis, design, system selection, and implementation.

4. Develop an information systems plan for the institution:
   - Link the information systems plan to the hospital's strategic business plan.
   - Establish institution-wide priorities for the development of information system resources.
   - Determine appropriate costs and commit the funds required to achieve information management objectives.
   - Update the plan at least once a year.

In order to ensure that systems are developed properly in accordance with hospital priorities, information systems planning is essential. An information systems steering committee (Figure 13-1) should guide the construction of a hospital master plan for information systems development. The steering committee should be chaired by the CIO or a senior executive designated by the hospital administrator. Representatives from the major patient care and administrative departments should be included as members. Typical responsibilities are outlined in Exhibit 13-1.

Exhibit 13-2 summarizes the major elements to be included in the information systems master plan. The plan should be directly linked to the hospital's strategic planning process, and priorities for information systems should be determined by the strategic imperatives of the organization. Correlation with the hospital's financial plan is essential in order to establish the appropriate percentage of the operating and capital budgets to be devoted to systems design, operation, and maintenance.

The master plan should establish priorities for individual computer applications and should specify the overall approach to be fol-

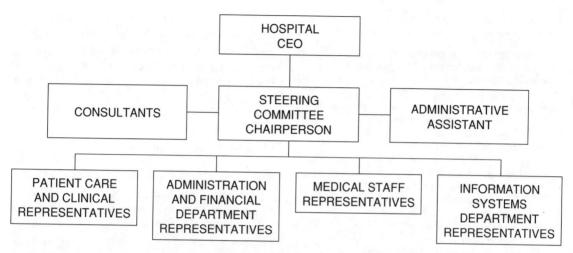

Figure 13-1 Information Systems Steering Committee Organization Chart

lowed for integration of systems (centralized processing or distributed processing following institution-wide data definition standards). The plan should include an analysis and evaluation of alternative approaches to systems analysis, systems design, and computer programming. (A more detailed discussion of systems integration and development alternatives occurs later in this chapter.)

The master information systems plan should include cost analyses and forecasts along with a

Exhibit 13-1 Information Systems Steering Committee Responsibilities

- Development and approval of information systems strategic plan
- Approval of information systems policies and procedures
- Establishment of information systems cost recovery and allocation policies
- Prioritization of major information systems projects according to hospital business plan
- Monitoring of major information systems projects with respect to schedule and budget

schedule of target dates for implementation of major applications. The plan should be updated at least once a year or whenever major changes in strategic direction occur.

5. Define information requirements before acquiring systems. Guided by the information systems master plan, careful analysis of information requirements should precede specific hardware and software selection. Users should be actively involved in this process. Individual computer applications must be planned so that system integration is achieved (i.e., the capacity for logical tracking and communication of information among related applications). The ability to combine clinical and financial information from different applications is essential for cost control and evaluation of patient care quality.

ORGANIZATIONAL ROLE

History and Background

Computer systems began to come into general use in hospitals during the 1960s. Most computer programs were developed by in-house staffs consisting of systems analysts and programmers and

Exhibit 13-2 Information Systems Master Plan

- Statement of Institutional Objectives
  - Priorities for Information Systems Relative to Strategic Priorities of Hospital
  - Correlation with Hospital's Financial Plan
- Statement of Priorities for Individual Applications
- Evaluation of Systems Architecture Alternatives
  - Centralized Database
  - Distributed Processing
  - Modified Distributed Processing (Central Database Linked to a Network of Microcomputers)
- Evaluation of Alternative Approaches to Systems Analysis, Systems Design, and Computer Programming
  - In-house Development
  - Contract Services
  - Use of Predesigned (Packaged) Software
  - Combinations of the Above
- Cost Analysis and Forecasts
  - Design and Development
  - Implementation
  - Operation and Maintenance
  - Postimplementation Review and Evaluation

were geared toward financial functions such as payroll, general ledger accounting, and patient accounting. Applications generally employed batch processing of transactions on a daily, weekly, or monthly basis; and data were not available for immediate retrieval at user work stations because of limitations of the technology. There was little system integration, and most applications were operated as independent departmental data processing systems.

Advances in telecommunications, mass electronic storage, and central processors led to direct user access to computerized databases during the 1970s and 1980s. Commercial firms began to develop generalized computer programs (applications software) for administrative and clinical departments, and hospitals began to move away from in-house design and programming of systems. Applications software packages are available for patient admissions/discharges/transfer (ADT); order entry and results reporting; patient accounting and accounts receivable; laboratory, pharmacy, and radiology systems; and several other functions.

Rapid advances in minicomputer and microcomputer hardware made decentralized or distributed processing throughout the hospital more attractive, and the technology came into the financial reach of even the smallest of hospitals by the beginning of the 1990s.

Organizational Policies

As mentioned previously, development of a strategic information systems plan is the first step in effective information management in hospitals. The plan should include key policies on information systems that reflect the long-term goals of the organization and major challenges facing the organization within the next five to seven years.[1]

There are at least four key policy decisions an organization must make to determine the appropriate information systems strategy:[2]

- whether to use commercial or internally developed software
- whether to use in-house or shared-service processing
- whether to use multiple or single-vendor supplied software systems
- whether to have centralized or decentralized control of computer and information systems and staff

Commercial versus Internally Developed Software

The first key policy decision, whether to use commercial or internally developed software, will have major implications. For example, the data processing staff required for in-house development of software is considerably different (in terms of the number and type of staff members) from the staff required for installation of commercial software (assuming the software vendor will have the primary responsibility for maintenance of the software). Due to the cost of developing software today, most health care institutions are moving toward obtaining commercial software.

In-House versus Shared-Service Processing

The next key policy issue is whether the hospital will process its own information on an in-house computer or process its data using a shared-service company. A hospital can either buy or develop software and yet operate that software on another organization's computer. The primary advantage of using shared-service processing is that the hospital does not have to maintain a computer facility and the associated staff needed to run the hardware. The primary disadvantage is that the hospital loses processing schedule flexibility.

Multiple- versus Single-Vendor Supplied Software Systems

Once a hospital has decided to use commercial software, it must next decide whether to obtain all its software from a single vendor or from multiple vendors. Generally, single-vendor systems are more highly integrated, and the application packages have been designed to complement each other. A major disadvantage with the single-vendor approach is that a single vendor cannot have strong functionality in all application areas within a hospital. This means that some departments may have highly sophisticated software and other departments only very basic, mediocre software. By using multiple vendors, the hospital has the opportunity to select the best software to meet each particular need. The major disadvantage of the multiple-vendor approach is the number of complex interfaces that must be developed to make this approach work. In addition, in a multiple-vendor environment, anytime a vendor upgrades its software, the interfaces may need to be updated or even rewritten. Thus, the maintenance and cost associated with these interfaces becomes a major issue.

Centralized versus Decentralized Control of Computer and Information Systems Staff

A final key policy decision a hospital must address is whether to use a centralized or a decentralized approach to data processing. In a centralized approach, the hardware and data processing staff are generally located at a single site. In a decentralized approach, the data processing staff and hardware can be distributed throughout various departments or business units of the organization. Some organizations have centralized their hardware components, but have decentralized the information systems staff within the various departments or business units. This approach allows the support staff to be intimately associated with each department and yet maintains the economies of scale associated with a centralized computer facility.[3]

In addition to these major decisions, several other factors or issues will influence an organization's policies regarding its information systems, including the following:

- organizational structure and controls
- technical simplicity versus interfacing complexity
- shared services support
- information systems requirements of the organization and each business unit
- access to a common database
- institution-wide information systems standards
- consolidated reporting
- uniform standard reporting
- current information systems
- space requirements
- costs and discounts

The organizational structure and controls associated with the information systems must reflect the management style of the organization and the related information requirements. If the organization is highly centralized, then the information systems structure should similarly be centralized. If the management style of an organization is highly decentralized, the information systems structure will most likely be decentralized. A policy on who reviews and approves all hardware and software purchases and information systems budgets must also be established.

Technical simplicity is another factor that may influence overall information systems policies. As the number of software vendors increases, the number of complex interfaces also increases. The technical complexities and risks associated with maintenance of these interfaces must be taken into consideration in determining the overall information systems approach.

Some hospitals and organizations will provide some centralized support services for evaluating hardware, software, telecommunications, and other related functions. Sharing services may also involve sharing of the actual central processing units (mainframe or minicomputers) among several different business units within the organization.

The information system requirements of the hospital and each business unit must be considered in determining the appropriate information systems strategy. Teaching hospitals may have some unique information systems requirements that a commercial vendor will not typically be able to meet. On the other hand, a smaller community hospital may find the software available from a commercial vendor adequate to its needs.

Access to a common database requires preplanning of key information systems–related standards. Executive management and departmental directors in a hospital generally need access to a common administrative database. The administrative database will include patient demographic information, financial information, and profit and loss information by department, DRG, and physician. Physicians, on the other hand, need access to a common clinical database. This means that if a patient moves from an outpatient setting through the emergency room to become an inpatient, then moves back to the outpatient setting, the information system must be able to track clinical data throughout all the episodes of patient care. This may mean the hospital and its associated physician group practices may have to utilize a common medical record number and common computer system in order to create this longitudinal clinical database and track the data.

The establishment of institution-wide information systems standards is extremely important for developing a more integrated system. The lack of standards will create many disparate software systems and associated hardware platforms. Having such disparate hardware-software systems makes it very difficult to link the systems together, both from a technical and software (i.e., user) point of view. Lack of standards will require development of complex interfaces that are costly to develop and maintain, may be "one of a kind," and will contribute nothing to the overall functionality of the system.

The information systems standards in a hospital typically include data element definition, data element coding system, file structure, hardware, patient care software, and personal computer software and hardware standards. Creation of institution-wide standards will greatly facilitate establishment of a common management or clinical database and improve access to multiple databases in a more distributed environment. Other evolving health care information systems standards include those being developed by the Health Level-7 group (an organization of hospitals, vendors, and consulting firms that devises health care data definition standards) and Medical Data Interchange (MEDIX). Government entities such as the U.S. Veterans Administration and the Canadian Health Care System have established uniform health care standards to be used within their patient care systems.[4]

An information system with a consolidated reporting capability can combine financial or clinical data from different sections within the hospital into a single report. This capability requires establishment of the institution-wide information systems coding and data definition standards mentioned above.

A system with a uniform standard reporting capability can produce reports for a particular function that are uniform in appearance and standard across all business units of the hospital. For example, all lab reports would be uniform in appearance regardless of which inpatient, intensive care, or outpatient clinic they supported. If the hospital establishes uniform standard reporting as an organizational policy, then the information system must be able to produce uniform reports.

In establishing information systems policies, the current information system and the support staff must also be taken into consideration. If the hospital has recently invested in new hardware, it may choose to establish a policy requiring future systems to operate on the existing or compatible hardware. Also, if the information systems staff are highly trained in a particular set of technical skills, the hospital may establish policies that do not allow a department to purchase hardware or software that cannot be supported by its own internal information systems staff.

Space requirements may also have an influence on information systems policies. A decentralized approach may require a computer room and support staff space in each facility, building, or other clinic area. On the other hand, if a hospital desires to move from a decentralized to a centralized approach, the space and environmental requirements for a new computer system may exceed what is available. This means that the hospital will have to develop a new computer facility in order to adopt a more centralized approach.

Information systems policies must also reflect costs or discounts associated with different approach alternatives. Generally, a centralized approach, when all the cost factors are taken into account, is less expensive than a decentralized approach. Also, discounts can be greater with centralized purchasing of hardware and software. Therefore, a hospital may establish a policy on centralized purchasing of all hardware and software even if the information system operates in a more decentralized manner.

ORGANIZATIONAL RELATIONSHIPS

The management policies and other related factors mentioned above will ultimately determine the organizational relationships of the information system. In particular, the choice of centralization or decentralization of computer systems will be of crucial importance. The trend today is toward centralized management of a highly complex, distributed data-processing environment that encompasses everything from the traditional centralized computer system to totally decentralized personal computers. The information system in tomorrow's hospital must be capable of managing this broad spectrum of computer systems in a well-controlled, highly integrated manner.

The advantages of centralization are that it

- facilitates development of a plan to meet major long-term system needs
- facilitates system integration
- promotes development of a "corporate" or institution-wide database
- maximizes the availability of technical staff expertise
- minimizes costly duplication of data entry and storage
- helps control cost

The advantages of decentralization are that it

- fosters innovation and creativity at the user level
- maximizes local flexibility in the selection of software and hardware
- facilitates satisfaction of short-term system needs
- maximizes user control
- promotes utilization of good department-level software
- avoids backlogs of demand at a central facility

In summary, analyzing various alternatives is a complex process. The business goals of the hospital and the various factors that influence information systems policies must be evaluated for each approach or option. The conditions or assumptions under which the hospital is willing to operate will set the stage for the evaluation and selection of the most appropriate approach.[5] The hospital must then collect as much factual information as possible on all alternatives and do a cost-benefit analysis to determine which is best for the organization. Once the hospital's approach is determined, an information systems organizational structure can then be developed to support the chosen approach.[6]

The Chief Information Officer

The CIO is the person in an organization mainly responsible for the information system. Typical titles include the chief information officer, vice-president of management information systems, management information systems director, and data processing manager.[7] Regardless of title, the CIO typically is a member of the executive management team or the executive cabinet, is considered an equal within the executive management team (with equal voting power), and reports to the CEO or top executive within the organization.

In a large organization, the position of CIO is generally a full-time, distinct position. However, in smaller hospitals, the chief financial officer (CFO) or chief operating officer (COO) may fulfill this function. A smaller organization would still have a director of data processing or management information systems as the primary person responsible for daily information systems functions, but this person would not be part of the executive management team.

The general roles and responsibilities of the CIO are listed in Exhibit 13-3. In general, the CIO is responsible for the planning, coordination, implementation, operation, and maintenance of all information systems–related activity within the hospital.[8]

Given today's health care environment, the CIO will need to be involved in every department. Therefore, the CIO must possess excellent management and technical skills in order to fulfill the responsibilities of the job.[9] These skills include communication, personnel management, strategic and tactical planning, and project management skills. The CIO must also have a thorough knowledge of the health care environment.

Exhibit 13-3 CIO Responsibilities and Estimated Time Percentages

- Planning (30%)
  —Strategic hospital business plan
  —Strategic information systems plan
  —Hospital and information systems budgets
  —Disaster recovery plans
- Coordination (30%)
  —Information systems committees
  —Information systems policies and procedures
  —Evaluation and selection of software
  —Information systems with hospital operations
- Implementation (20%)
  —General guidelines
  —Implementation plans
  —Vendor relations
- Operations (10%)
  —Setting of operational policies and procedures
  —General guidance of managers
- Maintenance (10%)
  —Establishment of user training and support functions
  —Monitoring of system functionality
  —Establishment of regular system updates

The CIO must possess excellent oral communication and writing skills and be able to communicate at both an executive and a staff level. The CIO also must be able to communicate all information systems–related activities to individuals in the organization in nontechnical English. The CIO must be able to manage personnel effectively by demonstrating clear and consistent goals, a decisive attitude, and a team approach to problem solving.

Since the strategic information systems plan is a key element in development of a successful information system, the CIO must possess excellent strategic as well as tactical planning capabilities. The CIO also must demonstrate strong project management skills. It is the CIO's responsibility to ensure that all projects thoroughly outline what is going to be done, when it is going to be done, who is going to do it, the total hours required to accomplish the project, and the total cost associated with the project.

The CIO must possess an excellent knowledge of the health care environment in general. The CIO must understand that the priorities and pressures involved in running a patient care facility are very different from those for non-health-care organizations. The knowledge of health care can then be incorporated into the implementation process for all new systems without having a major negative impact on patient care.

In addition to the management skills noted above, the CIO must also possess excellent technical skills as well as implementation and operations experience and general technical knowledge about information systems.

The CIO must have sufficient implementation experience to be able to monitor and evaluate general problems associated with the implementation of a complex information system. Operations experience related to hardware, software, operating systems, backup, and security is essential. The CIO must also possess an understanding of the capabilities and limitations of computer systems and a general knowledge of telecommunications, office automation systems, and personal computers.

In a recent survey, respondents cited the personal attributes they thought were necessary for a CIO to possess in order to be successful. The results are summarized in Table 13-1.

The functions commonly reporting to or coordinated by the CIO include information systems, telecommunications, and management engineering. Other functions sometimes reporting to the CIO include medical records, admitting, quality assurance or utilization review, materials management, ancillary services, planning and marketing, the business office, and other smaller functions.

The CIO is rapidly becoming a key executive in successful health care organizations. This individual must lead the executive management team in the development of information management systems, which are among the key assets of any organization.

PLANNING AND MANAGING INFORMATION SYSTEMS

Hospital Computer Applications

As mentioned earlier, system integration is essential for any hospital computerization program. Individual applications must be planned and implemented so that they can communicate and share information with one another.

Hospital computer applications can be grouped into three categories: administrative and financial support, clinical support, and strategic decision support. Administrative and financial applications are designed to support day-to-day operations in the financial and administrative areas of the hospital. Clinical applications involve the processing of information to support patient care. Strategic decision support systems assist with strategic planning, management control, and program evaluation at the executive level of the organization.

A hierarchy of systems is shown in Figure 13-2. The administrative and financial systems are at the base and are linked to the clinical systems; all of these provide information for use in the decision support systems, which assist management at the strategic level.

Administrative and Financial Applications

Accurate and timely financial information is essential for the effective operation of a modern hospital. Financial applications were the first to be de-

---

Table 13-1 Ranking of CIO Attributes

Attribute	Percentage of Respondents
Leadership Ability	83.1
Vision/Imagination	79.4
Business Acumen	49.3
Knowledge of Hospital Systems	44.1
Record of Success	15.4
Decisiveness	14.7
Hard Work	6.6
Technical Competence	3.7
Miscellaneous	4.4

Source: Data from *Health Care Chief Information Officer* by American Hospital Association, Center for Health Care Information, Andersen Consulting and Heidrick & Struggles, 1990.

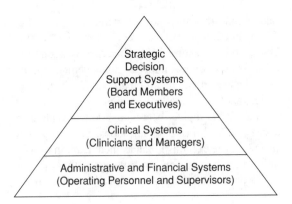

Figure 13-2 Computer Systems and Their Main Users

veloped in most hospitals. Computer systems can support the following financial functions:

- payroll preparation
- accounts payable
- patient accounting, billing, and accounts receivable
- cost accounting
- general ledger accounting
- budgeting and budget control
- financial reporting (including DRG analysis)

A large number of vendors offer financial software for hospitals. A good accounting system must be in place first before these systems will be effective in supporting hospital financial management.

Human resources information systems assist hospital managers and supervisors in work force planning and productivity. Functions include maintenance of computer-based employee records, position control linked to the budget, labor analysis, skills inventory, problem analysis (including turnover and absenteeism), labor cost allocation, and productivity reporting.

Hospitals must use their facilities in the most efficient manner in this era of cost and quality control. Computer systems are available to assist in the scheduling and monitoring of utilization (e.g., outpatient clinic visits, operating suite visits, and preadmission testing) in order to minimize daily fluctuations in census and optimize staffing levels throughout the hospital. Others can assist in scheduling of preventive maintenance, processing of work orders, and controlling energy utilization.

Materials management systems support cost control and service quality in the modern hospital. Systems are available for automated requisitioning, purchasing, and receipt of materials; inventory control; menu planning and food service management; and automated linkage of purchases to the accounts payable system.

Office automation has become commonplace in the modern hospital. Typical computer applications include word processing, electronic mail, meeting scheduling, maintenance of calendars, and management project reporting.

Clinical Applications

Clinical applications are described in detail in Chapter 14. The benefits of clinical computer systems include improved communication of physician's orders, more standardized protocols for diagnosis and treatment, improved recordkeeping for medical audit and quality control purposes, and establishment of a medical database linked to demographic data of patients for planning and evaluation of services.[10]

The major types of clinical applications include

- medical records management
- nursing applications
- medical decision support
- computerized instrumentation
- biomedical research applications
- clinical education applications
- physician office–hospital linkages
- clinical department applications (e.g., applications in the laboratory)

Strategic Decision Support Systems

Hospital managers require timely and relevant information in order to plan and evaluate services and control the use of resources. Although decision-support and executive-information systems are not used extensively today, the development and use of such systems will be critical in the decade to come. These systems are needed to support decision making at all levels of the organization as well as total quality management efforts.

Planning and marketing systems combine internal information from hospital administrative and clinical systems with external information about the community. These systems can generate planning projections of inpatient and outpatient activity by service (diagnosis related) and geographic area in the market served by the hospital.

Software is available for financial modeling and case mix analysis. These programs are capable of investment analysis, analysis of major capital purchases, simulation and modeling of the effects of price discounts given to major purchasers of care, and analysis of the effects of changes in third-party reimbursement.

Health care delivery is very labor intensive. Productivity management systems monitor employee performance against pre-established standards to help managers gain control over salary expenses.

Decision support systems in hospitals must provide data on the units of service produced, the resources consumed in providing these services, the quality of services rendered, and the effectiveness of services in meeting community health needs. It is important to note that decision support systems require well-integrated feeder systems and are difficult to install.

Evaluating and Selecting Systems

Vendor Selection Process

The vendor selection process must be based on careful planning and on defining user requirements. As mentioned earlier, the information systems plan must take into account the global requirements for information management in the organization as well as the detailed functional user requirements. These two sets of requirements will provide the

foundation for evaluating vendor products and ultimately selecting a system.

The vendor selection process generally can be either an informal process or a formal process. An informal process tends to involve a smaller group of individuals and less documentation, and generally a request for proposal (RFP) is not prepared. It may, however, include the use of a request for information (RFI) as a way of obtaining some detailed information. The RFI can be a valuable tool for screening software vendors and their products and reducing the number of vendors that need to be evaluated. A third-party consultant can also be hired to assist in planning the overall project or to provide outside expertise.

A list of potential software vendors can be obtained from major trade journals and vendor guidebooks, such as *Computers in Healthcare, Healthcare Informatics, Hospital Software Source Book,* and *R. L. Johnson Reports,*[11] as well as from professional meetings, consultants, and other hospitals.

A formal vendor selection process generally involves a larger team of individuals, requires more documentation, and includes a formal RFP. A third-party consultant is usually hired to assist throughout the process.

A model formal vendor selection process is presented in Figure 13-3. The process begins with the development of global system requirements. These global requirements reflect the overall purpose of the vendor selection process and, in a very general way, identify the kind of software application packages that are going to be obtained. Once the global system requirements have been developed, the hospital can begin development of detailed functional requirements. The object is to list the functions and features required by the hospital as a whole and by each department that is obtaining software during the selection process. Normally, detailed function requirements are developed by each individual department and then consolidated into one document, which then becomes part of the RFP.

As part of the selection process, the hospital must prepare the formal criteria by which it will evaluate vendors. The vendor evaluation criteria can gener-

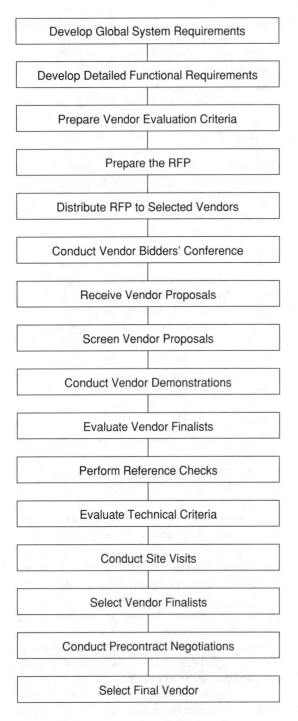

Figure 13-3 Formal Vendor Selection Process

ally be grouped into five categories: functionality, flexibility, integration, vendor stability, and cost. The hospital must identify what characteristics under each of these categories are going to be used to evaluate the vendors, and it must then determine the appropriate weight each of the categories will have in the overall evaluation. Thus, the hospital will produce a set of evaluation criteria that are quantifiable and will assist in the overall vendor selection process. It is important that the hospital determine vendor selection evaluation criteria before looking at or examining any of the vendor products. The selection criteria should truly reflect the values and needs of the hospital and not the marketing literature provided by the vendors.

The hospital can then prepare the formal RFP. The RFP should contain not only the detailed functional requirements developed earlier but also sufficient information about the hospital for each vendor to appropriately answer the questions. Most vendors require certain statistical volume data as well as projected growth data in order to correctly size the hardware for the institution. The RFP should state a deadline for receipt of the proposal and identify a single individual to deal with vendor questions. This individual is responsible for coming up with the answers and forwarding them back to the vendors.

Once the RFP is finalized, it can be distributed to a select group of vendors that generally meet the initial global requirements of the hospital. It is recommended that the RFP be sent to no more than five or six vendors. Not only does keeping the number down simplify the evaluation process, it is also fair to the vendors, because it is expensive for the vendors to respond to RFPs. The hospital should allow at least four weeks for the vendors to respond to the RFP. This will allow time for the vendors to get their questions answered and produce a quality proposal.

After the RFP has been distributed, the hospital may wish to conduct a vendor bidders' conference. The purpose of a bidders' conference is to answer questions the vendors may have in a public forum. All vendors should be invited to the bidders' conference, and all questions asked during the conference should be answered in writing, and the responses should be distributed to all vendors. If the RFP is organized well enough and contains sufficient detailed information, a vendor bidders' conference may not be necessary.

After the vendor proposals have been received, the hospital must begin an initial screening of the proposals. The screening will involve a formal evaluation of each vendor's proposal based on the vendor evaluation criteria established previously. Depending on the vendor responses received, some of the vendors may be eliminated at this time. If the hospital has previously determined that some of the requirements are mandatory, the hospital may wish to eliminate at this point vendors that are unable to meet these requirements.

Once the vendor proposals have been screened and inadequate proposals have been eliminated, the hospital can invite the remaining vendors to conduct product demonstrations. Prior to conducting these demonstrations, the hospital should determine exactly what it wants to see from all the vendors. The hospital can then develop a formal script that can be sent to each vendor, with instructions for each vendor to conduct their demonstrations according to the script. By having all vendors follow the same demonstration script, the hospital will be able to evaluate the demonstrations in a more quantifiable and thorough manner. Without any formal script, the vendors will tend to demonstrate only those portions of their product that they desire to show (i.e., the product's strengths). However, this will not allow the hospital to evaluate the overall strengths and weaknesses of each software product.

After the product demonstrations have been conducted, the hospital can perform reference checks and evaluate the technical specifications. The hospital may also be able to eliminate some of the vendors at this time. Once the reference checks and technical evaluations have been completed, the hospital will need to determine the vendors for which it wants to perform site visits. Since site visits take a long time to schedule, are expensive to the hospital, and may be highly influenced by the vendors, it is important that the site visit team have a checklist prepared before going to a new site. The

site visit checklist will allow the team to evaluate the vendor's product in a more rational manner. It will also allow the team to ask the same questions at different sites and therefore be able to compare the same functions and features across all vendors.

At this point, the hospital should select two vendor finalists. Generally, there are still many unanswered questions, even in the case of the top two vendors. As the hospital begins to conduct some precontract negotiations, some of the outstanding issues, technical and otherwise, will become clarified. By conducting precontract negotiations with two vendors, the hospital has maximum leverage in terms of negotiating and pricing issues. Once the precontract negotiations have been completed, the hospital should be able to determine a preferred final vendor. Again, it is recommended that the hospital continue to deal with two vendors until contract negotiations are complete.

It is important throughout the vendor selection process to document all findings quantitatively wherever possible. The selection committee discussions, recommendations, and key decisions also need to be thoroughly documented. Since the selection process may require 6–12 months to complete, the documentation will become an important reference source for the selection committee as it proceeds through the process.

Contract and Performance Requirements

Once the hospital has selected a preferred vendor, formal contract negotiations can begin. Because of the detailed nature of this work and the importance of developing a good solid contract, it is important that, if the hospital does not have appropriate expertise, a third party be hired to assist in the contract negotiation process. The hospital should attempt to hire a consultant who has just negotiated a contract with the hospital's preferred vendor. Such a consultant will have a thorough knowledge of the vendor's contract and the areas open to negotiation and the areas not open.

There are several key points to keep in mind when negotiating a contract. First, do not accept the standard vendor contract as presented. The standard vendor contract is constructed and phrased in such a way as to be highly favorable to the vendor. Second, as mentioned above, hire a consultant who has just negotiated with the preferred vendor. This consultant will know those areas of the contract that are negotiable. Finally, include the entire vendor proposal, which contains the vendor's responses to the hospital's detailed functional requirements, as part of the contract.

Another contractual area that is difficult to address is response time guarantees. Most vendors that offer response time guarantees define the boundaries of those guarantees so rigidly that any variation caused by the hospital automatically voids the guarantees. It is important to tie the response time guarantees to the vendor's responsibility to take corrective action, including adding any additional hardware needed to maintain the response time guarantees. If the software vendor is unwilling to be financially responsible to maintain a response time guarantee and add appropriate hardware accordingly, then the software response time guarantee is really of little value to the hospital.

Another important point is to separate out all costs and payment issues and deal with them in a separate attachment. Many vendors will spread payment and other financial issues throughout the contract. In this case, it is very difficult, as the contract negotiation process evolves, to keep track of all the financial issues.

Before beginning contract negotiations, the hospital must

- identify the contract negotiation team and designate an official spokesperson
- identify and list all points to be negotiated
- categorize all points to be negotiated as high, medium, or low priority
- determine the role of each contract negotiating team member

During the actual contract negotiations, the hospital should

- lead the contract negotiation process
- present all negotiating points as of "high" importance to the hospital
- be willing to give ground regarding some low-priority issues as necessary
- be prepared to take as many breaks as necessary to allow hospital team members to discuss negotiating issues (especially issues they do not agree on)

Contract negotiations constitute one of the most important steps in developing a hospital information system. If the implementation of the new hospital information system is successful, then the contract becomes almost unnecessary. If, however, the implementation is not successful and a problem arises between the hospital and vendor, the only remedies or courses of action are those that are clearly specified in the contract. Any verbal promise made by any marketing representative during the sales cycle will have absolutely no significance.

Use of Legal Counsel

It is important that legal counsel be used at appropriate points throughout the contract negotiation process. The lawyer may come from the hospital's own legal department. However, it is important that the individual reviewing the contract has experience with computer systems and with the general operation of a health care institution. The lawyer's first job is to review the initial RFP before it is sent to the vendors. The lawyer should focus on legal issues and not be concerned with functional and technical issues related to the information systems function. It is important that the lawyer review the RFP at this stage, since the response to the RFP of the winning vendor will become a legal part of the final contract.

The lawyer should also review the initial standard contract presented by the vendor. This review should be done early on in the vendor selection process so that any key issues identified at that point can be brought to the attention of the vendor. The lawyer can come up with a list of issues to be subsequently negotiated during the actual contract negotiation process.

The lawyer should be used throughout the contract negotiation process to review the various revisions of the contract. Again, this review should focus on legal issues and not functional and technical issues, which are the responsibility of the information systems department and the users. All outstanding legal issues not resolved prior to beginning formal contract negotiations will then become part of the contract negotiation issues list. The legal department also needs to prioritize the various legal issues so that the contract negotiation team can respond accordingly.

Use of Consultants

Outside consultants can be used throughout the vendor evaluation, selection, and contract negotiation process. However, effective use of consultants requires that their role be clearly identified ahead of time. An open-ended consulting arrangement can be very expensive for a hospital while offering little assistance. However, consultants can benefit a hospital by providing outside expertise and field experience, functioning as a "neutral party," countering the influence of internal politics, and providing direct assistance to keep the overall process flowing.

Cost-Benefit Analysis

As part of the vendor evaluation and selection process, a hospital may wish to do a cost-benefit analysis. The cost-benefit analysis can be separated into two parts: the cost analysis component and the benefit analysis component. At a minimum, the hospital should always complete the cost analysis portion.

The initial cost-benefit analysis may actually be performed during the strategic information systems planning process. In developing a strategic plan, it is important that the cost associated with each alternative approach to implementing a new hospital information system be identified. Once these costs have been identified, the expected benefits or cost savings associated with each alternative can then be determined. If part of the cost savings is expected to be the

result of a reduction in personnel, it is extremely important to have every department manager participate in the analysis process and "buy in" on the the reduction. Some institutions actually have each department manager sign a document agreeing to a certain reduction in staff associated with the implementation of a new hospital information system.

Some hospitals already have hospital information systems they want to replace because of obsolescence. These institutions typically have old, home-grown systems that are no longer cost-effective to maintain. In addition, many of the old systems lack the ability to accept software changes. In such a case, a hospital may decide to obtain a new hospital information system without performing a total cost-benefit analysis. However, as mentioned above, the hospital still needs to determine the overall costs of replacing its information system.

A hospital may also decide that a primary goal of obtaining a new system is to develop additional and better management information. This additional information may, ultimately, be used to help control or reduce costs.

Regardless of the motives for obtaining a new hospital information system, it is imperative that a hospital clearly understand the total costs associated with a new system. Whether or not a hospital will be able to obtain a projected benefit depends on how well the hospital can manage its overall resources. It is important to keep in mind that a hospital information system is merely a tool that can be used in the overall management of a hospital. A hospital information system by itself will not reduce costs.

Security and Confidentiality

Types of Security

Security in hospital computer systems can be divided into two major types: physical security and system security. Physical security refers to the actual physical security of the terminals, personal computers, paper records, printouts, diskettes, and other electronic equipment associated with the system. Due to the large increase in the use of personal computers today, it is important that all personal computers, associated diskettes, and other equipment be well secured. The personal computers should also have a security package that requires some type of initial ID and/or password in order to use them.

System security encompasses both hardware and software security. The typical hardware security system involves protection of local area networks as well as protection against unauthorized dial-in access. A network security system monitors each individual node on the network and controls access to nodes. A remote dial-in security system is used in institutions where many users dial in through the telephone to the computer system. This front-end security system requires all users to dial into the computer, identify themselves, then hang up. The security system keeps a log of appropriate IDs, passwords, and home phone numbers and will dial the user back and make the connection. A dial-back system is especially helpful in preventing unauthorized personnel from getting into the computer system.

A software security system includes user IDs, passwords, system audit trails, and antivirus utilities throughout the information system. Most software security systems require the user to enter a user ID followed by a password. The combination of ID and password will identify what application areas the user is authorized to access. In management of a software security system, it is important to change passwords for all employees on a regular basis. It is also important to remove user IDs and passwords for all employees who leave an organization. In a large institution, the responsibility of adding and deleting user IDs and passwords can be handled by a few key groups of individuals. Each group, however, will only be able to handle the user IDs and passwords of certain classes of users. The finance department may handle all of the user IDs and passwords for finance employees, and the nursing department may handle all user IDs and passwords for nurses.

In addition to user IDs and passwords, the hospital computer system should maintain an audit trail of all transactions occurring in the system. The "invisible" audit trail should identify all users of the system and the transactions they initiate, along with dates and times. The audit trail logs are extremely valuable in identifying potential sources of security breaching.

Another factor to consider is the existence of computer viruses. Computer viruses are software programs that "attach" to other programs; may duplicate themselves and spread; and may destroy user programs, user data files, and even the computer operating system programs. Several antiviral packages are available that can be installed on personal computers and network computers in order to both detect computer viruses and prevent them from entering the system.

Data Recovery

Data recovery systems must include all types of data, including paper documents. Users must have some type of backup system in place prior to initiating the use of any new hospital information system. Every hospital unit should have a procedures manual readily available to follow in case of computer failure. The backup procedures manual should contain the "forms" necessary for continuing normal operation.

Backup of personal computers is extremely important. It is generally the responsibility of the individual user to back up his or her own personal computer. The backups are recorded on tape cassettes or diskettes. Depending on the nature of the work, the backup tapes or diskettes should be stored offsite.

As local area networks increase in number, backup of these networks becomes another important factor. Generally, a single network administrator is responsible for backup of the network system. However, as the networks continue to multiply, the ability to back up local area networks from a central site assumes greater importance. Ultimately, hospitals will need to design a network system that will allow backup of all local area networks from a central location.

Today, the backup of central computer systems is a fairly standard process. The backups are conducted on a daily, weekly, and monthly basis. Duplicate sets of records are stored both onsite and offsite. For some large systems, important data are stored electronically on two different mass storage devices. This allows a total backup of all transactions on a real-time basis. However, due to the cost of this approach, most hospitals do not use a dual on-line backup approach. In the future, as the price of mass storage devices decreases, it will be feasible for hospitals to use a dual on-line backup mechanism for their vital information. Hospitals should also have an uninterruptable power supply system to protect the central data-processing equipment from "going down" in case of a power outage.

Disaster recovery plans need to be developed for each major and satellite computer facility operated by a hospital. Each site must have its own specific disaster recovery plan. The plan must identify the appropriate disaster levels and the actions to be taken for each level. It must be updated at regular intervals and whenever a new piece of hardware is added to the computer facility.

The disaster recovery plan must also be tested periodically. The extent to which a plan is tested will depend on the degree of criticality of the computer systems that may be affected. It is expensive to test a disaster recovery plan, however testing the plan can be considered an important form of insurance. In the event of a real disaster, proof of testing could aid in the recovery of damages from the hospital's insurance company.

Security Policies and Procedures

In order to develop effective policies and procedures regarding security, a hospital should establish a security committee. This committee should be composed of individuals from various departments within the hospital, such as administration, medical records, risk management, and information systems, as well as physicians, nurses, and internal auditors.

The hospital security committee should consider all types of information, including paper records, electronic data, printouts, patient medical records, and all other forms of information. The security committee, on behalf of the hospital, must develop a policy statement that clearly identifies and out-

lines the institution's policies and procedures with regard to security. These policies and procedures must be officially adopted. The policy statement on security must be worded so that it applies to all types of information regardless of form and is easily understood by all employees. Once the statement is developed, it must be signed by all employees at regular intervals. The security committee should review and update the security policy statement annually or even more frequently.

Hospitals are especially vulnerable when it comes to the actual patient medical record charts. These charts are generally accessible to many individuals throughout the hospital. Due to legal implications, access to patient information will become more restricted in the next decade. Even though computer systems have the ability to transmit information around the world, increased restrictions will continue to be placed on patient information. Therefore, any hospital considering a new information system should carefully evaluate the system's security subsystem.

Hospitals must follow good management practices and principles for handling confidential information. They must take a more aggressive posture toward security in the future. Good security systems, policies, and procedures enable hospitals to guard against possible breaches of security and the potential liability associated with these. (For more information on the use and regulation of health care information, please refer to Chapter 15.)

RESOURCE REQUIREMENTS

Information Systems Components

The selection of the components for a hospital information system should be based on an analysis of user requirements and system design functions for each health care division. As mentioned previously, development of a strategic plan is the key to determining the specifications for a hospital information system. A tactical plan can then be developed as a natural outcome of the strategic plan. The tactical plan will include a list of applications to be added or replaced, the order in which applications are to be added or replaced, and the estimated cost to add or replace each application. The tactical plan, therefore, outlines what the hospital is going to do, when it is going to do it, who in particular is going to do it, and the approximate cost of accomplishing the desired goals.

In acquiring any new software package, the hospital must make the decision to develop the package in-house or to acquire it from a commercial software vendor. Once the make versus buy decision has been made, the software selection process can proceed. If the decision is made to acquire a commercial software package, the final software package selection will usually drive the associated hardware decisions. However, if the hospital has recently purchased hardware or favors a certain type of hardware, then this factor must be taken into account in the software selection process. In that situation, only software that will run on the specified hardware will even be considered in the selection process.

Another option in the development of a hospital information system is to acquire the data-processing software and all support functions from a shared service vendor. This option does not require the hospital to make a large capital investment in the overall information systems functions, but the hospital must be willing to accept the software capabilities on offer. Another advantage of this approach is that the hospital does not have to maintain a large in-house information systems department. Therefore, this approach is particularly attractive for small rural hospitals, since they may have difficulty hiring appropriate staff.

Hardware Components

The hardware components associated with a hospital information system include the central processing unit, input and output devices, electronic storage devices, and the network support systems. In today's complex information systems environment, central processing units include mainframe computers, minicomputers, and personal computers. Primary input devices include both nonintelligent terminals (dumb

terminals that cannot operate without being connected to and controlled by the central computer) and intelligent terminals. Today, most intelligent terminals are personal computers. Output devices include the terminals (intelligent and nonintelligent) and printers. Data storage devices include magnetic disks, magnetic tapes, and, more recently, high-density optical recording devices. Magnetic storage can be written to and read from many times, whereas optical storage devices can be written to only once but read from many times. Therefore, optical storage devices are used for longer-term storage of data.

The network system consists of all the telecommunication components necessary for transmitting data throughout an organization—the cable in the walls, the various devices to receive and transmit data at both ends of the cable, and the sophisticated operating system. Many of the newer hospital information systems are based on local area networks. However, local area networks require sophisticated hardware and software and supporting technical staff. Therefore, an institution needs to carefully consider whether it really wants to use local area networks in the development of its information system, since they are difficult to support.

Staffing

The design, implementation, operation, and maintenance of hospital information systems requires highly trained technical staff. If an information system is network based, telecommunications expertise will also be required within the hospital.

The recruiting and retaining of competent information systems staff is becoming more difficult, especially for small to medium rural hospitals. Because of the difficulty, these hospitals need to consider an approach that involves more vendor support and less dependence on in-house staff.

Finally, information systems and other staff must be identified for training on the hospital information system. Vendors typically provide the initial training for the hospital trainers. In addition, some vendors offer computer-based training packages that can supplement the instructor taught courses.

Regardless of size, a hospital must allocate sufficient resources to train users on any new system and to continue to train new employees as they join the organization. Without this training, efficient use of the information system cannot be maintained. Overall, training is an essential ingredient for the success of any hospital information system.

Information Systems Budget

The cost of handling information in a health care organization is substantial. It is estimated that a hospital spends up to 40 percent of its total operating budget in just handling information.[12] Nursing alone spends approximately 15 percent of a hospital's total budget in handling information. These high spending percentages make it essential that appropriate dollars be budgeted for information systems.

Hospitals presently spend approximately 2–3 percent of their operating budget on information systems.[13] Other service organizations, such as insurance banking, spend 7–15 percent of their operating budget on information systems. Hospitals must be willing to make larger investments in information systems if they expect to realize the potential quality improvement, cost-containment, and management control benefits.

Computer Facilities

An appropriate computer facility must be available to support a hospital information system. This facility must be designed to take into account some of the special requirements of data processing operations, such as security systems; smoke, fire, and water detection systems; power conditioning and protection units; and chilled water and air conditioning units. The data processing facility must also include special rooms, such as a cold room to house the central processing unit and disk drives, a printing and production room to handle the large volume of printouts from the data center, a special telecommunications room to house the network and communications equipment, and uninterruptable power

supply and battery rooms to house the power backup equipment. Appropriate break and eating areas for staff should be accessible 24 hours a day, seven days a week. In addition, if users are to be trained in the computer facility, adequate user training rooms must be incorporated.

All construction of new buildings or remodeling of old buildings must take into account the telecommunications closets and cabling required to support complex networks as well as the computer equipment that will be installed throughout the hospital. A new hospital facility should be prewired for data and voice communications in every room of the hospital (i.e., there should be a telephone outlet and a data outlet). Also, when remodeling or planning new nursing stations, it is essential to consider the number of power outlets and data lines that will be required for the computer equipment. Most nursing stations today are not designed to support adequate computer equipment.

Another essential ingredient in the development of a hospital information system is a long-term telecommunications plan. A telecommunications plan will outline what networks, cabling, and other hardware will be necessary to support the hospital information system. This plan becomes the blueprint for wiring new and existing buildings in the future. In addition, the telecommunications plan permits the hospital to revise its data processing architecture in a gradual stepwise manner and to spread the cost of a new sophisticated telecommunications system over several years without rendering the current system useless. The telecommunications plan sets standards for the operation of current and future networks. Such standards greatly facilitate the connection over time of different local area networks and computer systems.

The resources required for development of a hospital information system are substantial. Careful planning by the hospital will permit more effective utilization of the dollars available to invest in the system. Furthermore, as the cost of handling information increases in health care, investing more in information systems becomes more feasible. Therefore, hospitals can expect to spend considerably more resources on information systems in the future. This increased expenditure, however, should be offset by a reduction in the cost of handling information per transaction.

QUALITY MANAGEMENT

Assessing Information System Performance

All hospital information systems should be periodically evaluated. Computer applications should be evaluated on two parameters: (1) how well they satisfy objectives established by users and (2) their efficiency of operation (timeliness, costs, minimum error rates, etc.).

Each system must be evaluated on the basis of its own specific objectives. However, general questions to be used in an evaluation protocol might include the following[14]:

1. What impact has the system had on direct patient care?
2. To what extent has the system brought about beneficial changes in internal operating procedures?
3. To what extent has the system improved strategic information for management?
4. What is the economic impact of the system?

Computer system evaluation should be a responsibility of the CIO. Formal evaluation protocols should be established to guide the review process. New systems should be reviewed six to twelve months after they have been installed and have settled into routine operation. Users should participate in the evaluation process, and consultants might be used to assist in major system evaluations.[15]

Information Systems Support for Total Quality Management

The major indicators of quality improvement related to effective use of information systems in hospitals include the following:

- improved strategic planning through the availability of timely, relevant information for
  —projection of operating trends
  —identification of environmental threats and opportunities
  —analysis of competitor actions and future plans
  —portfolio analysis (setting of priorities through comparative performance projections for different business areas or product lines)
  —analysis of opportunities for diversification of products and services
- improved medical outcomes at the lowest possible costs
  —enhanced quality of care
    —treatment patterns for individual patients planned and compared against regimens for a large number of similar patients in a clinical database
    —risk reduction through demonstration that medically necessary and historically mandated procedures have been followed
  —cost control
    —clinical justification for tests and procedures that go beyond patterns suggested by the clinical database
    —development of generalized protocols for nursing care, medical treatment, and follow-up that are clinically effective and cost-efficient
  —medical effectiveness (outcome) analysis
    —comparative analysis of alternative treatment protocols
    —problem analysis (complications, infections, complaints, etc.)
- more efficiency in hospital's daily operations resulting in improved patient satisfaction and containment of costs
- demonstration of management efficiency through
  —evaluation of products and services

—measurement of the impact of services provided to hospital clients, including individual patients and the broader community

—cost and revenue analysis measured against "bottom line" financial performance standards

THE FUTURE OF INFORMATION SYSTEMS MANAGEMENT

Emerging Trends

Emerging trends in hospital information systems and computer technology include the following[16]:

- There will be continued movement toward use of purchased applications software rather than software designed and developed in-house.
- There will be a continued trend toward open system architecture, with computing distributed to multiple users linked together by communications networks.
- Improvements in system integration will occur as a result of the development of health industry standards for information sharing across hardware and software products from different vendors.
- There will be increased availability of generalized clinical knowledge bases in all of the major medical specialties and increased use of information systems to support clinical decisions (computer-aided diagnosis and treatment planning).
- Information technology will be used by hospitals to gain competitive advantage in the marketplace.
- Management information systems will be able to generate organizational performance indicators to assess quality and measure accountability.

New Software and Hardware Technologies

Advances in information technology have consistently outstripped the ability of hospitals to use that technology effectively. New developments on the horizon in computer hardware, software, and telecommunications will dramatically impact the way hospitals plan and organize their information systems in the next 10–15 years. Below are described a small number of technologies that are currently in development but are predicted to become operational in many hospitals by the year 2000.

Voice Recognition Systems

These systems will be able to translate the spoken word into digital signals for computer storage and processing. They will permit the replacement of cumbersome and error-prone dictation systems used in the emergency room, the operating suite, the laboratory, the radiology department, and other clinical departments. They will help make the total electronic medical record more feasible.[17]

Electronic and Optical Storage Systems

Movement toward the paperless medical record will require continued advances in the electronic and optical storage of information. Optical laser disk storage systems combined with electronic indexing will permit storage and retrieval of digitized images of documents and medical images. Hospitals are beginning to employ this technology in their medical records departments, and it should be commonplace by the end of the century.[18]

Noninvasive Medical Procedures

Computer technology will continue to have substantial impact on medical diagnostic and treatment procedures. More noninvasive procedures will be available to physicians, offering the triple benefits of improved quality of care, reduced patient discomfort, and lower cost. Examples include computerized image enhancement, radiation treatment, and continuous drug infusion systems.[19]

Artificial Intelligence and Expert Systems

Generalized databases of current medical knowledge will become available in computer form for all of the major medical specialties by the year 2000. Physicians and other patient care personnel will use these expert systems routinely for combining patient-specific information with a generalized knowledge base to support diagnosis and treatment planning. Hospitals will promote the use of this technology to gain competitive advantage in the marketplace.[20]

All of these new information technologies will be subjected to close scrutiny and careful economic analysis before they are adopted by hospitals. Key variables in these analyses will include technical feasibility, equipment costs, software costs, training costs, implementation costs, effects on employee productivity, documented quality improvements resulting from use of the technology, and savings in overall information processing costs.

Information technology will not solve all the problems we face. Computer systems cannot replace the judgment and experience of seasoned managers. However, better clinical and managerial decisions will result from improved availability of information. Patients and society in general will be the ultimate beneficiaries of the improved services that result from effective information management.

ADDITIONAL RESOURCES

Austin, C.J., and J.M. Trimm. Information technology and the clinical laboratory: Agenda for the '90s. *Clinical Laboratory Management Review,* July-August 1990, pp. 254–262.

Computers in Healthcare. Monthly journal published by Cardiff Publishing, 6300 S. Syracuse Way, Suite 650, Englewood, Colo. 80111, 303/220-0600.

DeLuca, J. *Health care information systems: An executive's guide for successful management.* Chicago: American Hospital Publishing, 1990.

Healthcare Informatics. Monthly journal published by Health Data Analysis, Inc., 2902 Evergreen Parkway, Suite 110, Evergreen, Colo. 80439, 303/674-2774.

Heidrick and Struggles. *Health care chief information officer.* Chicago: Heidrick & Struggles, 1990.

Hospital information systems: State of the art. Chicago: Dorenfest & Associates, 1992.

Kropf, R. *Service excellence in health care through the use of computers.* Chicago: American College of Healthcare Executives, 1990.

Lichtig, L.K. *Hospital information systems for case mix management.* New York: Wiley, 1986.

Matson, T.A., and M.D. McDougall, eds. *Information systems for ambulatory care.* Chicago: American Hospital Publishing, 1990.

Person, M.M., III. *The smart hospital: A case study in hospital computerization.* Durham, NC: Carolina Academic Press, 1988.

Schmitz, H.H. *Managing health care information resources.* Gaithersburg, Md.: Aspen Publishers, 1987.

Trends and assessment of the hospital systems industry. Danville, Calif.: R.L. Johnson & Associates, 1986–1991.

U.S. Congress. Office of Technology Assessment. *Hospital information systems at the Veterans Administration.* 100th Cong., 1st sess., 1987. Special Report No. OTA-CIT-372.

NOTES

1. R.C. Howe and V. Oestreicher, Corporate Information System Strategies, *Computers in Healthcare,* October 1987, pp. 47–49.

2. Ibid.

3. R.C. Howe and V. Oestreicher, Corporate Information System Strategies: Alternatives, *Computers in Healthcare,* January 1988, pp. 22–25.

4. U.S. Congress, Office of Technology Assessment, *Hospital Information Systems at the Veterans Administration,* 100th Cong., 1st sess., 1987, Special Report No. OTA-CIT-372; MIS Group, *Guidelines for Management Information Systems in Canadian Health Care Facilities* (Ottawa: MIS Group, 1985).

5. Howe and Oestreicher, Corporate Information System Strategies: Alternatives.

6. R.C. Howe and V. Oestreicher, Corporate Strategies: Organizational Structure, *Computers in Healthcare,* June 1988, pp. 24–28.

7. R.C. Howe, CIO, VP MIS, MIS Director, DP Manager— Who Cares? *Healthcare Computing and Communications,* September 1987, pp. 44–45.

8. Ibid.

9. American Hospital Association, Healthcare Information Management, Andersen Consulting, and Heidrick & Struggles, *Health Care Chief Information Officer* (New York: Heidrick & Struggles, 1990), 7.

10. C.J. Austin, *Information Systems for Health Services Administration,* 4th ed. (Ann Arbor, Mich.: Health Administration Press, 1992), 215–218.

11. *Computers in Healthcare* (Englewood, Colo.: Cardiff Publishing); *Healthcare Informatics* (Evergreen, Colo: Health

Data Analysis, Inc.); *Hospital Software Source Book* (Gaithersburg, Md.: Aspen Publishers, 1985); *R.L. Johnson Reports* (Danville, Calif: R.L. Johnson).

12. S. Dorenfest, Future of Health Care Administration, panel at the fall meeting of the ECHO, September 23, 1986.

13. American Hospital Association, *Guide to Effective Health Care Information Management.*

14. Austin, *Information Systems,* 182.

15. Ibid., 182.

16. C.J. Austin, Information Technology and the Future of Health Services Delivery, *Hospital and Health Services Administration* 34, no. 2 (1989): 157–165.

17. Ibid., 159.

18. Ibid., 159.

19. Ibid., 161.

20. Ibid., 160.

Edward J. Hinman

Clinical Data Systems

14

Purpose: The purpose of clinical data systems is to acquire, analyze, retain, and retrieve the data needed to provide, monitor, and evaluate patient care services.

INTRODUCTION

Clinical data may be defined as organized elements of data concerning the health care needs of individuals, diagnostic and therapeutic interventions, and the outcomes of those interventions. Clinical data include the administrative, financial, planning, and evaluative data used in providing health care services. Clinical data are usually recorded electronically or in paper-based files.

Traditionally, clinical data systems have been primarily historical documents, but they are being used increasingly to support immediate decision making. Clinical data systems have expanded to include reminders to perform certain procedures, alerts to potential problems with drug combinations or laboratory findings, treatment assistance using artificial intelligence, and matching of patient information

to diagnostic and therapeutic paradigms. Future systems are expected to link individual patient data to structured knowledge files from the medical literature in both outpatient and inpatient settings. This chapter focuses on the functions, management principles, and applications associated with managing clinical data using current technologies, although it discusses new developments as well.

Clinical data systems provide the fundamental information for all patient–care related activities in health care institutions. Following is a list of the principal functions that are dependent upon these systems:

1. patient care
2. management
3. reimbursement
4. epidemiology
5. reporting and regulation
6. quality assessment
7. utilization management
8. risk management
9. teaching and research

MANAGEMENT PRINCIPLES

The following principles must be kept in mind in managing clinical data:

- All information gathered from patients, including data derived from their body fluids and tissues, should be accurate and available to health care providers to use in providing timely care.
- All information generated through the provision of patient care should be available to management to assist in planning, controlling, and evaluating the institution's clinical activities.
- Clinical data systems must have the capability of providing longitudinal information (entire history) about individual patients regardless of the site of their care within the institution or individual clinical department.
- Clinical data systems must be capable of supporting the long-range goals and objectives of the organization.
- Clinical data systems must satisfy reporting and regulatory requirements while protecting the right to privacy of patients and providers.
- Clinical data systems must be an integral part of the quality management process, including quality assessment and assurance, utilization review, total quality management, and risk management.
- Clinical data systems should be structured in such a way that teaching and research activities are supported.
- Clinical data systems must be part of the total information system of the institution.

ORGANIZATIONAL ROLE

Health care information systems have traditionally encompassed historical clinical information contained in paper-based medical records, clinical and administrative data from the ancillary clinical departments, and business information from the administrative departments. All of the information sources were typically managed separately, which resulted in gaps in or duplication of data.

History and Background

The first hospital medical records contained information only on the care rendered to patients during their stay at the hospital. Records were filed by individual admissions. Over time it became apparent to physicians and hospital administrators that past medical information was critical to understanding a patient's current problems and the impact on the hospital; therefore, a longitudinal inpatient medical record became the standard. As hospitals began to provide outpatient care, records of that care were developed. The unit medical record, containing both inpatient and outpatient data, was the next step. This is the current method of storing information about individual patients in most health care institutions. Over the past two decades, four academic institutions pioneered developments in automated medical records—Duke University, Harvard University, Indiana University, and the University of Utah. Development of these systems has progressed to the point that other hospitals have begun to use them.[1]

One of the first automated information clinical systems to be developed was the registration, admission, discharge, and transfer system. This system was developed during the 1960s for registering patients and for census and bed control purposes.

Automated systems were next introduced into the pharmacy, laboratory, and radiology departments. These systems were used to manage work assignments and information flow in these departments and to provide reports on patient care activities. By the end of the 1970s, physician and nurse order entry systems linking these three departments had become essentially complete information management systems. The next major developments included nurse staffing models to analyze patient care severity and to project nursing hours for each unit, nursing care plans, and critical care monitoring systems.

Clinical decision support system prototypes have been under development for the past 30 years and are just beginning to become commercially available. The purpose of these expert systems is to assist clinical decision making by matching patient information with diagnostic and therapeutic probabilities and other data from the published medical literature.[2] Integration of clinical and administrative data systems is also being actively pursued at a number of institutions, often in collaboration with vendors.

The Relevance of Clinical Information

To understand the role and importance of clinical data systems, the users and their expectations must be understood (see Table 14-1).

Individual providers use clinical data systems in all tasks involving direct patient care. These users include physicians, nurses, technologists, pharmacists, therapists, nutritionists, and other health care providers. Providers practicing both outside and inside institutions expect the information contained in the clinical data systems to be current (i.e., all known data are recorded). They expect the reports contained to be complete and accurate. The speed of availability expected depends upon the severity of illness of the patient. For example, in emergency cases there is an immediate need for information, whereas information for patient follow-up can be provided with several weeks' delay. At all times, the information must be legible and in a readable format or be easily transferable to a readable format.

Individual providers expect clinical data to be retained for at least the minimum length of time legally required, but in most cases they want the data to be retained indefinitely. Ensuring security of the information from unauthorized release and from alteration or theft is considered to be of paramount importance.

Institutional providers such as skilled nursing facilities, free-standing ambulatory surgical centers, day treatment centers, and home health agencies have similar clinical data needs as hospitals, although there are quantitative variations. For example, nurses practicing in a general hospital will have the same qualitative data needs as nurses practicing in a home health agency, but the amount of detail and the speed of availability needed differ markedly.

Payers for health services, whether individual patients or third-party payers, require selected information from clinical data systems so they can reimburse physicians and institutions appropriately.

Health care institutions are subject to various forms of regulation. Some of this regulation is mandatory (e.g., licensing and safety requirements) and some is voluntary (e.g., the standards that must be

Table 14-1 Clinical Data System Users and Their Expectations

Users	The Data Are:						
	Current	Complete	Accurate	Available	Legible/ Readable	Retained	Secure
Individual Providers	H	H	H	H	H	M	M
Institutional Providers	H	H	H	H	H	M	M
Payers	M	M	H	H	M	L	L
Regulators	L	M	L	L	L	M	H
Patients	H	H	H	H	H	M	H
Legal Systems	L	H	H	M	M	H	H
Institutional Managers	L	H	H	H	M	H	H

Key: H = high expectations; M = medium expectations; L = lower expectations.

met for Joint Commission on Accreditation of Healthcare Organizations accreditation or Medicare and Medicaid certification). Both mandatory and voluntary regulation require the provision of information about the facility, such as the number of beds, types of clinical services provided, number of admissions, number of patient days, and number of operations (see Chapter 15 for more detail).

Patients need access to clinical data for purposes of continued care. The information may be sent directly to a new provider of services or may be carried by the patient. Further, patients need data to assert claims for employee benefits such as short- or long-term disability and workers' compensation or to support requests for sick leave. Patients who feel that they have sustained an injury due to professional negligence use the records to strengthen their claims. Patients may also request copies of the records concerning their care to verify the completeness and accuracy of the information. Although there is still resistance on the part of some health care providers to make this information available to patients, it has been clearly established that patients have a right to the information.[3]

Legal systems use information from health care institutions for both criminal and civil purposes. Criminal purposes include documentation of child or adult abuse, substance abuse, gunshot wounds, and other criminal trauma. Civil purposes include determination of competence and custody and evaluation of workers' compensation claims and personal injury cases, including product liability and professional negligence (malpractice) cases.

Institutional managers use clinical data to augment administrative data in planning, organizing, controlling, and evaluating the activities of the institution as discussed in Chapter 13.

FUNCTIONS OF CLINICAL DATA SYSTEMS

Clinical data are acquired from and input by patients, physicians, and the institution's providers. The data fall into three general categories. First, there is the historical information that the patient provides; second, there is the information obtained from the physical examination; and third, there are the results of the tests or procedures performed on the patient or the patient's tissues or body fluids. Data gathered by the physician and the institutional provider are the result of observation or examination. These data may be directly entered by any of the three sources (patient, physician, or other health care provider) by a series of different techniques. Input methods include selecting items from a computer screen menu; typing; and using light pens, bar code readers, a "mouse," optical scanners, monitors connected to patients, and voice recognition systems as well as traditional hand-written in noncomputerized systems.

Data is stored in the memory of the clinical data systems or on paper, microfiche, computer tape, computer disk, optical laser disk, or "smartcards." Primary data are data collected from a source that has not been analyzed. Data analysis allows summarization, linkage to other data elements, and interpretation. Primary data or analyzed data may be transmitted.

Transmission of data may be through hard-wired direct connections, disks, audiotape or videotape broadcast, microwave fiber optic links, or hard copy. Retrieval of data may be by automated prompts, query, search programs, or human memory. The output may be in a typed format, an audio format, or a visual format (e.g., pictures, graphs, and tables), or may consist of x-rays or electrocardiograms.

The input and retrieval functions may be performed by the patient, a member of the family, a physician, or the institutional provider.

The nature of the institutions using the data determines the total scope of the clinical data systems. A vertically and horizontally integrated system of hospitals and other health care facilities requires the most detailed and complex clinical data systems. A single physician's office would usually operate with a simple type of data system.

Clinical Information Requirements

The integration of clinical and administrative data systems requires significant philosophical reorientation as well as systems development leading to open access between the data systems. The principal purpose of administrative data systems has been to generate bills and the principal purpose of clinical data systems has been to provide care to individual patients. If clinical data systems are now to support all of the functions listed previously in this chapter, access to the data contained in the administrative systems becomes imperative. Furthermore, increasing sophistication in the administrative data systems requires access to individual and aggregate clinical information. For example, imagine an operating room supervisor wishes to schedule surgical cases for the following day. The age, diagnosis, severity of illness, planned procedure for each patient, and name of each attending surgeon need to be available. Information concerning the average length of time it has taken each surgeon to perform the relevant procedure, as well as clinical information, is also critical in devising an optimum schedule.

Organizational Location

In hospitals, the medical records department was traditionally the place where clinical information was collected and stored. With the advent of computerized clinical information systems, the role of the medical records department changed, and the data collection, storage, and retrieval functions were transferred to the health information system. Medical literature was contained in the medical library. Both the medical library and the medical records department usually reported to the assistant administrator in charge of ancillary clinical or administrative services (Figure 14-1). Because of computerization and the increasing sophistication of the clinical data systems, management information system departments were developed to deal (primarily) with administrative data. Developing health information system departments that incorporated certain clinical data systems and the management information systems was the next logical step, and this occurred in the late 1970s and early 1980s.

Management information and health information system departments have generally reported to the chief financial officer (Figure 14-2). The current interest in information systems as a means of managing larger institutions is leading to the use of a chief information officer (CIO), who serves at the same level as the chief financial officer, the chief operating officer, and the vice-president for medical affairs (Figure 14-3).

Resource Requirements

The requirements for operating clinical data systems include personnel, hardware and software systems, space, maintenance, and updates of system and financing.

Personnel

There are two groups of personnel who must be properly trained if the clinical data systems are to be effective: the technical experts and the actual users. The first group includes medical (health) records administrators and medical library science experts. Their skills are needed to oversee the medical records and medical literature components of the clinical data systems. Programmers, systems analysts, computer operators, and information system managers are needed to design and keep the systems running.

Each hospital will need at least one certified health record administrator to advise on the details of diagnosis and procedure coding. Such administrators are similarly expert in the content required for patient care and in regulation and reporting requirements. With the current availability of medical bibliographic material to anyone with a personal computer and modem, a medical librarian is not needed on the staff of many community health institutions.

The second group of personnel requiring training includes all of the care providers in the institution who will be inputting or accessing information. They must have sufficient training to operate the data systems and preserve the security of the systems.

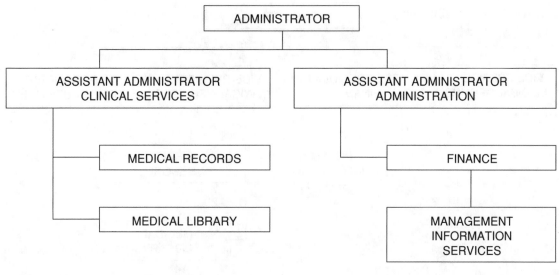

Figure 14-1 Early Organization of Hospital Data Functions

Types of Clinical Data Systems

Clinical data systems may be divided into six types, which are discussed below.

Individual Patient Medical Records

The first and most important type of clinical data system is the patient medical record system, which contains all of the data concerning individual patients. Ideally, each medical record should be a continuous inventory going back to the time of birth and up to the current interaction with the health care delivery system and should be available wherever the patient is seeking care. Most health care managers feel that the problem-oriented medical record approach described by Weed has significant merit, because it orients the information around a problem list and outlines all current and past problems.[4] Each encounter is described, and the information is organized into subjective and objective assessment by the physician, and the plan is developed for further diagnosis and treatment for each active problem (the "SOAP" note).

Summaries of Clinical and Administrative Data

Some clinical data systems are summaries of clinical data used by providers, third-party payers, managers of the clinical departments, and affiliated institutions for communication purposes. Summaries of administrative data include daily, weekly, monthly, and yearly information, such as the number of admissions by patient classification, by payer classification, and by diagnosis and number of operative procedures.

Disease Registries

Information can be organized into disease registries (e.g., cancer registries) for specific purposes, such as tracking the incidence and prevalence of problems of concern to health planners and policy makers.

Department-Specific Data

Department-specific information is used to manage the individual departments, such as the phar-

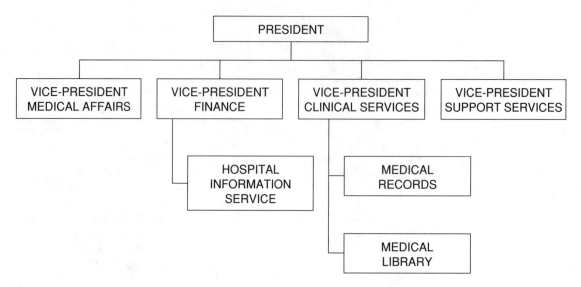

Figure 14-2 Recent Organization of Hospital Data Functions

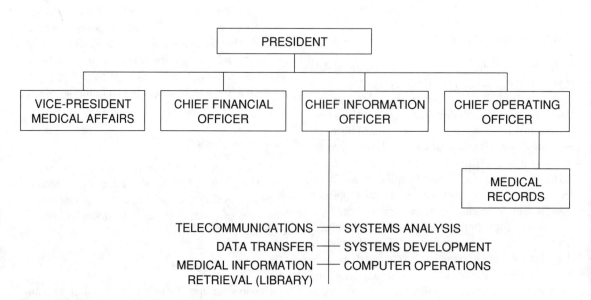

Figure 14-3 New Approach to Organizing Hospital Data Functions

macy, the laboratory, and the radiology and nursing departments.

Medical Literature and Decision Support Systems

Medical literature information and clinical decision support systems are necessary to assist physicians and other health care providers in keeping abreast of new developments. These systems are helpful for information management, focus the attention of physicians on specific problem areas, and develop patient-specific recommendations.

Patient-Carried Records

Patient-carried records allow individuals in our mobile society to have medical information about their past and current problems and treatments available wherever they may travel. These records may be in a paper, microfiche, or smartcard format.

Data Elements

The data elements in clinical data systems include the kinds of patient-specific data listed below:

- demographic
- historical
- occupational
- environmental
- social
- physical findings
- results of diagnostic procedures
- treatments (including health education)
- follow-up
- outcomes
- consent

Clinical data systems also contain the following types of institutional data:

- services performed
- individuals who performed the services

- results of the services
- resources utilized

Ideally, there should be a linkage between the patient and institutional data elements that would make it possible to determine for each patient what services were performed and who performed them and also to determine for each kind of service which patients received it.

CLINICAL INFORMATION APPLICATIONS

Clinical data system applications are of two principal types: applications for managing patient care and applications for managing the health care delivery system. Specific applications include performance documentation and monitoring, cost determination and reimbursement, reporting and regulation, research and teaching, and epidemiology.

Using the Medical Record To Manage Patient Care

The reason for the existence of any health care institution is to provide patient care. Each medical record must contain enough information to accurately identify the patient and to document the diagnostic and therapeutic plan (and the rationale behind the plan) for the problem that brought the patient to the institution. It should also note the response to treatment and any modifications made in the treatment plan.

Details of projected follow-up, including health education information to be provided to the patient, need to be included as well. If the case is clinically difficult, the record should reflect the complexity. The medical record represents the documentation of services provided to the patient and the results of those services. A properly organized medical record can identify preventive services provided to the patient previously and serve as a reminder when additional services are needed.

Documentating and Monitoring Performance

Clinical data systems provide management with information to be used in planning, making resource allocation decisions, and analyzing the productivity and profitability of the institution. They also provide management with information on the types of patients cared for, the severity of their illnesses, the intensity of the services provided to them, and the short-term outcomes. Administrative data systems provide information on staffing, hours worked, supplies consumed, and space and equipment utilized. Together, these systems provide management with an overview of all institutional activities.

Cost Determination and Reimbursement

To ensure prompt reimbursement for services rendered, clinical data systems must be able to provide a list of the diagnoses and the diagnostic and therapeutic procedures performed and the charges for these procedures. Because health insurance plans have specific limitations and exclusions, payers frequently need to review clinical data to determine the medical necessity, under the insurance contract, of the services provided. They also need to be able to verify that the services for which they are billed were indeed rendered and that the diagnoses and procedural codes assigned relate directly to the patients' problems and the amounts of the claims.

Reporting and Regulation

Clinical data systems provide the information necessary for fulfilling reporting and regulatory responsibilities. The most common forms of mandatory reporting are births, deaths, occurrences of certain diseases, and cases of suspected abuse of children or adults. Reporting of sexually transmitted diseases is a major part of the battle to reduce their frequency (see Chapter 15).

Research and Teaching

The research and teaching activities conducted in any health care institution need clinical data systems to provide detailed information concerning the types of patients, the nature of their illnesses, the diagnostic procedures performed, the treatments provided, and the outcomes of those treatments.

Epidemiology

Summaries of clinical information provide the basis for epidemiologic evaluation of patient care needs, such as the occurrence and frequency of problems and the response to various interventions. A specific example is the evaluation of nosocomial (hospital-acquired) infections to determine the source so that corrective actions may be instituted. Epidemiological techniques supported by clinical data assist in the evaluation of the quality of care provided and the results of changes in treatment patterns.

QUALITY MANAGEMENT

Quality management includes quality assessment, utilization management, and risk management. Next to direct patient care services, these are the most important activities that rely on clinical data systems. The data needed for clinical data systems to assist these three functions include clinical indicators, severity of illness indicators, intensity of service indicators, incident reports, and occurrence reports. Clinical indicators are instruments that measure some aspect of patient care that can guide providers in monitoring and evaluating the quality and appropriateness of the care given.[5] Indicators serve as flags that suggest that an event has occurred or is about to occur, or that some problem is present. Indicators should be used for high-risk, high-volume, or problem-prone aspects of care. An example of a clinical indicator is postoperative mortality of patients following cholecystectomy (gallbladder removal). Other data needed are severity of illness indicators, which are items that indicate the degree of illness of a patient. Examples include abnormal blood pressure and abnormal body temperature. Intensity of service indicators are measures of the resources being used by the patient.

Examples are intravenous medications and frequency of dressing changes. Incident reports are prepared by staff following events that could result in injury or illness.

Developing clinical data systems to become part of total quality management requires that they be used for the six activities discussed below.

Setting Clinical Standards

Ensuring that patients receive the same level of care regardless of their geographic location and their care providers requires that acceptable clinical standards be established and met. Currently, there are a number of organizations developing clinical standards using the method of consensus. These include the National Institutes of Health, the Agency for Health Care Policy and Research, the American Medical Association, and professional medical organizations such as the American College of Physicians, and the American College of Obstetricians/Gynecologists. Some standards are based upon hard research, but most of those currently in use were arrived at through consensus.

When properly utilized, clinical data systems are ideal for collecting information used for developing clinical standards, since they can record what was done for patients with different problems and what were the results of the treatments. Once standards are developed, they must be adopted by authoritative professional groups and then put into practice.

Detecting Exceptions

Sophisticated clinical data systems allow the use of clinical standards to detect exceptions. The presence of an exception alone does not necessarily indicate that an improper action has been taken or that a bad outcome will occur.

Clinically Evaluating Exceptions

There must be a clinical evaluation of each exception to determine whether the exception repre-sents a deviation from the standard of care. This kind of evaluation, of course, is the basis of peer review quality assessment.

Instituting Corrective Actions

If the deviation (exception) appears to be clinically significant, a corrective action should be taken. This action may be a simple reminder, counseling, a prescription for continuing medical education, or a disciplinary action of some type.

Monitoring Improvement

Following the corrective action, the clinical data systems can be used to monitor improvement and determine whether further exceptions occur. If they do, the cycle should be repeated.

Evaluating the Impact of Using Clinical Standards

Periodically, the impact of this use of clinical standards must be evaluated to determine whether the system is working appropriately.

LEGAL AND ETHICAL ISSUES

Clinical data systems contain and process information that is inherently sensitive and which may have legal and ethical implications. A number of these implications are discussed below and in Chapter 25.

Consent

The purpose of informed consent is to document that the patient was informed of the nature of the problem, the proposed treatment, the anticipated results and likelihood of success of that treatment, any risks or complications associated with that treatment, alternative treatments, and the consequences of no intervention. The fact that a discussion about these issues occurred and that the patient agreed to the proposed treatment needs to be documented in the patient's record. This documentation consists of (1) a record of the discussion and the patient's acceptance of the recommendation by the physician and (2) the patient's signature confirming the discussion.

Record and Information Ownership

For a number of years there was a major debate as to who owned the medical record and who owned the information contained in the record. It is well established at this point that the actual medical record itself is owned by the hospital, physician, or other health care provider who created the document. However, the information about the patient is solely owned by the patient. Therefore, to meet the needs of patients and providers, methods for maintaining privacy and security and determining when to release records must be in place.

Record Authenticity

The authenticity of paper-based records is established by the contemporaneous signature of the person entering the information. There should be no alteration of the record. In the event of an error, a line should be drawn through the incorrect item and a dated, corrected entry made. Both the deletion and the new entry must be signed or initialled by the person making the correction.

Given that records are increasingly being automated, the issues surrounding electronic signatures are now of major importance. For an electronic signature to be accepted, it must be contemporaneous. The person entering an electronic signature must be identified through the computer by some type of user identification, such as an ID card plus alphanumeric code, an alphanumeric code alone, an optical analysis of signature, voiceprints, or fingerprints.

The signature must indicate approval of the information preceding it and must be time dated, and there must be sufficient system security that alteration cannot be made without a clear audit trail of what was changed and who made the change.

Subpoenas and Discovery Requests

Legal demands for medical information occur during litigation involving a patient. Generally, health care institutions will have legal counsel determine whether and how much of the record must be released given the nature of the court request. Requirements vary from jurisdiction to jurisdiction and depend substantially upon the type of litigation.

Litigation

Medical records must usually be provided for review when a patient sues a physician or the institution, when a patient alleges product liability, following a motor vehicle accident or other trauma, or in some job-related situations.

Preservation of Data

Records must be preserved in such a way so that they may be retrieved and read whenever needed. Because of the large volume of information about each patient that accumulates, especially during hospitalization, the problem of storing paper-based records became severe. Now that more and more information is computer based, the problem of storage space has lessened. However, finding information is now becoming a much more important issue than previously.

Records must be retained at least for the period of time during which there is a legal need. In most jurisdictions, this period is felt to be a minimum of three years. However, the record of a pregnant woman or newborn child might have to be retained for as long as 21 years (until the child reaches majority at 18 years plus a period of time after that in which any problem that resulted from the pregnancy or the infancy of the child is legally allowed to be recognized). Methods of storage become important from a legal standpoint, since the records must be secure and there must be identification of the information by the individual.

Release of Information

Concern for the protection of privacy of individual patients and providers led to legislation and a subsequent major study commissioned by Congress.[6] A significant result of the study was the identification of issues involved in releasing information, including the following.

Primary versus Secondary Release

A simple request by the patient to have information released to him- or herself, another health care provider, a third-party payer, or an attorney must be honored when made in written form. This release is considered to be primary. However, there are circumstances in which the person receiving the information might deliberately or inadvertently release it to a secondary source. Generally, this is inappropriate without the express consent of the patient. Therefore, release forms should contain statements concerning what is to be released, to whom it is to be released, and for how long the consent for release remains in effect. Individuals receiving the information should not release it again without additional specific consent from the patient.

Release to Other Providers in the Same Institution

It is generally accepted that information may be released to other health care providers within the institution treating the patient without explicit patient consent. Release to institutional colleagues is defensible on the grounds that it can contribute to direct care, institution peer review, quality of care assessment, research, and education. In the case of release for research or educational purposes, identification of the patient should be removed from the record if the information could possibly be used secondarily.

Release to Other Institutions

Information may be released to other providers in other institutions only upon the consent of the patient unless the patient presents a threat to someone in the institution or to him- or herself.

Release to the Patient

In most states, the patient has an absolute right to the information contained in the record. The only exception is in certain cases of mental illness, and in those circumstances the patient has the right to have the information released to someone else of his or her selection.

Release to Third-Party Payers

Third-party payers need to have information about the patient and his or her treatment in order to adjudicate insurance claims. Most third-party payers obtain a general release upon insuring the individual. In some states, an additional consent is needed for each episode of care.

Release to Public Officials

Certain information must be released to public officials and agencies, particularly the health department, if an infectious disease is diagnosed. Possible additional justifications for release of information include criminal injury and child and adult abuse.

Release to the Legal System

Finally, information may be released as the result of a subpoena or discovery request in certain types of litigation; these were briefly discussed earlier.

Confidentiality, Privacy, and Security

The protection of privacy of patients and providers requires that records be kept confidential and secure. The basic criterion for accessibility is need to know: Information should only be provided to those individuals who have a need to know about the patient's condition in order to provide further care or to adjudicate insurance claims. Most health care institutions require that employees sign confidentiality statements that contain a provision for automatic termination if there is violation of confidentiality. Information system departments must monitor confidentiality carefully and must maintain the security of their systems from unwarranted access or alteration of documents (see Chapters 13 and 15 for more on security and confidentiality).

Standard Nomenclature

To achieve effective use of clinical information, it is becoming more and more important that there be standardization of the medical nomenclature and standardization of information system files and operating systems or translators so that one system can communicate with another. The National Library of Medicine is developing a unified medical language intended to help standardize the nomenclature. The American Society for Testing Materials has established several standards for a number of the elements in registration, admission, discharge, and transfer systems and laboratory systems, for example.

Ethical Issues

Minors

Whether minors can independently receive health care, consent to that care, and release information concerning that care varies between jurisdictions. In a number of states, minors become emancipated (i.e., treated as adults) when they get married or live away from home and are self-supporting. In those circumstances, a minor has the right to request care, give consent to care, and control release of information. In a number of states, a minor has the right to receive assistance from family planning services, including getting an abortion, as well as receive treatment for sexually transmitted diseases without parental consent or notification.

Managers should become familiar with the laws and practices in their individual jurisdictions.

Incompetent Patients

Some of the same consent and release of information issues that arise in the case of minors also arise in the case of patients who are deemed to be incompetent to make decisions concerning their medical care. Documentation of incompetency is imperative in the medical record. Each state has specific rules for defining and dealing with these patients.

Mental Health Records

Mental health records are subject to special confidentiality regulations, although these vary from state to state. Security for these records and special consents is more rigorous than in the case of routine medical problems.

Human Immunodeficiency Virus (HIV) Testing

In many jurisdictions, ordering a test for HIV infection requires informed consent by the patient and pretest counseling. In such cases, the consent must be clearly documented in the clinical data systems.

Workers' Compensation Cases

Patients must allow the release of their records in order to be covered by workers' compensation programs. This may present certain ethical problems, since during treatment additional information not directly related to the alleged injury is sometimes obtained.

THE FUTURE OF CLINICAL DATA SYSTEMS

The transition from paper-based medical records, paper-based medical literature, and partially automated administrative and other data systems to fully integrated information systems that support the entire institution will occur in the decade of the 1990s.

The ability to link clinical data systems in one health care institution to those in another is becoming more important as the mobility of our society continues to increase. Local area networks and distributed networks are means of achieving linkage. Standardization of data elements and standard nomenclature must be addressed to facilitate the creation of networks. Protection of privacy of patients from unwarranted release of information through networks is a significant issue facing managers in the 1990s.

Recently, an Institute of Medicine committee recommended that a computer-based patient record exist for every single person by the end of this decade.[7] At least part of the information would likely be carried by the individual so that any health care provider in the United States would be able to read it and receive the details from a centralized databank. This would result in significant improvements in patient care and in a significant reduction in the duplication of tests and diagnostic procedures. Safeguards to prevent unauthorized uses will have to be developed.

Expected developments in technology will include improvements in voice inputting and increased miniaturization, which will facilitate transportation of clinical data system devices and enhance remote monitoring capabilities.[8] Continued development of expert systems and linkages between clinical data systems will provide unlimited access to "medical consulting" for all physicians. Direct linkages between health care providers and third-party payers will result in faster and more accurate payment for services. (See Chapter 13 for more information on computer hardware and software developments.)

Information networks will continue to develop. Academic medical centers, including academic medical libraries, will be at the center and will be linked to community and specialty hospitals and practicing physicians. These networks will facilitate data management and promote high-quality patient care.

ADDITIONAL RESOURCES

Organizations

American Health Information Management Association (formerly American Medical Record Association), 919 N. Michigan Avenue, Suite 1400, Chicago, IL 60611.

American Medical Informatics Association, 4915 St. Elmo Avenue, Suite 302, Bethesda, MD 20814.

American Society for Testing Materials, 1916 Race Street, Philadelphia, PA 19103.

Institute of Medicine of the National Academy of Sciences, 2101 Constitution Avenue, N.W., Washington, DC 20418.

Joint Commission on Accreditation of Healthcare Organizations, 1 Renaissance Boulevard, Oakbrook Terrace, IL 60181.

Public Health Services, 5600 Fishers Lane, Rockville, MD 20857. Includes the Agency for Health Care Policy and Research, the Food and Drug Administration, the National Institutes of Health, and the National Library of Medicine.

Books and Articles

American Hospital Association. *Integrated quality assessment: A model for concurrent review.* Chicago: American Hospital Publishing, 1989.

American Medical Association, Council on Ethical and Judicial Affairs. *Current opinions.* Chicago: American Medical Association, 1989.

American Medical Association. *Defining, measuring, and assuring quality of care.* Chicago: American Medical Association, 1989.

American Medical Record Association. Confidentiality of patient health information: A position statement of the American Medical Record Association. *Journal of the American Medical Record Association* 53 (1982): 51–64.

Barnett, G.O., et al. DXplain: An evolving diagnostic decision-support system. *Journal of the American Medical Association* 258 (1987): 67–74.

Berwick, D.M. Continuous improvement as an ideal in health care. *New England Journal of Medicine* 320 (1989): 53–56.

Brennan, T.A., et al. Identification of adverse events occurring during hospitalization. *Annals of Internal Medicine* 112 (1990): 221–226.

California Medical Association. *Report on the Medical Insurance Feasibility Study.* San Francisco: Sutter Publications, 1977.

McDonald, C.J., and W.M. Tierny. Computer-stored medical records: Their future role in medical practice. *Journal of the American Medical Association* 259 (1988): 3433–3440.

Rasinski, D. *Risk management in practice.* No. 353R5M. Washington, D.C.: American Society of Internal Medicine, 1983.

Shortliffe, E.H. Medical informatics and clinical decision making: The science and the pragmatics. *Medical Decision Making* 11 (1991): 512–514.

U.S. Department of Health, Education and Welfare. *Quality assurance of medical care.* DHEW HSW 73-7021. Washington, D.C.: U.S. Government Printing Office, 1973.

Weed, L.L. *Knowledge coupling.* New York: Springer-Verlag, 1991.

NOTES

1. W.W. Stead, A Quarter Century of Computer-Based Medical Records, *MD Computing* 6 (1985): 75–81.

2. E.H. Shortliffe, Computer Programs To Support Clinical Decision Making, *Journal of the American Medical Association* 258 (1987): 61–66.

3. E.J. Hinman, The Patient-Carried Personal Health Record, in *Advanced Medical Systems: The 3rd Century* (Miami, Fla.: Symposia Specialists, 1977).

4. L.L. Weed, Medical Records That Guide and Teach, *New England Journal of Medicine* 278 (1968): 593–600, and 652–657.

5. R. Lehman, Forum on Clinical Indicator Development: A Discussion of the Use and Development of Indicators, *Quality Review Bulletin,* July 1989, pp. 223–227.

6. Privacy Protection Study Commission, *Personal Privacy in an Information Society* (Washington, D.C.: U.S. Government Printing Office, 1977).

7. Institute of Medicine, *The Computer-Based Patient Record* (Washington, D.C.: Institute of Medicine and National Academy Press, 1991).

8. C.J. McDonald, Medical Information Systems of the Future, *MD Computing* 6 (1989): 82–87.

Homer H. Schmitz
Charles A. James

15

External Information Management

Purpose: The purpose of external information sources and applications is to monitor changing environmental conditions; to monitor economic, political, social, and ethical trends; to update knowledge of laws and regulations; to investigate the needs and expectations of constituents, the community, and the broader society; to learn about new technical and professional advancements; and to provide information to external parties in a manner that is accurate, informative, and ethical and protects confidentiality.

INTRODUCTION

Health care organizations are being held to increasingly higher standards of accountability by patients, the community, and government. In turn, they are becoming increasingly sensitive to their environment—monitoring changing conditions; economic, political, social, and ethical trends; laws and regulations; and new technology and professional advancements. While protecting confidentiality and the rights of individuals and institutions, they must furnish appropriate, valid, timely,

and accurate information to a variety of outside organizations and agencies that monitor their performance.

Health care organizations derive their information from a variety of internal and external sources. This chapter primarily addresses the external sources of information. It is important for decision makers to be aware of these sources and to take them into account in their strategic-planning and decision-making processes so that they will be able to accurately assess health care issues and trends and thus better predict the future health care needs of the communities in which they operate. This chapter also discusses the circumstances in which institutional information must be provided to external organizations.

This chapter identifies four significant external health information issues that impact a health care organization:

1. The availability of health information and where it can be found.
2. The regulation of health information. Access to the information by individuals and the public is often a key issue.

3. Health care legislation. Organizations attempt to influence legislation prospectively and respond to its requirements retrospectively.
4. The use of health information. Once the information is identified and obtained, organizations must determine how it should be used. Use of the information often triggers conflicts between individuals and institutions.

These issues must be addressed before it can be understood how to use health information effectively.

In the 1990s, health information will be a major building block of strategic and tactical planning and also of good clinical management. The object of this chapter is to provide the reader with insights concerning the use and regulation of health information. It also intended to familiarize the reader with where needed information can be found.

When discussing health information, special attention must be given to confidentiality and other ethical issues. Issues of confidentiality frequently arise in situations where health information is being communicated. Patient, physician, institutional, and public rights must be considered, but in some instances the rights of various constituents are at odds with one another.

MANAGEMENT PRINCIPLES

There are several management principles that should govern an organization's use of external information.

- The organization should continually monitor its external environment to ensure that its strategies, programs, and services are appropriately focused on community needs and economic, political, and social realities.
- External and internal information must be handled in a manner that not only ensures confidentiality but also addresses the legitimate requirements of those who need the information to provide individual services or monitor organizational activity.

- The organization should understand what information is needed and how it is to be used so that appropriate information sources can be identified and appropriate data collected while unnecessary or irrelevant information is discarded.
- The organization should set up a process for identifying new sources of relevant information and integrating them into the information management of the organization.

PUBLIC ACCOUNTABILITY

A health care organization has a responsibility to the community it serves. This responsibility encompasses many obligations, such as the obligation to measure the amount of charity care provided or the obligation to monitor its economic performance, including its pricing policies and profitability levels. If the organization does not recognize its responsibility or fails to act appropriately, it is likely to find itself in difficulty with its constituency.

Thus, a health care organization not only must be aware of the existence of external needs for information but also must design and maintain an information system that can respond to these information needs appropriately. The institution must have a mechanism to make it aware of these requirements on a timely basis so that they can be taken into account in management decision making.

History and Background

Health care organizations have not always been particularly sensitive to their environments. Prior to the 1980s, competition was practically unheard of, consumer pressures were virtualy absent, regulatory agencies provided information to the organizations and trade associations, and the legislative climate was much more serene than presently. Thus the need for aggressive external information-gathering activities was not acute.

In the past, external information was mainly used to monitor operational measures vis-à-vis regional and national performance norms. The Hospital Administrative Services (HAS) report was perhaps the most common vehicle for comparing actual operations with external norms. The object of this kind of comparison was to motivate improvement of the statistical and economic performance of the organization.

In the 1970s and 1980s the legislative climate was monitored by industry associations and a few institutions. In some cases this monitoring was more a defensive than an educational measure, with a focus on influencing pending legislation that was expected to have an adverse impact. Monitoring was rarely viewed as a way of learning about public expectations.

Historically, most health care organizations have not investigated public attitudes except for the purposes of market analysis and new product development. Public opinion was rarely solicited as a means of discovering the degree of organizational accountability expected by the public or the extent to which organizations were responding appropriately. There is currently much more recognition by organizations that they are accountable to the public and that communication mechanisms with the external environment must be created in order to be able to behave in a responsible and proactive way. (See Chapter 1 for more on community accountability.)

Government Regulation

Federal and state government entities are attempting to make health care institutions more publicly accountable for financial and clinical outcomes. Several states are or are about to begin releasing hospital-specific data relating to patient outcomes. California, for example, "will [publish] yearly reports on mortality and other patient outcomes at 528 acute-care hospitals statewide."[1] In those states where such information is released, the impact could be enormous. While some might regard outcome data as internal data, they are being made external by public policy, at least in the sense

of the timing and form of their release and the requirement that they be released. Outcome data are a new type of external data that health care organizations must deal with. The public can identify the organizations from which the data come, but the organizations exercise little control over their release, use, or interpretation.

Another type of accountability is related to tax-exempt status. The IRS is questioning whether the appropriate amount of charity service is being rendered by tax-exempt health care organizations. Its position is that, since nonprofit health care organizations do not pay taxes, they have obligations to provide benefits to the community, including an obligation to provide charity service in an amount roughly equivalent to the taxes that would have been incurred if they were for-profit organizations. The IRS is also evaluating the levels of unrelated business income accruing to tax-exempt entities and assessing whether profits are being used to benefit individuals—a practice prohibited for tax-exempt organizations under section 501(c)(3) of the Internal Revenue Code. Obviously, any institution wishing to respond to IRS inquiries in a meaningful way must have an information system that can accurately document the information relating to services and actions for which the organization is being held accountable.

A third area of accountability relates to the Medicare "fraud and abuse" regulations and interpretations. These regulations, and especially their interpretations, change rather frequently. The intent of these regulations and interpretations is to ensure that all financial transactions between the government and health care providers are legitimate and free of any conflict of interest. The regulations are primarily focused on financial accountability.

Public Expectations

The public also has expectations regarding health care institution accountability. In contrast to governmental expectations, those of the public are not backed by regulation and penalties. This does not make them any less important, since unmet public expectations may eventually be reflected in legislative proposals. Public feedback is a critically important source of external information for an institution. The institution must learn what the public's expectations are and adjust its actions so that the needs of the public and the needs of the institution are all being met.

The public expresses itself through the news media, the formation of business coalitions, and the complaints of patients. Health care institutions must be careful not to mistake the communication of public expectations for confrontation. For example, a health care institution could confuse the message of the stereotypic patient "who is always complaining about costs" with public expectations that the rate of health care inflation should be reduced.

The public generally holds health care institutions accountable for costs, access to care, quality, dignity, integrity, and confidentiality. The messages are being sent. It is not always the case that the receiver is tuned in. Even if it is, there is the question of what response is most appropriate.

Institutional Accountability

In those cases where an institution receives an external message and understands it, the key question is what it does in response. This is at the heart of institutional accountability. The most desirable situation is where an institution voluntarily accepts full accountability, thereby negating the need for external criticism. A well-regulated organization understands the parameters within which it operates (internal and external standards) and takes steps to ensure that it has timely and reliable information for determining when it is operating outside those parameters. When the proper boundaries are crossed, it is necessary to take managerial action to bring operations back into alignment with organizational standards.

One way an organization can learn it is not meeting relevant standards is to be cited by a legal or regulatory agency. A more proactive method is to have timely and reliable information in the hands of institutional decision makers that will allow them to know when operations are outside of the operational norms.

Comparison Shopping in the Health Care Marketplace

One factor that could encourage recognition of accountability is patient comparison shopping in the health care marketplace. Although comparison shopping is not widespread yet, it has the potential to make health care providers more willing to accept accountability in the areas of quality, service, and finance.

There are a number of interested parties, including government, managed care organizations, corporations, and individuals that are concerned about the costs of health care and the relationship between the costs and the product being offered. There is growing interest in shopping for medical services on the basis of price.

Organizations are also being held accountable for the quality of care they provide. The public wants the best health care available. There are few institution-specific empirical data available that would allow the public to draw meaningful conclusions about quality. Even in those states where hospital-specific data will be published, misinterpretation of the data by the public is a potential problem. Nevertheless, the public is interested in quality, and it will draw conclusions.

Similarly, the public is interested in service and will be drawn to those institutions that are able to meet the perceived needs of patients. Service encompasses everything from the quality of the food to the friendliness of the staff and the timeliness of their responses to the needs of patients and families.

In all three areas—finance, quality, and service—organizations will find themselves being held accountable by the patients and families they serve. They must put information systems in place that provide reliable information that allows them to meet public expectations and, where deviations exist, to take action to bring institutional performance into alignment.

Public Sanctions

Poor performance carries with it the potential for sanctions. To date, the only public sanctions have been those instituted for infringements of regulations. For example, health care providers are barred from serving Medicare or Medicaid patients as a result of inappropriate actions. The public has not yet acted in a concerted manner to punish poor performance, although the corporate sector is beginning to flex its muscles. In particular, business coalitions have sometimes been formed for the express purpose of providing the corporate sector with a greater voice in the allocation of health care services.

Although it is not possible to predict the future with any degree of certainty, public boycotts or other kinds of sanctions could well be used against health care organizations that fail to meet public expectations.

MONITORING THE EXTERNAL ENVIRONMENT

Most health care organizations have more data, but not more information, than they can effectively use. Data are of little use if not transformed into meaningful information.[2] Given the current degree of competition, it is necessary for organizations to be well informed about the dynamics of their environment. There is an enormous quantity of health care data available. The difficulty is discovering what types of data are available, how to access the data, and how to transform the data into useful information. Information resource management is the process of turning enormous amounts of data into a form that institutional decision makers can use.

External Data Requirements

In order to respond to the public, an organization must first be able to identify issues of importance to its constituency. For example, the organization can-

not respond to consumer preferences if it has no mechanism for gathering relevant information and therefore is unaware of the options. It must deploy its information resources so that responsible and well-documented answers can be arrived at. Its resources must be able to provide the following types of information.

Strategic Planning and Marketing Information

To some extent, this category of external information encompasses all of the others. It includes information about community and physician needs and expectations and economic, political, legal, and technological factors. When an organization is unaware of how these factors are driving public expectations, there is little reason to expect that the institution's strategic planning process can be appropriately focused. (See Chapter 17 for more on planning and marketing.)

Information on Patient and Community Needs and Expectations

This type of information provides the organization with insights into expectations within its service area. In general, the result of not paying attention to this type of information is declining market share. It should be noted that the community includes employers and payers, not just the individual patients the institution seeks to attract.

Information on Physician Needs and Expectations

Just as an institution must seek to become aware of patient and community needs, it must try to gather information on the expectations of the physicians associated with it. This kind of information partially overlaps information on technological and professional advances, but the primary focus is on practice needs at the institution. The consequence of not seeking this type of information is often a declining market share, since the physicians will begin to doubt the institution's willingness to assist them in their practice of medicine.

Information on Changes in the Economic and Political Climate

This type of information needs constant updating because of the rapidity of changes. It is no longer possible to speak of a domestic economy. We are all part of a global economy, and the health care sector is no exception. To some extent, the political climate reflects public expectations, but it is more than that. The political climate also reflects economic factors as well as politicians' perceptions of expedience. Failure to keep informed about new developments can result in suboptimal operational performance and declining market share.

Information on Laws and Regulations

Laws flow from the political environment. Regulations can have their origin in government agencies, such as the Internal Revenue Service, or in accrediting and credentialing bodies, such as the Joint Commission on Accreditation of Healthcare Organizations. The infringement of laws and regulations can result in sanctions, so information about them is of critical importance.

Information on Technological and Professional Advances

This external information is important because it provides insights about options that the organization has. One likely effect of ignoring this kind of information is decline of market share, since the organization will not be perceived as providing state-of-the-art health care.

External Data Sources

In order to collect the data required to satisfy the external information requirements outlined above, an organization must be tenacious and innovative. Some specific sources of external data are discussed below.

Centers of Health Care Data Research

There are several centers of health data research. Local libraries, especially medical and law school libraries, will have addresses for these centers. Principal centers include the U.S. Public Health Service, the U.S. National Center of Health Statistics, the U.S. Health Resources and Services Administration, the Centers for Disease Control, and the National Institute for Occupational Safety and Health. Of course, the American Medical Association, the Joint Commission on Accreditation of Healthcare Organizations, the Catholic Health Association, and the American Hospital Association can also provide useful resources and direction. (This list of centers is not intended to be exhaustive.)

Computerized Databases

There are also numerous computerized database vendors in the health care market today (see Exhibit 15-1). A computerized database provides access to health-related information via a direct computer link between the institution and the data file. Most of the databases currently available provide access to biomedical and clinical information much like a medical library. An organization needs to consider several issues before determining which database (or databases) can provide the information that will be most useful. An article in *The Internist* suggests a variety of issues to consider before choosing a database:

- The actual nature of the database. Exactly what type of information will it supply the manager (e.g., biomedical, statistical)?
- What type of options are available? How user-friendly is the database? What are the mechanics of using it?
- Is the system search through menus or is it command driven?
- What type of support system is provided with the database?
- What type of cost is involved? In addition to initial cost, on-line charges and annual membership fees are considerations.

Exhibit 15-1 Representative Computerized Medical Databases

BRS Information Technology	**DIALOG Info Services**
1200 Route 7	3460 Hillview Avenue
Laytham, NY 12110	Palo Alto, CA 94304
800/345-4277	800/334-2564
800/468-0908	
(Marketing)	**BACS/MEDLINE**
	Washington University
	School of Medicine
MEDLARS	660 S. Euclid
National Library of	St. Louis, MO 63110
Medicine	314/362-7085
8600 Rockville Pike	
Bethesda, MD 20209	**PaperChase**
800/638-8480	Beth Israel Hospital
	330 Brookline Avenue
AMA/NET	Boston, MA 02215
GTE Telenet	
Medical Info Network	
8229 Boone Boulevard	
Vienna, VA 22180	
800/368-4251	

- What are the hours of availability? Some databases are available to the subscriber 24 hours a day, while others have considerable restrictions on the hours of availability.[3]

Other Sources

In addition to databases that provide predominantly biomedical information, there are databases that provide demographic information. The National Center for Health Statistics (NCHS) produces data tapes available for public purchase. The NCHS offers more than 500 data files containing National Health Interview Survey data; National Health and Nutrition Examination Survey data; data on vital events such as natality, mortality, divorce, and fetal death; data on health resources utilization; and other health-related data. The NCHS has a data release policy that protects the confidentiality of the respondents who supplied the original data, and at the same time allows statistical data to be disseminated to all interested consumers in a prompt manner. Most of the data files contain microdata, which is useful to researchers because it allows them to aggregate the findings in a format that facilitates analysis.

The NCHS publishes the *Catalog of Electronic Data Products,* which provides background information on the NCHS data-gathering and data-disseminating process, general descriptions of the available data tapes, and information on how to order the data tapes.[4]

In 1986, Congress authorized the National Practitioner Data Bank (NPDB) for the purpose of increasing the efficiency of quality assurance in medical care. The *National Practitioner Data Bank Guidebook* states that the intent of Title IV of Public Law 99-660 is

> to improve the quality of medical care by encouraging physicians, dentists, and other health care practitioners to identify and discipline those who engage in unprofessional behavior; and to restrict the ability of incompetent physicians, dentists, and other health care practitioners to move from State to State without disclosure or discovery of the practitioners' previous damaging or incompetent performance.[5]

The *Guidebook* lists numerous types of health care practitioners and organizations that must be aware of the legislation and abide by its provisions. The list includes state licensing authorities, medical malpractice insurers, hospitals and other health care entities, professional societies, physicians, dentists, and other licensed health care practitioners.

The NPDB's collection and release of information activities focus on four areas:

1. medical malpractice payments
2. adverse licenser actions
3. adverse actions regarding clinical privileges
4. adverse actions regarding professional society memberships[6]

Table 15-1 lists reporting requirements, and Table 15-2 indicates which individuals and organizations may request information.

The NPDB has established regulations relating to confidentiality of the reported information. Civil

Table 15-1 National Practitioner Data Bank Reporting Requirements

Entity/Action	Physicians and Dentists	Other Licensed Health Care Practitioners
Medical Malpractice Insurers	Must report	Must report
Payment resulting from written claim of judgement		
State Licensing Boards	Must report	No reporting requirements*
Licensure disciplinary action based on reasons related to professional competence and conduct		
Hospitals and Other Health Care Entities	Must report	May report
Professional review action based on reasons related to professional competence or conduct, adversely affecting clinical privileges for a period longer than 30 days; or voluntary surrender or restriction of clinical privileges while under, or to avoid, investigation		
Professional Societies	Must report	May report
Professional review action, based on reasons related to professional competence or conduct, adversely affecting membership		

*Must report when the requirements of Section 5 of P.L. 100-93 are implemented.
Source: The National Practitioners Data Bank Guidebook, U.S. Dept. of Health & Human Services Publication No. (PHS) 90-1213, July 1990.

Table 15-2 Release of National Practitioner Data Bank Information

Entity	Information Request (Query) Status
Hospitals	Must request
Screening applicants for medical staff appointment or granting of clinical privileges; every two years for physicians, dentists or other health care practitioners on the medical staff or granted clinical privileges	
Hospitals	May request
At other times as they deem necessary	
State Licensing Boards	May request
At times as they deem necessary	
Other Health Care Entities	May request
Screening applicants for medical staff appointment or granting of clinical privileges; supporting professional review activities	
Professional Societies	May request
Screening applicants for membership or affiliation; supporting professional review activities	
Plaintiff's Attorney	May request
Plaintiff's attorney or plaintiff representing himself or herself (pro se) who has filed a medical malpractice action or claim in a State or Federal court or other adjudicative body against a hospital when evidence is submitted which reveals the hospital failed to make a required query of the Data Bank on the practitioner(s) also named in the action or claim	
Physicians, Dentists, and Other Health Care Practitioners	May request
Regarding their own files	
Medical Malpractice Insurers	May not request

Source: The National Practitioners Data Bank Guidebook, U.S. Dept. of Health & Human Services Publication No. (PHS) 90-1213, July 1990.

penalties of up to $10,000 can be imposed against each responsible individual, entity, or organization that is in violation of the confidentiality regulations.

Some external information is not readily available in compiled form. As a result, it might be necessary for an organization to set up its own data-gathering mechanism to acquire the information. For example, if the organization wishes to ascertain the expectations patients and the community have for its performance and service, it must construct an information-gathering mechanism that produces the appropriate data. Similarly, information about physician needs and expectations is not readily available unless specific information-gathering mechanisms are constructed. In general, this kind of external information does exist, but it must be gathered and analyzed.

ETHICS AND CONFIDENTIALITY

As mentioned in Chapters 13 and 14, health care organizations have the responsibility to handle information in a way that does not jeopardize individual or institutional rights of privacy and confidentiality. Confidentiality, besides being morally obligatory, promotes the physician-patient relationship. The general injunction to preserve confidentiality has become codified in legal requirements specifying the kinds of information being protected from intentional or unintentional breaches of security. Maintaining the confidentiality of specified individual and institutional information is central to an organization's management of its information resources. In addition, it helps to engender open communication and trust between patients and the health care community.

Ethical Foundations

Ethics is involved in every aspect of health care, from the most basic level of doctor-patient confidentiality to institutional versus public rights of access to information. The Council on Ethical and Judicial Affairs of the American Medical Association has five established *Current Opinions on the Principles of Medical Ethics and Rules,* which provide a useful starting point for establishing institutional policies and expectations. These guidelines specifically apply to privacy and confidentiality. Their underlying message is that all patient information should be kept private and confidential unless the patient has otherwise consented, there is potential third-party harm, or the release of the information is required by law or contract.

However, in today's health care environment, the controversies that surround diseases such as AIDS have necessitated the application of ethical principles to the issues of physician-patient confidentiality, physician-industry confidentiality, insurance company representative confidentiality, computer confidentiality, and attorney-physician confidentiality.[7] It is critical to understand the importance of balancing the right to individual privacy with the community's right to be protected from dangers.

Confidentiality is an issue that is grounded in ethical concern. In the practice of medicine, physician-patient confidentiality has a dual purpose. First, it shows respect for the patient's privacy and autonomy and gives dignity to the relationship. Second, it promotes trust and permits honest communication between the patient and physician. Obviously, breaching confidentiality can create barriers that might ultimately lead to less-than-optimum clinical results.

Since confidentiality issues are basically ethical issues, it might be useful to focus on certain specific ethical considerations associated with AIDS as a basis for appreciating the current debate about confidentiality. AIDS-related issues are particularly helpful in this regard because they involve not only patient rights but the rights of physicians, institutions, and other involved third parties. It should be noted that the following discussion focuses on the physician-patient relationship because this has been the focus of most of the literature. However, the issues are similar in the case of other health care relationships, such as the institution-patient relationship.

In addition to its set of five current opinions, the American Medical Association published in 1989 the *AMA Policy Compendium*. This text includes a discussion of policies specific to physician-patient confidentiality as it relates to AIDS. It also outlines numerous topics that concern the physician-patient relationship, including the following[8]:

- counseling
- HIV test consent
- discrimination laws
- confidentiality laws
- contact tracing and partner notification
- sanctions for willfully infecting others

While each of these topics lends itself to ethical discussion, the focus below will be on confidentiality laws and contact tracing and partner notification.

Confidentiality and the Right to Privacy

The AIDS epidemic has necessitated a re-evaluation of the application of some ethical principles used by physicians and other health professionals in their practice of medicine. In particular, two claims about confidentiality have been challenged: that there must be respect for an individual's privacy and that breaches of confidentiality render individuals unwilling to share openly and honestly. Even if medical confidentiality is regarded as a duty, there is still the question of whether it is an absolute duty.[9] Some norms have evolved that allow the revealing of confidential conversations in certain situations, such as when there is reason to believe harm will occur to the patient if the confidence is not broken, when there is reason to believe harm will occur to other parties, and when there is reason to believe that harm will occur to society. Some legal precedents have also been set along these lines.[10]

The complex nature of AIDS-related ethical issues is reflected in various journal and newsletter articles. According to one article, "As it becomes clear that AIDS is not a fleeting crisis but is here to stay, the medical profession is being forced to alter one of its most strongly held ethical positions—doctor-patient confidentiality is not as sacred as it once was."[11] This article makes the point that, although patients have a right to the protection of privacy and confidentiality, involved third parties have a right to be made aware of and protected from possible infection. However, the right of third parties to be informed must be balanced against the associated risks of revealing patients' HIV status and the social stigmatization that might result.

As pointed out by another article, physicians have certain responsibilities when handling cases of contagious disease. "The patient has a moral and legal responsibility to prevent harm to others. The physician has the duty not only to attend the patient, but, more important, to prevent dissemination of the infection to the public. However, legal patient confidentiality restraints severely hamper his or her ethical duty to protect the public."[12] Physicians often face the dilemma of deciding between an individual patient's right to privacy and the right of society to be protected from the spread of disease.

The ethical guidelines published by the AMA in its HIV policy compendium, while emphasizing the patient's right to confidentiality, also assert that involved third parties must be made aware of the risk of infection. The compendium includes guidelines on contact tracing and partner notification that should be familiar to all health care practitioners. These guidelines recommend

- establishing a system for contact tracing and partner notification for unsuspecting sexual or needle-sharing partners
- making provisions in any contact tracing and notification program for adequate safeguards to protect the confidentiality of seropositive persons and their contacts
- supporting legislation on the physician's right to exercise ethical and clinical judgment regarding whether or not to warn unsuspecting and endangered sexual or needle-sharing partners
- promulgating the standard that a physician should attempt to persuade an HIV-infected

patient to cease all activities that endanger unsuspecting others and to inform those whom he or she might have infected

- supporting the reportability of HIV seropositive patients to the departments of health of the fifty states for the purpose of contact tracing and partner notification[13]

Tarasoff v. Regents of the University of California (No. 551, p. 2d 334) established as legal precedent that the third party's right to know can override the patient's right to privacy. In this case, a young woman was not notified by the therapist that his patient had threatened to kill her. The young woman was killed by the patient, and the family sued the doctor for not having warned her. The family won the ruling in the California Supreme Court.[14]

Medicine and society continue to evolve, as do medical ethical issues. Some physicians now accept that the changing environment in which they practice medicine necessitates a re-evaluation of how traditional ethical principles should be applied. Although some principles are adhered to because they appear in the Hippocratic oath (Exhibit 15-2), other principles and guidelines flow from an understanding of human well-being and the physician-patient relationship. Thus, confidentiality is viewed as a good because it encourages the patient to be honest with the physician. It helps establish a trust. It also promotes the patient's relative right to privacy.[15] Following is one view expressed by a rural practicing physician of how changes in society require a re-evaluation of the way ethical principles are applied:

> The Hippocratic Oath is some 2,000 years old. Some hold it to the same conviction and with absolute obsession not to let it mature and develop along with the institutional development of society and therefore it is usually quoted as a truism with little adaptation to the changes in time. The fundamental ethical moral principles espoused in the Hippocratic Oath remain as much a validated commitment by health care professionals but it is only natural to recognize the application of the document has to also meet the workable translations of the soci-

Exhibit 15-2 Hippocratic Oath

> I swear by Apollo the physician, by Aesculapius, Hygieia, and Panacea, and I take to witness all the gods, all the goddesses, to keep according to my ability and my judgement of the following Oath:
>
> To consider dear to me as my parents him who taught me this art; to live in common with him if necessary to share my goods with him; to look upon his children as my own brothers, to teach them this art if they so desire without fee or written promise; to impart to my sons and the sons of the master who taught me and the disciples who have enrolled themselves and have agreed to the rules of the profession, but to these alone, the precepts and the instruction. I will prescribe regimen for the good of my patients according to my ability and my judgement and never do harm to anyone. To please no one will I prescribe a deadly drug, nor give advice which may cause his death. Nor will I give a woman a pessary to procure abortion. But I will preserve the purity of my life and my art. I will not cut for stone, even for patients in whom the disease is manifest; I will leave this operation to be performed by practitioners (specialists in this art). In every house where I come I will enter only for the good of my patients, keeping myself far from all intentional ill-doing and all seduction, and especially from the pleasures of love with women or with men, be they free or slaves. All that may come to my knowledge in the exercise of my profession or outside of my profession or in daily commerce with men, which ought not to be spread abroad, I will keep secret and will never reveal. If I keep this oath faithfully, may I enjoy my life and practice my art, respected by all men and in all times; but if I swerve from it or violate it, may the reverse be my lot.

etal structure in which they are being applied. This doesn't mean that the Hippocratic Oath can be interpreted one way in one society and one way in another society, but means that each society has the obligation to take the truisms of the document and translate them into a truism within their societal structure.[16]

Ethical issues frequently face managers as they access, process, and use information. Because of the pervasiveness of such issues, several additional views about ethics in health care are offered here. According to Dr. Leon R. Kass, "Ethics is first and foremost seen as a field of theorizing. Though ethics is eventually concerned with matters of conduct—with what we do and how we live—most scholars of ethics and theorists . . . do not begin concretely with real actors and deeds but abstractly with theories about action and its proper justifications."[17] In Kass's view, ethics is basically an interpretive activity in which abstract theory is applied to human actions.

Larry R. Churchill states that "our culture is well on its way to reducing medical ethics to legal requirements, general citizen ethics, or personal values. A distinctive ethic for medicine provides critical distance and moral meaning for the profession and an enriched societal ethic."[18] Churchill advocates that confidentiality not be seen merely as a legal requirement or an abstract good. In his view, correct understanding of confidentiality can help protect and promote the health of patients, third parties, and society.

Confidentiality and Proprietary Rights

Data must be protected from unauthorized access and use. Security and confidentiality therefore become a primary focus for the management of information in any institution.

There can obviously be breaches in security and confidentiality in the case of both paper and electronic documents. The result is the same but the approaches to dealing with it might be different. Methods for dealing with paper documents have been practiced for many years and are relatively well documented. Therefore, the focus of the following discussion is on security and confidentiality in an electronic system.

Confidentiality

A breach of confidentiality can be viewed as a breach of security. It can involve unauthorized access to or disclosure of confidential information, and, like other breaches of security, can result from intentional or unintentional actions.

A breach of confidentiality is more than the disclosure of information about an individual—it is an unauthorized disclosure. The distinction is subtle but important. Many organizations have access to information about individuals and can use that information without specific consent. In these cases, the consent is gained by regulation or contract. However, information about individuals generally should not be disclosed to a third party without documented authorization by the individuals or releases authorized by court proceedings or contracts.

The results of the various types of threats can have an effect on security or confidentiality, or both (see Table 15-3).

QUALITY MANAGEMENT

An organization's information resources must be organized in such a way that the data needed for quality management are gathered and disseminated. Further, the data must be of the highest quality.

Characteristics of Good Data

It has been said that the only thing that is worse than no information is bad information.[19] When decision makers have no information, they are fully aware of the riskiness of the decision. However, when decision makers have unreliable information that is thought to be valid, a false sense of security invades the decision-making process and the results can be more serious than if the decision makers were properly wary.

When an organization assembles information (internally or externally generated) for decision-making purposes, it is imperative that the information be "good." Good information has certain characteristics, including timeliness, accuracy, and reliability.

Timeliness

The necessary information must be available to the decision makers at the time that the decision is being made.[20] If the information exists within the organization but is not available when the decision

Table 15-3 Results of Threats to Information Systems

Threat	Security	Confidentiality
Unintentional Physical and Intentional Physical	Destruction of hardware Destruction of software Destruction of data	
Intentional Physical	Modification of hardware Modification of software Modification of data	Modification of software Modification of data
Unintentional Nonphysical and Intentional Nonphysical	Disclosure of software Disclosure of data	Disclosure of data

Source: Adapted from *Hospital Information Systems* by H.H. Schmitz, p. 146, Aspen Publishers, Inc., © 1979.

is being made, it might as well not exist at all. The time frame of the information must also be known. For example, information from a previous fiscal year inadvertently substituted for the current information is not timely. In addition, it is not accurate and can have a devastating effect on the organization if it is used as the basis for a decision.

Accuracy

Decision makers normally assume that the information they are given is accurate. When it is not, the consequences for the organization can be significant.

The relationship between timeliness and accuracy can be illustrated by what sometimes occurs in billing patients. When checking out of a hospital, a patient might be asked to pay his or her portion of the bill. This necessitates telling the patient what services were rendered and which ones he or she is required to pay for. In some cases charges arrive after the patient has paid the amount calculated at the time of checkout, and therefore the patient might be asked to pay an additional amount. When it becomes apparent that the information given by the hospital representative does not match what is ultimately expected, the patient is likely to conclude that the information was inaccurate, not that it was merely incomplete because it was not timely.

Information accuracy depends on the design of the information system and the procedures used to produce the information. A poorly designed system or faulty operation of the system has the potential to produce inaccurate information. Proper procedures and controls help to minimize the occurrence of inaccurate information, although a certain amount of strictness is also necessary, since even a well-designed system with proper procedures can be undermined by indifference or casualness on the part of the users.

Reliability

Although reliability is related to timeliness and accuracy, there is an additional dimension that warrants mention: It is possible for the same facts to generate different information or interpretations. The information as presented to decision makers may have been unintentionally influenced by the perspective of the persons managing the data. It is therefore important for the decision makers to recognize that alternative interpretations of the data are possible and to try to understand the basis of the interpretation that is offered.

Cost-Benefit Analyses for Health Services

It is not enough that the information be timely, accurate, and reliable—its acquisition and use must be cost-effective. In the present competitive health care environment, cost is an important factor. If two organizations have the ability to produce information at approximately the same levels of accuracy, reliability, and timeliness but one information system is significantly more costly than the other, the organization with the more costly system is placed at a competitive disadvantage.

An extension of the idea of cost-effectiveness relates to the use of information for cost-benefit analyses of health services. Both internal and external information is often used to evaluate the economic performance of health care providers. Here, cost-effectiveness relates not to the cost of producing the information but to the economic performance of the organization. Case mix analysis and the evaluation of the performance of health care programs within institutions are examples. Of course, it goes without saying it is crucially important that this information be timely, accurate, and reliable, for otherwise any conclusions drawn would be suspect.

Accountability and Total Quality Management

The concept of total quality management must be applied at several levels. First, the information that is produced and used within an organization must be timely, accurate, reliable, and cost-effective. The extent to which the organization is successful in gaining an accurate understanding of the quality of its operations and the care it provides is directly related to the quality of the information it uses. Some member of the organization must be given responsibility for the quality of the information and must be held accountable for maintaining the specified level of quality.

The issue of what organizational structure is most conducive to managing information resources is beyond the scope of this chapter, but much has been written on this subject and on the role of the chief information officer. In some cases, this role embraces the management of the entire decision-making process.[21]

THE FUTURE OF EXTERNAL INFORMATION MANAGEMENT

To be effective in the years ahead, an organization must identify future trends and construct policies and objectives that will increase its chances of meeting future community needs and expectations in an economically responsible manner. This is a continuous process, because the evolution of the environment requires that the organization continually monitor its constituency and make appropriate changes in direction.

Emerging Trends

The health care market is in a state of vigorous change. There are numerous forces, including political, economic, religious, and social forces, that are driving this change, and they all have their own focus. Combined, they are creating the current trends in U.S. health care. Organizations must not only identify these trends but also be responsive to the subtle gradations of special needs that are often unique to individual local settings.

As in the case of any open system environment, the trends are constantly changing in minor ways in response to stimuli received from the public. It is therefore important to identify major areas of focus, because organizations must fashion their information systems to address these areas, which include the following:

- rising health care costs
- universal access to care
- methods to finance the health care system
- methods to measure the quality of services offered
- epidemiological issues such as AIDS

Proactive Communication

As organizations identify future trends and develop information systems that allow them to measure and respond to environmental changes, it is also important that they establish communication systems (one part of an information system) that interact with the environment.

Historically health care providers have been in a reactive mode. They have found themselves in the position of having to respond defensively to criticism from the public. Taking a proactive stance would be more desirable, because it would allow the providers to be among the forces shaping the environment. Therefore, as health care organizations identify the interests of their constituencies and gather information in response, they should proactively communicate this information so as to help fashion the future.

Developing Valid Measures of Performance

If health care organizations are to be effectively proactive, valid measures of performance must first be identified and agreed upon. The parties that need to agree on the measures include not only health care providers but other stakeholders in the system, such as the government, the business sector, and the general public. Although coming to a consensus has thus far been a laborious process, it is nevertheless important that it continue. Without agreement from all the stakeholders, it is not likely that any measures of performance will be useful.

ADDITIONAL RESOURCES

American Medical Association. *AMA policy compendium: Current policies of the AMA House of Delegates through the 1989 interim meeting.* Chicago: American Medical Association, 1989.

American Medical Association. Council on Ethical and Judicial Affairs. *1989 current opinions: Principles of medical ethics and rules.* Chicago: American Medical Association, 1989.

Appelbaum, P.S., et al. Researchers' access to patient records: An analysis of the ethical problems. *Clinical Research* 32 (1984): 399–403.

Beauchamp, T.L. The management of medical information. In *Contemporary issues in bioethics,* eds. T.L. Beauchamp and L. Walters. 3d ed. Belmont, Calif.: Wadsworth, 1989.

Blake, D.C. State interests in terminating medical treatment. *Hastings Center Report* 19, no. 3 (1989): 5–14.

Christoffel, T. Review of 'The health of the republic: Epidemics, medicine, and moralism as challenges to democracy'. *Journal of Health Politics, Policy and Law* 15 (Spring 1990): 232.

Churchill, L.R. Reviving a distinctive medical ethic. *Hastings Center Report* 19, no. 3 (1989): 28–34.

Crisp, R. Autonomy, welfare and the treatment of AIDS. *Journal of Medical Ethics* 15, no. 15 (1989): 68–73.

Curran, W.J. Protecting confidentiality in epidemiological investigations by the Centers for Disease Control. *New England Journal of Medicine* 314 (1986): 1027–1028.

Fleetwood, J.E. Giving answers or raising questions: The problematic role of institutional ethics committees. *Journal of Medical Ethics* 15, no. 3 (1989): 137–142.

Gilbert, J. Philosophical, ethical, and legal aspects of resuscitation medicine. *Critical Care Medicine* 10, suppl. 17 (1989): 1085–1086.

Gillett, G.R. Informed consent and moral integrity. *Journal of Medical Ethics* 15, no. 15 (1989): 117–123.

Greaves, D. The future prospects for living wills. *Journal of Medical Ethics* 15, no. 15 (1989): 179–182.

Havard, J. Medical confidence. *Journal of Medical Ethics* 11, no. 6 (1985): 8–11.

Holm, S. Private hospitals in public health systems. *Hastings Center Report* 19, no. 5 (1989): 16–21.

Kars-Marshall, C., et al. National health interview surveys for health care policy. *Social Science and Medicine* 26 (1988): 223–233.

Kass, L.R. Practicing ethics: Where's the action? *Hastings Center Report* 20, no. 2 (1990): 5–11.

Kluge E.W. Designated organ donation: Private choice in social context. *Hastings Center Report* 19, no. 5 (1989): 10–16.

Kottow, M.H. Medical confidentiality: An intransigent and absolute obligation. *Journal of Medical Ethics* 12, no. 15 (1986): 117–122.

Lowey, E.H. Teaching medical ethics to medical students. *Journal of Medical Education* 61 (1986): 661–665.

Nowell-Smith, P. Euthanasia and the doctors: A rejection of BMA's report. *Journal of Medical Ethics* 15, no. 15 (1989): 124–128.

Ross, M.W. Psychosocial ethical aspects of AIDS. *Journal of Medical Ethics* 15, no. 15 (1989): 74–81.

Schmitz, H.H. *Managing health care information resources.* Gaithersburg, Md.: Aspen Publishers, 1987.

Stanley, J.M. The Appleton consensus: Suggested international guidelines for decisions to forego medical treatment. *Journal of Medical Ethics* 15, no. 15 (1989): 128–132.

U.S. Department of Health and Human Services. *Catalog of electronic data products.* Publication No. (PHS) 90-1213. Washington, D.C.: U.S. Department of Health and Human Services, 1990.

U.S. Department of Health and Human Services. *National practitioner data bank guidebook.* Washington, D.C.: U.S. Department of Health and Human Services, 1989.

Winston, M., and Sheldon H. Landesman. AIDS and a duty to protect. *Hastings Center Report* 17, no. 2 (1987): 22–23.

NOTES

1. News at Deadline, *Hospitals,* November 5, 1991, p. 10.

2. H.H. Schmitz, Decision Support: A Strategic Weapon, in *Healthcare Information Management Systems,* ed. Marion J. Ball et al. (New York: Springer-Verlag, 1991), 42–48.

3. Computer Databases, *The Internist,* October 1985, p. 24.

4. U.S. Department of Health and Human Services, *Catalog of Electronic Data Products,* Publication No. (PHS) 90-1213 (Washington, D.C.: U.S. Department of Health and Human Services, 1990).

5. U.S. Department of Health and Human Services, *National Practitioner Data Bank Guidebook* (Washington, D.C.: U.S. Department of Health and Human Services, 1989), 2.

6. Ibid.

7. American Medical Association, The Council on Ethical and Judicial Affairs, *1989 Current Opinions: Principles of Medical Ethics and Rules* (Chicago: American Medical Association, 1989), 9.

8. American Medical Association, *AMA Policy Compendium: Current Policies of the AMA House of Delegates through the 1989 Interim Meeting* (Chicago: American Medical Association, 1989).

9. T.L. Beauchamp, The Management of Medical Information, in *Contemporary Issues in Bioethics,* ed. T.L. Beauchamp and L. Walters, 3d ed. (Belmont, Calif.:Wadsworth, 1989), 375–376.

10. Ibid.

11. *AIDS ALERT: A Monthly Update for Health Professionals* 3, no. 8 (1988): 133.

12. *A Physician's Guide to Medical, Legal, Confidentiality and Ethical Issues* (Prepared on Behalf of the Risk Management Committee, The Doctors' Company, 1989).

13. American Medical Association, *AMA Policy Compendium.*

14. *Tarasoff v. Regents of the University of California* (No. 551, p. 2d 334).

15. Correspondence with Father Patrick F. Norris, O.P., Center for Health Care Ethics, St. Louis University Medical Center, St. Louis, Missouri.

16. Interview with Dr. Donald L. James, Phelps County Regional Medical Center, Rolla, Missouri.

17. Leon R. Kass, Practicing Ethics: Where's the Action? *Hastings Center Report* 20, no. 2 (1990): 6–7.

18. Larry R. Churchill, Reviving a Distinctive Medical Ethic, *Hastings Center Report* 19, no. 3 (1989): 28.

19. H.H. Schmitz, *Managing Health Care Information Resources* (Gaithersburg, Md.: Aspen Publishers, 1987), 89.

20. Ibid, 90–91.

21. Ibid, 97–142.

David J. Fine
Rohn J. Butterfield

Financial Planning and Management

Purpose: The purpose of financial planning and management is to accurately record and report the financial performance of the organization and to project and plan for performance in future operating periods.

INTRODUCTION

This chapter provides an overview of the history and current landscape of health care financing in the United States; a brief discussion of the role and structure of the finance function in health care organizations; an examination of tools and techniques for budgeting, reporting, monitoring, and analyzing financial data; and a survey of financial trends likely to affect managers in the 1990s.

MANAGEMENT PRINCIPLES

Certain financial management principles apply to any business endeavor, and these features are worth reviewing before beginning our examination of topics specific to the health care setting:

- For-profit businesses exist to provide, in economic terms, maximum sustained wealth for their owners. Similarly, nonprofit organizations strive to maximize funding to ensure that they will continue to be able to provide needed services or products to the community served.
- Wise decision making regarding the development of sources of funds and the efficient use of funds is fundamental to achievement of the economic goals of any business.
- The finance function of a business enterprise provides the management team with the financial information necessary for making resource-maximizing choices. As a result, the finance function is integral to the operation of all businesses.
- While the finance function is necessary to the healthy status of any organization, it is not sufficient for decision making. The mission, goals, objectives, investor needs, and many other factors often temper the strictly economic motivation for operating a business. Each manager's experience base and sometimes his or her intuitive hunches merge with colleagues' expertise and objective data to yield the final decision on any issue. It is the rare decision, however, that does not need the support of finance inputs.

- Structurally, the finance department of an enterprise is a staff function supporting all other operational aspects of the organization, including top management. Therefore, given the pervasive impact of the finance function and its critical importance to decision making, a chief financial officer (CFO) is typically found at the highest level of management. He or she is charged with providing leadership to an extensive host of staff services. It is not unusual to find health information systems, materials management, and even telecommunications reporting to the CFO in addition to the more traditional accounting, billing, receivables/payables, and reporting/analysis functions of the finance division.

Finally, the authors assume that the reader is familiar with the basic principles of financial and managerial accounting. While these tenets will not be made explicit herein, they always operate in the background of any discussion of financial management. No manager without a working knowledge of accounting can fully benefit from the content of this chapter.

There are certainly many financial management practices common to all organizations, and the above management principles apply to health care as well. In general, however, the similarities end here. From patient billing and receipts to the sources of revenues and price setting, the health care organization is different from almost every other business. The next section will trace the evolution of these differences and the effect they have on day-to-day decision making in health care organizations.

THE EVOLUTION OF HEALTH CARE FINANCING

Early History

Medical care in the United States has made enormous strides during the twentieth century. Before this century, hospitals provided primarily palliative care for the indigent sick and dying. Funding for these activities derived from voluntary public contributions, philanthropic efforts, and religious organizations. Staffing before the latter part of the nineteenth century drew from the lower strata of society, sometimes from prisons and poorhouses. Professional nursing did not exist then, and recommendations to train nurses academically were met with derision. Renovation of hospital facilities was virtually unknown, and conditions were often grim.

The conditions in hospitals contrasted sharply with the highly personalized home care service provided by physicians to those who could afford to pay out of pocket. The model of care provision for these wealthier individuals was family oriented, though the medicine practiced may not have been any more curative than that supplied in the hospital setting.[1]

Major advances in hygiene, public health, and surgery in the late nineteenth century prompted the hospital to evolve into the primary site of care for most acute illness. Physicians began to view the hospital as a laboratory or workshop for conveniently and efficiently maximizing the benefits of these advances.[2] Technological developments throughout the twentieth century further solidified the role of the hospital as the primary site for inpatient care. Because more and more paying patients wanted the advantages of this setting, the recovery of costs for services, which had largely depended on philanthropy, now hinged upon billing and reimbursement.

During the same period, routine ambulatory care moved from the home to the physician's office, where technological advances could be more easily used and access to the hospital was more convenient. Outpatient care, however, was still largely attainable only by those who could pay.

Early in this century, social reformers in the United States, mostly outside the government, recognized the need for some form of medical insurance. Many European nations had incorporated medical care into their social insurance programs by this time. Early U.S. efforts failed because of the lack of political influence of the reformers, the decentralized nature of the American government, and the low cost of health care at the time.

As the cost of health care increased, the pressure for medical insurance expanded. Hospital care, in particular, began to materially affect the pocketbooks of the middle class in the 1920s. The evolution of the medical profession into a powerful political coalition occurred during this period. Physicians began to cluster around the hospitals in urban areas, reducing the previous emphasis on rural care.

Committee on the Costs of Medical Care

These developments spawned the establishment of a privately funded commission, called the Committee on the Costs of Medical Care, in 1926. This was a blue-ribbon committee, composed of economists, physicians, and other experts and chaired by Stanford University president Ray Lyman Wilbur.[3] In its final report, published in 1932, the committee proposed a voluntary program of health insurance but stopped short of recommending compulsory insurance. At the time, this proposal did not satisfy any major constituency on the committee. The reformers wanted compulsory insurance, and the physicians not only opposed compulsory efforts but objected that voluntary insurance was a step along the way to completely socialized medicine.

The Depression also contributed to the recognition of the need for a different system to finance health care. Physician's office visits declined, and those who did seek care were often unable to pay their bills. Hospital census dropped, philanthropy fell, and payment defaults rose.

Blue Cross, Blue Shield, and Commercial Insurance Plans

Efforts to move toward any type of national insurance plan failed, even during these difficult times. The hospital industry, therefore, took action on its own in the late 1920s. Individual hospital service plans were established that guaranteed complete hospital coverage in exchange for a predetermined fee. After some intervention from the American Hospital Association, regionally based third-party plans replaced individual hospital plans. Hospitals continued to underwrite these broader plans financially, although the regionally based plans were separate corporate entities. By 1939, most states had legally recognized these service plans. Collectively, these plans are now known as Blue Cross insurance.

Late entries to the insurance market, Blue Shield plans were established in the late 1930s to help cover the cost of physician services. The first such plan, the California Physicians Service, was introduced in 1939 and covered both inpatient and outpatient services.[4] Blue Cross, although prevented from covering physician services, played a large role in the development of Blue Shield, and both plans often operated out of the same office.

Commercial indemnity plans developed alongside these hospital plans, but paid hospital and physician charges at reduced levels and required copayments from patients. Indemnity insurance directly paid patients only for specified services on a charge basis and based their premiums on experience ratings consistent with their other insurance products. Hospital service plans had typically reimbursed hospitals on a charge basis for a broad range of services, with premiums based on community ratings.[5] Indemnity insurance attempted to control actuarial risk by limiting the services patients could demand and by requiring out-of-pocket cost sharing. Service plans had attempted to control provider behavior to limit risk exposure. The insurers often used fee schedules, provider service contracts, and other similar methods to achieve these goals.

Direct Service Plans

The final major type of health insurance to emerge during these early years was the direct service plan, which integrated physicians and facilities into a unified corporate entity. Payment for services took the form of fixed subscription or membership fees paid by the patients. In exchange, the patients had unlimited access to care, and the plans managed insurance risk by controlling provider behavior and patient choices within the plan. This arrangement allowed direct service insurers to control billing costs as well. Using salaried physicians and maintaining hospital ownership significantly reduced the need for detailed itemized bills.

An early example of this type of insurance was the Ross-Loos Clinic in Los Angeles. In 1929, two physicians contracted to provide comprehensive care for the employees of the Los Angeles Department of Water and Power. Included in the package was complete hospital coverage. By 1935, enrollees totalled nearly 40,000, and the fee was a little over two dollars per month per member.[6] Perhaps the best-known direct service insurance plan is the Kaiser-Permanente health plan, which began in 1935. Collectively, these plans, commonly known as health maintenance organizations (HMOs), constitute the fastest growing segment of the private health care funding market. (For more on managed care, see Chapter 8.)

Medicare and Medicaid

Continued medical advances, rising costs, reorganization of the hospital as the primary site of acute care, and union efforts to include comprehensive health care service in benefit packages characterized the post-Depression years. Unions, almost single-handedly, changed the way health services were paid for. Out-of-pocket reimbursement declined, replaced by employer-sponsored insurance. By the mid-1950s, over 50 percent of Americans had some form of hospital and surgical insurance.[7]

The combined effect of medical and technological advances, continued rising costs, and general optimism about the future peaked in July 1966 with the enactment of Medicare and Medicaid legislation. At this point, the U.S. government and the states became major partners in the financing of health care. Federal, state, and local governments account for over 40 percent of the total health dollar expenditures. This contrasts sharply with the 1960 figure of 22 percent.[8] Given their importance to the financing of health care, Medicare and Medicaid will be examined in greater depth.

Medicare covers Americans over the age of 65 and younger citizens with specialized needs, such as those with renal disease or certain disabilities. Funds for Medicare derive from employee payroll taxes. Coverage consists of two parts: Part A for hospital services, and Part B for inpatient and outpatient physician services.

Originally, Part A made payments to providers based on *cost plus,* meaning actual cash expenditures plus noncash items such as depreciation on equipment and bad debts.

This method of payment was meant to ensure that hospitals receiving funds from the government would not realize a profit from providing services to claimants. This was in sharp contrast to the initial charge-based reimbursements made by indemnity and Blue Cross plans. Ironically, over the next decade or so, Medicare accounted for the steepest rise in health care expenditures in U.S. history. A number of contributory factors can be identified.

First, access to care was extended to a large portion of society that had previously been unable to afford insurance. Care for the elderly also required a higher cost per case than that for other age groups. Therefore, the absolute volume of health services delivered expanded dramatically and immediately, and the expansion has continued because of growth in the population of persons over 65 and the lengthening of life spans.

Second, and no less important, the cost-based reimbursement scheme adopted by Medicare provided strong incentives for hospitals to exploit an economically protected niche. Unlike other segments of the economy, except perhaps the defense and aerospace industries, payment for services provided in the health care sector was underwritten by the U.S. government and large insurance firms. Although hospitals provided some charity care, it was not unusual for a community hospital to have total write-offs and contractual adjustments between 5 and 10 percent of gross charges.

Beyond this insulation from the marketplace, hospitals received funds above costs to ensure the continued growth of technology and facilities. Under the Medicare payment methodology, costs essentially were no object, so unlimited expansion in the number and quality of services provided was possible. True to the economic theories of Adam Smith, the hospital industry took full advantage of these incentives.

Medicaid provides comprehensive health care services to the poor. Persons falling below certain income levels are eligible. Funding derives from the states, with matching funds provided by the federal government. Administration of Medicaid is at the state level, and therefore program organization varies widely.

Although this is an oversimplification, hospital financial management strategies from 1966 to the early 1980s seemed focused on maximizing reimbursement from Medicare and Medicaid, setting pricing policies for charge-based payers, ensuring collection from persons still paying out of pocket, and delineating investment strategies for the incoming flow of dollars. Such behaviors did nothing to restrain health care demand, nor was there any real incentive to pursue cost-reduction or cost-accounting strategies. In addition, concern for competitive issues was negligible, except perhaps with respect to physician recruitment efforts.

Cost Containment

Although insurers in the late sixties and the seventies adjusted their payment schemes in various ways (e.g., most of the Blue Cross plans switched from charge-based to cost-based reimbursement), it was not until the eighties that the next set of dramatic changes occurred. After Medicare helped to push health care expenditures from $19 billion in 1960 to $275 billion in 1980[9] and employers experienced double-digit increases in the cost of health care benefits, the total cost of health care became a national issue—and has remained so to the present. Figure 16-1 shows the enormous growth in national health expenditures and the change in payer mix just before Medicare implementation and for the most recent period for which data are available.

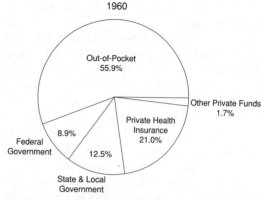

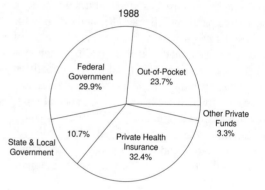

Figure 16-1 A Comparison of Personal Health Care Expenditures in the United States in 1960 and 1988, Excluding Prepayment, Administration, and Government Public Health Activities. *Source: Health United States 1990,* U.S. Department of Health and Human Resources, 1990.

Prospective Payment and Diagnosis-Related Groups

Medicare responded to the issue first and introduced a prospective payment system at the national level in October 1983. While not an entirely new idea, the system changed the economic incentives for hospitals permanently. Unlike the past, hospitals became partners in risk sharing within the Medicare program.

Based on a methodology developed at Yale University, Medicare originally established 468 diagnosis-related groups (DRGs). These groups organized diseases by body organ systems. Based on the average historical costs for reimbursing each DRG, Medicare set prices prospectively on a per-discharge basis for every DRG. Medicare then paid these prices to hospitals for each discharge regardless of the actual cost of care delivered.

Medicare phased in its prospective payment system during the rest of the 1980s, allowing hospitals time to adjust to the extensive implications of switching from cost-based reimbursement to a price-based payment scheme. The methodology for establishing payments was complex and vestiges of the complexity remain today. In addition, the system has created continuing political competition among the teaching, urban, and rural provider sectors, each of which seeks to maintain special reimbursement considerations (e.g., "indirect medical education," "sole community provider," "disproportionate share," and "urban wage indices"), and also among niche providers, which seek to maintain "exempt" units.

To illustrate, suppose that, for a given hospital, reimbursement for a discharge under the cost-based system was $5,000 but that under the prospective payment system Medicare set the price for this discharge at $4,000. If hospital costs remained at the same level under the prospective payment system, the hospital would lose $1,000 for every discharge in this DRG. Likewise, if costs could be lowered below the $4,000 threshold, the same hospital would experience a surplus of funds. In short, hospitals now bear the responsibility for their economic viability: A cost-controlled hospital will profit, but a high-cost hospital will probably experience financial losses.

Medicare payment as a percentage of total collections from all sources also greatly influences fiscal viability. For example, a high-cost hospital with few Medicare patients could raise prices, relying on private payers to offset the Medicare shortfall through cost shifting. A cost-controlled hospital with a high Medicare volume will have few opportunities to offset any Medicare losses.

Many state Medicaid programs have taken the Medicare lead and use DRG-based payment systems. A number of Medicaid programs have contracted with or established their own HMOs. Others have contracted directly with providers for discounted charges or other economically favorable terms.

Preferred Provider Organizations and Health Maintenance Organizations

Many private insurers now contract with or own HMOs or have established preferred provider organizations (PPOs). PPOs contract with providers at favorable rates and set up strict utilization criteria for patient access to services within the contracted panel of providers.

As noted earlier, such direct service providers have achieved a strong economic position within the current health care marketplace. These organizations are usually categorized under the rubric of managed care. A primary care physician who works for or contracts with the HMO acts as a gatekeeper for all services used by patients. Generally all care costs are covered, and preventive outpatient care is encouraged, but the primary care physician's permission must be obtained for any care provided outside that physician's office. This controls patient access to the more expensive forms of care, such as surgery.

HMOs have financial incentives to keep members out of the more expensive care channels. HMOs receive a certain amount of money per month per member, termed a capitation payment. Using the capitation payments, the HMO generally pays for all primary care office costs and outpatient ancillary testing plus referrals to specialists and hospitalization. To realize a profit, the HMO must ensure that the total cost of these integrated services is less than total capitation payments. HMOs have a strong economic incentive to emphasize outpatient and preventive care rather than the use of specialists and hospitals, which costs substantially more.

Physician Reimbursement under Medicare

Part B payments can be made either to the physician, based on reasonable and customary charges, or directly to the patient on the same basis. In the former case, physicians accept assignment, which means they agree to accept Medicare reimbursement as payment in full. In the latter case, physicians can charge the patient more than the reasonable and customary amount and make an effort to collect the difference. Medicare provides incentives for physicians to accept assignment.

Currently, Medicare is phasing in a resource-based relative value system (RBRVS) for reimbursing physicians. Developed at Harvard University, categorization of outpatient visits and surgical procedures is based primarily on effort and time estimates. Patient care activities are assigned a value based on these factors, with payments made based on the derived values. This methodology is perhaps best described as primarily an instrument of public policy, with Part B cost reduction as a byproduct.

By basing payment on time and effort, the government seeks to shift reimbursement from high-cost, procedure-oriented surgical specialties to medically related specialties and thereby make nonsurgical specialties like general internal medicine and family medicine more attractive to prospective physicians.

The Blues and the indemnity insurers mimicked the Medicare changes of the early 1980s. Charge-based payments are still basic to indemnity plans, but most of the Blue Cross plans eliminated these payments long ago. However, even the charge-based payers have increased the deductible and coinsurance payments required from patients. Discounted contracts with hospitals are now the rule, not the exception.

Financial Planning and Management

As managed care options have grown and American health care system dollars have become scarcer, the tasks performed by the finance department have increased in complexity. Chief financial officers now must focus more attention on cost accounting, reporting, systems, decision support, and other internal resource management functions. As a result, the role of the finance department in any health care enterprise has assumed greater importance over the years. There is no reason to expect that future changes in reimbursement, such as managed competition, will change this trend.

ORGANIZING THE FINANCE FUNCTION

This section examines generic organizing principles of the finance function. Thoughtful organization is the key to fulfilling the role of the finance department and the goals of the enterprise.

The board of trustees is the starting point for organizing the finance function, since the board is responsible for all aspects of business operations, including fiscal affairs. In order to monitor the financial activities of the business, the board typically establishes a finance committee.

The committee, whose membership includes the CFO and chief executive officer (CEO) oversees the operating position of the organization, the adequacy of capital resources, and the status of all investments. Serving in a staff capacity to the board, it then reports to and advises the board on recommended actions. Responsibility for providing information to the committee and board and for carrying out decisions of the Board is delegated to the CEO. It is not uncommon to find budget, audit, investment, or other specialized subcommittees operating as subunits of the finance committee or the board.

The CEO is ultimately responsible for the financial resources of the hospital. Typically, the duties related to financial resource management are delegated by the CEO to the CFO. The CFO typically reports directly to the CEO, along with hospital operations management personnel.

The duties of the CFO drive the way the finance department is organized. First, the CFO develops, coordinates, and monitors the financial plan of the enterprise. He or she coordinates preparation of the budget for the organization, helps to set performance standards, educates management regarding the internal and external financial environment, and provides operations personnel with the information necessary for monitoring budget compliance.

Second, the CFO oversees the collection and recording of financial data and resources. This typically is termed the general accounting function. It includes general ledger maintenance, establishment of policies, internal auditing, billing, receivables/payables management, payroll, cashiering, and inventory control.

Third, the CFO sets up routine and special reports for management that, among other things, measure actual performance against predicted performance. Financial results frequently are interpreted orally for management and the board. Standard accounting financial reports are also prepared and external audits of them coordinated. Given the multitude of external agencies and payers affecting internal business operations, the CFO and his or her staff are increasingly involved in advocacy reporting.

Finally, the finance department usually has a section that provides decision support and advice. Management engineering studies, productivity or cost-accounting standards development, and even quality measurement are components of this function. Decision support services can be invaluable to the operations manager, especially when confronted by specialized requests arising from the total quality management process or program evaluation.

Other management functions often grouped with the finance department include information services, such as computing and telecommunications. In the hospital setting, departments involved in financial data gathering, such as the medical records, admitting, and materials management departments, sometimes report to the CFO.

A new duty of the CFO that has arisen in the last few years bears mentioning because of the growing emphasis on managed care. Finance staffs now spend a significant proportion of their time preparing for and presenting competitive bids for exclusive or shared rights to specified patient populations. Winning or losing contractual service agreements with insurers and managed care firms can mean financial success or failure no matter what the type of organization.

In staffing each of the functional areas of the finance department (see Figure 16-2), the CFO must be mindful of the expertise required for each. Certified public accountant credentials may be required for the internal auditor and the manager of the accounting section, among others, whereas the analysis section might be staffed by industrial engineers.

As with all departments of an organization, careful hiring practices should be exercised to ensure that appropriate persons, with sufficient skill levels, are assigned to each activity. Although staffing should be efficient, there must be enough personnel to guarantee effective performance of the finance activities required by the enterprise. Productivity standards can be developed for the billing staff (e.g., bills processed per day) and others performing routine duties, but the manager's experience, in concert with other senior staff input, will often be the basis for choosing the number of persons to perform certain tasks.

Electronically automating certain finance functions is an excellent method for improving staffing and expanding the capabilities of the finance department. Financial and managerial accounting, billing, budgeting, payroll, inventory management, admitting and discharge, and financial analysis are commonly automated in large organizations. The types of information systems range from simple general ledger or payroll systems used in small physician group practices to the very large mainframe or networked systems used in multihospital entities. Organizations may also opt to contract with outside service bureaus for some of these functions. (See Chapter 13 for more information on automating financial services.)

THE FINANCE FUNCTIONS

Budget Planning

The operating budget of an organization provides guidance for planning and controlling revenues and

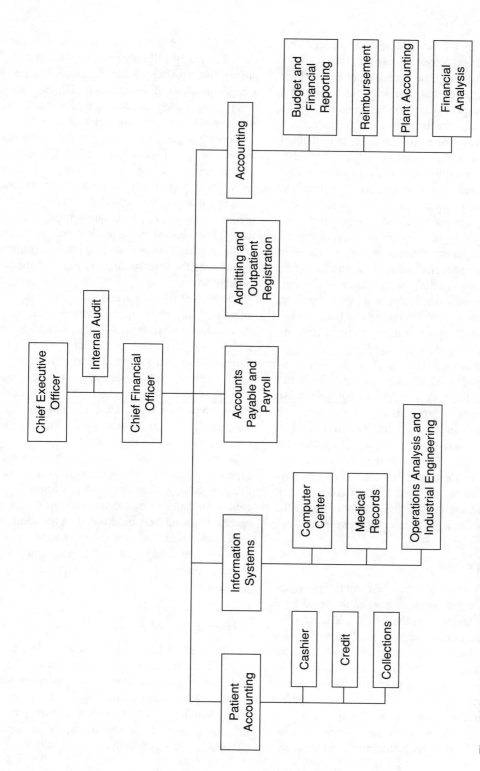

Figure 16-2 Finance Department Organization Chart

expenditures by predicting expected financial performance. Budgets cover a one-year period called a fiscal year. Longer time frames may be used for analytical purposes, but they will still consist of a series of one-year periods. The longer the time frame, the greater the likelihood that the budget will be inaccurate, based as it is on information about the organization, the external economy, and other factors that are highly speculative. Consequently, budgets are used most often for near-term planning.

Budgets are utilized to measure actual financial performance against predicted (budgeted) performance. The ability of operations managers to meet or exceed budget expectations is a crucial factor in the evaluation of management performance. Thus, the budget serves as the basis for financial accountability and control. The budget is so important that, once approved by the organization's board, it becomes essentially a performance contract between the organization and the manager.

Budgeting has not always had the primacy it enjoys today. Prior to Medicare's requiring a budget as part of its conditions of participation, hospitals used a simple matching of expenditures and revenues, with no real forecasting. Given that hospital costs or charges were usually reimbursed fully, incentives for forecasting expenditures were minimal. It was only as the pressure for cost containment grew and payment mechanisms changed to emphasize prudent buyer considerations that the budget assumed the same importance it has in other business sectors.

Budget Types

Hospitals can use one of these budgeting approaches: the appropriation budget, the fixed forecast budget, and the variable or flexible budget.[10]

The appropriation budget is used most often for government health care service units. A fixed number of dollars are assigned to an institution and its departments based on the previous year's expenditures. Because the budget is fixed, there is often no incentive for the manager to economize.

For example, the manager who effectively manages resources below budgeted levels must return excess dollars to the central authority. The next year the central authority will only grant the previous year's amount to the manager's department, plus an amount for inflation. Should service levels rise, the manager will be caught short, and the overage will count as a negative in his or her evaluation.

Somewhat greater flexibility exists in the fixed forecast budget. This budget, still used in most organizations, allows for yearly forecasts of activity levels. It also allows for adjustments to expenditures based on services provided and relies upon the predictive abilities of the management team. Although adjustments to the original budget may occur during the fiscal year, there is often a significant lag between the actual activity change and the budget adjustment.

The budget that is far and away most useful in today's rapidly changing financial environment is the variable or flexible budget. This budget requires a highly sophisticated cost accounting function. Expenses that change little year after year, regardless of service level changes, are held fixed, much like the appropriations budget. The expenses that vary with service levels are each converted to an expense per unit of service and are forecast on a monthly basis for the fiscal year.

In automated systems, where timely reporting of expenses is possible, a continuous form of the flexible budget may be instituted. As each month concludes, the budget's estimate of variable costs is replaced with a new estimate based on the additional information provided by the previous month. As a consequence, budgeting occurs essentially on a monthly basis. Of course, revenues must be adjusted as well.

Preparing the Budget

Since the budgeting process consists of forecasting expenses and revenues, a sound method for collecting and reporting accurate financial and service level data is crucial to successful budgeting. In addition to historical trending of activity, organizational goals and objectives must be considered. Finally, anticipated changes in activity levels must be estimated.

All these efforts require excellent cooperation from managers, physicians, and employees. The entire health care team should be involved if possible, and the recent advent of total quality management serves to highlight the desirability of maximum employee involvement in such efforts. Predicting the future is never easy, especially in these times of great change. Therefore, as many relevant information resources as possible should be used. Consensus regarding the budget should also be a major goal of the process. Although not everyone will be pleased with budget expectations, senior management should be comfortable that as much input as possible has been considered in constructing the final budget.

Since personnel expenses are more than half of the expenses of the typical health care organization, wages and salaries must be budgeted and controlled judiciously. If possible, it is best to separate existing staffing levels from consideration of budget needs. Often termed zero-based budgeting, this method requires the manager to predict service levels and the inputs (personnel) needed to efficiently produce the required outputs (services). Then and only then does the manager set the budgeted amount to be requested. Zero-based budgeting, which can also be applied to resources other than personnel, encourages the manager to stringently review inputs without regard to historical staffing practices and prejudices.

Budgeting is often the only time the manager gets to take a step back and create an ideal department staffing plan. Staffing should therefore be based on actual services provided and the time and effort required to perform the units of service as efficiently as possible. Capable cost accounting and management engineering resources, available in the finance departments of large organizations, as well as creative budgeting of overtime and part-time resources, can be invaluable in helping to determine appropriate staffing levels objectively. In smaller enterprises, determining the most productive staffing may be more intuitive, but every effort should be made to use objective methods as much as possible.

Once the staffing needs are determined, they are translated into dollars based on wage and salary rates. Benefits are often calculated by the finance department as a percentage of wages and salaries. Opportunities to economize on benefits are more difficult, since historically based benefits may be viewed as inviolable by employees. Therefore, care must be taken when adding new benefits, as they often become entrenched over time.

One method of reducing benefit costs is to institute cafeteria-style selection of benefits. In this method, a certain amount of employer-provided benefit dollars are allocated to each employee. Employees may select benefits based upon their specific needs up to the amount of the dollars provided. If an employee desires additional benefits, he or she may pay for them out of pocket. This helps the employees and the employer. Employees can choose only those benefits needed, and the employer has the potential to limit benefit costs more effectively. (See Chapter 18 for more on employee benefits.)

Budgeting for supplies and other nonpersonnel expenses requires the manager to have detailed knowledge of the materials needed to produce units of service. An x-ray or lab test each uses specific supplies, and these supplies should be enumerated and costed. Then, based on the predicted units of service, the manager simply adds the costs to yield a total expense for each procedure. These costs are aggregated based on the predicted units of service. After estimates of price inflation for the materials are made, the total cost is placed in the budget.

There are many categories of nonpersonnel expense in a budget to help the manager better track changes in usage of discrete materials. A sample classification of these categories, including personnel categories, is presented in Exhibit 16-1.

Once the operational expense budget is completed, the manager should expect timely reports of actual versus budgeted performance, usually on a monthly basis. The best reports present workload data, such as service units provided during the period, along with trended financial performance during the current and previous fiscal years. Productivity reports on the work force should also be

Exhibit 16-1 Classification of Expenses

Salaries and Wages	Job-applicant expense
Professional personnel	Gas and heating fuels
Regular pay	Electricity
Supplemental pay	Water
Technical personnel	Heating and cooling
Regular pay	Building rental
Overtime pay	Office equipment rental
Shift differential	Data processing equipment rental
Supplemental pay	Other rentals
Office and service personnel	Building repair and maintenance
Regular pay	Medical equipment repairs and rentals
Overtime pay	Other equipment repairs and rentals
Shift differential	Travel expense
Supplemental pay	Legal services
	Medical and clinical contracts
	Accounting and auditing services
Employee Benefits	Other consultants
FICA	Laboratory fees
Retirement plan	Custodial contracts
Health insurance	Office supplies
Life insurance	Household and institutional supplies
Workmen's compensation	Food
	X-ray film
	X-ray tubes
Operating Expenses	Sutures
Postage	Cylinder gas
Communication	Chemicals and reagents
Freight and cartage	Instruments
Data processing	Drugs
Publishing, printing, photography	Disposable packs and instruments
Insurance	Reusable sterile service items
Awards	Prostheses and implants
Dues, subscriptions	Other supplies
Conference registration	Research and laboratory supplies
Employee relocation	

Source: Reprinted from *Administration and Supervision in Laboratory Medicine* by J.R. Snyder and D.A. Senhauser (Eds.), p. 420, with permission of J.B. Lippincott Company, © 1989.

produced monthly; these should compare service units, productive time, overtime, and dollars as compared with budgeted amounts.

Financial Reporting and Analysis

Berman et al. divide financial reports into two types: stock reports and flow reports.[11] Stock reports include those that describe the management's performance in managing assets and liabilities at any one point in time. These reports are often referred to as snapshot reports, since they hold the flow of business constant for a moment to assess where the organization stands. Such reports include the balance sheet, receivables, and cash reports.

Flow reports relate performance to daily business activities. The *profit and loss statement* serves as a global report for evaluating financial performance of the enterprise. This report, produced monthly, contains information about revenues, expenses, and surpluses (profits) versus budgeted amounts, and it trends these data over time. The profit and loss statement defines the bottom-line net income so often referred to in business circles.

In the case of any report, stock or flow, certain requirements of financial reporting must be met. The report must be timely, clear, and accurate. Management must have the report in time to make effective operational changes, it must be readily understood by management, and the data must not be presented in a misleading way. In addition, the report should be internally consistent and therefore comparable from period to period.

Finally, the report should contain expert analysis that represents the finance department's best interpretation of the financial data. The data should be packaged in a concise manner, and highlights of significant results should be reviewed by finance staff, although enough data need to be presented to allow independent interpretation by operations managers. Good report analysis can often mean the difference between a wise or unwise decision.

The *balance sheet* (Exhibit 16-2) is the primary stock report. It presents all of the organization's assets and liabilities at one point in time. It is usually prepared on a quarterly or annual basis. The difference between assets and liabilities is the firm's net worth or financial value. The report gets its name from the balance that is struck between assets on one side of the ledger and liabilities and net worth on the other.

Analysis of the balance sheet involves a thorough examination of ratios drawn from the elements of the balance sheet and compared with industry standard values. These ratios are used to gauge the fiscal viability of the organization. Exhibit 16-3 presents basic ratios and describes their significance.

Other reports supplement the balance sheet and are composed of subsets of the data contained therein. *Cash reports,* drawn from detailed daily reports, are prepared frequently and describe the sources and uses of cash between two dates. Generally, cash holdings should be kept to a minimum, just enough to cover short-term payroll needs in most cases. Cash that remains uninvested actually devalues over time, because the organization forgoes interest that could be earned on investments in the marketplace or the business itself.

The *accounts receivable report* measures the organization's ability to collect outstanding cash debt owed to the business. The days' receivables statistic tells management how many days of revenue are still uncollected. The more days' revenue outstanding, the less cash is available for other purposes. This statistic measures the liquidity (the availability of cash) of the organization. The *aged accounts receivable report* tells the manager the length of time each outstanding receivable has been on the books, presented in thirty-day segments. The older the debt, the more likely it is to be written off. This report indicates the success of the collections department in collecting outstanding debt. Thus, the sheer number of receivables and the timeliness of their collection are communicated to management in this and the preceding report.

Inventory reports provide material turnover data and inventory turnover rates. The inventory turnover rate is calculated by dividing supplies and other materials used in a specified period by the inventory on hand at the end of that period or by an averaged inventory on hand for the period. The higher the rate, the lower the carrying or storage costs. This is generally the result wanted, although stockouts may occur at very high turnover levels.

Fixed asset, depreciation, and accounts payable reports round out the set of reports generally provided to management. These reports will not be described, not because they are unimportant, but because they are less applicable to the daily management of the enterprise.

Revenue Generation and Third-Party Relationships

The sources of revenue for health care enterprises have been discussed in detail in the section on the evolution of health care financing. This sec-

Exhibit 16-2 Sample Statement of Financial Position, June 30, 1991 and 1990

Assets	1991	1990
General Funds		
Current assets		
Cash and short-term investments	$ 9,096,852	$ 3,675,088
Receivables (less allowances for uncollectible accounts)	27,172,521	29,351,436
Due from governmental agencies	13,392,435	7,433,891
Inventories	2,546,310	2,216,872
Self-insurance trust (current)	1,180,000	1,060,000
Prepaid expenses	1,379,390	1,825,184
Total current assets	54,767,508	45,562,471
Assets whose use is limited		
Debt reserve funds	4,186,126	4,172,608
Designated by board for capital improvements (certificate of deposit)	3,018,319	2,778,109
Property acquisition funds	15,259,844	22,308,984
Self insurance trust fund	7,041,418	5,996,420
Total assets whose use is limited	29,505,707	35,256,121
Investment (at cost)	152,000	150,000
Deferred charges and other noncurrent assets (net of accumulated amortization)		
Financing costs	1,518,459	1,609,438
Property, plant, and equipment		
Land	4,260,758	4,260,758
Buildings and improvements	60,005,439	49,349,751
Equipment	29,565,136	26,268,312
Total	93,831,333	79,878,821
Less accumulated depreciation	(34,013,416)	(29,286,607)
Property, net	59,817,917	50,592,214
Total assets	$145,761,591	$133,170,244
Liabilities	1991	1990
Current liabilities		
Current portion of notes payable	$ 842,497	$ 660,053
Current portion of bonds payable	2,162,690	2,039,683
Accounts payable	8,546,212	9,233,909
Accrued expenses	2,851,930	2,098,191
Accrued bond interest	1,697,463	1,729,079
Current portion of accrued malpractice claims	1,180,000	1,060,000
Due to restricted funds	134,849	262,495
Total current liabilities	17,415,641	17,083,410
Accrued malpractice claims	13,076,305	10,309,366
Notes payable	2,812,500	54,171
Bonds payable	62,550,885	64,430,049
Fund Balances		
Designated for property, plant, and equipment	3,018,319	2,778,109
General	46,887,941	38,515,139
Total fund balances	49,906,260	41,293,248
Total liabilities	$145,761,591	$133,170,244

Exhibit 16-3 Basic Financial Ratios

Liquidity Measures

$$\text{Current Ratio} = \frac{\text{Current Assets}}{\text{Current Liabilities}}$$

Ratio of current assets to current liabilities. It is the basic index of financial liquidity. The higher the ratio value, the better the hospital's ability to meet its obligations.

$$\text{Acid Test Ratio} = \frac{\text{Cash + Marketable Securities}}{\text{Current Liabilities}}$$

Ratio of the sum of cash and marketable securities to current liabilities. It is the most rigorous test of liquidity, taking into account the composition of current assets and recognizing that accounts receivable and inventories—while current assets—are not cash. The higher the ratio value, the better the hospital's ability to meet its obligations.

$$\text{Collection Period} = \frac{\text{Net Accounts Receivable}}{\text{Average Daily Operating Revenue}}$$

Ratio of accounts receivable net of uncollectables to daily operating revenue (total revenue divided by 365 days); a measure of the length of time accounts receivable are outstanding. Increasing values for this measure indicate a lengthening of the collection period and can signal future liquidity problems. The collection period should also be kept in balance with a similar ratio measuring payment period. Separate collection period ratios can be calculated for patient care and nonpatient care accounts receivable as well as for accounts receivable by class of payer.

Capital Structure

$$\text{Long-Term Debt to Fixed Assets} = \frac{\text{Long-Term Debt}}{\text{Net Fixed Assets}}$$

Ratio of the proportion of fixed assets financed through long-term debt. The higher the ratio the less relative security perceived by a lender and the more difficult it will be for the hospital to secure future loans. Also, as the ratio increases, the hospital should examine its profitability position so that it is better able to support existing debt and flexible enough to acquire additional debt. This examination should consider not only operating efficiency but also rate structure matters.

$$\text{Long-Term Debt to Equity} = \frac{\text{Long-Term Debt}}{\text{Unrestricted and Board Restricted Equity}}$$

Ratio of the two long-term sources of the hospital's financing. As this ratio increases, the hospital becomes more highly "leveraged," and its ability to acquire future debt financing is reduced.

$$\text{Debt Service} = \frac{\text{Net Income + Depreciation}}{\text{Debt Principal Payment + Interest}}$$

Ratio that measures the ability of the hospital to pay its debt, both principal and interest. The higher this ratio, the more secure the lender and the greater the hospital's future debt capacity. This ratio identifies the relationship of debt capacity to earnings and cash flow. Commonly used variations of this ratio are:

$$\frac{\text{Net Income + Depreciation}}{\text{Interest}} \quad \text{and} \quad \frac{\text{Net Income + Depreciation}}{\text{Total Liabilities}}$$

The first is the measure of the hospital's ability to pay interest expenses and the second is an indicator of the cash available to meet all obligations.

continues

Exhibit 16-3 Continued

Activity

$$\text{Total Asset Turnover} = \frac{\text{Total Revenue}}{\text{Total Assets}}$$

Ratio that is used to indicate the relative efficiency of the use of assets. Typically, high values for this measure are viewed as indicating higher levels of performance. The denominator of this ratio should be net of depreciation. Variations of this ratio include fixed asset turnover and current asset turnover. While these activity ratios can be used as surrogate measures of efficiency, other indexes and factors must also be considered, for example, occupancy rates, plant age and design, and payer mix.

$$\text{Inventory Turnover} = \frac{\text{Total Operating Revenue}}{\text{Inventory}}$$

Ratio that measures the hospital's investment in inventories. Low values typically imply overstocking—an excess investment and an inappropriate use of assets.

Operating Margin

$$\text{Operating Margin} = \frac{\text{Total Revenue} - \text{Total Expenses}}{\text{Total Revenue}}$$

Ratio of net income to total revenue. It is a measure of profitability. Operating margin can be calculated in aggregate as well as for patient care services and non-patient-care services (nonoperating revenues). In this measure, the revenue figures should reflect net revenue, that is, revenues less contractual adjustments.

$$\text{Return on Assets} = \frac{\text{Income} + \text{Interest Expense}}{\text{Total Assets}}$$

Ratio of net income to total investment in the hospital. It is a measure of the relationship of operating margin (total revenue − total expense) to the assets, that is, the investment in the hospital. Interest expense is added back to eliminate bias due to the method of financing the assets. The ratio can also be calculated net of interest expense.

$$\text{Nonoperating Income Contribution} = \frac{\text{Nonoperating Net Income}}{\text{Net Income}}$$

Ratio of non-patient-care services (nonoperating) net income to total net income. It provides a measure of the importance of nonoperating revenues to the hospital's overall financial status.

Source: Reprinted from *The Financial Management of Hospitals* (7th Edition) by H.J. Berman, L.E. Weeks, and S.F. Kukla, pp. 689–690, with permission of Health Administration Press, © 1990.

tion will examine how the revenue budget is prepared and how rate setting is done.[12] The revenue budget forecasts expected cash receipts for the organization. Components of the forecast include gross patient charges, deductions from gross charges, and cash from investment interest and non-patient-related services.

While historical trending of patient mix is important, since it provides information about what pay-

ers reimburse for specific segments of the patient population, financial managers must be even more cognizant of changes in the rules for reimbursement. Has an insurer switched from cost-based reimbursement to DRG-based prospective payments? Has Medicare changed its rules for calculating house staff costs? Has an HMO negotiated a change from per diem to per discharge payment terms? These and many other types of changes must be carefully monitored by the finance department staff.

The staff must also be adept at predicting changes in federal and state regulations. If possible, it is wise to have someone from the organization personally involved in helping to make or at least monitor and comment on proposed policy changes.

Based upon the best information available, the finance staff consolidate data on service levels of the enterprise, the patient mix, and known and predicted changes in payer reimbursement policies into a forecast estimate of revenue, deductions from revenue, and cash collections for the entire organization. This estimate should be worked out early in the budget process to provide a rough target for operations expenses. Of course, any budgeted net surplus or income should also be part of the target setting.

Once the expenditure budget is completed, including proposals for new programs or enhancements to old ones, an iterative process begins. New revenue from program changes is incorporated into the revenue budget.

Intense scrutiny of proposed program changes is required to ensure that estimates of revenue and expense are accurate. The finance department's analysis section is crucial to this examination. Operations managers should also be able to provide simple break-even analyses for their proposals.

If financial goals can be achieved solely through a balancing of net revenues on the one side and total expenditures and net surplus or income on the other side of the ledger, then the budget is complete. If net revenue does not meet expenditure and bottom-line goals, the organization must consider price increases. If the revenue exceeds expenditure and bottom-line goals, then the enterprise can consider reducing current prices, as a function of marketplace conditions.

Pricing strategies have changed over time. For many years, setting rates in hospitals was an integral part of the budgeting process. So-called revenue-producing departments, those that issued charges for their services, were called upon to subsidize other departments that did not issue charges, such as housekeeping, admitting, and the laundry.

In effect, revenue-producing departments had to set prices high enough to cover their own expenses plus those of the other departments.

Briefly, there are three common methods for setting prices in hospitals. The hourly rate method is used for departments like the operating room and labor and delivery. The rate is established by calculating the total costs and dividing them by projected hours of facility use. The cost-plus (or surcharge) method is used in departments where supply costs are high relative to personnel costs. Personnel costs and other nonsupply costs are spread over the total number of products, and the variable product costs are then added to the base personnel costs. The pharmacy and central supply typically use this method.

Finally, the weighted value (or relative value pricing) method is often used in departments such as the laboratory and radiology. This method involves finding the direct cost of each test and assigning weights to all costed tests based on the magnitude of the direct costs. Each test's weight is then multiplied by the predicted number of tests to be performed to yield the total number of weighted units for that test. Next, the weighted units for all tests performed are added to produce the total weighted units for the department.

The total costs of the department, including direct and indirect costs, and the institutionally required surplus contribution are added together and then divided by the total weighted units for the department. The result is the total cost per weighted unit. The total cost per weighted unit is then multiplied by each test to yield the price for the test. Exhibit 16-4 illustrates this calculation method for a laboratory.

Although these pricing methods are still in use, the changing marketplace for health care has altered these "textbook" methods considerably. Competition, particularly in the outpatient and managed care settings, has required significant discounting that many times does not allow the hospital to cover all costs plus the required surplus/profit contribution. These losses are then shifted to other payers who still pay based on costs or charges. Prices are

Exhibit 16-4 Weighted Value Method of Rate Setting

Test	Number Performed	Relative Weight	Weighted Units
Irregular antibody screen	300	1.2	360
Complete blood count	750	0.8	600
. . . .	. . . .	. . . .	. . . .
Chemistry, profile	1,000	2.3	2,300
Luteinizing hormone and follicle-stimulating hormone	325	4.5	1,462.5
Total number of weighted units produced			47,220.0

Financial Requirements		
Direct costs	$435,000	
Indirect costs (28%)	121,800	
Required contribution (10%)	55,680	
		$612,480

Cost per Weighted Unit
($612,480/47,220) $ 12.97

Test	Relative Weight	Cost per Weighted Unit	Price
Irregular antibody screen	1.2	$12.97	$15.56
Complete blood count	0.8	12.97	10.38
. . . .	. . . .	. . . .	. . . .
Chemistry, profile	2.3	12.97	29.83
Luteinizing hormone and follicle-stimulating hormone	4.5	12.97	58.37

Source: Reprinted from *Administration and Supervision in Laboratory Medicine* by J.R. Snyder and D.A. Senhauser (Eds.), p. 437, with permission of J.B. Lippincott Company, © 1989.

raised even higher to cover these losses, requiring even deeper discounts. This pricing spiral has continued over the years, with the result that those who pay based on cost or charges and their business customers have instituted discounted, managed care, or prospective payment systems themselves.

As the market has matured and more alternative payment systems have been established, the opportunities for hospitals to use cost-shifting pricing strategies to cover costs and contribution have dwindled. For instance, a price increase of one dollar may only yield twenty-five cents in actual collections, because many payers make a fixed payment regardless of price.

More often, payment increases are now negotiated between the hospital and the payer on a contractual basis. The result is that the emphasis in the finance revenue generation function has shifted from simple price-setting methods to extremely complex contractual negotiations. Further, controlling costs so that they fall below contractual payment amounts is now the only truly useful way to manage the organization successfully.

There are certain niches still remaining that accommodate standard pricing strategies, such as home care and other forms of outpatient care, but these already highly exploited areas are also being restrained rapidly by payers.

Many of these reimbursement issues also apply to physician practices, though not to the same degree. The fee-for-service (or charge-based) system still dominates, and pricing relates less to the actual costs of operating a practice than the reasonableness of fees as compared with those of other practices. Generally, practice costs run between 40 and 60 percent of collections. Historically, as practice costs have risen, fees have been increased accordingly. In recent years, in fact, physician fees have increased at a higher rate than hospital charges.

During the past few years, the new cost consciousness of hospitals has collided with the physicians' understanding of their financial world. Still reimbursed largely based on charges, physicians may find it difficult to understand why hospitals are so concerned about reducing costs, sometimes to the point of reducing service levels as well. Economic incentives that used to be coincident have been transformed into opposing incentives.

As payers have begun to turn their attention to physician costs, the incentives are slowly becoming coincident again. The next section discusses methods for monitoring and controlling costs, in ways that allow the needs of both physicians and hospitals to be met.

Managing Costs

There are two basic ways to categorize costs in an organization: by management responsibility and by product line.[13] That is, costs are gathered by manager or by product or service. Management responsibility costing is best for businesses organized around functional departments, as are most hospitals and group practices. Product line costing is ideal for enterprises organized by product or service lines or for evaluating the financial performance of a service within a functionally organized business.

Under responsibility costing, direct costs are collected and assigned to the department. The accounting entities set up to collect these costs are called cost centers. Direct costs are those that can be directly linked to the department's products or services. These costs, including personnel and supply costs, are those most controllable by the manager.

Indirect costs (or overhead) are those expenses not specifically tied to the products or services but necessary for the operation of the department as a whole. Such costs include expenditures for laundry, housekeeping, depreciation, utilities, and maintenance.

Responsibility costing assigns indirect costs using a mathematical allocation method that approximates the actual usage of overhead services by each department. Indirect costs are less controllable by the department manager than direct costs, since the former are out of the specific span of control of the department manager. Department profit and loss and other performance reports often separate direct costs from indirect costs as a result.

Product line costing, on the other hand, requires some method for ascertaining all costs (direct and indirect) and assigning them to a defined product or service. This is often called full costing. The mechanisms commonly used for accumulating these costs are job order costing and process costing.[14]

The job order costing system attaches costs to a particular job (in a hospital, the equivalent of a job might be a patient or a DRG). In manufacturing settings, the job would literally accumulate tickets signifying work accomplished during the job process. In the health care setting, this sophistication does not exist. For instance, the exact full costs of producing an x-ray or a test are rarely known. Consequently, a method for calculating the ratio of cost to charges has been developed to estimate costs for revenue-producing departments. Overall direct and allocated indirect costs for a cost center are determined and then divided by the total gross charges for the department to yield a ratio that is then applied back to a specific test. For routine daily nursing care, the direct and allocated indirect costs are simply added.

Ancillary charges accumulated for a patient or DRG are translated into costs using the ratio of cost to charges method, with routine nursing care costs added to yield the total cost of the "job." Since the method is crude (costs are often not related to charges accurately), management engineering resources are often used to determine actual test or procedure direct costs. Following Pareto's Law, these studies are usually performed on the most used tests or procedures first.

In process costing, tests or procedures of a like nature are grouped and are assigned an average total cost value. The weighted or relative value method discussed earlier regarding pricing is often used to calculate differential group costs. In terms of accuracy, this mechanism lies somewhere between actual costing and the ratio of cost to charges method, and it is often combined with the job order costing method to improve accuracy and avoid having to perform actual test-by-test costing.

In sophisticated cost accounting systems, which often require a significant investment in staff and computing hardware and software, these costs are compared against standard costs. This comparison helps determine the efficiency of operations in terms of dollars.

Standard costs are set in the following way. All tests and procedures are microcosted at the department level using productivity studies developed by management engineering to achieve the most efficient cost per unit of service possible. Once established, these standards are used in the budgeting process to estimate cost center expenses for the coming year. The operating manager simply predicts the number of procedures of each type and applies the standard cost to each of the procedures. Total costs for each procedure are then added to yield total departmental cost.

Throughout the year, reports are issued regularly to compare actual versus standard costs, and variances must be explained by the operating manager. The standard costs should be updated frequently to account for changes in technology or work flow that affect the cost of producing a unit of service.

If standard costing can be implemented and properly maintained, it is possible to replace the productivity management systems commonly in use today, since the management of dollars implies effective management of workload and hours. However, cost accounting systems that include standard costing are extremely difficult to establish

in service-oriented businesses, and they are costly to implement and maintain. Therefore, many health care enterprises still use some form of productivity management to control costs.

Instead of standards based on ideal costs, a productivity management system sets standards for the ideal effort that should be expended to produce a product or service. Although the cost accountant establishes direct and indirect expenses, the management engineering staff examine each procedure carefully to determine the time required to perform each task involved in the procedure as efficiently as possible. The total time for all procedures is translated into total full-time equivalents (FTEs), and this standard is used to budget personnel expenses. As workload fluctuates through the fiscal year, productivity standards can be used to increase or decrease personnel resources accordingly. Productivity management systems fall short of cost accounting systems because they take into account only personnel expenses, not all costs. However, many health care businesses find productivity management systems effective for controlling the costliest portion of their budgets.

Managing Inefficiency

While cost accounting and productivity management systems have proven helpful, they do not address all aspects of inefficiency. For example, since standard costs and productivity standards are established on a micro basis within departments, these methods do not address the inefficiencies that result from the interaction among departments. It is these systems' inefficiencies that often add the most to cost and subtract the most from the quality of service. Unfortunately, they are very difficult to deal with for many organizations.

Several approaches have been taken to address systems problems. Management engineering techniques were the first to be used. Queuing studies told managers how to relieve long patient waiting times and more effectively move patients within the institution. However, disagreement between departments regarding whose behavior should change often compromised implementation. In addition, in the hospital setting, other nonemployee groups (e.g., physicians or vendors) were sometimes part of the problem and could not be effectively integrated into the problem-solving process.

Next came quality circles, which attempted to put line employees together to solve their own problems. While these had some effect within departments, cross-departmental issues were rarely resolved.

Concurrent with quality circles, product line management came into vogue. Once implemented, this approach to management had the advantage of including employees and physicians from multiple departments in the problem-solving process. In addition, financial and operational responsibility for the components of the product or service was unambiguously identified, yet team methods were used for overall management.

Today, total quality management has replaced these strategies but incorporates parts of all of them. The primary thesis of total quality management is that an organization can never reach perfection yet must always strive for it. Achieving a climate in which active striving for excellence occurs depends on empowering first-line employees to solve problems, providing them with the necessary tools to analyze issues, and ensuring that the right constituencies are involved. Upper management must commit to participation in the problem-solving process and implementation of the solutions recommended. A team approach is used to organize the effort.

This is not a process with an end, because no problem is ever solved. Nor is it a fad that dies with waning enthusiasm. It must be a permanent change in the way the company does business—a permanent change in the culture of the organization. It is based on the tenet that the employees who do the work can solve the institution's operational problems on a continual basis if they have access to the right analytical tools.

The role of the finance department is to help employees understand that the best solutions to systems problems are those that not only provide higher quality service but improve efficiency as well. The finance department must also provide support and education for the analytical and technical aspects of problem solving. The question to ask is not "How do we cut FTEs?" but "How do we perform this service so that it satisfies patients and makes our job easier and simpler?" Cost reduction then becomes a byproduct of the total quality management process, not the goal itself.

Whether or not one chooses to use the label *total quality management,* cost management has matured to the point of recognizing the value of maximizing all human resources in achieving institutional goals. The authors believe that the total quality management approach, or a home-grown version of it, will yield not only cost-efficiency, better systems, and greater patient satisfaction but improved work force morale as well.

Managing Working Capital

Most of the reports related to managing cash or near-cash assets have already been reviewed. Here, working capital will be defined, and some basic methods for handling cash, investments, accounts receivable, and inventories will be reviewed.

Working capital comprises the total current assets of the business, including cash, short-term investments, accounts receivable, and inventories. The current ratio is a reflection of net working capital, since it expresses the excess of current assets over current liabilities as a percentage.

One of the three primary reports prepared for external reporting purposes is the *statement of cash flows* (the other two are the profit and loss statement and the balance sheet). Basically, this statement shows where cash has been received from and where it has gone. This is of interest to management because cash only passes through working capital accounts, and the path cash takes is often difficult to trace effectively without such a report.

The minimum cash requirement for an organization for any period is that cash inflows equal cash outflows. Management of cash must ensure that sufficient cash is available for obligations requiring cash but that the amount is not so large as to cause significant carrying costs. Excess cash at the end of any period should be invested in short-term investments to ensure interest income until the cash can be used for higher-return investment in long-term (fixed) assets or, in a for-profit organization, for paying dividends.

The above discussion suggests that it is better to minimize cash holdings. This is in fact true, because if cash were better held in short-term investments, then the profit maximizing company might well become a market investor in preference to being in the health care business.[15] Therefore, the cost of working capital is the interest rate received on short-term investments.

Investments in the enterprise, then, should always have a better return on investment than that of short-term securities. The difference between these two returns is the opportunity cost, since this is the value of opportunity lost by investing in securities versus the firm.

Inventories and Accounts Receivable

The investment in inventories requires equal attention. There is also an opportunity cost to holding inventories, and this cost is "equal to the highest alternative rate of return that could have been obtained times the average amount of funds that are invested in inventories."[16] The goal of inventory management is to minimize the opportunity cost of holding inventories while minimizing stockouts at the same time.

Accounts receivable have an obvious opportunity cost. They are essentially payer obligations waiting to be converted to cash. Accounts receivable are similar to a cash shortfall for the relevant period. Receivables can be charged interest for the time they are outstanding, but few health care organizations practice this method of recovering the opportunity cost because of their public service mission. Credit cards are often accepted by health care businesses because the handling charges paid to the credit card companies are often less than the costs of collecting the bills.

Debt may also be used. Factoring is the method whereby the receivables are sold to a lender who bears the risk of collection. Receivables may also be discounted to provide collateral for a loan, but in this case the hospital is still responsible for collections. Generally, discounting is cheaper than factoring, but neither method should be used if at all possible. Lending rates for each method are often higher than the minimum cost of working capital.

Because receivables are intangible, they are inherently the riskiest component of working capital. The best strategy for minimizing opportunity costs with receivables is still to minimize the time between the issuance of the charge and the receipt of the payment.

Many payers reimburse on their own schedule, so the best method for accelerating payment is to tighten internal controls on the billing and collection functions. Charges must be issued promptly and accurately, either manually or electronically. Paperless billing is also available from some payers, including Medicare. Collections can be enhanced by a good preadmission process, when accurate information can be collected about insurers or other payment arrangements can be made through counseling services. Some insurers, including Medicare, also offer advance payments on their accounts, paid and reconciled on a periodic basis.

QUALITY CONSIDERATIONS: THE AUDIT FUNCTION

There are two forms of control exercised over the quality of financial records, practices, and policies. The purpose of external (or independent) audits is to ensure the reliability and consistency of financial statements so that they may be confidently used for comparative or other purposes by agencies and organizations outside the firm. The statements verified most commonly are the balance sheet, the statement of revenues and expenses (or profits and losses), and the statement of cash flows, all of which have been discussed in this chapter. Operationally, an independent audit provides a check on the quality of finance department performance.

At minimum, an external audit should be conducted by an outside certified public accountant who has been selected carefully to ensure that there is no possible conflict of interest. Payment of the auditor should not be contingent upon the results of the audit. Further, the auditor should be selected by the board. and the audit itself should be monitored and reviewed by the board or a committee of the board. This practice will enhance auditor independence. The individual or firm selected should have experience with health care organizations.

An audit uses standard accounting methods to test the accuracy of the financial statements. Instead of reviewing each transaction, sampling techniques are used. If reliability is established, the opinion states that the financial statements were prepared in accordance with generally accepted accounting principles and fairly represent, in all material repects, the financial position of the organization. If there are issues affecting the reliability of the statements, these are generally included as qualifications to the opinion.

In unusual cases, the auditor may issue an adverse opinion or a disclaimer indicating that the statements were either unreliable or that not enough information was provided to issue an opinion. Such an outcome will have obvious negative effects on the standing of the organization, and corrective actions should be instituted immediately.

The other type of audit, the internal audit, differs from the external audit in focus and concept. Internal auditors are employees of the organization and report to the CFO, CEO, or board. They examine financial and operational matters in order to reveal incorrect practices, the need for policy or organizational revision, incompetent personnel, fraud, theft, or other irregularities. Consequently, they focus on meeting the needs of management instead of the needs of outside agencies. Finally, their work is ongoing, whereas an external auditor is typically hired to perform a yearly review.

Some practices that might be reviewed in the course of an internal audit include competitive bidding procedures, the separation of the cashiering and accounting functions, the matching of

packing slips with purchase orders, and ledger reconciliation.

Internal and external audits imply a less-than-trusting view of human nature. Practical experience, however, has turned the authors into firm believers in the value of auditing.

MANAGING AND PLANNING FOR CAPITAL INVESTMENT

The Capital Budget

The process by which capital assets are acquired is equal in importance to operational budgeting. In addition, both types of budgets are symbiotic. Effective operational budgeting supports the achievement of cash contribution goals, which in turn help in financing capital acquisitions. The capital budget also provides equipment and facilities that can improve the likelihood of financial success.

On the other side of the coin, poor capital acquisition decisions can be even more disastrous than unwise operational decisions, since their effects will be incurred over a much longer period of time. Since capital items are purchased to enhance the return on investment from operations, equipment that is underutilized or is not operated efficiently may negatively affect revenue and expense streams far into the future.

Capital items are defined as fixed assets expected to have useful lives greater than one year. While there are some caveats, this definition will serve our purposes.

The capital budgeting process begins with the determination of a budget period. Based upon the goals and objectives of the organization, short-term and long-term periods are established. The short-term budget covers equipment and facilities for a period of one year. The long-term budget plan covers a three- to five-year period. The long-term plan is particularly important, as should be clear from the cautionary note above, but the same prediction risks that were discussed regarding the operational budget apply here as well.

In large organizations, the capital budget is often the subject of greater debate than the operational budget. The capital budget is the "reward" for excellent operations, and many in the organization are willing to temper operational excesses in anticipation of the capital payoff. Thus, there is often great competition for inherently limited capital dollars. Although the manager can establish and implement a capital budgeting process that is highly rational and straightforward, he or she should also be aware that political leverage within the organization will be marshalled during the final phase of decision making. Organizational politics are not inherently positive or negative, simply a fact of life that should be factored into the budgeting process.

The capital budget may be divided into two categories. First there are the low-cost items falling below some dollar threshold, perhaps $5,000. For these items, analysis needs are minimal. Each item should be classified as new, replacement, renovation, or improvement. The items may simply be given numerical rankings based upon perceived value to the organization or placed into broad priority categories such as the following (in order of importance):

1. items that are necessary to continue or increase service levels
2. items that will produce cost savings or profit at present service levels
3. items that will improve the quality or effectiveness of present services
4. items that will contribute to new services or the improvement of existing programs

Low-cost items may then be individually purchased by ranking or group purchased based on category. Often a combination of the two methods is used.

For major capital purchases, a more complex process is required. Although the basic categorization of capital remains the same, the level of analysis increases dramatically. For items in the last two categories in the list above, some form of benefit analysis should also be performed, and the two

types of analysis should be combined to yield a single ranking. Cleverley provides a good description of benefit analysis and the capital decision-making process.[17]

To mitigate the effects of competition on capital resources, the authors have found it beneficial to establish a committee of major stakeholders to help evaluate and prioritize items prior to budget finalization. In hospitals, this generally means a committee of influential medical staff members.

During this process, the administration completes its analysis and prioritization based upon the best information possible and tells the committee the amount of projected capital funds available. Minor capital is then approved as a lump sum by the stakeholder committee, and major capital is presented to the committee on an item-by-item basis by those requesting the items. The committee then prioritizes the items again, provides each presenter with reasons for approval or disapproval, and passes the new capital budget on to the administration for further action.

This process helps ensure that key clinicians are aware of the limits of capital resources; informs them of the total scope of the plan; involves them in the evaluation and approval process; and, hopefully, creates a consensus among all parties, or at least helps those not receiving items to understand the institution's reasoning better. A similar internal process is also helpful for the operating budget.

Capital Analysis Techniques

Prior to applying any analytical techniques, the following information should be gathered for each major capital item[18]:

1. the purpose and importance of the item, including patient care benefits (in narrative form)
2. the expected utilization of the item, including an evaluation of competitive modalities available elsewhere and demand for the service
3. the expected life of the item and estimates of the total costs of the item, including delivery and installation; the yearly incremental cash

outflows, or cash expenses, associated with operating and maintaining the item; and the yearly incremental cash inflows or cash savings resulting from the purchase

4. the net cash flows for each year in the life of the asset, calculated by subtracting incremental cash outflows from incremental cash inflows

5. the operational rate of return expected from use of the item based on the firm's requirements

There are four techniques commonly used for analyzing capital projects; two are simple and two are complex. The pros and cons of each will be discussed.

The *payback* method calculates how many years of net cash flows it takes to recover the total costs of the original purchase. This method does not account for any return on investment or cash flows beyond the payback point. However, it is useful for rough comparisons of items having like purchase prices and useful lives. Since it favors the earliest payback, the measure indicates the level of risk assumed, albeit in a rudimentary manner.

The *average rate of return* method attempts to provide the manager with an indication of the average yearly return on the investment. First, the sum of all yearly net cash inflows is calculated for the life of the item and divided by the useful life of the item in years. The result is termed the average annual investment return. The initial cost of purchase is then discounted by the depreciation for each year in the life of the item. These discounted yearly figures are then summed and divided by the useful life of the item in years. The result is termed the average annual investment. The average annual investment return is then divided by the average annual investment to yield the average rate of return. A more conservative calculation leaves the numerator intact but changes the denominator to the original purchase cost and does not calculate an average.

Projects are then prioritized based on average rate of return. This technique gives a very crude picture of return on investment because of its dependence on averages. Averages do not allow for a determination of which projects pay off earliest.

The next two methods of analysis require an understanding of the concept of the time value of money (e.g., it is worth more to a person owed money to receive the money sooner than later). The notion of present value is central to this concept. Precisely defined, "The present value of an amount that is expected to be received at a specified time in the future is the amount which, if invested today at a designated rate of return, would cumulate to a specified amount."[19]

The first method depends on the calculation of *net present value*. In this method, the present value of the sum of net cash inflows is calculated using the specified rate of return. This has the effect of bringing all future cash flows back to the present, discounted by the specified rate of return, so that the resulting present value can be compared to the original purchase cost.

The net present value results from subtracting the original purchase price from the present value. If the net present value, expressed in dollars, is zero, the original investment in the equipment or project will yield exactly the rate of return specified. If the net present value is positive, then the item provides a higher rate of return than expected by the amount of dollars expressed. If the net present value is negative, the enterprise will not receive the expected rate of return on the investment by the number of dollars expressed. Items are then prioritized based on net present value.

The advantages of the net present value method are many, but the primary advantage is that the manager is given a true evaluation of items or projects based on the firm's required return on investment. The method does not take into account differences in initial investment sizes among projects, however, nor does it control for differences in useful lives. There are methods for alleviating these shortcomings and the reader is referred to any comprehensive finance text for further guidance.

Although we believe that the actual method for calculating present value may help clarify the concept, we have concentrated on the decision rules instead.

There are pocket calculators readily available that will calculate present value and net present value.

The final method, which uses the *time-adjusted return,* is a variant of the preceding approach. In this method, complex mathematical iterations are applied to yield the rate of return that results in a net present value of zero dollars, called the internal rate of return. Capital projects are then prioritized based on the internal rate of return (the greater the rate, the higher the priority). Again, pocket calculators are available that will calculate this rate.

Because no required rate of return is specified at the beginning, as in the preceding method, the time-adjusted return method makes the implicit assumption that all net cash inflows are reinvested at the internal rate of return, which is not always the case. This shortcoming makes the net present value method, which adjusts for differences in investment size and useful life, the analytical tool of choice.

A comparison of the different techniques is presented in Table 16-1.

Financing Capital Acquisitions

Before discussing the best way to finance capital items, the reader should be familiar with the basic methods of financing. Capital leases or purchases are financed by contributions from operations or debt. Operating leases are financed from operating expenses.

The differences between the two types of leases is relatively simple. A capital lease cannot be cancelled during the term of the lease, and there is an option to buy at the end of the lease. For accounting purposes, the capital lease is treated like a purchased item. The operating lease is cancellable during the leasing period, it is treated as an operating expense, and there is no option for purchase.

In general, operating leases should be avoided for major capital items, because these leases drain dollars from the bottom-line contribution for an extended time and there is no residual (salvage) value when they end. Hence, the manager faces the choice of using internally generated operating surpluses (profits), capital leases, or debt.

Whether to use internal or external funds for capital acquisition is analytically similar to the "make or buy" decision that often faces manufacturing firms. The same analytic techniques can be used to evaluate, for example, whether it makes more sense to maintain a hospital-based food service or to contract for various components of the service with outside vendors.

The present value method reviewed earlier is the best way to choose the least costly method for acquiring capital items. For example, say an item's total purchase cost is $125,000 and the firm's required rate of return is 15 percent. For the lease, annual lease payments are $30,000 over a five-year period. The present value of these payments is $100,565, discounted at 15 percent. For the loan, the interest rate charged on the $125,000 loan by the vendor is 12 percent over five years. The annual loan payment for the item is therefore $30,961. Discounted at 15 percent, the present value of this financing method is $103,786.

Since present value, not net cash inflows, has been used to evaluate the options, the method with the lowest present value is the best way to finance the item. In this case, the lease option should be chosen, assuming no differences in salvage value at the end of the five-year period. Using future value, a component of the present value calculation, financing methods with and without salvage value can be evaluated to further refine the decision-making process.

THE FUTURE OF FINANCIAL PLANNING AND MANAGEMENT

Many trends have already been identified in this chapter: the continuing concern for health care costs expressed by the public and private sectors of the economy; the increasing variety of alternative health care systems under development in response to the rapid escalation of health care costs; the change from fully financed care to managed care; the movement of health care from a sickness-oriented inpatient industry to a prevention-oriented

Table 16-1 Data Analysis Techniques

Method	Calculation	Ranking System	Decision Rule	Benefits	Deficiencies
Payback	Years until original investment recovered from cash flows	Shortest to longest payback in years	Shortest payback best	Useful for comparing projects with similar useful lives A crude measure of risk	No recognition of time value of money Ignores cash flows beyond payback
Average Rate of Return (ARR)	Average yearly return as percentage of average yearly investment	Highest positive to lowest positive ARR	Highest ARR best	Accounts for all cash flows	No recognition of time value of money Blurs differences in timing of cash flows
Net Present Value (NPV)	Present value minus initial investment	Highest positive to lowest positive NPV	Highest NPV best	Accounts for time value of money Evaluates projects at same required rate of return	Ignores differences in investment size Comparison of projects with different useful lives difficult
Time-Adjusted Return (TAR)	Rate of return at which NPV equals zero is calculated; result is internal rate of return (IRR)	Highest to lowest IRR; reject if below required rate of return	Highest IRR best	Accounts for time value of money	Usefulness questionable if IRR is substantially different from actual expected return on reinvestment

Source: Reprinted from *Administration and Supervision in Laboratory Medicine* by J.R. Snyder and D.A. Senhauser (Eds.), p. 431, with permission of J.B. Lippincott Company, © 1989.

outpatient industry; and the evolution of national health policy.

The delivery and financing of health care are clearly in transition, and we posit that the transition will continue throughout the nineties. What will the health care landscape look like in the twenty-first century? Immodestly, we offer a snapshot of our vision of the future.

First, health care financing will be completely based on prospective payment, managed care, and managed competition. Successful hospitals will concentrate only on the sickest of patients and will diversify into outpatient and other vertically and horizontally related businesses, including retirement homes, insurance, home care, and long-term care. Greater consolidation of health care providers will yield a dozen or so companies that will dominate the clinical and insurance markets.

As the number of uninsured persons grows and the middle class reacts to increasing out-of-pocket expenses, the federal government will be pressured to institute some form of national health insurance using market-based models that are designed to control costs and discourage demand for services. Such reforms are already underway.

Technological development will continue, but there will be fewer buyers. Some method, perhaps hospital closings and consolidations, will be found to reduce the amount of duplication of technology.

Finally, it is our belief that, while market forces will continue to help rationalize a very ponderous and disorganized health care industry, there will also need to be a re-evaluation of the purpose of health care services. For example, the goal of Great Britain's National Health Service is to ensure the health of the nation. The United States has no such Holy Grail. By establishing one, the United States might, for the first time, be able to establish market incentives that lead us to better health rather than greater consumption of services after health has already deteriorated.

ADDITIONAL RESOURCES

Organizations

American Hospital Association, 840 North Lake Shore Drive, Chicago, IL 60611. 312/280-6000.

Healthcare Financial Management Association, #2 Westbrook Corporate Center, Westchester, IL 60154. 708/531-9600.

Books and Articles

American Institute of Certified Public Accountants. *Hospital audit guide.* 6th ed. New York: American Institute of Certified Public Accountants, 1987.

Carver, J. *Boards that make a difference.* San Francisco: Jossey-Bass, 1990.

Cleverly, W.O. *Essentials of health care finance.* 2nd ed. Gaithersburg, Md.: Aspen Publishers, 1986.

Cleverly, W.O. Financial Ratios: Summary indicators for management decision making. *Hospital and Health Services Administration,* special issue, 1981. Vol. 26, pp. 26–47.

Dowling, W.L. Prospective reimbursement of hospitals. *Inquiry* 11, no. 3 (1974): 163–180.

Herkimer, A.G. *Understanding health care accounting.* Gaithersburg, Md.: Aspen Publishers, 1989.

Kukla, S.F. *Cost accounting and financial analysis for the hospital administrator.* Chicago: American Hospital Publishing, 1986.

NOTES

1. P. Starr, *The Social Transformation of American Medicine* (New York: Basic Books, 1982), 155.

2. V. Fuchs, *Who Shall Live?* 2d ed. (New York: Basic Books, 1983), 80.

3. Starr, *Social Transformation of American Medicine,* 261; R. Stevens, *In Sickness and in Wealth* (New York: Basic Books, 1989), 123.

4. Starr, *Social Transformation of American Medicine,* 307.

5. P.J. Feldstein, *Health Care Economics* (New York: Wiley, 1983), 155.

6. Starr, *Social Transformation of American Medicine,* 301.

7. Feldstein, *Health Care Economics,* 152.

8. U.S. Department of Health and Human Services, *Health United States, 1990,* Pub. No. (PHS) 91-1232 (Hyattsville, Md.: U.S. Department of Health and Human Services, 1990), 193.

9. D.S. Rothman, *Strangers by the Bedside* (New York: Basic Books, 1991), 12.

10. D.J. Fine et al., Budgeting Laboratory Financial Resources, in *Administration and Supervision in Laboratory Medicine,* eds. J.R. Snyder and D.A. Senhauser (Philadelphia: J.B. Lippincott, 1989), 419.

11. H.J. Berman et al., *The Financial Management of Hospitals,* 7th ed. (Ann Arbor, Mich.: Health Administration Press, 1990), 399–419.

12. Fine et al., Budgeting Laboratory Financial Resources, 434–438.

13. Berman et al., *Financial Management of Hospitals,* 652.

14. Ibid., 659.

15. Ibid., 283.

16. Ibid., 319.

17. W.O. Cleverley, *Essentials of Health Care Finance* (Gaithersburg, Md.: Aspen Publishers, 1986), 342–369.

18. Fine et al., Budgeting Laboratory Financial Resources, 427–431.

19. R.N. Anthony and J.S. Reese, *Accounting Text and Cases,* 7th ed. (Homewood, Ill.: Richard D. Irwin, 1983), 614.

Trevor A. Fisk

Strategic Planning and Marketing

17

Purpose: The purpose of strategic planning and marketing is to ensure that the organization is sensitive to its social, economic, and political environment; anticipates and responds to major environmental changes; prepares and implements effective approaches to improving its operational performance; and develops and retains its client sources.

INTRODUCTION

Most managers in any health care organization focus upon immediate and short-term needs and tasks. Yet their organization functions within an external environment that is in constant flux, bringing new opportunities and threats. If the leadership of the organization is to steer a course that responds to environmental opportunities and threats, it has to *plan*. Some time must be spent looking beyond short-term issues.

The value of planning lies not only in the definition of a set of longer-term objectives but also in the internal consensus that the planning process helps to create. Complex organizations cannot function if every decision must be made by the board or the CEO. A shared plan allows initiatives to be decentralized while maintaining a common sense of direction.

The organization's client constituencies form part of its external environment. These constituencies and their relative importance to the organization's effectiveness vary among health care providers. However, the needs, preferences, attitudes, and satisfaction of client groups are important to the organization's future. Their opinions can change and therefore cannot be taken for granted. The organization must maintain a systematic *marketing* relationship with its clients.

FUNCTIONS

Because planning and marketing are both directed at keeping the organization responsive to its external environment, their activities interrelate and can overlap. As a result, there is considerable variation in how these two functions fit within the organizational structure and how they relate to each other and to the allied functions of public relations, community relations, and facilities planning. As illustrated in Figure 17-1, marketing can be treated as

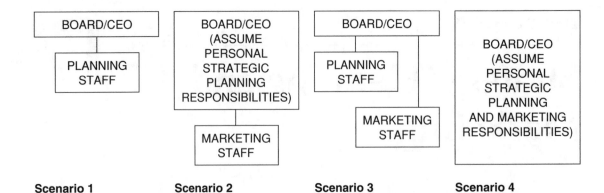

Scenario 1
Highly regulated
organization with little
competition

Scenario 2
Strategy-focused
leadership see need for
special marketing
support

Scenario 3
Leadership see need
for specialist support in
both functions (note: in
this scenario, planning
and marketing may
report to the CEO
through a shared senior
executive)

Scenario 4
Undifferentiated
strategic leadership

Figure 17-1 Alternative Ways of Organizing Strategic Planning and Marketing

an incidental activity of planning, planning and marketing can both report to a common senior executive but each have defined roles, or planning and marketing can be treated as components of the larger function of strategic management.

There is a reason to expect the structure, relationship, and precise roles of these functions to vary among institutions. Since their purpose is to ensure an appropriate response from an organization to its environment, different environments (or different perceptions of them) should give rise to differences in the location and scope of planning and marketing functions.

A private hospital or hospital system in a metropolitan area of the United States may, for instance, legitimately perceive itself as being in a more competitive local marketplace for health services than a municipal hospital in the same city, a rural community hospital, or a hospital functioning in the regulatory setting of a Canadian province.

There is also a reason to expect the structure, relationship, and roles of these functions to change

within any one institution over time: Environments change.

For instance, many U.S. hospitals thrived in the 1950s and 1960s in a local environment characterized by a shortage of inpatient beds. Planning for additional capacity, as well as obtaining the necessary state approvals, was a major preoccupation of senior managers. Many of the same hospitals, however, found there was a shift in the 1970s and 1980s toward excess inpatient capacity, and thus marketing to attract a larger market share of hospital admissions assumed a new importance.

In other words, all health care organizations devote some time and effort to planning activities and to marketing activities, but the form, scope, and relationship of these efforts vary widely. For each organization, the main determinant is its perception of the nature of its environment (e.g., the degree of competitiveness, regulation, etc). Moreover, its perception is likely to change over time.

Because strategic planning and marketing activities are so closely related in concept, practice, and organizational structure, they are sometimes viewed as indistinguishable. However, despite their common focus on the organization in its environment, each has a distinct perspective:

> Health planning is preparing for tomorrow's health management. Planning is the process of making decisions in the present to affect future outcomes . . . to move a system from a present state of affairs to a future more valued state of affairs.[1]

> Marketing is the analysis, planning, implementation and control of carefully formulated programs to bring about volunteer exchanges with target markets for the purpose of achieving organizational objectives, and using effective pricing, communication and distribution to inform, motivate and service the market.[2]

It makes sense to consider planning and marketing activities together, but it is important to bear in mind their distinct purposes and processes. Otherwise, the intellectual discipline that each offers—planning with its focus on systematically preparing the organization for its future in all of its key dimensions, marketing with its focus on present and future organizational relationships with client constituencies—may not be able to benefit the organization's strategic management to the extent that it could.

Strategic planning often involves the following seven tasks:

1. *Coordination of strategic information.* The object is to ensure that the organization is consistently informed of significant developments in its external environment.

2. *Definition of the organizational mission.* The organization must periodically determine whether its central purpose (or purposes) remains valid or requires adjustment.

3. *Coordination of strategic responses.* An ongoing process is needed for deciding how the organization will respond to major external developments in order to sustain its mission.

4. *Space and facilities planning.* The organization must systematically consider its future physical plant needs (major decisions in this area of planning often need to be made well in advance because of the long lead time that can be required for facilities construction; facilities planning and construction is covered in depth in Chapter 22).

5. *Program development and project review.* The organization must use a systematic approach for assessing significant individual projects and tracking their progress.

6. *Regulatory planning.* The organization must establish and maintain an active relationship with external agencies whose approval is needed for significant projects.

7. *Establishing and maintaining relationships with other provider institutions.* A growing number of health care organizations are combining into health care systems or joint venturing in particular programs, which adds interinstitutional negotiations and relations as factors in the planning process.

Typical marketing responsibilities include the following:

- *Market research.* The organization must keep informed about the attitudes, preferences, and opinions of its client constituencies.

- *Strategic marketing analysis.* This involves assessing and advising on opportunities or threats in the organization's marketplace and on the likely market response to new projects under consideration. (Strategic market analysis apparently overlaps with planning, but marketing as a discipline focuses on assessing market response whereas planning is concerned with a broader range of strategic aspects of new projects.)

- *Program design.* The marketing staff are responsible for assessing and advising on ways of enhancing the appeal of a program to its potential clients.

- *External communications.* Public media are used to educate potential clients about available services and their distinctive benefits.

- *Internal communications.* The object is to develop an internal consensus regarding the organization's mission, goals, action plans, and standards of service.
- *Fulfillment.* It is important to ensure that potential clients can easily access the organization and its services and that the services meet their expectations.

MANAGEMENT PRINCIPLES

The following management principles are basic to effective strategic planning and marketing in health care:

- Organizations must anticipate and adapt to changes in their environment.
- In a successful organization, there is typically a high level of internal consensus about its mission, future vision, and the main strategic issues it must confront.
- Any organization must try to distinguish between external factors that it can influence and external factors that it cannot but that may limit its freedom of action. It is easy to waste time trying to alter the inevitable rather than adjusting to the inevitable.
- A health care organization must try to identify those programs that it can viably sustain given the foreseeable changes in its environment (e.g., changes in regulation or marketplace competition).
- Every organization has target markets with which it must sustain effective communications and relationships and whose satisfaction with the organization is important to its future strength.

ORGANIZATIONAL ROLE AND FUNCTION

Recognition of the need for comprehensive regional health planning in the United States can be traced back to the 1927 creation of the Committee on the Costs of Medical Care, which had some success in stimulating joint planning by hospitals, doctors, and public health officials.[3] Regional health planning became more firmly established in the 1940s.[4] The 1946 Hill-Burton Act provided federal funding for hospital construction projects that had been demonstrated to meet a public need (approval was gained through a formal state health facilities planning process).

By the 1960s, further federal statutes had reinforced this concept of health planning. In particular, the 1966 Public Health Service Act Amendments provided for two tiers of health planning organizations. Each area or region was to have a health systems agency consisting of a small secretariat of health planners and a council of provider and consumer representatives, with consumers in the majority. This model was to be replicated at the state level. Starting with New York in 1964, many states strengthened this process by requiring a positive endorsement from these agencies for all hospital major capital projects before issuing a certificate of need. By 1974, the National Health Planning and Resources Development Act made it mandatory for all states to have such certificate-of-need processes as a condition of receiving support under various federal funding programs.

The coming of the Reagan administration, with its philosophical commitment to deregulation and scaling back government activities, led to a withdrawal of federal funding for health system agencies, which largely disappeared at both state and local levels. With renewed discretion over their certificate-of-need laws, some states effectively abandoned them; others maintained them but with higher dollar thresholds for the capital cost of projects requiring prior state approval.

In parallel with these legislative changes, American doctors and hospital administrators, since the early 1970s, have increasingly perceived a growing competition among themselves for patients. In previous decades, the supply of physicians in most specialties and the supply of hospital beds in most regions were insufficient to serve the population adequately. One frequent symptom of inadequate supply was that many patients needing a non-emergent hospital admission were put on a waiting list (such lists often extended several months into the future). Increases in the physician supply, continued construction of hospitals, reduced lengths of stay, changes in treatment philosophy, and greater use of outpatient surgery gradually alleviated this undersupply of health care resources and, by the early 1980s, had replaced it with a situation of excess capacity, at least in many areas of the country.

Thus, health planning itself in the United States has been profoundly altered, at several key periods in its development, by significant changes in its own environment. The American hospital planner of 1970 would almost certainly have cited developing liaisons with regulatory agencies as the most important of the activities listed above. Much of this planner's time would have been devoted to relations with health system agencies and state officials and to steering the hospital's projects through their approval processes. The most respected and experienced hospital planners could be found serving as provider representatives on health system agency committees, helping to review proposals from surrounding institutions. By 1990, hospital planners, in most states, still had to work with state officials in order to receive certificates of need, but less frequently and without the time-consuming involvement of health system agencies.

Because of the increased competition among hospitals and the greater riskiness of new projects and programs in a typically oversupplied market, there is a new emphasis on the use of strategic planning activities. Like executives who work in other high-competition sectors of the economy, senior health care administrators now tend to see their organizations' future viability as dependent upon the quality of their assessment of the environment and the wisdom of their planning decisions. This orientation is often reinforced by the presence on hospital boards of trustees from other industries with experience in competition.

These changes have not eradicated the need for hospital planners to maintain relationships with lo-cal grass-roots organizations, local health officials, and others who can both advise on needs and aid with program grants or community support for projects still requiring state approval. Liaisons with regulators have not disappeared as a priority for health planners, but they have become one facet of a wider concept of effective planning.

The accepted role of planning in health care organizations has also been influenced in recent years by research and publications exploring the nature of planning activities in successful enterprises. One major emphasis of such scholarship has been on the internal benefits of the planning process. Complex enterprises cannot be run effectively by detailed top-down commands but require an internal consensus regarding their strategic priorities and objectives. This means that departments and individuals are given a large measure of autonomy but act to achieve shared goals (i.e., they are flying in the same direction but not necessarily in formation).[5] A systematic planning process provides one mechanism for building an internal consensus among relatively autonomous health care professionals and their departments or across the sites of a multiunit healthcare system.

The presence of a coherent strategic plan can be equally indispensable to a health care organization's external credibility (i.e., how it appears to capital funding sources, vendors extending credit to the organization, or contract purchasers of health care services). As the chairperson of the board of one academic medical center stated in his organization's annual report,

> If an organization is to inspire confidence in its sense of direction it must pass three tests. It must be able to articulate its vision. If it cannot, it may not have one. It should be able to express that vision succinctly, because lack of brevity may well reveal lack of focus. Finally, that vision should clearly manifest that the organization is committed to responding to the expectations of the various communities and constituencies that it serves, for, otherwise, its plans may be founded solely in its own introspective concerns.[6]

Thus, the tripartite role of institutional planning is to ensure that the organization anticipates and adapts to its changing environment, helps develop an internal consensus, and contributes to building external confidence in the organization.

The emergence of a strongly competitive environment for many American hospitals has also led to the growth of formal marketing activities. The first hospital marketing staffs were introduced by the large for-profit hospital chains in the early 1970s. By the mid-1980s, most U.S. hospitals had a mechanism for the marketing function in place. Since then, the scope of activities of some marketing staffs has expanded beyond marketing communications to the wider set of functions listed above.

In Canada, although most hospitals are private entities, they derive much of their reimbursement via global prospective budgets from provincial public insurance programs, with separate regulatory controls on capital spending and consequently on major programmatic or physical plant modifications. Often those capital spending controls are extensive, requiring, for instance, that a hospital seek provincial or local approval at several strategic planning stages. In Ontario, to take one example, a hospital's leaders may have to participate in a role study that examines the functions of each institution in the region; then seek endorsement of a master program that describes the individual hospital's intended role in detail; then obtain subsequent agreement to a master plan for the hospital, a physical planning document, and a functional program that outlines the hospital's policies, organization, and proposed workloads.

While there is patient choice in Canada, few parts of the country have the "excess" hospital capacity present in many U.S. communities. Canadian health organizations thus have as much, if not more, need for strategic planning as a basis for their dialogue with official funding sources, but, because of the absence of significant competition, they have less need for formal marketing efforts. Nevertheless, they can still usefully apply specific aspects of the managerial science of marketing. Market research can illuminate the reasons behind physician referral patterns and patient behaviors and thereby enhance institutional planning. Marketing communications can more fully inform client constituencies and help to ensure that services are well regarded and well utilized.

In Canada and in some other countries where health care is heavily government funded and regulated, there is interest in how U.S. hospitals cope with a strongly competitive environment because of the possibility that elements of competition may in the future be introduced into their systems. Official efforts to create more of a health care marketplace in other countries where health care is even more directly provided by the state, such as France and the United Kingdom, have stimulated more interest in health care marketing theories and methods.[7]

In any country, therefore, the role in the 1990s of each planning and marketing activity has to be understood in the context of a current but changing external environment that could include new elements of government regulation and competition among providers.

PLANNING ACTIVITIES

As noted earlier, seven principal activities are essential to any comprehensive approach to strategic planning. Their implications are reviewed below.

Coordination of Strategic Information

Through planning activities, health care organizations and their leadership strive to remain informed about six critical external issues:

1. health care technologies
2. public health care policy
3. health care economics
4. competitive organizations
5. social or demographic changes
6. epidemiological issues

Health organizations gather information about these six areas in the following ways:

- They regularly scan relevant publications looking for new information about issues that could have significant impact. (This scanning is purposeful. The best planners have developed lists of potentially important issues and systematically build up information files on them, either on paper or in a computer).

- They subscribe to special information services (e.g., a service that provides information about emerging advances in health care technology).

- They keep in touch with outside contacts who may have advance knowledge of changes in public policy or local public health priorities.

- They gather information from their own staff (e.g., physicians attending professional association meetings may hear of incipient developments in their fields of expertise).

- They gather insights from their own clients (e.g., referring physicians, patients, and payers). The task of gathering this kind of input overlaps with marketing's monitoring of the views, reactions, and preferences of clients using market research.

It is essential for organizations to be systematic and disciplined in seeking and analyzing information so as to avoid reacting to anecdotal and only partly accurate input.

In any organization, those involved in strategic planning should look for evidence of trends (processes that have already started and seem likely to gain momentum) and discontinuities (environmental factors that seem to be undergoing a radical change). Through the strategic planning process (Figure 17-2), the organization tries to categorize these trends and discontinuities as opportunities or threats.

A strategic opportunity arises if some environmental factor seems likely to create more demand for some service that the organization either provides or has a better prospect of being able to provide than competitors. A strategic threat exists if some environmental factor seems likely to depress demand for one of the organization's services. For instance, in many older metropolitan areas, the inner city tends to lose population while the suburbs grow. This trend presents an obvious opportunity to

suburban hospitals but is a threat to those at the city core. It may not, however, constitute a real opportunity for a suburban hospital that is not particularly adept at serving the specific needs of those groups responsible for the local population growth.

Definition of the Organizational Mission

Although the organizational mission is treated in Figure 17-2 as a predetermined starting point for planning, in reality the mission should be periodically reassessed. The main purpose of defining a mission is to provide the organization with a clear focus. The mission is an internal motivator. It summarizes what the individuals in the organization collectively aspire to achieve—their vision of what the future should be.

The ideal mission statement is neither so narrow as to inhibit the organization from responding to significant changes in its environment, nor so wide-ranging that it leads the organization away from its field of institutional competence (see Figure 17-3). Theodore Levitt, a student of marketing, wrote an influential article warning against the dangers of defining a mission that is too narrow (myopic).[8] In response to Levitt, many organizations have developed mission statements that define their purpose in terms of the generic service that they perform (e.g., "health care") rather than the way in which they currently choose to perform it (e.g., through hospital-based care). Thus, a good mission statement indicates the ongoing service, not the current method of delivery, and it opens up institutional strategic thinking to new ways of delivering the same service.

More recently, however, it has been recognized that organizations can run into trouble by being too far-sighted (presbyopic).[9] By focusing excessively on longer-term roles and needs, some organizations pay insufficient attention to short-term or intermediate-term opportunities to sustain and expand existing activities and programs. They may also be tempted to diversify into fields that appear close to their current areas of expertise but, in fact, call for different managerial paradigms and experience.

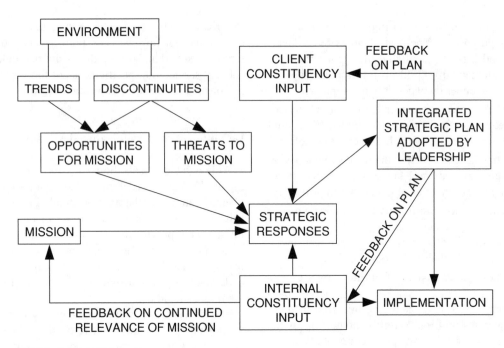

Figure 17-2 The Strategic Planning Process

For instance, in the United States a number of hospitals and hospital systems reacted to the changing pattern of health care delivery by diversifying into fields such as home care, medical equipment leasing, and patient transport. Some of these hospitals saw disappointing results from such diversification and have subsequently retrenched, narrowing their focus to hospital-based services. Other hospitals that also diversified succeeded in maintaining a viable balance between diversification and the continued evolution and adaptation of their more traditional services.

Coordination of Strategic Responses

Planners do not dictate organizational responses to perceived opportunities and threats but manage a process involving a broad representation of organizational leadership to reach a consensus.

Most commonly, organizations plan strategic responses with two time horizons in mind, the one

relatively long-term, the other more immediate. The traditional approach is to devise a long-term plan, updated annually and supplemented by annual goals and objectives for the next 12 months. Re-

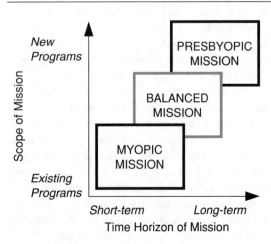

Figure 17-3 A Comparison of Balanced, Myopic, and Presbyopic Missions

cently, that approach has fallen into some disfavor, both in health care and in the business world.[10] It may, however, still be required of health care institutions, such as public hospitals, accountable to government agencies committed to the concept of somewhat detailed long-range planning. Health institutions with the flexibility to determine their own approach to planning may see the rate of environmental change as precluding detailed multiple-year forecasts.

The alternative approach is to develop a less detailed strategic plan (or strategic agenda or vision statement). This kind of plan lists the major environmental issues the organization may face over the next several years and describes in broad terms how it intends to respond.

Under both approaches to strategic planning, therefore, the organization seeks to look at least several years forward and to define where it intends to be. The critical difference is the degree of specificity about long-term objectives and action plans.

Just as importantly, the ideal long-term or strategic plan defines or implies what the organization does not intend to be.[11] The organization can thereby avoid expending time and energy on ideas that may have some merit but are not critically important to realizing its strategic vision.

Space and Facilities Planning

The traditional five-year plan usually integrates space and program planning, which produces the appearance that facilities and programs are being planned in a sychronized manner. However, the need for greater flexibility in program planning (due to rapid changes in the environment) makes it hard to dovetail program plans with facilities plans. A major building project may take three years or longer from initial discussion to completion, during which time the programmatic assumptions that formed part of the original decision will probably be modified by further environmental changes.

Contemporary planning tends to recognize, therefore, that some incongruity between planned facilities and actual future program needs is unavoidable. It attempts to minimize the gap by giving even more attention to space and facilities planning as an activity in its own right and by attempting to plan facilities that can be used in various ways or easily altered (see Chapter 22).

Program Development and Project Review

Because the environment is dynamic, it constantly creates new or amended program concepts for the organization to consider. They may be identified through scanning the environment, or they may be suggested by a physician or some other person within the organization or by someone external to the organization (e.g., a consultant, a potential joint venture partner, or someone with an existing program for sale).

One study of project review methodologies in successful business enterprises provides a useful model of the process that many health organizations also strive, in differing degrees, to follow.[12] Figure 17-4 depicts that process and identifies some of the major planning and marketing issues that can arise at each step. Guidelines for using the process include the following:

- Once programmatic ideas surface, from whatever source, they should be rapidly screened by the organization's leadership to determine if they fit closely enough with the five-year or strategic plan to merit a detailed feasibility assessment.

- If an idea passes that initial screen, a subsequent thorough feasibility study advises whether the proposal has enough market potential and financial viability to be worth pursuing.

- If the organization's leadership, after such a study, agrees that the idea is feasible, it should then proceed to a service development analysis, which addresses practical issues such as where the service or program will be located, what hours it will operate, what features may

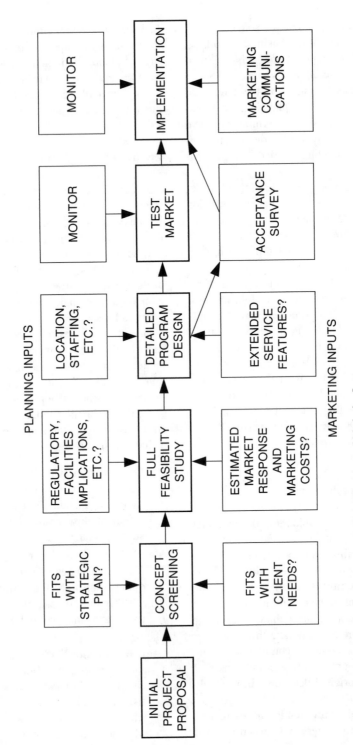

Figure 17-4 Project Review Process, Including Major Planning and Marketing Issues

be needed to maximize its appeal to patients or physicians, how it will be priced, and so on.

- If the proposal still looks attractive after that step, it should ideally be tested in some limited fashion before being fully resourced and implemented. If actual test marketing is infeasible, one alternative is to do an acceptance survey, presenting the concept as now fully defined to a sample of potential clients and assessing their likelihood of using it.

A health care organization depends upon the initiative of a large number of physicians, other health care professionals, and administrators. As already noted, one purpose of developing institutional plans is to build a consensus among individuals in the organization. The organization's process for considering proposals for new programs and projects should involve the internal sponsors or champions, keep them informed of the progress of their proposals, and if the proposals are rejected, provide reasons for the decision.

The ideal institutional process for evaluating and making progress on proposed initiatives should include well-defined and consistently applied criteria for project evaluation, a tracking system that thoroughly documents the progress of each proposal as it moves through the process of review (and possibly implementation), and timely communication of the reasons why certain projects will not be pursued.

Regulatory Planning

As well as requiring hospitals to obtain certificates of need for projects above a designated cost threshold, some states regulate the growth of specific hospital services that they perceive as likely to proliferate unnecessarily. Therefore, in addition to certificates of need, the inspection and approval of various state agencies may be required before, during, and after the construction of new facilities.

As previously noted, even more rigorous processes for obtaining governmental approval may well become the norm for public health care institutions in the United States and for health care organizations generally in other countries. Consequently, planning staff will probably be increasingly involved in preparing documentation; seeking advice from consultants, lawyers, hospital associations, and others; and dealing with the officials responsible for reviewing projects.

The parallel existence of internal and external regulatory approval processes for planning decisions contains the potential for confusion in an organization's approach to strategic decisions. Success in obtaining external approval for a plan or project should be regarded as the key step in the organization's own decision to proceed only if the regulatory source of that approval effectively guarantees to hold the organization harmless should the project fail to reach forecast levels.

A separate and more rigorous process of internal approval is necessary to ensure that the potential risks and returns of the plan or project have been comprehensively and realistically assessed and tested. It is easy for regulated enterprises to mistake regulatory approval for plans or projects as an endorsement of their business potential; in reality, the regulators evaluate such plans and projects from the standpoint of their societal impact, not their financial viability.

For instance, a state certificate of need approving a new service does not imply that the institution can successfully organize the service, attract sufficient patients, or achieve financial viability at whatever price various payers may be prepared to accept.

Thus, a health care organization may have to review projects internally, much as commercial enterprises do in their planning. It must not confuse the two processes of internal and external review.

Relationships with Other Provider Institutions

An increasing number of health care organizations are involved in joint ventures with one or more other institutions. A significant number of American hospitals are also now members of a hospital system.

The planning and development of a joint venture typically raises issues not present with purely internal projects (e.g., division of costs and revenues, allocations of overhead, formal written definitions of the responsibilities of the separate parties, and provisions for unilateral termination). An even wider range of such issues can arise in the case of a formal agreement between two or more organizations to merge or to associate in a manner short of full merger.

Planning within a single health care organization can involve elements of negotiation (e.g., with physicians, among departments), but the range of issues requiring a negotiated and legally documented resolution multiply when two institutions—each with its own governing body and its own management—seek to combine their efforts and resources. There are, of course, compelling reasons for mergers, lesser forms of association, or joint ventures. Organizations that join together can often contain costs through the realization of economies of scale, achieve a greater combined market share, and increase quality and cost-efficiency by pooling resources and expertise (see Chapter 9).

In many health care organizations, all or some of the physicians upon whom they depend for professional staffing and direction are not employees but self-employed practitioners. A joint venture, association, or merger between two organizations may well, therefore, depend upon the active endorsement of more than just the governing bodies. As a result, contemporary planning in health care organizations, particularly in the United States, has acquired a new dimension—alliance building and maintenance.

MARKETING ACTIVITIES

Market Research

The groups that a hospital or other health care organization would be well advised to survey periodically include patients, the local public, local business leaders, and those physicians who are affiliated with the organization or refer patients to it.

National surveys are also reported from time to time in health care journals, but care must be exercised in verifying that national attitudes reflect local attitudes.

Market research is useful for exploring

- the health care organization's image (both positives and negatives)
- the level of public awareness of the organization, and its mission, capabilities, and services
- the preferences of potential clients when choosing among local health care providers
- the desires of potential clients regarding the delivery of health care services
- the actual behavior of potential clients when accessing health care services
- the levels of satisfaction among those with direct experience of the health care organization
- the responses of client groups targeted specifically by communications from the health care organization

The leadership of the health care organization tends to form its own impressions of the various opinions and behaviors of client constituencies. However, random comments and observations may not be fully representative, and systematic surveys can provide a more thorough understanding of the marketplace. Thus, the organization must strive to ensure that its surveys employ a valid methodology and that findings are reported and assessed in an objective manner.

In addition to formal quantitative surveys, market research often employs focus groups drawn from the target audience for a program to explore qualitative issues in more depth. Perhaps even greater care must be taken in impartially summarizing and reporting the in-depth discussions in these groups. They can, however, provide insights not readily attainable in large-scale surveys.

Strategic Marketing Analysis

Just as the health care organization's planning activities can range from strategic reassessment of mission and defining its strategic agenda to detailed review and development of new programs, so too can its marketing analysis activities.

No institutional strategic plan is fully comprehensive unless it addresses how the organization "can differentiate itself effectively, capitalizing on its distinctive strengths to deliver better value to its customers."[13] When the leadership of the organization focuses on how to differentiate itself, it brings strategic marketing analysis to bear on its strategic planning.

Some health care organizations function as monopolies, as sole available suppliers of health care or some health care service for a specific client constituency, but they are the exception. More typically, local physicians have choices of where to practice or refer, local patients have choices among health providers, and some payers can opt to contract only with selected providers. In such circumstances, each health care organization's strategy should include planned actions to differentiate itself from competitors. The strategy of seeking to be an exact replica of other providers, can rarely, if ever, succeed. Each provider usually possesses some distinctive attributes, and the only realistic choice is whether to formulate a deliberate strategy for differentiation that seeks to exploit or modify them or instead to passively accept whatever distinguishing image circumstances happen to yield.

One basic approach to developing a marketing strategy is to pay attention to "the four Ps" of marketing (product, pricing, promotion, place). Since being originally described in 1964 by Jerome McCarthy, the four Ps have been referred to by many other authors as a general model of marketing.[14] McCarthy, however, appears to have used the concept more precisely—as a way of indicating the four critical decision variables to be considered in defining any organization's distinctive marketing mix.[15] A health care organization may differentiate itself from alternative suppliers in terms of the *products* or services provided, the *pricing* for the services, the *promotion* of the services, the *places* the services are provided (and access routes), or some combination of these.

Although the first three Ps are largely self-explanatory, the fourth P, place, can be misinterpreted. It signifies not merely location but the entire strategy for the distribution of the services.

Most commercial products are distributed to consumers from the point of manufacture or assembly via retailers or other intermediaries. By contrast, many services attract desired clients to the point of service. That is true of most health services, although there are exceptions, such as home care or house calls. Typically, patients must travel to the doctor's office, hospital, or other health care facility. Not only that, but they often gain access to some services via other services. For example, a primary visit to a doctor's office might be followed by a hospital visit arranged for by the doctor. Thus, the differentiating strategy of a health care organization might include developing unusual ways of providing or facilitating the use of various pathways to its services.

At the level of programmatic planning of specific services, client constituencies can be one of the sources of information about opportunities for new services. For instance, it may be through a dialogue with community physicians that a hospital discovers a medical need not currently being addressed by any local provider.

During the feasibility study stage of a project review, critical issues include the likely patient volumes for the proposed program and the marketing costs that may be required and should therefore be built into the financial analysis. The marketing staff should thus be a key supplier of input into feasibility studies to ensure that unrealistically high volumes or unrealistically low marketing costs are not assumed. There are a variety of established methodologies for assessing market potential and marketing costs of a proposed program (see Figure 17-4).[16]

Program Design

Marketing theory distinguishes between the *generic service* (the benefit that a service confers on a client), the *tangible service* (the process by which the service is delivered), and the *extended service* (the additional features that add value to the service and give it a competitive edge).[17] The object of the marketer in program design is to determine the extended service features essential to the program's competitive capability. Specific market research, surveys, and other sources may provide insights that can be extremely helpful in making decisions on such matters as the opening hours, acceptable waiting times, appointment scheduling systems, and amenities.

External Communications

External communications is frequently equated with advertising in printed or electronic media, but advertising is just one of an array of available marketing communication tactics. Institutions may seek publicity through media coverage, personally sell to client sources, and offer sales promotions, such as open houses or free screenings.[18] The appropriate mix of tactics for any particular need is partly determined by the organization's policies and formal or informal codes of behavior. For example, health care organizations still vary in their readiness to engage in paid advertising, even if that is the most cost-effective communication tactic.

Hospitals and doctors in the United States made frequent use of media advertising prior to the 1890s. By 1900, however, the frequent abuse of advertising by unqualified competitors led most hospitals and branches of the medical profession to declare such practices unethical.[19] Only with the emergence of excess capacity and competition in the 1970s did significant health provider advertising reappear. This trend was further stimulated after the 1980 election of Ronald Reagan. In particular, the Federal Trade Commission insisted upon the removal of any ban against advertising in the rules of medical societies, arguing that such bans could constitute a restraint of trade.

Organizational philosophies aside, there are a range of decision-making rules to aid in determining the appropriate level and mix of promotional tactics to use in any set of circumstances. Common to all of them are the five concepts discussed below.

The first two key concepts are *reach* and *frequency*. To be effective, a communication must, in fact, reach a critical mass of potential clients. The task of developing a communication cannot be logically divorced from the task of ensuring its effective delivery to a large enough audience.

Consider an announcement of screenings for prostate cancer. The sponsoring institution usually has in mind some minimum target number of participants in a screening program for it to be regarded as a success. If, for instance, the goal is to attract between one and two hundred males over 40 or with a family history of prostate cancer, the announcement may have to reach many thousands of such males, since only a small percentage of those reached by any announcement are likely to respond.

Typically, a communication must also be repetitive to achieve maximal impact, making frequency a further critical factor. Repetitions of a communication to the same audience usually achieve more than just arithmetic increases in response, at least until the saturation point, after which response rates decline as further repetitions occur.

For example, a single announcement letter to physicians about a new service is less likely to be effective than a planned series of announcements. Thus, effort and money can be wasted on communications that are either inadequate or excessive in their reach or frequency.

Another critical concept is hierarchy of effects. The idea here is that an effective message must capture the intended audience's attention, create awareness of the service, create a preference for the service, and motivate some fairly immediate response.

A communication that fails to move the audience through this full hierarchy not only may be a waste of effort but may actually do the organization more harm than good. If, for instance, it arouses interest in a service and stimulates response but does not create a provider preference, it can aid other organizations at the expense of the organization that originated the message.

Finally, *segmentation* and *positioning* are key concepts in marketing communication. Segmentation is the classification of potential clients for a program or service into subgroups, each of which possesses distinct demographic characteristics or attitudes, values, and behaviors. One goal of segmentation is to identify one or more client subgroups that the organization may be better able to serve than its competitors (by virtue, for instance, of its location, reputation, or resources). The object of positioning is to develop communications that effectively portray the organization as meeting the needs and preferences of those target segments.

Often the concepts of segmentation and positioning are applied only to the development of marketing communications. However, marketing logic suggests they could be employed beneficially in the design of services, shaping them to cater to the desired market segments more effectively than the similar services of competitors.

Indeed, they are also relevant to the basic process of defining institutional strategy. In a situation with multiple providers of services, there are segments of the public for which each institution has a comparative advantage as a supplier, and therefore there are positions within the array of locally available services that each institution should optimally occupy.

With these concepts in mind, for any given communication challenge, the organization should attempt to answer the following questions:

1. Which segment of the client base do we most wish to communicate with?

2. What is known about how that target audience thinks and behaves?

3. What are the most cost-effective tactics to communicate with that target segment with adequate reach and frequency?

4. Which creative approach to and positioning of the communication will best accomplish the full hierarchy of effects?

Fulfillment

Fulfillment is the process through which an organization ensures that it delivers what its clients expect of it. In any successfully established enterprise, the majority of customers are not generated

through current marketing efforts. The majority comprise repeat users and new clients attracted by the recommendation of past clients.[20] The role of current marketing communications is to add some first-time clients and to reinforce the positive opinions of satisfied previous clients. Thus, organizations typically depend at least as much on fulfillment as on proactive marketing to potential clients.

For health care organizations, fulfillment often has three critical aspects: access, service delivery, and follow-up to service. Marketing in health care is increasingly involved in facilitating access to health care and hospital services. Traditionally, patients have usually gained access to a hospital as a result of being in the care of a physician on its staff, being referred to one of its specialists by a primary practitioner, or coming to its emergency room or clinics. The quest for more patients by many health care organizations has led them to place more emphasis on ensuring that these mechanisms work well and, if necessary, on supplementing them with new means of public access such as contracting with managed care organizations (see Chapter 28).

Many hospitals, for instance, have now developed telephone referral services for members of the public to call for help in arranging an appointment with one of their doctors. Many tertiary centers have similar services to make it easier for community doctors to refer to one of their specialists. Various health care organizations have created satellite centers to improve access.

The second major aspect of fulfillment is service management. Within recent decades, the advent of advanced survey methodologies has made it possible to measure client satisfaction, to assess the relationship between satisfaction with individual components of service and intent to reuse, and to set priorities for operational actions to improve reuse rates. Consequently, many health care organizations are engaged in surveying referring physicians and patients themselves and in amending procedures and amenities to maximize satisfaction.

Service management has increased in importance in recent years because of the enhanced focus within health care organizations on quality and productivity. Some widely advocated approaches to total quality management and productivity enhancement have been imported from other types of industry, where they incorporate an emphasis on customer satisfaction as one (not the only) important measure of the quality of tangible product or intangible service outcomes. "Service quality is not a separate discipline from services marketing. Companies with poor service cannot succeed at marketing."[21]

Many health care organizations are now paying added attention to client retention. Since much health care is provided episodically (for many patients, substantial time may lapse between one episode of care and the next), more health care organizations are seeking to maintain a bond with recent patients or referrers by using various formal follow-up mechanisms. The reminder card that many doctors send to patients whom they have not seen for some time is one simple example.

RESOURCE REQUIREMENTS

By 1990, U.S. hospitals were devoting an average of between 1.5 and 2 percent of total budget to marketing, planning, and public relations activities combined. A small hospital may have some 2 or 3 people responsible for these several related functions, a medium-size hospital may have up to 7 or 8, while the largest major medical centers can have upward of 20. Typically, the larger staffs perform certain tasks that are contracted out by smaller organizations but may be more economically conducted in-house when a certain scale of production or effort is reached (e.g., feasibility analyses in planning and graphic design in marketing).

Organizational policy can be another important factor influencing the size of planning or marketing staffs. A major commitment to contracting with managed care plans, for instance, may necessitate the addition of payer relations personnel, who might be located in the planning or marketing function, in the finance department, or in a joint venture entity with the medical staff. As another example, various hospitals have decided to seek contracts

from employers for workers' compensation services, industrial wellness programs, and so on, necessitating the added presence of a sales team.

For these reasons, it is impossible to present one archetypical organization chart showing the placement of planning and marketing at a large number of hospitals.

Many health care organizations, both large and small, make significant use of outside consultants and services in their planning. The role given to external consultants varies with the size and sophistication of the internal staff. Planning consultants may help the organization's board, CEO, and other senior leaders to construct and document the organization's strategic plan itself. They may also help in drafting certificate-of-need applications or provide specialized knowledge of potential investments that may have worked well elsewhere but present inherent risks for a new and inexperienced entrant. For this reason, some health planning consultants offer specific competence in such areas as HMO contracting, women's health centers, or physical rehabilitation programs.

Outside consultants and services may also be asked to assist in such marketing activities as market research (to provide anonymity or independent analysis), publications (to supplement internal resources that may be overloaded or inadequate for a particular project), and media advertising (outside agencies may have more knowledge of media buying and a higher level of creative capability than the organization may be able to sustain internally).

Where to draw the line between making and buying is a source of continuous debate in all organizations, but there is always some point beyond which it does not make sense to staff for tasks that vary in their intensity or require talented people in short supply.

An area in which there is growing dependence on outside vendors for planning and marketing and many other organizational functions is computer support, particularly innovative software. The most common areas of computer application now include the following:

- analysis and mapping of local demographics

- storage of attitudinal survey data for future retrieval, reanalysis, and longtitudinal comparison
- analysis of patient databases for geographical origin and payer mix to determine relative profitability, areas appropriate for marketing efforts, and characteristics for future positioning and segmentation strategies
- storage of medical staff profiles for physician referral services and of data on individuals who call these services for assistance
- matching referral service caller information with subsequent patient data to identify revenues generated by responders to advertising
- desktop publishing
- computer-aided graphic design
- local area networking for paperless sharing of information

Certainly at the larger health care organizations, marketers and planners are now among the most extensive users of personal computers and mainframe databases (see Chapter 13).

QUALITY MANAGEMENT

Since strategic planning is concerned with the organization's effective response to its environment over time, the ultimate judgment as to its effectiveness can only be made after a period of years. The long-term question is: Has the organization succeeded in maintaining its strength and viability by adapting prudently to changing circumstances?

There are, however, several more immediate indicators of the quality of any enterprise's strategic planning:

- Does the organization have a documented strategic plan or agenda that identifies likely new opportunities and threats and indicates how it intends to respond?
- Does that documented agenda show evidence of realism? The strategic objectives should

seem within the organization's competence to accomplish over a period of several years, and the focus of the agenda should indicate, explicitly or implicitly, what the organization will not attempt to do as well as what it will attempt.

- Is the strategic plan or agenda a "living" plan? In other words, is the plan being used to shape key decisions as they arise?
- Is there evidence of a high level of internal consensus that the strategic plan or agenda is a good one?
- Are major capital and programmatic decisions being reviewed systematically and thoroughly?
- Does the organization's leadership really use planning data in its strategic discussions? In other words, is it looking at facts as well as concepts and opinions?

The quality of marketing activities is similarly identifiable both over time and more immediately. Marketers distinguish between the *communication effects, sales effects,*[22] and *transformational effects*[23] of their activities. All three may be quantifiable on a short-term and long-term basis.

A communications effect occurs when there is firm evidence (most frequently from before-and-after market research) that a marketing message has in fact been received and understood by the intended audience.

A sales effect occurs when there is firm evidence of an actual response to a marketing communication. Most immediately, this effect may be quantifiable in terms of volume (e.g., callers to a referral service or attendees at an event). Subsequently, it may be possible to track the actual revenue attributable to the response (i.e., the money spent by responders who wound up using the organization's services).

A transformational effect occurs when the rate of reuse by past clients increases as a result of specific communications targeted at that audience or of planned internal service efforts to increase client satisfaction. Uncovering evidence of this effect may require both analysis of usage patterns and some attitudinal research (e.g., patient surveys) to demonstrate a relationship between improved satisfaction and any increased reusage.

In practice, it is seldom if ever possible to track and quantify all of the communication, sales, or transformational effects resulting from marketing initiatives. Some of the effects may be delayed well into the future, some may be almost impossible to trace, such as increased visits to the offices of associated physicians by individuals the organization has little chance of interviewing. However, if the marketing function can track and identify marginal added revenue greater than the cost of the marketing activities, it has shown that the organization is better off as a result of these activities.

THE FUTURE OF STRATEGIC PLANNING AND MARKETING

The strategic planning and marketing challenges facing health care providers seem certain to grow in complexity. Perhaps the two most important trends will be the accelerating rate of change in medical technologies and the likelihood of reforms in the regulatory and financial environment.

Significant changes in technology, in any sector of the economy, can reshape products and services, the marketplace for those products and services, and, ultimately, the structure of the sector itself. In other sectors dependent upon high technology, the average corporation tends to be large, and much of the technological innovation affecting it emanates from its own research labs. Telecommunications, computers, pharmaceuticals, and chemicals are four examples.

By contrast, health care is provided by hundreds of thousands of self-employed professionals and thousands of relatively small institutions, whereas much of the innovative technology is developed by outside enterprises or in the labs of a small number of academic medical centers. Clearly, it is somewhat easier for an organization to anticipate technological advances when they are being pursued by

scientists directly employed by the organization itself or by one of a limited number of competitors than when, as in health care, they originate from just a few provider institutions or from sources outside the provider community. Yet, anticipating and responding to innovation in clinical methods will be increasingly important for the strategic planning and marketing of health care organizations.

Competition among U.S. providers seems certain to increase further, and failure to respond effectively will result in more health care organizations facing bankruptcy and in more mergers (by hospitals in pursuit of greater combined market share and economies of scale). Even as the United States moves toward some significant reform in its financing of health care, competition among providers for resources, physicians, and patients is unlikely to disappear. The form that competition has taken over the last decade or so is at least partly due to health insurance mechanisms that make some patients worth more than others to doctors, hospitals, and other providers. However, it is unclear that a reformed system will result in equal payment to providers for all patients with a similar medical need.

Even if it does, the root causes of competition lie elsewhere—in a relatively abundant supply of physicians, particularly of specialists; in excess hospital capacity in many communities; and in a rapid rate of medical discovery and innovation that requires providers to continually make substantial investments so as to keep their practices state of the art. Indeed, even where the available supply of physicians and hospital beds is currently close to actual societal needs, as in many parts of Canada, the changing nature of health care technologies may well create a greater sense of competition among providers as more services formerly within the domain of hospital inpatient programs shift to ambulatory settings, including doctors' offices.

Some of the planning techniques now employed in health care originated in approaches designed and developed within and for government agencies charged with seeking to meet multiple societal needs using a predictable but finite stream of tax revenue. Other planning techniques originated in the approaches to strategic planning and major capital investment analysis of successful commercial businesses whose survival as profit-making enterprises depends upon determining the right corporate response to foreseeable environmental changes. This duality of planning perspective will remain, but the trend to import proven advanced methods from other sectors of the economy may accelerate.

In the United States, in addition to the internal imperatives to reduce risks in decision making by more thorough planning, external sources of capital (e.g., banks, bond-rating agencies, and underwriters) will scutinize the health care organization's plans and planning processes more critically if continued reimbursement reform lowers their operating margins. In an era of rapidly advancing medical technologies and limited societal resources, more stringent standards of justification of institutional plans and capital acquisitions are likely to be adopted. Even in countries, including Canada, where institutional plans and capital investments require government approval, the methods used by regulators to assess project feasibility are likely to be further influenced by the methods used by leading business enterprises.

It is also conceivable that countries other than the United States will experiment with introducing at least some element of provider competition into their health care systems.

Whatever the degree of regulation of the health care system of any country, its providers must also contend with the phenomenon of expanding consumerism. Patients are increasingly convinced that they not only have a right to informed involvement in clinical decisions affecting their own care but are entitled to a certain quality of service and certain amenities. Such expectations may seem at variance with their equally strong interest in cost containment, but consumers do not necessarily accept that fast, high-quality service and moderated rates of price inflation are mutually exclusive goals.

At the same time, government and private payers are demanding that providers demonstrate the quality of their health services by establishing quantifiable and comparable outcome measures and maintaining appropriate databases. As data on the interrelation-

ship of costs, service standards, quality, and clinical outcomes increase and multiply, health marketing will be challenged to develop effective and ethical methods to communicate such information truthfully to payers and the larger public.

Health marketing must also adapt to advances in communication technology, which is changing as rapidly as medical technology. The continuing decline in the number and readership of newspapers, the continuing proliferation but relatively high failure rate of new special-interest magazines, the fall in network TV audiences, the uncertain future scope of cable TV, the potential telecommunications revolution that could ensue from a fiberoptic cable network or greater access for individuals to telecommunications via satellites, the increased viewing of videotapes, the continuing growth of personal computers, and the emergence of database marketing are current trends that suggest future changes in how clients and client sources will access information.[24]

More stringent standards of truth in marketing are likely to be applied in the health care sector. Historically, there has usually been a delayed response between the emergence of widespread marketing communications in an industry or sector of the economy and the definition (by legislative, judicial, or regulatory bodies) of the boundary between truth and deception in making claims about that category of product or service.

Specific areas of strategic planning and marketing in which greater sophistication may, therefore, be expected include:

- Technology assessment
- Competitive pricing models and methodologies
- Project feasibility assessment models and methodologies
- Building quality into the organization both in its response to consumer expectations and its ability to quantify and describe its comparative clinical performance
- Adapting to rapidly changing mass media technologies that will present new challenges for effective marketing communication

- Maintaining high ethical standards in communications

Whatever changes occur in the mechanisms used to pay hospitals, doctors, and other health providers, the forces of rapid technological innovation, an abundant supply of many health resources, cost containment, and pressures on operating margins will combine to make each health care organization more critically dependent upon the quality of its own strategic planning and marketing.

ADDITIONAL RESOURCES

Health Organizations, Societies, and Agencies

Academy for Health Services Marketing, American Marketing Association, 250 S.Wacker Drive, Chicago, Ill. 60606. 312/648-0536

American Group Practice Association, 1422 Duke Street, Alexandria, Va. 22314. 703/838-0033

American Management Association, 8655 W. Higgins, Chicago, Ill. 60631. 312/693-5511

American Marketing Association, 250 S. Wacker Drive, Chicago, Ill. 60606. 312/648-0536

The Conference Board, 845 3rd Avenue, New York, NY 10022. 212/759-0900

Health Care Advisory Board, 501 C Street, N.E., Washington D.C. 20002. 202/544-2700

Healthcare Forum, 830 Market Street, San Francisco, Calif. 94102. 415/421-8810

Medical Group Management Association, 104 Inverness Terrace E., Englewood, Colo. 80112. 303/799-1111

Society for Healthcare Planning and Marketing, American Hospital Association, 840 North Lake Shore Drive, Suite 5E, Chicago, Ill. 60611. 312/280-6086

Society for Marketing and Public Relations for Healthcare, American Hospital Association, 840 North Lake Shore Drive, Suite 9E, Chicago Ill. 60611. 312/280-6359

Periodicals

American Demographics, PO Box 68, Ithaca, NY 14851. 607/273-6343

Harvard Business Review, Soldiers Field Road, Boston, Mass. 02163. 617/495-6800

Health Care Marketing Report, 3050 Presidential Drive, Suite 111, Atlanta, Ga. 30340. 404/457-6105

Health Care Strategic Management, 770 N. La Salle Street, Suite 701, Chicago, Ill. 60610. 312/943-3200

Health Management Quarterly, The Baxter Foundation, One Baxter Parkway, Deerfield, Ill. 60015. 708/948-4556

Hospitals, American Hospital Publishing, Inc. 737 N. Michigan Avenue, Suite 700, Chicago, Ill. 60611. 312/440-6800

Journal of Health Care Marketing, American Marketing Association, 250 S. Wacker Drive, Chicago, Ill. 60606. 312/648-0536

Journal of Marketing, American Marketing Association, 250 S. Wacker Drive, Chicago, Ill. 60606. 312/648-0536

Modern Healthcare, 965 E. Jefferson, Detroit, Mich. 48207. 313/446-0499

Sloan Management Review, M.I.T. Sloan School of Management, 292 Maine Street, E 38-120, Cambridge, Mass. 02139. 617/253-7170

Books and Articles

American Board of Family Practice. 1987. *Rights and responsibilities, part 2: The changing health consumer and patient/ doctor partnership.* Lexington, Ky. Author.

Brown, M., and B. McCool. 1980. *Multi-hospital systems: Strategies for organization and managment.* Gaithersburg: Aspen.

Coddington, D. (ed.). 1990. *The crisis in health care: Costs, choices and strategies.* San Francisco: Jossey- Bass.

Fisk, T. 1988. What is excellence in health care marketing? *Topics in Health Care Financing:*14 (3).

Griffith, J. 1987. *The well-managed community hospital.* Ann Arbor: Health Administration Press.

Levey, S. and T. McCarthy (eds.). 1977. *Health management for tomorrow.* Philadelphia: J.B. Lippincott.

Meterko, M., E. Nelson, and H. Rubin (eds.). 1990. Patient judgements of hospital quality. *Medical Care,* 28 (9).

Porter, M. 1985. *Competitive advantage.* New York: The Free Press.

Reibstein, D. 1985. *Marketing: Concepts, strategies and decisions.* Englewood Cliffs, NJ : Prentice-Hall.

Tilbury, M., and T. Fisk. 1989. *Marketing and nursing: A contemporary view.* Owings Mills, Md.:Williams & Wilkins.

Vichas, R. 1982. *Complete handbook of profitable market research techniques.* Englewood Cliffs, NJ: Prentice-Hall.

NOTES

1. S. Levey and T. McCarthy, *Health Management for Tomorrow* (Philadelphia: J.B. Lippincott, 1980), 11.

2. J.K. Simon, Marketing the Community Hospital: A Tool for the Beleaguered Administrator, in *Strategic Planning in Health Care Management,* eds. W. Flexner, E. Berkowitz, and M. Brown (Gaithersburg, Md.: Aspen Publishers, 1981), 56.

3. E. Saward, ed., *The Regionalization of Personal Health Services* (New York: PRODIST, 1976).

4. S. Jonas, *Health Care Delivery in the United States* (New York: Springer, 1986).

5. T. Peters and R. Waterman, *In Search of Excellence* (New York: Warner, 1982), pp 318–325.

6. J. Stratton, *Annual Report 1991* (Thomas Jefferson University, Philadelphia, 1991), 1.

7. Health Care Survey, *The Economist,* July 6, 1991, pp. 1–18.

8. T. Levitt, Marketing Myopia, *Harvard Business Review,* July-August 1960, pp. 45–56.

9. L. Hrebiniak and W. Joyce, The Strategic Importance of Marketing Myopia, *Sloan Management Review* 28, no. 1 (1986): 5–14.

10. See, for instance, J. Quinn, Strategic Change: Logical Incrementalism, *Sloan Management Review* 30, no. 4 (1989).

11. M. Porter, *Competitive Strategy* (New York: The Free Press. 1980).

12. Booz, Allen and Hamilton, *New Product Management* (New York: Booz, Allen and Hamilton, 1982).

13. M. Smith, *Pharmaceutical Marketing* (Binghamton, N.Y.: Pharmaceutical Products Press, 1991), 160.

14. J. McCarthy, *Basic Marketing: A Managerial Approach* (Homewood, Ill.: Richard Irwin, 1964), 38–40.

15. P. Kotler, *Marketing Management* (Englewood Cliffs, N.J.: Prentice-Hall, 1972), 44.

16. M. Bradley et al., The Finance/Marketing Interface in Hospitals, *Health Care Strategic Management* 5, no. 5 (1987).

17. P. Kotler, *Marketing Management,* 424–425.

18. D. Reibstein, *Marketing Concepts, Strategies and Decisions* (Englewood Cliffs, N.J.: Prentice-Hall, 1985), 389–391.

19. P. Starr, *The Social Transformation of American Medicine* (New York: Basic Books, 1982).

20. T. Fisk et al., Creating Satisfied and Loyal Patients, *Journal of Health Care Marketing* 10, no. 2 (1990): 5–15.

21. L. Berry and A. Parasuraman, *Marketing Services: Competing through Quality* (New York: The Free Press, 1991), 175.

22. K. Panda, *The Measurement of Cumulative Advertising Effectiveness* (Englewood Cliffs, N.J.: Prentice-Hall, 1964).

23. R. Westbrook, Product Consumption Based upon Effective Responses and Postpurchase Processes, *Journal of Market Research* 14 (1987): 79–81.

24. S. Brand, *The Media Lab: Inventing the Future at MIT* (New York: Viking Penguin, 1987).

Part IV

Resource Management

Laura Avakian

Human Resource Management

18

Purpose: The purpose of the human resources department is to enhance the quality of the institution's services by hiring and contracting with qualified staff; developing its leadership; recommending strategies for organizational effectiveness; and fostering employee satisfaction, teamwork, fairness, legal compliance, and productivity in the work environment.

THE FUNCTIONS OF THE HUMAN RESOURCES DEPARTMENT

The management of human resources is the responsibility of every manager and supervisor in the organization. It is the human resources department's role to serve as a consultant to the organization's leadership and its line managers and to help them perform their role in directing the work of staff. In this capacity, the human resources department is responsible for the following functions:

- *Recruitment and Placement.* The purpose of this process is to identify candidates for available positions. Employment staff conduct re-

cruitment and advertising programs and facilitate internal promotions and transfers.

- *Pay and Benefits Administration.* Direct and indirect compensation must be delivered in ways that are legal, are internally equitable, and keep the organization competitive with other employers. Performance appraisal and incentive pay programs also need to be developed and monitored.

- *Labor Relations.* In organizations with collective bargaining agreements, the department is involved in the negotiation and administration of union contracts. In nonunion organizations, the department provides counseling, supervisory training in fair employment practices, and assistance in the internal resolution of employee grievances.

- *Legal Compliance.* The department must ensure that federal state laws and regulations concerning pay, benefits, conditions of employment, and the safety and rights of workers are complied with.

- *Effective Management of the Changing Workplace.* The department develops programs and processes that elicit and resp[...] opinions, enhance internal [...] unications, create a positive work environment, and recognize employee accomplishments.

- *Work Force Planning, Employee Education, and Career Development.* Based on the organization's future staffing needs and the availability of workers, the department may need to establish linkages with schools and vocational programs in addition to creating in-house training programs and career paths and supporting job-related external education. It also must develop and conduct supervisory and leadership training programs.

MANAGEMENT PRINCIPLES

In directing the human resources of the organization, managers accept responsibility for adhering to these principles:

- Management should ensure that there is sufficient staff to perform the work, the employees are given reasonable workloads, the performance expectations are reasonable, and the employees have the resources to do their jobs properly.
- Compensation and benefits programs must be competitive, meaningful to employees, and appropriate to the organization's financial position and objectives.
- Any contract governing employee matters should be adhered to in the spirit as well as the letter of the agreement.
- Interpersonal and organizational problems should be given attention and resolved in ways that are legal, positive, and timely.
- Individuals should be treated fairly, and the organizational climate should promote dignity, courtesy, and respect.
- Cultural diversity should be valued and respected in addressing particular issues that arise in regard to certain segments of the work

[...].g., people of color, older workers, parents, women, disabled, illiterate, and non-English-speaking workers).

- The organization should establish standards for and evaluate the quality and efficiency of employees' work and ensure that processes are in place for continuous improvement and reward.
- Management should educate and develop employees to keep pace with changing technology and to maximize the talents of the work force.

ORGANIZATIONAL ROLE AND FUNCTION

The Role of the Human Resources Department

The human resources department, whose responsibilities were traditionally restricted to record-keeping and payroll monitoring, now plays a multidimensional role in the development of strategies for addressing change (see Table 18-1). It plays a major role, for example, in advancing employee productivity and quality management in ways that enhance work life and contribute positively to the bottom line. Human resources professionals are now called upon to participate in the planning of innovative and cost-effective programming. Additionally, they are functioning more as consultants and facilitators as multisite organizations seek centralization of policies and as community linkages grow in importance.

The vice-president of human resources brings a unique perspective to organizational decision making. He or she offers expert opinion, based on data and analyses, on such things as the costs of changes in labor distribution or the impact of changes on employee morale. The human resources leader is also knowledgeable about the organization's finances, mission, facilities plans, and corporate structure. Today's human resources leader is a "big picture" thinker, a true peer of other health care administrators.

Although human resources has found its way into the board room as a partner in the strategic

Table 18-1 Hospital Personnel Management Models

	Simple Personnel Model (pre-1965)	Labor Relations Model (1965–1975)	Human Resource Model (1975–1985)	Matrix Model (1985 to early 1990s)
Approach to Personnel Management	Benign neglect Indifference	Containment of external forces	Human resources perspective (emphasis on people as the most important resource)	Modified human resources perspective
Role	Recordkeeping	Cope	Intervention (for change)	Intervention (for organizational survival)
Process	Simple functional (not integrated)	Fully functional	Integrative functional	Creative functional
Organizational Philosophy about Employees	Neutral (employees are just another resource)	Conflict and confrontation	Collaborative-cooperative (organization and employees have mutual interests)	Competitive-participative
Predominant Strategy	Inactive compliance	Reactive	Proactive	Innovative
Influence on Organizational Policy	Minimal	Increasing	Enhanced	Greater
Acceptance by Managers and Staff	Minimal	Necessary	Enhanced	Greater

Source: Reprinted from *Hospital and Health Services Administration,* Vol. 31, p. 26, with permission of Health Administration Press, © 1986, Foundation of the American College of Healthcare Executives.

management of the organization, it has not abandoned its responsibilities to maintain records, develop pay policy, and solve labor relations problems. On the contrary, human resources staff must be more knowledgeable than ever in each area of specialization.

Whereas once the delivery of each program or policy was an end in itself, the contemporary human resources department integrates its services and approaches with those of the larger organization's systems and mission. As an example, a hospital's decision to expand its ambulatory services may be strongly influenced, if not determined, by the availability of nurses or other staff; the costs of recruitment, wages, and training; or the effects of the expansion on the morale and retention of current employees. Analyzing these issues and making recommendations about possible approaches are appropriate tasks to assign to human resources staff. Although such functions as recruiting nurses or determining salary costs are not new to human resources, this kind of forecasting and integration with business planning is a far more sophisticated activity than was expected of personnel departments in the past. The organization chart in Figure 18-1 shows a common arrangement of key human resources functions.

The top human resources manager in a health care organization today typically reports to the chief executive officer or chief operating officer. He or she is usually one of five to ten key administrators forming the principal leadership group of the institution. In organizations that use corporate titles, the head of human resources is typically a vice-president or senior vice-president.

As a partner with other senior administrators, the human resources manager looks at the new challenges faced by the health care industry: greater financial risk, greater competition, diversification, downsizing, mergers, and alternative delivery systems. As the authors of a recent article state,

The personnel function will be increasingly called on to support new strategic initiatives. These will include implementation of human resources acquisition and maintenance programs to ensure an adequate supply of labor, both in terms of quantity and skills, as well as outplacement of displaced workers. The personnel function will be a partner in the formulation of such strategies and will be required to focus on labor productivity and organizational climate as it relates to overall productivity. It will be given the task of integrating the hospital's human resources into the new organizational structures and work systems. This change will be a challenge, requiring a more sophisticated personnel function.[1]

TASKS AND RESPONSIBILITIES

Recruitment and Placement

Once the organization's position complement—the number of jobs and the types of work needed to be performed—is established, the human resources

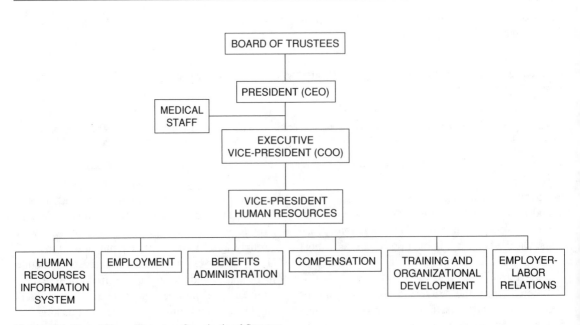

Figure 18-1 Typical Human Resources Organizational Structure

department plays a critical role in seeing that these positions are appropriately staffed. Following are the tasks performed by the human resources staff in fulfilling this role.

Staffing Planning

On a periodic basis, the employment specialists within human resources assist line managers in developing strategies for meeting anticipated staffing requirements. Armed with data about the projected supply of health care workers, employment staff can develop a plan that targets recruitment of particular specialists and identifies the most likely and cost-effective sources of potential applicants. This activity is an important component of a health care institution's strategic planning. The availability and affordability of nurses, radiology technicians, cardiac perfusionists, or other skilled workers could make a significant difference in an organization's decision or timetable for expansion or redesign of patient services. Where severe labor shortages are predicted, the staffing plan may call for alternative strategies for meeting the organization's needs, such as redesigning jobs, developing internal training programs, or forging alliances with external agencies or schools to do skills training. Data on available workers may be obtained from the U.S. Department of Labor, the American Hospital Association, and various professional societies.

Recruitment

Given the increasing demand for health services, there is an ongoing need to recruit workers into health care jobs and students into various fields of relevant study. To fill existing vacant positions or those where turnover is high, human resources staff develop advertisements for local or area newspapers, professional journals, and, with increasing frequency, radio and television. The recruitment staff of most hospitals maintain ongoing relationships with area vocational and technical schools and colleges that train health care specialists. Such schools often have career fairs, interview days,

placement offices, and other means of connecting students to potential employers. Another popular recruitment tactic is to hold an open house. A hospital, for example, might invite nurses, secretaries, or other job seekers to a reception where they could meet prospective coworkers and tour the facilities.

In times of extreme labor shortages, a number of employers have tried bold, attention-getting recruitment tactics, such as paying "bounties" to current employees who refer others for hire, paying moving expenses or signing bonuses, or offering paid vacations, cars, and other perquisites to new hires. These programs can be problematic, because they treat some employees in a privileged fashion and are difficult to retreat from once the shortage crisis is past.

As aids to planning, employment staff generally maintain records of responses to advertisements and recruitment events. They also perform cost-per-hire analyses to ensure that their efforts are as cost-effective as possible. Conducting exit interviews with employees leaving the organization, particularly those who leave with less than one year's service, can be valuable in determining effective recruitment and retention strategies.

Promotion and Transfer Programs

It has become customary to post publicly a notice internally that a job is available, thereby giving current employees an opportunity to apply before outside applicants are considered. Job posting is an effective means of identifying capable individuals who can present themselves as candidates and who might otherwise be overlooked in a more informal process. Job posting also helps an organization meet its affirmative action obligations, since it provides a fair, objective selection process rather than permitting arbitrary promotions. With this system, women and people of color are given greater opportunities for advancement. A job-posting program loses credibility if supervisors are allowed to bypass the process in promoting favorite employees or if a number of employees are repeatedly rejected when they bid for jobs. This kind of program is most effective when interviewers are skilled at career counseling and when time limits, reference checks, and other program mechanisms are used consistently and in a professional manner.

Career Ladders

Career ladders are formal programs that grant employees more pay and recognition for taking on new duties and responsibilities as they gain proficiency in their jobs. Progression up the ladder is generally contingent upon an individual's acquiring additional formal education, participating in workshops and on committees, serving as a preceptor or mentor to junior staff, perhaps doing original research or publishing, or otherwise demonstrating new skills. Career ladders are prevalent in nursing departments but are also used by other health professionals such as medical technologists, radiology technicians, pharmacists, and social workers. Human resources staff work with line managers in the design of such programs to ensure that the responsibilities at each rung of the ladder are sufficiently differentiated to justify different levels of pay. They also advise on the promotion process, ways of giving recognition, and the process for appealing a promotion decision.

Supplemental Staffing

When an organization has large numbers of vacancies or an activity level that requires additional staff, the human resources department may be called upon to locate temporary or supplemental staff. In most parts of the country, there are agencies that supply nurses, technicians, secretaries, laborers, and others on a per diem or project basis. Because agencies usually receive premium rates, many hospitals have developed in-house pools of workers on-call for temporary assignment. Not only are the rates of pay less than for agency workers, but in-house pool workers have the advantage of already knowing the practices and procedures of the organization and tend to have a greater degree of commitment than agency workers. The human

resources department ensures that pay and benefit policies are appropriately designed and administered and that work records and evaluations are maintained.

Alternative Work Arrangements

Due to shortages of needed personnel and to workers' changing life styles and expectations, health care organizations have begun to try a wide variety of scheduling and staffing methods. Fairly common now are workweeks consisting of four 10-hour shifts or three 12-hour shifts. One also may find many hospitals using variable schedules that include incentives for working shifts considered less desirable by staff. One common example is a plan that provides nurses who work 24 hours on the weekend with a pay and benefits package equivalent to that of nurses who work 40-hour weekday schedules. There are many variations on this theme. Nursing units certainly use variable schedules; however, laboratories, radiology departments, and other units that must staff evening, night, or weekend shifts have also begun to experiment with creative schedules.

Health care has long relied on part-time workers. However, new variations of part-time work are being utilized, such as job sharing, where two employees split the responsibilities of a single full-time position and also share the benefits afforded full-time workers. Job sharing differs from regular part-time jobs in that there is more coordination and cross-coverage. Work-at-home programs are also being tried—typically with jobs such as medical transcription or other computer or clerical work that can be done at another location if the equipment can be set up appropriately. Human resources departments design, facilitate, and administer such programs. However, new options are often generated by workers who have a particular scheduling need. Creating a climate of innovation and willingness to experiment may be the human resources department's greatest contribution to the flexible work arrangements as components of the employment system.

Pay and Benefits Administration

Health care organizations in the United States typically spend in excess of 50 percent of operating dollars on employee pay and benefits. Compensation is also a critical factor influencing employees' perceptions of the organization's fairness, and it is a key determinant for many job applicants in considering a new position. Pay and benefits administration is governed by extensive regulation and legislation and is monitored by a variety of government agencies. For all these reasons, the planning and administration of compensation programs is one of the most important functions of the human resources department.

Designing Pay and Benefit Programs

In simpler times, health care employers could determine pay practices by surveying area hospitals and checking on the movement of the consumer price index (CPI) once a year. These days, planning is more sophisticated and requires long-term strategies. Many organizations begin the process by defining a compensation philosophy. As an example, an organization may decide that it is appropriate to establish pay levels at the 75th percentile of the local health care market and to make individual pay increases contingent upon meritorious performance. Organizations continue to look at what their competitors pay, but they also see compensation as a strategy for ensuring competence and achievement of goals. In other words, they examine their mission and their financial objectives and then determine the kinds of reward systems that fit their particular philosophy and purposes. For some, incentive systems may be appropriate; for others, such systems could create tensions, be unaffordable, or be inconsistent with the organizational culture. Such factors as union contracts, union organizing activity, and economic downturns also affect an institution's compensation strategy.

Administration of Pay Programs

Once an organization's approach to compensation has been determined, two broad considerations typically influence the administration of the pay program: external competitiveness and internal equity.

External competitiveness is gauged by examining the competition (i.e., the organizations seeking to hire the same individuals or to entice away current employees) and going rates for jobs, including how quickly those rates are changing.

To investigate the competition, the compensation staff, working with recruiters and line managers, review the sources of applicants and hires. They may also look at data from exit interviews and other documents such as opinion surveys. Anecdotal information from employees and job applicants is important because the reputation an organization acquires for being a high payer or a poor payer strongly influences an individual's job decisions—even if that reputation does not correlate with reality.

Given the complexity of health care institutions today, they not surprisingly must consider many different markets whose pay practices are of interest. An organization will naturally look at similar, comparably sized organizations in the same geographical area to determine the wage rates paid to health care workers. However, it may also define the competitive market for pharmacists as including commercial pharmacies and pharmaceutical manufacturers. It may also want to see what insurance companies, banks, and other kinds of service companies are paying business office staff. The defined marketplace for computer analysts and operators may include area high-tech industries and so on. Geography may be a determinant as well. An organization may look at regional or national surveys for data on managerial, executive, or physician pay if the recruitment area is broader.

Once the markets of interest are defined, compensation specialists use survey instruments to capture the relevant data. Consulting firms and professional societies often supply surveys; others may be initiated by an individual organization. Such surveys range from comprehensive surveys covering many jobs to an informal "calling around" to determine current rates for a single job. Surveys are generally designed to provide information on benchmark positions—those that can be cleanly compared from one organization to another on the basis of similar job requirements and scope of responsibility. Positions such as "radiographer," "staff nurse," "data-entry clerk," and "medical records coder" are examples of benchmark jobs for many hospitals. Single incumbent jobs, such as "assistant to the director of marketing," or jobs that are not defined by their titles, such as "financial specialist," are usually omitted from surveys, since there may be no clear market or the information could be inaccurate or misleading.

The information one receives on benchmark jobs typically includes the minimum pay rate (sometimes called the starting rate) for a given job, the maximum pay rate, and the weighted average (the average of what incumbents in that job are actually being paid). From looking at high and low payers and at the averages for a given market, compensation specialists may then determine how they want to position their organization as a payer within that market. Because there is no one right rate of pay, it is important for an organization to articulate its philosophy or approach to compensation (e.g., aggressive or conservative, an average payer or "among the top five teaching hospitals," etc.). Articulating general guidelines can contribute to the creation of a targeted and more effective and competitive pay program.

Internal equity is an important concept, because the morale of an organization is frequently influenced by employees' perceptions of fairness of treatment, particularly in relation to pay. Whether pay rates are made public or not, employees generally know what each others' salaries are, and great distrust and unhappiness will surface if internal differences do not seem to correlate with clear differences in levels of job responsibility or requirements. A pay system that is seemingly arbitrary or that favors certain jobs or individuals may also lead to discrimination charges or a review by the U.S. Department of Labor.

To ensure themselves—and external auditing groups as well—that pay rates are equitable, employers typically use some form of job evaluation system to provide a basis for comparing positions. Formal job evaluation systems rank positions based on a variety of factors common to all jobs. The factors usually include the amount and kind of education required, the amount and kind of experience required, the degree of decision making, the consequence of making errors, the amount of responsibility for others' actions and results, the number of individuals supervised, and the extent of responsibility for budgets.

Smaller organizations may use fairly simple ranking methods to determine pay equity. Most larger health care institutions, however, have somewhat more elaborate mechanisms, often some form of point-classification system. In this kind of system, a given job is assigned a certain number of points for each factor, depending on its complexity and amount of responsibility. The total points accumulated from a review of all factors determine the classification of the job and its relationship to other positions. Jobs with similar point values are then grouped together in a single pay grade, and compensation specialists assign a salary range (i.e., minimum and maximum earnable amounts), making sure that pay relationships between job grades are appropriate.

One ongoing compensation responsibility is the evaluation of new jobs or the reclassifying of existing jobs if the duties change. This is done by reviewing a job description or questionnaire completed by the manager of the department where the job exists. The manager or the incumbent in the job may also be interviewed. Some organizations use job evaluation committees to assign the points or review the compensation analyst's recommendation.

Pay ranges are examined on a regular basis, generally annually, unless labor market conditions force a more frequent look. It is sometimes necessary to establish "market" or "exception" pay ranges for jobs when the going rates in the market are inconsistent with the range one would normally assign in order to maintain internal consistency among pay ranges. Such ranges should be viewed as temporary, and efforts should be made to get the salaries realigned relative to others in the job evaluation system.

Performance and Incentive Compensation

In addition to determining a base salary derived from job evaluation and market surveying, organizations often seek some means of rewarding individual competence and achievement. Some have "merit pay" systems that acknowledge varying levels of performance by employees with the same job expectations. Others offer "incentive pay" systems that grant additional compensation if employees reach performance targets beyond those that would be normally expected. Where jobs are covered by a collective bargaining agreement, individual pay raises are likely to be granted more for longevity than for merit, and the timing of such increases is established in the union contract. Where the contracts do not prescribe individual salary increases, raises may be granted based on pay-for-performance systems. At a predetermined time—often on the anniversary date of hire or at the conclusion of the fiscal year—the manager conducts a performance appraisal meeting with the employee and discusses the extent to which his or her performance has met previously established expectations and what goals have been achieved.

This conference is often used to set new goals or targets for the coming year and to identify what new skills, education, or experience the employee will need to fulfill the coming demands of the job. The rating on the performance evaluation guides the manager in deciding an appropriate pay increase.

The role of compensation specialists is to put forth guidelines for determining raises, taking into consideration the hospital's budget and organization-wide performance measures and objectives. Human resources staff also develop performance appraisal instruments and train managers to conduct meaningful performance reviews. Such training should communicate the expectation that the managers will give regular feedback and provide ongoing guidance to help employees achieve agreed objectives. A performance plan that comes out of a desk drawer only at annual review time will not be effective. The Joint Commission on Accreditation of Healthcare Organizations has established standards for review mechanisms to ensure that employees are rated and paid on their performance of job-specific criteria and not for ambiguous or irrelevant factors such as personality or appearance.[2]

Group Compensation

Increasingly popular are forms of group compensation. Bonuses or other kinds of rewards to a group of employees who collectively achieve goals or do a project exceptionally well can reinforce the importance of teamwork and promote collaboration in identifying and solving problems.

Gainsharing is a form of group compensation in which an amount of money is shared across an entire organization when certain budget objectives are exceeded. It is similar to profit-sharing in for-profit companies in that financial surpluses are shared with the employees based on a predetermined formula. Gainsharing differs, however, in that the amounts shared are not derived from the overall profitability of the company but are calculated based on productivity improvement that may come from cost savings achieved through worker efficiency or through improved quality. Gainsharing relies on some process of worker involvement in helping the organization achieve its goals and requires that employees are given sufficient information and support to influence financial and qualitative outcomes on an organization-wide basis.

Although still experimental in the health care setting, gainsharing plans like Rucker plans or Scanlon plans, which have been used in manufacturing industries for decades, are being tried in a variety of service sector areas, including hospitals.[3] A *Modern Healthcare* article reported that 11 percent of 618 hospitals surveyed have such incentive plans and 29 percent plan to start them.[4] They appeal to organizations that believe there is ample opportunity for continuous productivity and quality improvement and that workers, if appropriately empowered, will make suggestions for changes that benefit patients and the organization. Such plans appear to work best in places with strong cultures that foster employee participation and teamwork.

Gainsharing does not replace base compensation but offers the opportunity for some periodic monetary reward—generally paid in bonus form—as an incentive for achieving efficiencies and offering suggestions.

Benefits Administration

Fringe benefits are an important part of an individual's total compensation. Administering benefit plans has become an increasingly complex task for human resources staffs because the costs of such programs have escalated and the amount of government regulation has grown enormously. Further, because the demographics of the North American labor force have shifted to include more women and more dual-income families, traditional benefit plans do not meet the needs of many workers. Benefits administrators are responding with more contemporary plans.

Health and welfare benefits remain at the core of most programs. These include some forms of health insurance, life insurance, accidental death coverage, and sick pay or disability insurance. Retirement plans are generally provided by health care employers. And, of course, holiday and vacation pay have been standard fare as benefits for some time. Either as a result of union contract negotiation or a desire to add a competitive element, some employers provide such benefits as dental insurance and optical insurance; programs to assist with mortgage or student loans, legal expenses, or automobile and other transportation costs; and tuition reimbursement for job-related education. Many offer tax-deferred annuity programs and credit union affiliations.

Some organizations include as fringe benefits such offerings as employee assistance programs, which make counseling and referrals available to employees who have personal problems affecting their work; health promotion or wellness programs; recreational activities; preretirement counseling; and employee picnics or group outings to sport events.

It is more prevalent now for organizations to assist their employees with child care arrangements.

A comprehensive study of work force trends and issues showed that over one-third of the businesses surveyed offer programs to ease conflicts arising from work- and family-related problems.[5] Examples include child care referral systems, use of sick days to care for sick children or parents, and flexible spending accounts.

Hospitals have been pioneers in the development of onsite child care centers and the provision of assistance in subsidizing child care.[6] Although their efforts may have been in response to the changing needs of workers and the shortage of health professionals such as nurses and therapists, many organizations find that helping with child care gives them a competitive advantage in recruiting and retaining staff.

Programs to assist employees in the care of elders are also gaining attention. These may include information and referral services or leaves of absence to assist aging parents.

"Flexible benefits" or "cafeteria plans" have become popular because they provide companies with an affordable way to deal with the varied needs and desires of workers. Essentially, a flex plan offers a menu of options from which employees may choose different types and levels of benefits. Generally, such plans provide some core benefits—perhaps an individual health insurance plan with a deductible feature, a life insurance benefit equal to one year of pay, and a long-term disability plan providing 60 percent of annual compensation during the disability period. This core plan would have a dollar value and be provided to the employee at no cost. However, the employee might wish to select different levels of coverage—either more or less, depending on age, marital status, cost, or any variety of reasons—or purchase additional benefits. To extend the earlier example, an employee might opt for no health insurance if already covered by a spouse's plan and receive cash or benefits credits instead. That employee then might select a long-term disability plan providing compensation equal to twice the employee's annual salary. Additionally, he or she might opt for a family dental plan and a short-term disability policy and set aside money in a pretax reimbursement account to be used for child care expenses.

Cafeteria plans can benefit both employees and employers. Employees, obviously, are able to select benefits that are personally meaningful. Employers are able to add choices to the menu because the employees are paying for them at advantageous group rates.

Clearly, flex plans require extensive communication from benefits staff as well as cogent, accurate written materials that explain the options and consequences of selection. The administration of such a program takes more time, and employees must assume more responsibility for these benefits than under traditional programs.

Another innovation that extends the notion of partnership and shared responsibility between company and employee is "earned time" or "paid time off." In a paid-time-off program, each employee is granted a "bank" of paid hours from which he or she draws to receive pay during absences for any reason. The banked hours, accrued on a weekly or biweekly basis, may be expended in return for sick time, vacation, or holiday pay, as in traditional programs, but they can also be used when a child is ill, for any unplanned emergency, or for any other personal reason, planned or unplanned. Such programs often have provisions for cashing in hours rather than taking the time off. These programs are often perceived by employees to be fairer than typical sick-pay programs, since everyone is treated equally and no one is penalized for being healthy. They offer flexibility and promote trusting relationships. As accrued time-off benefits do affect an organization's balance sheet, however, employers must be careful to monitor the amounts carried forward from year to year. Like flex plans, paid-time-off programs require greater communication and new methods of administration.

The Future of Fringe Benefits

Fringe benefits, as a "second paycheck," continue to be important. Even more than salary, they are a maneuverable part of compensation that can be adapted to fit an organization's values and strategies. Benefits can significantly impact recruitment and retention, particularly since an employer can design specific programs targeted to appeal to doctors, executives, nurses, or service workers.

The IRS and other government entities have an increasing interest in benefit programs as well. One reason is the enormous potential revenue that could be generated if benefits were subject to taxation. Vast amounts of regulation in recent years have been directed toward issues of potential discrimination in the design and implementation of health and welfare plans. Retirement programs are undergoing major redesign due to government concern about plans that discriminate in favor of highly paid individuals but also because employees' work and retirement patterns have shifted, requiring new thinking about retirement benefits. With many older people in the work force and many who have changed jobs a number of times, there is no longer a clear definition of normal retirement, and many Americans are without sufficient savings to sustain them for a long period without income in an inflationary era. What are the roles and responsibilities of the government, the employer, and the individual? These are all being re-examined, and inevitably there will be more legislation and more costs affecting all concerned.

In the meantime, the creative design and application of fringe benefits can give health care organizations an advantage in attracting and satisfying workers.

LEGAL AND CONTRACTUAL RESPONSIBILITIES

Labor Contract Administration

Status of Union Organizing in Health Care

Since 1974, when health care employees were given the right to organize and bargain collectively for wages and benefits under the National Labor Relations Act (NLRA), about 20 percent of health care workers have joined unions. About the same percentage of U.S. hospitals have one or more bargaining units.[7] Most of the union organizing activity occurred in the late 1970s and early 1980s, and organizing activity has been on the decline ever since. In 1981 there were 206 elections held in hospitals, whereas in 1985 there were only 62.[8] The rate of union victories has remained fairly constant, however, with around 55 percent of elections being won by unions.[9]

There are indications that union activity may increase, however. The recent National Labor Relations Board (NLRB) rule that established eight categories of hospital workers as separate bargaining units is perceived as an opportunity for significant gains for unions.[10] The economic climate and the uncertainty of health care financing may also motivate employees to seek the protections promised by organized labor. These conditions will serve to exacerbate an organization's vulnerability to unionization. However, unions are still most likely to target organizations that have weak, insensitive supervision and arbitrary, inconsistent practices concerning pay, promotions, and grievance resolution.

The Role of Human Resources in Labor Relations

Where unions have successfully organized a segment of workers, human resources staff need to be specialists in collective bargaining and contract administration. Understanding the applicable laws, advising managers on appropriate actions relative to unionized employees, and maintaining effective union and employee relations are part of the labor specialist's role.

In the unionized organization, a key labor relations responsibility is negotiating the contract on behalf of the employer. Other key responsibilities include preparing the organization to handle work stoppages or strikes, administering the contract on a day-to-day basis, and dealing with grievances and arbitration. All of these are discussed below.

In a nonunionized setting, human resources staff must also be familiar with labor law and know legal, effective ways to respond to union organizing

attempts. When organizing efforts are underway, employee relations staff need to educate supervisors regarding their responsibilities according to the NLRA. In nonunionized organizations, key employee relations tasks include developing supervisory policies and writing employee handbooks that define fair treatment and the rules of the organization. Many of the policies are similar to those found in union contracts. The handbooks delineate conditions under which employees may be laid off, disciplined, or discharged and include policies on such subjects as overtime, uniforms, and lunch and break periods.

Many nonunionized institutions have developed grievance procedures that provide an opportunity for an employee to challenge a manager's decision. Some provide binding arbitration as the final step in the process, as do many union contracts; others place the final decision with the chief executive officer or a committee of managers and peers. Unlike union stewards, employee relations staff do not take sides in a grievance, but they may help the employee prepare a written position statement and may help the supervisors articulate their responses. They are the facilitators, ensuring that the process is timely, objective, and nonretaliatory.

Negotiating the Labor Contract

After an election has been held and a union is certified as the bargaining agent for a unit of workers, the employer and the union are obligated by law to meet and to participate in "good faith" bargaining. The duty to bargain does not constitute a duty to agree, however; and it is not uncommon during the negotiation process for both parties to accuse each other of bad faith bargaining when there is refusal to yield to the other's position. The NLRB reviews any formal allegations of refusal to bargain in good faith and determines whether unfair labor practices have occurred.

The NLRA defines the subject areas that must be negotiated: "rates of pay, wages, hours, or other conditions of employment." A number of NLRB and court rulings have resulted in the inclusion of a additional bargaining issues (Exhibit 18-1).

Exhibit 18-1 Union Contract Negotiation Issues

- Discharge
- Suspension
- Layoff
- Recall
- Seniority
- Discipline
- Promotion, demotion, and transfer
- Assignment within bargaining unit
- Safety
- Health practices
- Hours of work and overtime
- Vacations
- Holidays
- Leaves of absence
- Sick time and other benefits

As part of the bargaining process, the union will seek to include some provision in the contract that will require mandatory membership in the union. Such a clause offers security to the union. Contracts vary on the forms of union security included. Generally, the contract will have either an "open shop" provision, which gives employees the choice of joining or not joining the union, or a "union shop" provision, which requires all employees in the bargaining unit to join the union within a specified period of time after hire. Variations of these membership provisions occasionally occur, and states may have laws mandating certain membership requirements.

Just as unions seek to ensure maximum union security, management generally attempts to include a strong "management rights" provision in the contract. Sometimes such clauses are detailed, including specific rights of managers to hire, fire, determine job standards, and eliminate jobs. More often, they are as broad as possible to provide the latitude to take actions not specifically prohibited in the agreement.

Preparing for a Strike

The U. S. Congress recognized that a strike in a hospital or other patient care institution could create great concern, distress, and potential danger to patients and their families. In amending the NLRA

in 1974, it required that a union give management ten days' written notice of its intent to engage in a strike, picketing, or other work stoppage. Labor relations staff, however, should anticipate long before such threat occurs what the impact of a strike would be and help the organization prepare for it.

A written plan to deal with a strike situation should consider the following:

- whether the organization has the desire and ability to hire replacement workers
- the effects on nonunion workers and people in the community (are they likely to sympathize more with the striking employees or the hospital?)
- the organization's ability to transfer patients safely and legally to another facility
- issues of security—for employees, patients, visitors, and deliverers of goods
- the rearrangement of support services within the organization
- the length of time the organization can sustain operations and the length of time union members can likely stay out of work
- medical staff issues—their allegiances and concerns about income and their patients' safety

Administering the Contract

Once a union contract is in place, it is generally the responsibility of human resources staff to see that all agreements regarding wage actions and changes in benefits are implemented. They must inform others in the organization of any changes the contract might require in the management of employees. Since the contract deals with issues of discipline and discharge, human resources staff must advise supervisors on the appropriate process to be used in these matters and the kind of written documentation that is necessary.

Although the issues that lead to employee grievances may be similar in both union and nonunion institutions, there can be significant differences in their resolution. This is often true because the union representative, who views his or her role to be a vigorous defendant of the employees, will pursue any matter to the point where the head of labor relations, as representative of the hospital administration, must become involved—and even sometimes to the point of arbitration. A typical grievance process calls for a review of the challenged decision by the immediate supervisor and the next-level manager before the matter is taken to the labor relations official and is presented for arbitration. Union representatives, sometimes called shop stewards, will often seek to shortcut the steps and go directly to human resources staff with the aggrieved employee. Management may support this collapsed process if, in fact, labor relations staff have advised the supervisor on the action in the first place.

When management and union officials fail to come to agreement on the resolution of a grievance, it may be submitted to an outside arbitrator. Most contracts have this kind of provision so that both may be assured of an impartial review of the case. Generally, both the union and management review a list of arbitrators from the American Arbitration Association and agree on an individual to hear the case. The arbitrator's decision is final and binding on all parties.

Decertification

There are times when employees of a given bargaining unit may feel they are not well represented by the union that has organized them and may seek to abolish the union relationship altogether or join another union. The process of decertification is the same as the initial certification process: At least 30 percent of the employees in a bargaining unit must petition the NLRB to call an election, and a majority of those voting in the election must then vote for decertification if it is to occur. The NLRA specifies a window of time prior to contract expiration when a decertification petition may be filed.

Legal Compliance

Many federal and state statutes constrain an employer's actions relative to hiring, pay, benefits, and conditions of work. It is incumbent upon the human resources staff to know the laws and advise the organization accordingly to ensure that its employment practices are consistent with legal requirements. This section cites some of the more comprehensive federal laws that govern various aspects of employment in the United States. Additional information is presented in Chapter 27.

Equal Employment Opportunity and Other Discrimination Laws

Title VII of the Civil Rights Act of 1964 prohibits discrimination by an employer on the basis of race, color, religion, sex, national origin, or reprisal. Health care employers who are federal contractors also have affirmative action obligations imposed by Executive Order 11246. This order requires employers to take deliberate targeted actions to hire women and people of color so that the work force reflects the sexual and racial composition of the community. Appropriate records must be maintained that document these actions as well as those that affect the promotion, transfer, termination, and pay of women and people of color relative to other employees.

Job applicants and employees who are at least 40 years old are protected from discrimination on the basis of age in accordance with the Age Discrimination in Employment Act of 1967.

Discrimination against handicapped individuals is prohibited by the Americans with Disabilities Act, passed in July 1990. This act is more comprehensive in scope than previously enacted statutes on this subject (the Rehabilitation Act of 1973, sections 503 and 504).

The Vietnam Era Veterans Readjustment Assistance Act provides re-employment rights to an employee who leaves work to serve in the armed forces, and it also requires affirmative action by federal contractors in the employment of Vietnam era veterans.

The Immigration Reform and Control Act contains provisions regarding the authorization of immigrants and aliens to work in the United States. Employers are required to complete I-9 forms when immigrants and aliens are hired, and nondiscrimination provisions are also included.

The National Labor Relations Act prevents employers from discriminating against individuals who participate in unions or engage in protected concerted activity or who file charges or give testimony.

A number of other statutes prohibit retaliation and discrimination against employees for the exercise of rights under federal and state laws.

Laws Relating to Pay and Benefits

The Fair Labor Standards Act governs an organization's pay practices. It established the standard workweek to be 40 hours and provides tests for determining whether an employee is eligible for overtime pay (defined as one and a half times the regular hourly rate) for hours worked in excess of 40 in one week. Some jobs, including some paid on a salaried basis, are exempt from the overtime provision.

Employers are also required to follow federal minimum wage determinations. The U.S. Department of Labor issues information about minimum wage rates.

Comprehensive regulations affecting pension and welfare benefits are mandated by the Employee Retirement Income Security Act (ERISA), which was passed in 1974. Broadly defined, pension plans are those that provide some form of retirement income to employees, and welfare plans are insurances or other benefits available to participants or their beneficiaries in event of death, sickness, disability, or unemployment. Benefits such as vacation pay, leave-of-absence pay, employee discounts, and onsite recreation are among those excluded from ERISA coverage. ERISA addresses fiduciary responsibilities and sets forth reporting and disclosure requirements, participation rules, funding standards, and compliance and enforcement regulations.

Also affecting pension plans is the Tax Reform Act of 1986. The object of this legislation is to bring even-handedness to the provision of retirement benefits for high-paid and low-paid employees. In addition to requiring that certain tests be performed to determine compliance with its nondiscrimination provisions, this act also affects the tax-sheltered annuity plans made available to staff of nonprofit organizations.

The Comprehensive Omnibus Budget and Reconciliation Act (COBRA) requires employers to extend group health insurance plans to employees and covered dependents in certain circumstances for a period of time after coverage would ordinarily have ended. The qualifying circumstances are termination; the employee's death, divorce, or legal separation; the spouse's entitlement to Medicare; and the loss of dependency status of dependent children.

Laws Regarding Unionization and Collective Bargaining

The National Labor Relations Act, as amended, grants employees the right to organize and engage in concerted activity for the purpose of collective bargaining or other mutual aid or protection. Employers are specifically prohibited from interfering with these employee rights and from otherwise discriminating against employees in order to either encourage or discourage membership in a labor union. Hospital employees have been covered under the act since 1974. Although its provisions are most often considered in relation to union activity, the protection of the act extends to work stoppages and other concerted activity by nonunion employees.

The NLRB, which is charged with administering the act, issued a rule in 1989 that established eight specific bargaining units as appropriate for most health care institutions: registered nurses, physicians, all other professional employees, technical employees, skilled maintenance employees, business office clerical employees, all other service and maintenance employees, and guards. Although challenged by the American Hospital Association, the rule was upheld by the U.S. Supreme Court in a decision rendered in July 1991.

Laws Regarding the Workplace and Worker Safety

The Occupational Safety and Health Administration (OSHA) issues regulations regarding the safety of workers and the appropriate maintenance of facilities and handling of equipment and materials. Provisions for monitoring compliance with OSHA standards and penalties for noncompliance are included. Of great significance to health care institutions are recent changes to OSHA regulations regarding occupational exposure to hepatitis B virus and human immunodeficiency virus (HIV), hazard communications, and formaldehyde standards. Typically, the human resources staff work in conjunction with employee health services and safety officers to ensure compliance with the myriad regulations. They also work with line managers and employees regarding safety requirements.

The Federal Drug Free Workplace Act of 1988 requires employers to certify that they have drug-free workplaces if they are recipients of federal grants or contracts. The law requires policies and supportive programs, although it does not mandate drug testing.

In 1989, the Worker Adjustment and Retraining Notification Act was passed. The act deals with plant closings and layoffs and requires that employees of companies with more than 100 full-time workers be given 60 days' written notice prior to a plant closing or a mass layoff.

Human Resources Responsibility for Legal Compliance

The above mentioned laws are only some of the many that govern employment and conditions of work. Since most human resources professionals are not attorneys, how then can they ensure full compliance with the laws?

Certainly, human resources staff need to confer with legal counsel when they are presented with lawsuits or complaints from one of the regulatory agencies. Also, attorneys generally assist with labor contract bargaining and are needed in representations of the employer before the NLRB. Legal counsel should also review employment applications, supervisory and employee policy manuals, and other important documents. However, once policy guidelines are in place and contracts are approved, good judgment, personal sensitivity, and knowledge of how to use available resources become more important for their appropriate administration than a precise knowledge of law.

In organizations characterized by fair treatment, equal opportunity for advancement, and education and open communication about pay and benefits, there is far less contention and litigation stemming from employee-employer interactions. Human resources staff can do much to see that these elements are part of the environment.

Additionally, they can provide tools that will help managers behave legally and fairly, such as up-to-date policy manuals and training programs on interviewing, counseling, and corrective action; develop and monitor affirmative action goals; maintain appropriate employee records and safeguard confidentiality; and provide legal, standardized job and transfer applications, performance appraisal instruments, and other forms.

The interest of lawmakers and regulators in the world of work is not waning; on the contrary, it is growing in intensity. Thus the human resources professionals in every size organization have needed to become much more knowledgeable about legal matters.

ORGANIZATION AND EMPLOYEE DEVELOPMENT

Effective Management of the Changing Workplace

Human resources departments have traditionally been expected to arrange for special events to foster employee morale and positive employee-management relations. Common examples include receptions or banquets to honor long-service or retiring employees, holiday parties, picnics, and group outings to sports events. While scheduling such events remains on the agenda, the growing emphasis on employee participation and satisfaction has given new meaning to human resources management.

Employee participation and empowerment are now being built into business planning. One reason is that the individuals who have entered the work force since the early 1970s have had far different expectations than their parents. Today's professionals expect to be challenged and given a reasonable amount of autonomy. These expectations are quickly becoming the norm for nonprofessional employees as well. More importantly, organizations have recognized that capitalizing on the potential of their employees can result in higher productivity, improved quality, and better morale.[11]

Consequently, a large number of American companies are re-examining their work environments and management styles. According to a 1990 survey, 13 percent of U. S. companies were currently using "self-managed teams," and another 4 percent planned to adopt their use; 35 percent had employee involvement teams, and another 7 percent were intending to try them; and 28 percent taught supervisors how to promote greater employee participation, and another 8 percent were going to implement this kind of training.[12]

Figure 18-2, reprinted from the survey, shows the kinds of programming that organizations have undertaken to support employees' involvement in the workplace and their needs for more control, both on the job and in their lives outside the workplace. The survey noted the increase in the number of employee involvement programs in companies where there was some quality improvement effort in which employees participated. These companies, which represented over half of the survey group, tended to use employee participation programs and alternative work arrangements to a greater extent than survey participants as a whole.

As noted elsewhere in this chapter, the changing demographics in the workplace are also forcing the re-examination of organizational culture and management. Following are some of these significant demographic trends.

The work force is growing more slowly and is getting older. The average age of workers in 1987 was 36. It will rise to 39 by 2000 and to 41 by the year 2020. At the same time, the number of young workers (aged 16–20) entering the work force will decline by about 8 percent (two million workers) between 1987 and 2000.[13]

Women will continue to enter the work force in increasing numbers. They currently make up al-

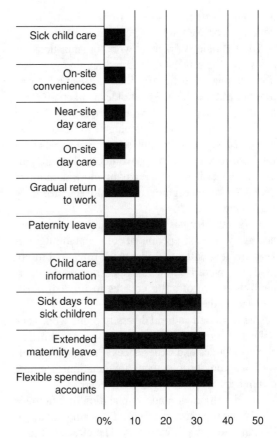

Figure 18-2 Programs for Dealing with Work and Family Conflicts. *Source:* Reprinted from *Workforce 2000: A Survey Report on Corporate Responses to Demographic and Labor Force Trends* with permission of the Hudson Institute and Towers Perrin, © 1990.

most half the work force, and two-thirds of new entrants between 1987 and 2000 will be women.[14]

Minority and immigrant workers will increase. The Bureau of Labor Statistics projects that 26 percent of all jobs in the year 2000 will be held by people of color and immigrants.[15]

The implications of these workplace trends for human resources management abound. As organizations address new workplace needs, they will look to their human resources staffs to advise on strategies and develop new programs. Following are some strategies and programs currently being developed or used in health care institutions.

To keep older workers at work, organizations are using flexible scheduling and redesigning jobs. Retirement and other benefit plans are being restructured to address the needs of older workers. For example, some plans allow employees to collect pension benefits while continuing to work part-time.

Job redesign and flexible scheduling are also being used to assist working women and single parents, and organizations are paying more attention to dependent-care programs and employees' needs for leave time.

A variety of types of training and retraining are necessary. To assist people of color and immigrants who are new entrants to the work force and to upgrade the overall skill levels of current workers, organizations are offering courses in English, reading, and mathematics.

The increased cultural diversity of the workplace holds the potential for conflict arising from differences in values and experiences. Programmatic efforts to promote tolerance, appreciation of ethnic differences, and teamwork are needed.

The development and organization of employee involvement programs require the sound advice of human resource professionals. The effects on total remuneration of gainsharing or other pay incentive systems need to be analyzed. Such programs call for a higher level of supervisory training and frequent, effective communications throughout the organization. Recruitment strategies, performance appraisal mechanisms, benefits administration, and new employee orientation all have to be rethought and possibly reshaped to support a participative culture. Additionally, new tools may have to be developed to measure and monitor the organizational climate. Possible tools include employee opinion surveys, exit interviews with terminating employees, focus groups or roundtable discussions—all of which can provide a wealth of data that will help management refocus and make decisions in support of a positive employee environment.

Far from merely creating good feelings, the strategies and programs described above are essential for improving the quality of patient care and the efficient management of organizational resources. Human resources professionals have a vital role in the development of employees and the use of organizational culture to influence positive outcomes for the employer and individual employees alike.

Work Force Planning and Education

A 1989 survey by the American Hospital Association to determine the extent of manpower shortages in health occupations gave the grim but expected news that vacancy rates for many occupations have not decreased and demand continues to rise.[16] Health care organizations know they must find other means besides the recruitment and compensation strategies noted in earlier sections to reduce employee turnover and develop workers to meet their future needs.

Training and educational programs, often created by human resources staff, are essential for worker development. To be effective, training must be designed for specific groups and tailored to their particular work settings. Cultural and organizational values must be considered, and evaluation methodologies should be established at the outset of the training (see Chapter 5).

Training the Entry-Level Worker

Bringing individuals with few skills or little education into the workplace poses special challenges. With meaningful support and encouragement, entry-level workers may acquire the education and skills necessary to be promoted to technical or professional jobs in the organization. Even if workers do not advance beyond entry-level positions, it is desirable that they become increasingly proficient in their work, function as team players, and contribute to making the work environment safe and harmonious.

Certain kinds of training may achieve these results. Some employers offer basic reading and math courses to workers. Some also offer assistance to employees in getting a high school diploma or qualifying for the GED examinations. For non-English-speaking employees, English as a second language courses are important, and supervisors who speak the native languages of the workers and who are sensitive to their cultural differences are critical.

Young people with no prior work experience may require basic job-readiness skills, including knowledge of job descriptions, work rules, performance standards, and appropriate communications. Having senior workers serve as preceptors or mentors can assist new employees by giving them positive role models.

Education for the Retention of Health Professionals

By the time an individual has succeeded in becoming a nurse, occupational therapist, clinical dietitian, or any type of health professional, he or she has had a significant amount of academic preparation for the job. Nonetheless, health professionals seek ongoing education to keep themselves current in their fields and to acquire new learning that may help them advance to other positions. Beyond traditional in-service education usually provided within departments, human resources staff can provide other learning experiences that serve to retain, encourage, and promote individuals.

Some of these may be courses offered onsite that teach management skills or serve as introductions to other disciplines such as hospital finance or medical records. Many institutions offer tuition reimbursement programs or other financial assistance to employees who go to a college or university for courses related either to their jobs or to other health care jobs.

Additionally, providing informational resources on topics such as "Adopting a Baby," "Planning for Retirement," or "Managing Stress," is very helpful to employees attempting to balance the demands of personal and professional life. Seminars or lunchtime discussions on these kinds of subjects demonstrate that the employer has an interest in the whole person and are highly valued by employees.

Developing Leaders

It is almost axiomatic that health care supervisors achieve that status by having been excellent nurses, technicians, physical therapists, accountants, and so on. While most individuals promoted to managerial positions have a strong desire to succeed, few have

been developed as managers per se. That is, they know little about the organization's overall business objectives and strategies, nor do they have the skills to delegate work effectively, appraise others' performance, interview job applicants, or counsel a failing employee.

Although not all leadership characteristics can be learned in a classroom—charisma, humor, and the ability to inspire, among others, appear to be innate—many skills can be acquired and perfected in a traditional learning environment. To retain excellent employees and simultaneously to develop strong leaders, many health care organizations invest considerable resources, both money and time, in management training. Countless materials are available from external sources, and many employers develop their own materials. Whether external, internal, or a combination of both, ongoing education for practicing and aspiring managers is an important tool for ensuring the effective functioning of today's complex health care institution.

What Do Executives Need To Learn?

Most health care executives realize that learning does not stop upon promotion to an administrative position. However, demands on time and other pressures often prevent senior administrators from continuing their education. Human resources staff can provide a great service to the organization's leaders by establishing forums where consultants, academics, or other business leaders can present their thinking on current issues and organizational development. They can also assist in arranging strategic planning sessions or hosting management retreats for the exploration of new business ideas or for group problem solving. The most effective organizations are learning organizations, and the human resources department has both the opportunity and the responsibility to support education for individuals at all levels of the organization.

RESOURCE REQUIREMENTS

The human resources of an organization are, for the most part, its employees, although trustees, physicians, volunteers, community groups, students, and external agencies are also sources of talent and assistance.

Labor Shortages

Historically labor intensive—hospitals spend 50–60 percent of their operating budgets on pay and benefits—the health care industry continues to rely on a variety of highly educated health profession-als, as well as a large group of workers with skills acquired through on-the-job training or vocational programs. The industry has been beleaguered in re-cent years by shortages of nurses, technicians, therapists, and other specialists such as pharmacists and medical record coders. Despite several rounds of wage escalations and a plethora of recruiting gimmicks, shortages of these personnel persist, and the future supply threatens to be insufficient.

Over the course of this decade, the demand for health care workers is expected to grow at a substan-tially greater rate than for other occupations. The U.S. Department of Labor projects that by the year 2005 all occupations will require a 20 percent increase in the supply of workers.[17] Health occupations will be among the fastest growing (see Table 18-2).

The greatest anxiety about shortages of health pro-fessionals has been focused on registered nurses, since nurses make up the single largest component of hospital work forces. A survey conducted by the

American Hospital Association in 1988 suggested that the shortage has eased. The survey of 813 hospi-tals across the country showed 13 percent of hospitals were experiencing a "severe" shortage of RNs in 1988, whereas 19 percent had reported severe short-ages in 1987. (Table 18-3 shows the severity of the shortage for hospitals of various sizes.)

Academic enrollments in nursing programs have also picked up somewhat. A survey from the Na-tional League of Nursing indicated that enrollments in associate degree programs actually increased from 1986 to 1987 (after two years of decreases in enrollment of more than 7 percent per year). Enroll-ment in baccalaureate programs continues to drop, but not as fast as it had. Enrollment dipped 9.8 per-cent from 1986 to 1987, compared to a decline of 10.3 percent from 1983 to 1986.

Even with some improvement in the severity of the crisis, the future demands loom large. Eli Ginzberg suggests that the nursing shortage is any-thing but short term. He cites the new technology and aging population as chief reasons. In the last 25 years, the ratio of nursing staff to patients doubled. Two out of five nurses are now assigned to critical care units.[18]

In addition to the nursing shortage, vacancies in other health occupations are also creating prob-lems. The highest vacancy rates, according to the 1988 AHA Survey of Human Resources, are for physical therapists (15.8 percent vacancy rate), oc-

---

Table 18-2 Fastest Growing Occupations, 1990–2005

Occupation	1990 (in thousands)	2005 (in thousands)	Numerical Change (in thousands)	Percentage Change
Home Health Aides	287	550	263	91.7
Physical Therapists	88	155	67	76.0
Radiologic Technologists and Technicians	149	252	103	69.5
Occupational Therapists	36	56	20	55.2
Medical Records Technicians	52	80	28	54.3
Respiratory Therapists	60	91	31	52.1
Registered Nurses	1,727	2,494	767	49.4
Nursing Aides, Orderlies, and Attendants	1,274	1,826	552	43.4
Licensed Practical Nurses	644	913	269	41.9

Source: Reprinted from *Monthly Labor Review*, November 1991, p. 81, U.S. Dept. of Labor, Bureau of Statistics.

Table 18-3 The Severity of the Nursing Shortage

Bed Size	No Shortage	Mild	Moderate	Severe
1–49	27.8%	24.0%	32.9%	15.2%
50–99	22.7	30.6	35.7	10.8
100–199	17.1	29.2	42.0	11.5
200–299	14.6	25.6	49.5	10.1
300–399	18.0	25.0	45.8	11.1
400–499	17.7	33.3	26.6	22.2
500 or more	7.1	24.2	45.7	22.9

Source: Data from *Hospitals,* May 5, 1989, American Hospital Publishing, Inc.

cupational therapists (14.6 percent), certified registered nurse anesthetists (10.2 percent), clinical perfusionists (10 percent), and speech pathologists (9 percent). There have been a number of responses to the shortages. The same survey reported that 22.4 percent of hospitals with shortages have reduced services they offer, 15.3 percent have closed units or beds, and 12.6 percent are diverting patients to other hospitals.

The shortages of needed personnel have also resulted in creative job redesigning. In particular, organizations have attempted to shift nonprofessional responsibilities to lesser skilled staff to maximize the effectiveness of nurses. The role of registered care technician, developed and encouraged by the American Medical Association in response to the nursing shortage, is an example of the shifting of responsibilities.

In addition to personnel shortages, other factors have also contributed to the creation of new definitions of work and new models of staffing. Many more women are in the work force, and many workers are eager to pursue other interests beyond work. Part-time, flextime, "mother's hours," and job sharing are but a few of the variable schedules offered by employers as a result.

Resources Required for Managing the Human Resources Department

The human resources department requires a variety of financial and material resources to administer the programs and processes for which it is responsible, including the following:

- recruitment supplies and expenses
  - —advertising (newspapers, journals, television, and radio)
  - —campus recruitment
  - —job fairs/conventions (such as student nurse association annual meeting)
  - —open houses
- temporary help agencies (supplemental staff, including nurses, clerical workers, and technicians)
- computerized information systems
  - —employee records
  - —applicant flow system
  - —affirmative action, immigration, pre-employment physicals, recordkeeping
- surveys (compensation, benefits, and employee opinion surveys)
- outplacement services
- legal services
- actuarial and other pension administrative services
- training and development resources (instructor salaries, classroom materials, and audiovisual equipment)
- employee health-related expenses
  - —wellness programs (fitness centers, aerobics, stress management, and smoking cessation programs)

—workers' compensation

—employee health services (pre-employment physicals and accident and illness treatment)

—OSHA requirements

—education materials (on workplace safety, AIDS, back injury prevention, etc.)

—employee assistance programs

- special events and celebratory activities (service award programs, retirement parties, holiday functions, and group outings)
- communications materials (management newsletter, policy and procedure manuals, personalized benefits statements, employee handbooks, orientation videos, non-English translations)
- conferences and seminars (education to keep staff abreast of trends in the field)

QUALITY MANAGEMENT

According to the literature on service excellence, quality services are services that meet or exceed the needs of the customers. Therefore, to determine whether the human resources department is providing quality services, it is necessary to consider who the various customers are and what they require. The customers have, of course, quite different reasons for coming in contact with human resources staff, and the department must have different ways of obtaining and evaluating feedback from them (including both external and internal customers).

External Customers

The majority of those outside the organization who have contact with the human resources department are job applicants. Because the pool of applicants is constantly shifting, their expectations may vary as well. Presumably, the needs of an applicant are met if she or he is offered and accepts a position. However, that is not necessarily true. Even someone who is satisfied with the outcome could be displeased with the selection process. Further, the reality is that most ap-

plicants are not hired, even in the tightest of labor markets. Therefore, the employment process must be designed in such a way that all job applicants feel their interest is valued while the organization's managers feel that only the most highly qualified applicants are referred for open positions. In other words, expectations must be managed as well as results.

There are both formal and informal means of testing the satisfaction levels of applicants and managers. Beyond assessing the subjective responses of the interested parties, the human resources staff must also develop objective measures to ensure that they are meeting the organization's needs. They might also periodically survey a selected sample of applicants, including some who were successful and some who were not. The survey might include questions such as these:

- Did the application receive prompt attention?
- Were the contacts cordial, professional, and helpful?
- Was the interview thorough? Did the applicant feel he or she had the opportunity to fully present his or her qualifications?
- Did the applicant receive sufficient information about the position and other aspects of employment?
- If not hired, did the applicant understand the reasons for nonselection? Would he or she still consider taking a position with the organization?
- If candidate declined an offer, why? What can be learned about the process or the organization from this experience?

The absence of negative feedback, such as complaints of discrimination or charges of favoritism, is also an indicator of quality service.

Employment staff must also identify and use objective criteria to ensure that they are achieving customer satisfaction in cost-effective ways. To that end, they monitor and evaluate the following data:

- amount and cost of advertising by position and department

- numbers of responses to ads and other recruiting methods and numbers hired from those sources
- ratio of applicants to interviews, ratio of interviews to referrals, and ratio of referrals to hires
- cost per hire
- affirmative action efforts (recruitment, interviews, and hires)
- length of tenure and successful performance on the job for those hired

Other external customers are the faculty and counselors from schools that train health professionals or influence students' career decisions. Employment staff are likely to have contact with individuals from a wide variety of colleges, technical and vocational schools, community training programs, high schools, and even elementary schools. Seeking regular feedback from the academic professionals and monitoring the relationships between students and the health care organization are valuable ways of determining the effectiveness of long-term recruitment strategies.

Internal Customers

Except in the employment arena, most of the human resources department's customers are internal—physicians, managers, and other employees. Again, there are both formal and informal ways of determining the effectiveness of the services provided.

One of the most informative tools is the employee opinion survey (or organizational climate survey). This instrument investigates employee attitudes about supervision, pay, benefits, recognition programs, safety, and effectiveness of communications, among other things. When conducted on a regular basis, employee opinion surveys uncover entrenched organizational strengths and weaknesses as well as improvements resulting from specific programmatic efforts.

There are numerous consulting firms that design and sell opinion surveys. In addition to tailoring the surveys to fit specific organizational interests, they generally provide a national database against which an individual organization can evaluate itself. The comparative data may help the organization decide how to allocate its resources and focus its attention.

Other formal but less elaborate feedback mechanisms produce valuable data as well. For example, if the organization is considering a change in its leave-of-absence policy or thinking of implementing a drug-testing program, the human resources staff might first meet with a variety of employees in a focus group to gauge their reaction and investigate the clarity of communications.

Advisory committees comprised of individuals representing special interests may also be excellent sounding boards for policy proposals and offer worthwhile feedback. Examples of such groups include older workers, those interested in workplace safety, parents, recovering alcoholics, minority supervisors, and clerical workers. Human resources staff must work effectively with these groups to see that they are heard (although they should not be allowed to dictate policy at the expense of other individuals or groups).

Again, unsolicited feedback should be monitored and given credence. Calls and letters of either praise or complaint are important indicators of the success of a program, policy, or staff member.

The human resources department should routinely and systematically gather data that reflect the volume and quality of work performed. The activities to be tracked include these:

- enrollments in benefits; utilization and claims
- requests for job evaluation; number of reclassifications
- number and type of grievances filed; data regarding resolution
- amount of participation in all programs (e.g., training, employee appreciation, and new employee orientation programs)
- promotions, transfers, and demotions
- number of transactions regarding personnel records

- amount and costs of nonproductive time paid (vacations, holidays, and sick leave)
- number and type of legal actions involving employees

Paying attention to trends and shifts in these areas aids human resources staff in planning programs and testing employees' receptivity to existing activities. Collection and analysis of these data is also vital to the strategic planning efforts of the organization as a whole, and human resources leaders have a responsibility to help other managers understand the implications of trends.

The human resource staff should also be cognizant of the absence of negative initiatives. The lack of union organizing activity, small numbers of grievances or complaints, and the absence of discrimination or legal suits may mean the environment is seen as fair and supportive to employees. Such quietness may also be the "calm before the storm," and the human resources staff should be alert to subtle shifts in the tone and temperament of the organization.

Once the measurement mechanisms are put in place, the human resources department should regularly assess the resulting data. Staff meetings to evaluate data and discuss the department's mission are necessary for ensuring that the department is delivering high-quality services and satisfying its many customers.

THE FUTURE OF HUMAN RESOURCE MANAGEMENT

Spawned in the 1980s by such books as *In Search of Excellence, Megatrends,* and *The Service Edge,* a set of related buzz-words are currently being heard in management circles: *total quality, human capital, patient-centeredness, values-driven management, corporate culture, empowerment,* and *participation.*

It is the era of maximizing human potential to gain a competitive advantage in a crowded marketplace. And the health care industry, which not so long ago would have rejected such terms as *competition, profit,* and *product line,* is today not only comfortable with that language but is scrambling for productivity and quality enhancements in order to deliver more sought-after services in more cost-effective ways.

At the very time the industry seeks to stretch its human capital, it also finds there are too few nurses, technicians, therapists, and other health professionals to satisfy its needs. Not only are the health care occupations suffering shortages, the country as a whole is experiencing the baby bust (which is currently causing declining numbers of college students and young professionals). The U.S. Census Bureau reports that the largest growing segment of the population consists of immigrants.

The changing demographics of the labor market, then, call for new strategies for recruiting and retaining employees.

In a recent Wyatt Company survey, chief executives in health care were asked how they perceive the environment of the next decade and how they plan to respond. It was clear that human resource issues command a dominant position in their thinking. The survey concludes, "Leading a changing work force through the nineties will require not only a recognition of changes in work force demographics, but more importantly, an understanding of how to manage effectively a work force characterized by such change."[19]

Retaining competent clinical staff and focusing on employee productivity go hand in hand. More than three-quarters of the CEOs who responded to the survey rated staffing problems as the primary difficulty they will face. These executives indicated their responses to these problems will include an emphasis on employee productivity and increasing the use of participative management.

In an effort to achieve efficiencies and enhance cooperation, survey respondents also suggested that organizations will need to include physicians in the planning and management of care as well as in its delivery. They will need to improve relationships between physicians and administrators and between labor and management. Education and training programs are seen as important aids in this endeavor, as are recognition and incentive programs. Many health care organizations are further enhancing their attempts at improving relations by applying the principles of total quality management developed by W. Edwards Deming or those of other proponents of continuous quality improvement such as Joseph Juran and Philip Crosby.

Essentially, though, one cannot separate human resources management from quality management, since the latter requires that all the people in an organization focus intently on quality improvement in their day-to-day actions. If top leaders convincingly express their commitment to quality improvement and managers provide the necessary training and coaching, employees will themselves identify and fix the system problems that are blocks to quality and efficiency. Such activity is at the core of human resources management.

Thus, a serious organizational attempt at quality improvement requires that all managers accept the importance of effective human resources management. This means that time and financial resources must be devoted to the development of leadership and coaching skills, quality improvement consultants must be hired or trained to teach managers and employees the methods of measuring quality, top managers must develop and articulate clear statements of purpose and direction, and communication strategies must be developed to ensure that all employees understand the value of achieving departmental and organization-wide missions.

In keeping with this thrust, organizational policies and practices as well as issues related to employee morale, such as pay, benefits, recognition, and advancement, must be reconsidered. To the extent that policies and procedures support teamwork and reward individual initiative, they will help the quality program. To the extent that there is dissatisfaction with conditions of work, low morale, or lack of confidence in management, any efforts to install systemwide quality improvement methods will be retarded and probably will not succeed.

In the next decade, with the whole organization focusing on its culture and means of problem solving, the human resources staff will have special jobs. For example, the employment staff will need to do more screening for applicants who fit the organization culturally (i.e., share its values). They will need to review job transfer and promotional practices to ensure that they support innovation and skill development. Compensation staff will need to make certain that job content descriptions include the employees' responsibilities for collaboration and problem solving. Are financial rewards consistent with what the organization is saying it values? Can salary and pay increase practices be openly discussed or are these subjects taboo? Too many corporate secrets or unexplainable practices will most certainly jeopardize a total quality management program.

The same kind of scrutiny must be used in reviewing benefits administration, labor relations, training and organization development, employee data administration, and the employee health, volunteers, and employee communications services, among others.

Human resources departments, in the final analysis, will need to let go of some of the control mechanisms that defined their activity in the past—many are now the responsibility of line managers. Human resources staff may instead provide much-needed expertise in assessing the organizational climate and advising programmatic approaches to enhance it. They are important teachers and role models for facilitation and coaching skills. Long the advocates for employee empowerment, human resources professionals now must welcome the paradox that such empowerment can be achieved only if they relinquish their ownership of this issue.

ADDITIONAL RESOURCES

Organizations

American Society for Healthcare Human Resources Administration, American Hospital Association, 840 North Lake Shore Drive, Chicago, Ill 60611, 312/280-6434.

Society for Human Resource Management, 606 North Washington Street, Alexandria, VA 22314, 703/548-3440.

Books and Articles

American Hospital Association. *Variable Staffing and Scheduling.* Monograph. Chicago: American Hospital Association, 1991.

Avakian, L. Human Resources. In the *Yearbook of health care management 1991,* ed. R. Heyssel. Baltimore: Mosby-Yearbook, 1991.

Crosby, P.B. *Quality is free: The art of making quality certain.* New York: McGraw-Hill, 1979.

Deming, W.E. *Out of the crisis,* 2nd ed. Cambridge, Mass.: Massachusetts Institute of Technology Center for Advanced Engineering Study, 1986.

Drucker, P.F. *Managing the non-profit organization: Practices and principles.* New York: Harper Collins, 1990.

McKeown, A.F., and M.L. Novak-Jandrey, eds. *Human resources management in the health care setting.* Chicago: American Hospital Publishing, 1991.

Peters, T.J., and R.H. Waterman, Jr. *In search of excellence.* New York: Harper & Row, 1982.

NOTES

1. S. Robbins and J. Rakich, Hospital Personnel Management in the Early 1990's: A Follow-up Analysis, *Hospital and Health Services Administration* 34 (1989): 395.

2. Joint Commission on Accreditation of Healthcare Organizations, *1992 Joint Commission Accreditation Manual for Hospitals* (Chicago: Joint Commission on Accreditation of Healthcare Organizations, 1992), 46.

3. C.S. Miller and M.H. Schuster, Gainsharing Plans: A Comparative Analysis, *Organizational Dynamics,* Summer 1987, pp. 45–46.

4. L. Perry, Gain Sharing Plans Aim To Boost Productivity, *Modern Healthcare* 20 (1990): 66.

5. *Workforce 2000: A Survey Report on Corporate Responses to Demographic and Labor Force Trends* (Indianapolis, Ind: Hudson Institute and Towers Perrin, 1990).

6. S. Cooke, Taking Care of Children—Daily, *Massachusetts Health Care,* October 1988, p. 8.

7. N. Metzger, The Union Movement: Dead or Alive, *Handbook of Healthcare Human Resources Management,* ed. N. Metzger (Gaithersburg, Md.: Aspen Publishers, 1990), 384.

8. C. Scott and J. Simpson, Union Election Activity in the Hospital Industry, *Health Care Management Review* 14 (1989): 21–28.

9. Metzger, The Union Movement, 384.

10. W.L. Becker and A.M. Rowe, Update on Union Organizing in Health Care, *Federation of American Health Systems Review,* September-October 1989, pp. 11–12.

11. Who Needs a Boss, *Fortune,* May 7, 1990.

12. *Workforce 2000 Survey Report.*

13. *The Wyatt Communicator,* Winter 1991, p. 6.

14. S.D. Nollen, The Work-Family Dilemma: How H.R. Managers Can Help, *Personnel* 66 (1989): 25–30.

15. *Wyatt Communicator,* 7.

16. American Hospital Association Survey (American Hospital Association, Chicago, 1989).

17. U.S. Department of Labor, Bureau of Labor Statistics, *Monthly Labor Review,* November 1991, p. 81.

18. E. Ginzberg, What Physicians Should Know about the Nursing Shortage, *Annals of Internal Medicine* 112 (1990): 319–320.

19. *Health Management USA . . . Leading a Changing Work Force* (Wyatt Company, New York, 1990) p. 320.

Walter J. Wentz

Materials Management

19

Purpose: The purpose of materials management is to acquire equipment, supplies, and services of the kind and quality and in the amount needed and to have them delivered when and where they are to be used—all at the minimum possible cost.

FUNCTIONS

The term *materials management* is commonly used to denote a centralized organization for the management and control of goods, services, and equipment from acquisition to disposition.[1] The term can be used, however, to denote six principal functions of materials management even in the case of a decentralized structure:

1. *Purchasing.* This is the process of acquiring supplies, services, and equipment. It includes the activities of product research, specifications definition, supplier selection, and order placement.

2. *Receiving and Stores.* These activities are related to receiving, warehousing, and inventory management as well as shipping out repairs and returns.

3. *Distribution.* This is the process of providing materials where and when they are needed. It includes requisitioning, stock replenishment, exchange cart systems, and posting charges for materials used.

4. *Processing.* The object of processing is to ensure that materials are in a form and condition ready for their intended use. It includes preparation, cleaning, sterilization, and disposal.

5. *Control.* Control is exercised at each stage of the materials management process. It involves policy and procedure definition, acquisition planning, and inventory control.

6. *Disposal.* Disposal or waste management is concerned with recycling and environmental protection issues, among others.

Materials management may be organized on a centralized or decentralized basis. In a centralized organization, all materials management functions are coordinated and directed through one department. A centralized approach is intended to provide an integrated system that contributes to the improvement of efficiency, cost-effectiveness, and control. Most organizations, however, maintain a degree of decentralization. Often departments with special needs, such as food service, pharmacy, and maintenance, retain the responsibility for some or all of their own materials management—such as the purchase of perishables or the processing and distribution of drugs or food. Whether organized on a centralized or decentralized basis, materials management is in large part a process, with its functional components flowing together as illustrated in Figure 19-1.

MANAGEMENT PRINCIPLES

The resources an institution devotes to materials management can be considerable. According to one study, a typical general hospital may spend 20–30 percent of its annual budget in buying materials and managing them after they are acquired.[2] Materials management plays a central role in ensuring that these resources are well used and is critical in supporting the activities of other departments, ensuring they have the supplies and equipment they need to perform their duties. The manager should keep in mind the following principles when organizing and directing materials management activities:

- Equipment and supplies should be acquired that are appropriate for their intended use.
- Materials should be acquired at the overall lowest cost consistent with specifications.
- Inventories should be maintained at the minimum level possible while ensuring supply availability.
- Materials should be made available at the time, in the amount, and in the location where they are required.
- Materials need to be in a form and condition for proper use.
- Materials must be handled and processed in a manner that ensures patients and employees are protected from harm and infection.
- The volume and quality of materials and their costs must be carefully monitored and controlled.

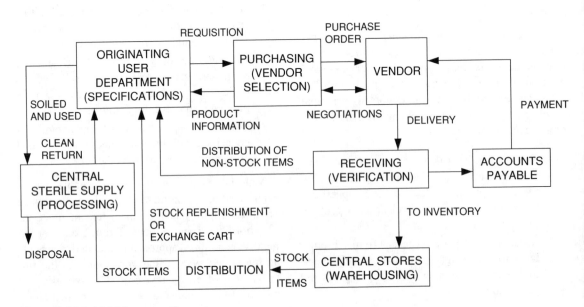

Figure 19-1 Materials Management Process

- Materials must be protected from damage, waste, and theft.

PURCHASING

Purchasing is the process of acquiring supplies, services, and equipment. It includes product research, specifications definition, supplier selection, and order placement.

In larger institutions purchasing activities are usually assigned to a purchasing department, which can be organized either as a separate department or as part of a larger materials management department or division. In a smaller organization, these activities may be assigned to an individual (a purchasing agent or buyer). Regardless of form or size, the purchasing department or agent has the following principal responsibilities:

- to provide information on available products, supply sources, and prices
- to assist all users in acquiring the supplies, services, and equipment they require
- to ensure materials are acquired in the amount needed and at an agreed price and are of a quality appropriate for their intended use
- to acquire materials at the lowest total cost to the organization and under favorable terms and conditions
- to design clear and well-documented procedures and controls for authorizing, acquiring, and distributing materials
- to ensure that all purchasing activities are conducted ethically and honestly and that material and financial resources are used appropriately and in a manner consistent with the organization's policy and budget.

Product Research

Product research, which is intended to provide current information on the availability and price of materials, involves three main activities: gathering product information, monitoring market conditions, and communicating with users and suppliers.

The purchasing department (or agent) should have access to current and accurate product information in order to ensure that the most appropriate materials currently available can be acquired at the most reasonable price. Product information is collected both on a general basis for a broad array of products and on a specific basis for selected equipment and supply items. On a routine basis, general product information is compiled—primarily from catalogues provided by manufacturers and vendors, trade publications, advertisements, and trade shows. The purchasing department should maintain a library of current product information.

In order to maintain current information, the purchasing department must continuously monitor market conditions for the introduction of new or modified products, current and future product availability, new vendors, price changes or competition, and changing patterns of use. Buyer's guides, for both industry and health care, are useful sources. The American Hospital Association's *Guide for Hospital Buyers* and *Health Care Product News,* published by Health Care Publications, are two good examples. A list of catalogues, periodicals, and other relevant literature is presented at the end of this chapter.

The purchasing department should maintain regular communication with users and suppliers. At the request of a user, the purchasing department may compile specific product information from specifications and promotional materials provided by manufacturers and sales representatives, product examination and trial, and reports from experienced users both inside and outside the organization. The purchasing department should establish an advisory or consulting relationship with all users to ensure that proper purchasing practices are followed. In addition, users are often an important source of information on changing market conditions.

Suppliers also need accurate information—on the needs of the organization and individual users—in order to recommend appropriate materials to the buyer. The purchasing department should help keep suppliers informed by arranging meetings between users and salespeople or manufacturer's representatives (if necessary).

Specifications Definition

The user is the focus of nearly all materials management activity. The entire process typically begins when the user initiates a decision to acquire a product or service. Specifications assure the user that the product or service will perform properly, will be of the quality needed, and will be acquired at a reasonable price. For many products that are widely available and are of a predictable quality, a standardized specification, a simple descriptive phrase, a product model or identification number, or even a brand name may suffice as a guide to purchasing. However, where a product is unique or expensive or where bids will be solicited, more formal specifications are essential. Specifications need to define both the detailed characteristics of the particular product and the general conditions that must be met by the supplier. Specifications should include the following basic elements[3]:

- *Physical Description.* A clear description of the item's physical and technical characteristics is needed. The description should be specific enough to avoid misinterpretation but include tolerances that allow for reasonable variation. It should relate to standard market specifications whenever possible.
- *Functional Description.* The functional description indicates the item's intended use and performance requirements. Defining a product's functional characteristics helps to prevent prejudicing the specifications so that they favor one supplier's product.
- *Quality.* The kind and quality of any required materials, workmanship, or finish should be specified.
- *Type and Size.* If there are types, grades, classes, and sizes that are required, these should be specified.

- *Shipping Requirements.* Packaging and labeling requirements, mode of transport, and time of delivery must be indicated.
- *Basis for Acceptance.* How and on what basis an item will be accepted or rejected needs to be defined.

It is the purchasing department's responsibility to work with the user to develop specifications that define the detailed characteristics of the product or service to be purchased. The following is an example of a simple but frequently occurring specification for surgical gloves[4]:

Product:	Gloves, surgical, latex rubber
Type:	Disposable
Description:	Cuff, rolled wrist, or other style
Material:	Latex rubber at ___ ozs.
Color:	Green
Sizes:	6½ to 9½
Packaging:	24 pairs per carton
Weight:	2¼ lbs. per carton

More complex equipment or supplies will require correspondingly more complex specifications, and at times the assistance of a specialized consultant might be needed.

Standardized specifications for a wide variety of products can be obtained from various government agencies, private testing companies, and trade organizations, such as those listed below[5]:

- National Bureau of Standards
- American Standards Association
- Bureau of Health Devices and Occupational and Health Act (U.S. Public Health Service)
- American Society of Testing of Materials
- Consumer Reports
- American Institute of Architects
- Health Industries Association
- Federal Bureau of Specifications
- American Surgical Trade Association
- General Services Administration
- Department of Defense
- American Institute of Electrical Engineers

In addition to defining the detailed characteristic of the particular product or service, specifications should also include statements that address the general conditions that must be met by qualified vendor, such as the following:

- format and time requirements for submitting bids
- inspection and testing procedures to be used in determining product or service acceptability
- shipping and/or installation instructions and requirements
- product servicing or maintenance requirements
- insurance, bonding, license, or legal requirements

A detailed index of general conditions like the sample presented in Exhibit 19-1 might be used in the preparation of specifications. For each condition listed, standardized language is available from the American Standards Association and other sources listed above. Conditions that are applicable to the items being purchased can be selected from the index, modified to meet the particular requirements of the organization, and included in the formal specification documents. As an illustration, if items 3–6 were selected from the index as relevant to the purchase of a major piece of equipment, the general conditions listed in Exhibit 19-2 would then be incorporated into the specification documents.

Supplier Selection

Supplier selection is intended to result in the choice of a qualified vendor who can provide the items specified at a reasonable price for each item and the lowest overall price for all acquisitions. It involves vendor identification and selecting prequalified and prime vendors.

The aim of vendor identification is to identify as many reputable and reliable vendors as possible for each product and product line in order to maintain price competitiveness and to ensure that materials are available from alternative sources on both a regular and emergency basis. Identification may be

---

Exhibit 19-1 Index of General Conditions

Paragraph	Condition Title	Paragraph	Condition Title
1.	Contents	11.	Prequalification of Bidders, Machinery, and Equipment
2.	Definitions		
3.	Contractor's Understanding	12.	"Or Equal" Clause
4.	Remedy of Defects, Deterioration, or Departure from Standards	13.	Major Equipment Stipulation
		14.	Return of Bid Security
5.	Notice and Service Thereof	15.	Rejection of Bids
6.	Proposals	16.	Award
7.	Irregular Proposals	17.	Contract Security
8.	Withdrawal or Revision of Proposals	18.	Contractor's and Sub-Contractor's Insurance
9.	Corporate Bidders	19.	Date of Contract
10.	Interpretations	20.	Failure to Execute Contract

Continued to Paragraph 80

Source: Reprinted from *Material Management and Purchasing for the Health Care Facility* by J.H. Holmgren and W.J. Wentz, pp. 48–49, with permission of the Association of University Programs in Health Administration, © 1982.

Exhibit 19-2 Sample General Conditions

3. Contractor's understanding: This paragraph reminds the contractor that he has read and agrees to all of the documents, studied all of the drawings related to the bid, and bids with full knowledge of his responsibilities and assurances to complete work satisfactorily.

4. Remedy of defects: The contractor agrees to remedy any defects in materials or workmanship discovered following completion. If he does not remedy the defect(s) within ten days of the notice of such defects, then the owner reserves the right to have the deficiencies corrected and the cost of such work be billed to the contractor.

5. Notice of service thereof: This provides for notice in writing to be given to the contractor by the owner for any information not given to the contractor in specification documents.

6. Proposals: Requires that proposals be submitted by the contractor in writing, legibly, on forms furnished by the owner and endorsed as provided in the contract documents.

Source: Reprinted from *Material Management and Purchasing for the Health Care Facility* by J.H. Holmgren and W.J. Wentz, pp. 50–52, with permission of the Association of University Programs in Health Administrations, © 1982.

done using informal and formal sources of information. Informal sources include other buyers in the health field, product users, and sales representatives.[6] Formal sources include trade catalogues, trade registers, and directories such as *The Medical Device Register,* Thomas's *Register of American Manufacturers,* MacRae's *Bluebook,* and Brady's *Hospital Consumables.* Trade journals, exhibits, and even the telephone yellow pages are also useful. The *Hospital Purchasing Guide,* published by Medical Business Services, Ambler, Pennsylvania, is a particularly noteworthy journal. Those vendors most qualified to supply a product or product line can be selected from the list of vendors identified. A process for vendor evaluation is discussed below in the section "Quality Management."

From the list of possible vendors, a few prequalified and prime vendors are selected—an approved list of suppliers with whom orders will be placed routinely. A number of prequalified vendors may be identified, some or all of whom may be invited to submit bids for a specified product or service. A prime vendor is a sole supplier or, more commonly, a major supplier of a particular product or product line and is expected to be a convenient and reliable source of supply at competitive prices, allowing the purchasing department to dispense with formal bidding.

Strategy Note: Using a prime vendor can cut down on paper work and still result in good prices if prices are routinely monitored to ensure competitiveness and the vendor selection process is periodically repeated.

Order Placement

The purchasing process culminates in a purchase order, a final commitment to buy a product or service from a selected vendor under specified conditions and at an agreed price. The process involves the development of a purchasing strategy, bidding, quotations, negotiations, and a purchase agreement.

The purchase department should develop a purchasing strategy that will be followed in acquiring supplies, services, and equipment at the overall lowest cost. An effective buying strategy begins with a commitment to obtain competitive prices in every case. In addition to the standard techniques of bidding, quotations, and negotiation discussed below, the purchasing department may wish to consider a strategy that involves the following:

- product standardization
- group purchasing
- consignment buying
- stockless purchasing
- capital equipment purchasing

Product standardization is intended to reduce the number of similar items purchased and stocked, thereby increasing the opportunities for savings through bulk purchasing. A product standardization committee, composed of administrative, nursing, physician, and other representatives, can help the organization identify product duplication, evaluate quality and performance, and help define standard specifications.

Product standardization is also a key to effective *group purchasing,* where the combined buying power of several organizations is used to gain lower prices than could be achieved by any single buyer. To make group purchasing worthwhile, the costs of participating in the group (membership fees, loss of institutional control, and the cost of group meetings) must be more than offset by reduced prices. Purchasing groups take several organizational forms, including consortiums, for-profit or non-profit corporations, federations, cooperatives, and associations. Whatever its organizational form, members of the group should be compatible (i.e., have similar needs and philosophies) and be well organized and efficient to ensure that savings are not eroded by high overhead costs.

Group buying, controversial as a concept from the 1950s to the 1970s, stabilized as a way of achieving savings. Through volume purchasing in the 1980s, the idea became so familiar to many health care management groups that independent industrial groups were formed to provide a vehicle for volume buying for small voluntary hospitals not a part of a system.

Since 1979, Voluntary Hospitals of America, Inc., the nation's largest health care alliance, has leveraged the vast purchasing strength of VHA hospitals to lower supply prices and improve availability. In the summer of 1985, VHA expanded its purchasing activities with the creation of VHA Supply Company, an innovative supply acquisition system. By 1990, VHA Supply's annual sales had reached $3 billion.

Through the process of supply chain management, VHA Supply brings value to VHA hospitals with new and improved approaches to hospital supply purchasing:

- For VHA hospitals, VHA Supply acts as a contracting agent, providing access to a range of products from alcohol preps to high-tech equipment through purchasing contracts.

- For manufacturers, VHA Supply serves as their representative to VHA hospitals, delivering efficiencies of increased volume and market share through high-volume participation.
- For distributors, VHA Supply maintains agency agreements that provide economies through increased volume, inventory control, prompt payment, and efficient automated order entry.

By bringing these business resources together with the purchasing volume of the VHA hospitals, VHA Supply provides a unique way of managing the purchasing and reducing the cost of products directly associated with hospital stays.

Other national competitors in volume health care purchasing include The American Health Care System (for-profit) in San Diego, California, and the Sun Health Enterprises in Charlotte, North Carolina. The trend toward group purchasing will continue throughout the 1990s.

In *consignment buying,* a product is delivered to the buyer but not paid for until it is used. Consignment buying is a useful strategy for reducing cash flow needs when acquiring expensive, highly specialized items whose use is infrequent but critical. Heart valves, intraocular lenses, and orthopedic implants are typical examples.

In *stockless purchasing,* the vendor maintains an inventory of the required items at its own site and delivers supplies directly to the user on demand. It is a useful strategy for nonurgent items that take up extensive storeroom space. Obviously, it requires the close proximity of a reliable vendor and well-disciplined users who conscientiously process the necessary paper work at the time of delivery.

Because of the potential investment involved, *capital equipment purchasing* poses a particular challenge to health care institutions. As with other purchases, a request for equipment usually originates with the user, but it could well go to the institution's chief executive officer or even the board of trustees before it is approved. The purchasing department, with the approval of administration, should establish clear purchasing guidelines that emphasize the importance of financial justification. A capital equipment evaluation form (Exhibit 19-3) can be useful in documenting the need for the equipment. A capital equipment committee, organized either administratively or as a board committee, can also be useful in reviewing all capital requests against overall institutional priorities and resources. In any case, the purchasing department should assist the user in developing appropriate functional specifications based on standards of performance. Care must be taken to avoid defining specifications so that only one supplier can provide the product.

Strategy Note: One piece of capital equipment can be equal in cost to a whole product line of small items. The purchase of capital equipment deserves special attention.

Bidding is a formal process for generating offers from competing suppliers. It is frequently used in the following circumstances:

- when buying standard items in large quantity
- when ordering an expensive item, such as radiology or laboratory equipment

---

Exhibit 19-3 Capital Equipment Evaluation Form

I. Costs

A. Estimated Cost of Equipment (including shipping) $ _____
B. Estimated Cost of Installation or Building Modifications $ _____
C. Depreciable Life of Project   _____ Years
D. Equipment To Be Replaced:
   1. Description _____
   2. Fixed Asset Number   _____
   3. Present Age   _____ Years
   4. Assigned Useful Life   _____ Years
   5. Current Book Value $ _____
   6. Current Market Value $ _____
E. Associated Increase in Expenses

Year	1	2	3	4	5	6	7	8
Training								
Labor								
Utilities								
Supplies								
Total								

II. Revenues and Decreased Expenses

Year	1	2	3	4	5	6	7	8
Revenue Increases								
Revenue Decreases								
Net Increase								
Expense Decreases								
Net Increase or Decrease								

- when ordering a wide array of equipment or furnishings, as when equipping a new or remodeled facility
- when ordering nonstandard items, such as custom-made or built-in furniture or unusual scientific equipment
- when contracting for a service, such as housekeeping or consulting
- when contracting for services related to construction or remodeling (e.g., architectural, engineering, or construction contractor services)
- when competition is strong

The bidding process is usually initiated by issuing a request for bid (RFB) or request for proposal (RFP), which includes all bidding documents, particularly specifications and general conditions. These specifications need to be clearly drawn to ensure comparability of the bids. Bids can be sought on an open or selected basis. Open bids are sought through public advertisement as well as invitations to prequalified vendors. Open bids are most often used where price competition is of greatest concern and service and other criteria are secondary. Selected bids are sought only from reliable, prequalified vendors, even though their products (e.g., x-ray machines) may not be directly comparable in all regards. Selected bidding excludes those vendors who are known to have inferior products or services. For construction projects, for the purchase of major capital items, or when government expenditures are involved, suppliers are often asked to provide sealed bids, which are then opened publicly. A bid is usually awarded on the basis of lowest total cost, with consideration given to installation, operating costs, warranties, and other cost-related conditions, as well as price. When a bid is awarded on some basis other than just price, or when a bidder is disqualified, the decision should be clearly explained and should be based on criteria included in the original bidding documents.

Strategy Note: To ensure active competition in the future (and as a matter of ethics), the details of one vendor's proposal should not be divulged to another vendor, and all unsuccessful bidders should be formally notified.

While bidding provides a formal process to ensure competition, as an alternative the purchasing department may solicit *quotations* from one or more vendors—usually prime vendors or others who have prequalified. A quotation is chiefly intended to provide price information, and although it may be the basis for an immediate commitment to buy, it may also be used for planning, price comparison, or other purposes.

Negotiations are used to reach settlement on price or other issues not specified in a bid or quotation. Negotiations are most appropriate in the following circumstances:

- where prices are fixed and other conditions are flexible
- when unacceptable bids have been received
- when precise specifications are difficult to define
- when an item is unique and expensive or only available from one source
- for large-volume or package orders for an array of similar products

In purchasing negotiations, the negotiators from the purchasing department should

- have a clear idea of what they hope to accomplish (lower prices, improved service, delivery, or whatever)
- be aware of what other buyers have obtained in terms of price or concessions
- be clear on their priorities, including the features or concessions that are most important
- anticipate and respect the concerns and positions of the vendor

A *purchase agreement* is the final step in the purchasing process and reflects a commitment, either informal or formal, by the buyer and the seller. An informal commitment may be made verbally, followed by a purchase order. A formal commitment is made by signature to a written document that spells out the obligations of the buyer and seller. Whether informal or formal, a purchase agreement is a legal contract and should address the following items[7]:

- date and place at which the contract is made, the names and addresses of the buyer, the buyer's agent, the seller, and the seller's agent
- description of the product or service
- price
- time and method of payment
- responsibility for paying shipping and insurance charges
- shipping instructions
- warranty of the seller as to kind, quality, and product life
- delivery date and place
- provision for claims

RECEIVING AND STORES

Receiving and stores activities include receiving, warehousing, and inventory management. Organizationally, these functions are usually attached to a purchasing department or are part of a larger materials management division. In a smaller organization, receiving and stores activities may be assigned to one individual, although some departments, such as pharmacy or food service, might handle their own materials. Receiving and stores staff have the following principal responsibilities:

- *Verification.* The staff must ensure that the materials received are as specified, in the quantity ordered, and in good condition.
- *Authorization.* They are responsible for approving payment for goods received.
- *Storage.* They are required to hold materials in a secure and orderly manner so that the materials are available, accessible, and in usable condition when needed.
- *Control.* They attempt to minimize the investment in excess inventory.

Receiving

Receiving is the point of entry for all materials used in the institution, and receiving staff ensure that the correct items, in proper condition, are accounted for and turned over to those responsible for their storage or use. Receiving staff

- expedite the unloading of deliverables to avoid demurrage charges
- inspect the condition of delivery containers and report damage
- check quantity and weights
- verify receipt of materials and identify discrepancies
- record shortages, overages, and incorrect or damaged materials
- record serial numbers on equipment deliveries
- distribute materials to appropriate department for storage or use
- notify accounts payable of receipt to ensure proper and timely payment

Receiving services may also include shipping or mailing correspondence and materials, including the return of damaged goods; mail receiving, sorting, and distribution; internal messenger services; and, occasionally, centralized duplication and printing services. These various services may be organized under a single shipping and receiving department or may be dispersed among two or more separate departments.

Strategy Note: For control purposes, receiving and warehousing activities should be functionally and physically separated.

Warehousing

Warehousing is the centralized storage of materials and supplies for the purpose of ensuring they are available, accessible, and in a usable condition when they are needed. Warehousing activities involve various materials-handling techniques and systems designed to move, sort, and store the institution's inventory of supplies and equipment until they are distributed to the end user. A list of materials-handling techniques, including required equipment, is provided in the section "Resource Requirements" later in this chapter.

Inventory Management

The goal of inventory management is to maintain the optimum level of stock required to ensure supplies are available when needed while eliminating unnecessary overstocking. Inventory management involves

- providing a well-organized storage system that ensures supplies are accessible when needed
- providing an efficient and secure system for adding and removing items from inventory and for monitoring inventory levels
- controlling the institution's investment in inventory by eliminating overstocking in dispersed storage areas as well as in centralized stores
- ensuring that stock is regularly rotated to minimize obsolescence
- minimizing the physical space and labor required for holding and processing inventory

A well-organized inventory system depends on two factors: an orderly storage system and clear stock identification. An orderly storage system requires that each inventory item be placed in a suitable area that is secure and accessible. Disorderly or haphazard storage contributes to misplacement, obsolescence, and theft. Accessibility requires clear and wide aisles, logical grouping of similar or related items, and clear stock identification. All stock and equipment should be clearly marked by name or description, stock or serial number, and delivery or expiration date.

Strategy Note: Changes in inventory are occurring constantly. The myriad transactions involved

must be constantly monitored. Well-designed computer systems are now available that can efficiently process these transactions.

Inventory control is essential. The aim of inventory control is to hold the least amount of supply while assuring availability. It involves six principal activities: (1) setting priorities, (2) conducting a physical inventory, (3) determining inventory value, (4) calculating turnover rate, (5) setting target inventory levels, and (6) developing strategies for adjusting inventory levels.

It is difficult and expensive to control every individual inventory item, and a set of priorities needs to be established to focus efforts on those items of greatest expense and vulnerability. As illustrated in Figure 19-2, the ABC approach categorizes all expenditures by rank order of dollar value invested. About 10 percent of all items, the A items, account for 70 percent of all expenditures. The B items amount to 20 percent of all items and account for 20 percent of expenditures. The C items amount to 70 percent of all items and account for 10 percent of expenditures.[8]

Obviously, the bulk of inventory control efforts are most profitably focused on the A items. From another perspective, in the hospital setting most supply costs are incurred in the following categories, representing either large volumes of inexpensive items or small volumes of very expensive items: surgical supplies and implants; anesthesia gases; pharmaceuticals and intravenous solutions; foodstuffs; linens; and dressings, kits, and patient supplies.[9]

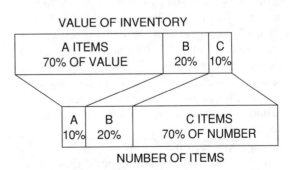

Figure 19-2 The ABC Approach to Prioritization

Based on the priorities identified, a physical inventory can be conducted with several objectives in mind: to measure actual stock against records; to adjust inventory valuation; to evaluate the efficiency of more routine inventory control systems; and to identify shrinkage, stock rotation, obsolescence, and security problems.[10] It is important to extend the physical inventory to the informal storage areas in user departments, since these areas may maintain inventories larger than those in central stores.

Strategy Note: If users tend to hoard excess stock in the work area, it may reflect lack of confidence in routine distribution systems, and a review of supply procedures may be warranted.

With a physical count of the items and recent price information, it is possible to determine the actual value of the inventory on hand—and to compare that value with records. Discrepancies should be identified and explained. Unusual shortages should be studied for possible theft or misappropriation. Disbursement systems may also need adjusting.

Comparing the value of supplies of a given item charged to a user in the last year with the value of inventory on hand results in a turnover rate for that particular item. The turnover rate can be calculated as follows:

$$\text{Turnover} = \frac{\text{Annual dollar value of issues}}{\text{Average inventory dollar value}}$$

While turnover is dependent on many circumstances, for most items a turnover rate of 12 (equivalent to one month's supply on hand) is considered acceptable. A lower rate of 8 or 10 (representing a somewhat higher inventory) may be more realistic in many circumstances, but a rate of 6 (two month's supply) or lower probably deserves attention and adjustment.[11] The turnover rate can be helpful in establishing target inventory levels for each of the categories studied. In setting targets, such factors as supplier accessibility, delivery time, criticalness of the item, and shelf life need to be considered.

Strategies for adjusting inventories include disposal of obsolete and slow-moving items and changing reorder cycles. Items can be disposed of by returning them to the vendor, finding another user, or selling, trading, or trashing them. Reorder cycles can be temporarily adjusted until stock is reduced or permanently adjusted to correspond more closely to patterns of use. Supplier delivery schedules may be altered to provide smaller deliveries more frequently.

There are several statistical methods that can be used in inventory control. In addition to the ABC priority ranking system mentioned earlier, the two most common methods are the reorder point method and the economic order quantity method. Both can be used for routine purchases. Calculating a reorder point can help determine when a particular item should be reordered on the amount left in inventory. It can be calculated as follows:

$$\text{Reorder point} = (\text{usage per day} \times \text{order lead time in days}) + \text{safety factor}$$

Average daily usage of an item is usually determined from a month's sampling of actual use. Lead time is determined from experience in processing orders, receiving items from the supplier, and placing them in inventory. The safety factor is the added amount of inventory needed to cover unusually high demands and unexpected delays in delivery. To illustrate, if the usage is determined to average 25 per day, the lead time is 21 days, and a safety factor of 250 (10 days' supply) is needed, the reorder point would be 775 [$(25 \times 21) + 250 = 775$]. In this case, when the inventory level reaches 775 items, a new order should be placed.

Calculating the economic order quantity is a way of determining the optimum amount or volume of an item to purchase at one time. The formula attempts to mathematically balance the cost of ordering with the cost of holding an item in inventory. Ordering costs are usually determined by dividing the yearly operating costs of the purchasing, receiving, and accounts payable departments by total purchase orders placed in that same period. Holding costs include the yearly operating costs of the central stores or warehouse (excluding supply costs) as a percentage of inventory value. The economic order quantity is calculated as follows:

$$\text{Economic order quantity} = \frac{2 \times \text{annual usage} \times \text{order cost}}{\text{unit cost} \times \text{holding cost } (\%/100)}$$

To illustrate, if the annual usage of an item is 2,400 units, there is a cost of ten dollars to handle an order, the price is one dollar per unit, and there is a carrying cost of inventory of 24 percent per year, then the calculation would be as follows:

$$\text{Economic order quantity} = \frac{2 \times 2,400 \times 10}{1 \times .24} = 447 \text{ units}$$

In this example, 447 units should be maintained in stock. Using the economic order quantity formula, a table can be developed that will help guide routine ordering policy. Precalculated economic order quantity tables are available from a number of sources, including the *Hospital Material Management Quarterly*.[12]

Finally, in any discussion of inventory, a clear distinction should be made between official and unofficial inventory. Official inventory is the amount recorded as an asset on the hospital's balance sheet. It is recognized as unexpended. Unofficial inventory is the amount of supplies that have been expensed but are still on hand in the departments. Unofficial inventory is the hospital's opportunity for savings. The goal should be to move unofficial inventory to official inventory, then reduce the amount using inventory control techniques. This provides more control over ordering, storing, and dispensing. Moreover, it will result in cash flow savings and expense savings.[13]

DISTRIBUTION

Distribution is the process of providing materials where and when they are needed. There are three basic approaches to distribution: requisitioning, stock replenishment, and exchange cart. In addition, the distribution process involves posting charges for materials used.

Requisitioning

Requisitioning is a direct ordering process initiated by the user. Whether it is for a supply item drawn from inventory or a piece of equipment to be secured by bid, requisitioning is the most simple and direct method of placing an order, requiring a minimal investment in support equipment or procedures. When used for routine purchases, requisitioning tends to place an excessive burden on the user. The user needs to constantly monitor available supplies, and every item that is needed must be specifically ordered. The system tends to encourage either more frequent ordering (requiring the user's constant attention) or hoarding (to avoid shortages). Since the user retains control over the process, requisitioning is more appropriate for ordering unusual, expensive, or nonrecurring items. In the requisitioning process, the actual delivery or transportation of the item to the user is on an ad hoc basis (i.e., in direct response to the requisition).

Stock Replenishment

In a stock replenishment (or PAR-level) system, a central stores clerk visits each user area according to a set schedule, in some cases daily. The clerk counts the supplies on hand, identifies shortages against a predetermined standard (or PAR level), writes an order, and provides the supplies needed, either from a traveling supply cart or from the central stores. A stock replenishment system requires a minimal investment in equipment, relieves the user from routine ordering, and directly links disbursements to usage. However, the system tends to be labor intensive, and because requisitioning and disbursement are handled by the same person, it provides weak control over misappropriation.

Exchange Cart System

An exchange cart system uses two transportable carts to serve each user area. One cart is kept on the user's unit. This cart is stocked to a predetermined level, and the user can draw supplies as required. A second cart is kept in the central stores area, where it is restocked to the prescribed level. According to a set schedule, the stocked cart is taken to the unit and exchanged with the depleted cart. The exchange cart system requires a greater investment in capital equipment supplies and the space to store and process the carts. Because it separates the process of ordering from distribution, it provides greater control over personnel.

Strategy Note: The most effective distribution systems are those that replenish supply levels to predetermined standards on a scheduled basis without the end user having to initiate a request. They reduce the purchasing time required by clinically trained staff, and they link the issuance of supplies to actual consumption.[14]

The selection of an appropriate distribution system—whether it be a requisitioning, a stock replenishment, or an exchange cart system or a combination—should be based on several factors:

- the design of the existing system, including its effectiveness and limitations
- the number of user departments and storage locations
- the quantity and mixture of supplies in each area
- existing storage and handling equipment
- available space
- the physical relationship of the departments
- internal traffic routes
- labor costs

Posting Charges

An essential component of the distribution process is the posting of charges to the user department or, in some cases, directly to the patient. The primary objective of posting is to assign the cost of materials to the ultimate consumer, which is essential for accurate cost accounting. A posting system involves two principal activities: cost determination and charge assignment.

Cost determination is intended to assign an appropriate cost for each item of supply. It is usually the responsibility of the accounting department but should involve the materials management department.

Cost can be calculated in several ways and may include the actual cost of the item, an average or estimated cost of the item or like items, an allowance for materials management overhead, and, in some cases, an allowance for general institutional overhead.

It is not practical to charge the patient for all individual items used. Some low-cost or routine items are more appropriately included in overhead charges or combined into a "package" or "kit." The assignment of a charge to a user can be accomplished in several ways. When a requisitioning system is used, the charge for the item ordered is made directly to the user when delivery is verified and notice is sent to the accounting department. In a stock replenishment system, charges are assigned to the department based on the record of items delivered by the stocking clerk. In an exchange cart system, charges are posted based on an inventory of returned items compared to those issued. For those items that are to be charged directly to the patient but are first delivered to the department, materials management typically attaches a "tag" or partially completed requisition. The tag is then removed by the department, completed with patient information, and sent to accounting. An effective charging system should incorporate automatic inventory control and minimize the amount of written documentation required.

PROCESSING

Processing, which is intended to ensure that materials are in a form and condition ready for their intended use, involves the activities of preparation, cleaning and sterilization, and disposal. The central sterile supply department plays an important role in processing activities.

The volume and variety of materials that need to be processed or reprocessed depends heavily on the use of disposables and reusables. A wide range of products are available in both a reusable or disposable form, including those shown in Exhibit 19-4.

The following advantages offered by disposables have led to their increased use[15]:

Exhibit 19-4 Disposable or Reusable Products

Aprons	Diapers
Bags	Dietary products
Blood collection	Gloves
Food storage	Gowns
Laundry	Handkerchiefs
Specimen	Kits
Trash	Catheterization
Utility	Irrigation
Bedpans	Peritoneal analysis
Blankets	Mops
Bottles	Needles
Catheters	Prep sets
Cloths	Sheets
Containers	Shirts
Coveralls	Syringes
Covers	Underpads
Examining table	
Mattress	
Tray	

Source: Reprinted from *Nonwovens and Disposable Soft Goods,* with permission of Rodman Publishing Co., © 1973.

- *Cost.* Disposables and nonwovens may be more economical, especially if the cost of reprocessing reusables is taken into account (although some would say this is changing because of the increased cost of dumping in landfills).
- *Safety.* Prepackaged, sterile products offer superior quality control and protection from infectious diseases (such as AIDS and hepatitis) for patients and employees.
- *Convenience.* The products are readily available, since there are no reprocessing delays.
- *Advances in Technology.* Advances can result from manufacturers' investment in product development and improvement.
- *Demand.* There is increased acceptance by and demand from users.
- *Legal Liability.* The manufacturers share the liability with the institution.

Preparation

Not all supplies and equipment are received in a form or condition ready for use. An item may need to be uncrated, sorted, assembled, and possibly tested prior to its distribution to the user. Items delivered in bulk may need to be broken down into units or sizes that are suitable for storage or distribution. Sorting is required for proper placement of items in inventory. Assembly may be required, especially with equipment and furniture. When furnishing new or remodeled facilities, a secured area may be needed to uncrate and assemble a large number of bulky items. Testing may involve determining if an item meets specifications but may also include calibration and adjustments required prior to use.

Cleaning and Sterilization

Cleaning and sterilization have traditionally been the responsibilities of the central sterile supply service, now often referred to as simply central supply. Historically, central supply was an adjunct service—reprocessing reusable instruments, utensils, supplies, and equipment in support, primarily, of the surgical suite and nursing services. Its primary role is unchanged, but its functions and activities have been substantially altered with the advent of disposable products, and it is now often incorporated into the materials management organization.[16] Even with the increased use of disposables, a substantial amount of material reprocessing is still required. Central service continues to decontaminate, clean, inspect, repackage, and sterilize operating room instruments, linens, and utensils. It usually combines reprocessed items with related disposable items, assembling a surgical case cart, for example. It may also be responsible for the collection and disposal of trash, especially contaminated materials.

Typically, within the central service area all soiled materials for reprocessing are transported to a decontamination area in enclosed carts. Contaminated items should be bagged by the user in water soluble bags and sent through a washer-sterilizer. Instruments and utensils are placed on racking tables and sent through an instrument utensil washer or an ultrasonic cleaning unit. Stripped carts proceed through a cart wash and then on to a restocking area. After cleaning and/or sterilization, instruments and utensils are sent to a preparation or repackaging area, where they are sorted, assembled into packs, wrapped, and placed on sterilization racks. After sterilization, they are stored in holding areas ready for distribution back to the user.[17]

The surgical suite is responsible for notifying central stores on the expected number and types of operations. Central supply then assembles the required procedure packs and other related supplies and makes up surgical case carts. The carts are delivered to the surgical suite and held in readiness. When an operation is completed, all instruments, utensils, linens, and used supplies are placed back on the case cart and returned to central supply, where the reprocessing cycle is repeated.

Disposal

Trash removal, including the disposal of contaminated and hazardous waste, is often the responsibility of a housekeeping or domestic services department but may also be organized under materials management.

Strategy Note: Health care organizations have a special obligation to properly control, handle, and dispose of contaminated materials and hazardous waste. Proper handling and disposal is vital to the safety of patients, employees, and the public.

CONTROL

Most health care institutions devote a sizable portion of their annual budget to the purchase and management of materials. Obviously, these expenditures require careful control. Control is exercised at each stage of the materials management process to ensure that materials

- are acquired at the agreed price
- conform to established standards of quality and performance

- are received in the amount specified and in good condition
- are not damaged, nor deteriorate during storage
- are secure from theft and pilferage
- are readily available for use

Control activities include defining policies and procedures, planning acquisitions, and monitoring materials and their related costs.

Policy and Procedure Definition

Materials management control requires clearly stated purchasing policies and well-defined operational procedures. If the institution is committed to purchasing supplies at the overall lowest cost, then appropriate policies are needed. For example, it might be required that comparative pricing be done on all purchases. Policies and procedures should be in writing, and there should be provisions regarding the following:

- *Authority*. The provisions should define who has the power to initiate and approve purchases of various value.
- *Accountability*. Documentation at each decision point in the purchasing process should be mandated.
- *Vendor Selection*. Procedures for prequalifying suppliers and protecting against arbitrary selection are essential.
- *Specifications*. Procedures for defining specifications and general conditions are also needed.
- *Standardization*. There should be a policy on standardization and procedures for implementation.
- *Contract Awards*. Procedures are needed that ensure the fair and honest granting of purchase contracts. Only purchase orders that have followed approved procedures should be honored.
- *Delivery and Inventory Control*. Also required are procedures for monitoring supplies.

- *Distribution.* Procedures for requisitioning, delivery, and posting charges should be established.

Strategy Note: To be effective, materials management policies and procedures must be endorsed by the administration and communicated and understood by all user departments.

Acquisition Planning

Acquisition planning involves the development of an overall purchasing approach (or strategy) for the organization and the design of a specific plan and budget for materials management activities. As with any other department, materials management should develop an annual operating budget detailing its salaries, department supplies, and other operating costs. In preparing its budget, it should project its expected workload in terms of number of purchase orders, volume of supply, and other measures. Materials management is also able to assist accounting in forecasting changes in the volume or cost of purchases during the next budgeting period. The annual budget is the primary planning document for the department and establishes the basic guideposts for measuring department performance. Actual performance should be measured against the budget periodically through the year.

Monitoring

Materials management processes large numbers of transactions involving substantial volumes of valuable supplies and equipment. Its operating systems need to routinely handle these critical resources while providing continuing documentation and protection against theft and misappropriation.

Documentation is important for making certain that appropriate procedures are followed and that costs are accurately assigned. While written documentation is still most common, automated procedures have been developed that permit documenta-tion to occur electronically (through code scanners and computer, for example). Whatever its form, documentation should occur at each stage in the acquisition process:

- *Requisitioning.* A numbered purchase order system helps to ensure that all purchasing is done centrally. Improperly numbered orders are refused.
- *Receiving.* A "blind" copy of the purchase order, excluding expected quantities, will force the receiving clerk to count the items delivered.
- *Distribution.* Exchange carts divide the responsibility for requisitioning (identifying shortages) and issuing supplies.
- *Accounts Payable.* Organizational separation, with independent verification, between accounts payable and materials management is beneficial.

The opportunities for theft and misappropriation are numerous but can be controlled through carefully designed procedures. Kickbacks are payments made by vendors to a buyer for placing an order (in the form of cash, favors, or concessions), and they invariably result in inflated costs to the institution. They are most prevalent where there is a direct and unsupervised connection between an individual buyer and the vendor. If the user both places the order and receives the goods directly, it is easy to overstate the amount received or remove part of the shipment and authorize payment of the invoiced amount. Theft or misappropriation is also a significant risk in the receiving area. A driver can deliver short, keep part of the shipment to sell elsewhere, and divide the proceeds with the receiving clerk. If unsupervised, the receiving clerk can verify a full shipment.

Theft can also occur within user departments, especially theft of routine stock items. Materials most susceptible to theft are those that are most marketable, such as meats, canned goods, linens, bulk paper supplies, and chemicals. Drugs (especially narcotics), syringes, and related supplies are also susceptible. Items in common daily use, especially inexpensive and easily transportable items, are often perceived to be inconsequential and are vulnerable to misappropriation by even honest employees. Pens, scissors, paper supplies, linens, and small food items are particularly vulnerable.

Strategy Note: To encourage honesty, the organization must first value honesty and communicate that value through its policies, through its management, and by example. In the end, dishonesty costs the institution, the patient, and the community.

Theft and misappropriation are the product of inclination and opportunity. Inclination, the propensity of an individual to be dishonest, can be controlled to some extent by proper personnel selection procedures. Proper training, clear work rules, and unambiguous disciplinary reinforcement can also reduce dishonest inclinations. Opportunity, access to tempting objects, is controlled through the development, communication, and enforcement of policies and procedures designed around four essential principles:

1. Documentation. Each transaction needs to be recorded.
2. Accountability. An individual must be held accountable for each transaction. In some cases, two organizationally separate individuals must independently document a transaction. The separation of requisitioning from receiving, the separation of receiving from central stores, and the separation of central stores from accounts payable are all examples.
3. Security. Access to vulnerable property must be restricted. Examples include limited access to storage areas, locked holding areas, wire cages, and documented release of goods.
4. Verification. Procedures must incorporate routine documentation, close supervision, and periodic verification. Physical inventories, random checks, and periodic review are all useful techniques.

ORGANIZATIONAL FUNCTION

Materials management developed in industry in the United States in the 1930s and expanded in the post–World War II area. Even though many factories had materials managers in the 1950s and 1960s, the new position was not fully accepted until the mid-1970s. Thus materials management has played an ever-growing role (and has had an ever-greater impact).

Industry acknowledges there have been pitfalls in the adoption of materials management, such as the lack of strong top management support and the refusal by personnel to discard old purchasing concepts. These are also possible pitfalls in hospitals and other health care facilities.

Materials management is organized differently in each health care facility depending on its size, physical limitations, management priorities, policies and procedures, and its staff and their qualifications. In larger institutions, typically larger hospitals, with a wide array of user departments and substantial annual expenditures for equipment and supplies, centralization offers the opportunity for improved efficiency, cost-effectiveness, and control. Benefits of centralization include greater product standardization, fewer purchase orders, quantity discounts, fewer burdens on users, and unified policies and procedures. A highly centralized department could include most or all of the following departments and activities:

- purchasing (including all purchasing for pharmacy, food service, laundry, maintenance, and other departments with specialized needs)
- receiving
- central stores
- central supply (sterile supply)
- mail and distribution
- shipping and transportation
- contract negotiation

Although still uncommon, in a few institutions, service departments that have a significant volume of regular supply purchases, such as pharmacy, food service, or laundry, may be organized under the direction of the materials management department. Obviously, to be effective, centralization requires clear objectives (the benefits of centralization), well-defined policies and procedures, and strong endorsement by the central administration. Figure 19-3 is a sample organization chart for a centralized materials management department in a large general hospital.

Decentralization allows for greater responsiveness to the needs of users departments. Departments with special needs, such as food service, pharmacy, housekeeping, and maintenance, remain responsible for some or all of their own materials management activities, such as the purchase of nonrecurring items, the purchase of perishables, or the processing and distribution of drugs or meals. Central sterile supply, radiology, laboratory, and other technical service departments also commonly handle their own purchasing needs. A smaller institution may not even have a purchasing agent, in which case purchasing is done directly by the user. A somewhat larger organization may have a purchasing agent, but the agent's primary role might be limited to assisting users in their purchasing activities. It is still common for even bigger institutions to maintain a largely decentralized organization, although the degree of centralization appears to be growing.

Personnel

Almost all hospitals and many other health care organizations have materials management or purchasing departments with some degree of centralization. The types of individuals that head these departments and the array of responsibilities and authority assigned to them varies widely, with the result that materials management is not yet a well-defined profession. The following are a few of the key positions commonly involved in materials management activities.[18] In smaller organizations, two or more jobs may be combined in one position.

Director of Materials Management. The director of materials management typically has overall managerial responsibility for a highly centralized organization. In addition to general management duties, the director has the following responsibilities:

- directing and overseeing centralized procurement of all supplies, equipment, and services
- developing standard specifications for invitations to bid
- organizing and overseeing receiving, storeroom, and distribution activities

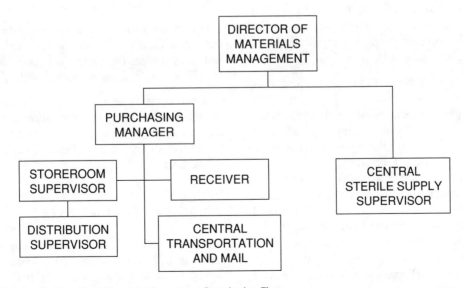

Figure 19-3 Sample Centralized Materials Management Organization Chart

- developing materials management policies and procedures and monitoring compliance
- serving as advisor and resource for all departments on materials management issues
- ensuring compliance with quality, safety, and environmental protection standards
- establishing and supervising systems for controlling inventory and costs

Broadly, the director should have

- basic management skills and aptitudes
- the ability to relate to other managers (including line and staff managers)
- knowledge of the basic concepts of purchasing and inventory control
- the ability to relate to vendors and negotiate successfully
- familiarity with medicochirurchical product lines and fair market prices
- familiarity with alternative distribution systems

The director should have a college degree, preferably in business administration or a related field, and have taken courses in bookkeeping, economics, marketing, mathematics, and business law. Postgraduate education is becoming more common, and some directors hold a master's degree in health administration.

Purchasing Manager. Typically, the purchasing manager performs various purchasing functions and activities. Responsibilities include interviewing sales representatives, securing bids and quotes, selecting suppliers, and placing orders for most materials, equipment, and services.

In a centralized organization, the purchasing manager would report to the director of materials management. In a decentralized (or less centralized) organization, the purchasing manager could be the most senior manager and be assigned a wide array of materials management–related activities. In either case, a college degree is highly preferred, with a postgraduate degree desirable.

Buyer or Purchasing Assistant. This individual performs a variety of purchasing activities (e.g., contacting vendors and preparing specifications and bidding documents), usually under direct supervision.

Stores Supervisor or Inventory Coordinator. This individual organizes and coordinates all receiving, stores, and inventory control functions.

Receiver. The receiver accepts incoming materials, verifies accuracy of shipment, inspects for damage, and delivers items to central stores or to users. A high school diploma and some experience are required.

Distribution Manager. The distribution manager coordinates requisitioning, ordering, and distribution of materials to ensure that inventory relates to usage. He or she supervises the distribution technicians, who assemble supplies for direct or cart distribution systems.

Central Supply Supervisor. This individual oversees the central sterile supply services. He or she works closely with nursing and the surgical suite to ensure that supplies and utensils are processed properly and safely and are available for use. The central supply supervisor is often a nurse.

Dispatcher. In an organization with a centralized transportation service, a dispatcher receives calls and assigns staff for patient transport, mail and messenger services, linen distribution, and the like.

A number of other kinds of employees are also commonly found in materials management, including central supply technicians, transporters, chauffeurs, truck drivers, messengers, and various clerical workers.

RESOURCE REQUIREMENTS

Health care organizations devote considerable resources to buying and managing materials. In a typical hospital, for example, materials management costs represent from 20 to 30 percent of total operational costs. Almost 27 percent of all hospital costs are spent for supplies and equipment, with another 19 percent spent for managerial support in the processing of materials, including labor, capital investment, and general overhead.[20] While the proportions are lower in nursing homes, long-term care facilities, and clinics, materials still represent a substantial cost for these organizations.

Facilities

The availability and cost of storage space will directly impact inventory management. On the average, the space required to house the central stores is estimated to be about ten square feet per bed for an acute hospital and about five square feet per bed for a skilled nursing home.[21]

Strategy Note: The criterion for determining need for storage space is as follows. Storage of an item is justified if it is more economical to maintain the item in inventory than to purchase the item on demand.

Specifically, facilities need to be provided for the following activities:

- delivery (delivery truck access, an unloading dock, dock plates for bridging between trucks and the dock)
- receiving (a covered and secured space adequate for uncrating and counting)
- central stores (a holding and sorting area [to hold goods delivered from receiving], a bulk storage area, and an active inventory area)
- distribution (an order processing or cart assembly area)
- management (office space for receiving users and sales representatives, for clerical processes, and for files and records)
- processing (may include separate areas for central sterile supply, mail and distribution, packaging, and other functions)
- dispersed inventory (storage space for shelving or cart storage on the user units)
- secured areas (caged storage, locked areas, and the like)

Equipment

Principal materials handling systems and equipment include these:

- automated systems (conveyors, overhead monorails, chain-drive trucks, pneumatic tubes, dumbwaiters, cart-washing equipment, and automatic cart systems)
- power equipment (cranes, trucks, forklifts, and power-lift trucks)
- hand equipment (handcarts, dollies, and a variety of special-purpose hand trucks and tools)
- shelving systems
  —pallet racks for large or bulky items stored on pallets
  —centilever racks for storing pipe, bars, and rods
  —bin racks for smaller items of various sizes
  —tier racks for lighter materials
  —flow-through racks for rapidly moving items such as pharmaceuticals and office supplies
  —frame racks for pipes and long items
  —rollaway racks (racks on wheels designed for portability)
  —double-deck racks to take advantage of high ceilings
- counters (large work surfaces for unpacking, sorting, order filling, and wrapping)
- security systems (automatic water sprinkler systems, smoke and heat detectors, environmental protection for weather and pest control, screened and caged areas, and burglar alarms)
- specialty storage equipment (walk-in refrigerators and freezers, refrigerated trash containers, and contaminated trash containers)
- disposal systems (trash carts and bins, compactors, incinerators, and garbage trucks)

Support System

Materials management involves large volumes of diverse transactions and is prime territory for the application of computer and other electronic technology. Well-designed dedicated computer systems are available that can handle the bulk of the required activities, including requisitioning, purchase order placement, inventory control, and usage monitoring. Electronic bar code readers are also finding broader applications, especially in inventory control and distribution. These systems do not appear to have any particular effect on personnel staffing requirements, but they do increase efficiency and accuracy. Where computerization or electronic wizardry does not seem practical, other well-designed manual and automated systems are available that can be adapted to the organization's needs and budget.

QUALITY MANAGEMENT

Broadly, the most basic measure of materials management quality is a whether the user is receiving the proper product when needed and at a reasonable price. Accuracy and promptness are key criteria.

Strategy Note: Quality begins with the establishment of performance objectives and clearly delineated policies and procedures, reinforced by training and supervision.

User Service

The supply-performance review is a means of evaluating how well materials management is meeting the needs of individual users. The specific supply and material needs of each unit or department must be delineated, including supply specifications, quantities, and delivery schedules. Care must be exercised to separate needs from wants, using actual patterns of use as a guide. Using the identified needs, supply standards and service criteria can be developed as the basis for performance review. Actual performance must be measured (including shortages, delivery delays, substitutions, and errors) and judged against the established standards. Discrepancies need to be evaluated and procedures and processes need to be adjusted as

needed. A supply-performance review should be conducted periodically (probably yearly) or in response to a special request or concern.

Supply Quality

In order to ensure the quality of its supplies and equipment, the organization must begin by designing appropriate specifications that emphasize product performance. A product standardization committee, described earlier in this chapter, can assist in establishing appropriate specifications. In addition, product testing and evaluation prior to purchase can give greater assurance that materials of poor or inappropriate quality will not be acquired. Even so, additional testing should be conducted after materials are delivered to make certain they actually meet the prescribed specifications. A value improvement program can help to ensure the quality of supplies. This type of program focuses on

- choosing standardized and compatible products and equipment whenever possible
- screening for the best-quality product in relationship to price, service, delivery, and other criteria
- evaluating product liability and safety and protection for patients, employees, physicians, and the institution
- testing products both before and after purchase

Vendor Performance

The purpose of vendor evaluation is to ensure that current and prospective suppliers are qualified on the basis of price, quality, reliability, honesty, delivery, and service. Existing vendors and, to the extent possible, potential vendors should be evaluated using performance data for a recent fiscal period. A comparison among vendors can then be made on the following basis[22]:

- prices for individual items and the overall price

- payment terms
- availability of local warehousing
- volume of purchase orders
- delivery schedule and reliability
- comparative transportation costs
- regularity of sales representatives, their visits, and their responsiveness
- evaluation of product quality by users
- competitiveness of bids when requested
- vendor's attention to cost-saving measures, such as combined shipments
- efficiency of vendor's order taking and processing
- accuracy of vendor's accounting and billing procedures

Here it should be noted that buying from the lowest bidder after playing one vendor against another in an effort to get one to cut the price is costly. This is the view of Deming, who also postulates the buyer should make a long-term commitment to work with a single supplier in an effort to help the supplier improve quality and reduce costs.[23] Thus a gain can be achieved by both the institution and the vendor as well.

Managerial Performance

The impact of managerial performance on quality depends on the level of centralized management authority and responsibility and the control exercised over acquisition and distribution. The following are indicators that managerial performance is satisfactory[24]:

- the existence of clear policies and procedures that are understood and followed throughout the organization
- documented receipt and accountability for all supply transactions
- reduction and control of both central and dispersed inventories

- maintenance of stock levels adequate to meet user needs
- prevention of lost patient charges
- control over disposition of obsolete and excess supplies and equipment
- reduction of the user's burden for acquisition, including elimination of excess paper work
- contribution of overall cost-containment activity

More specifically, managerial performance can be measured through supply-price comparisons, cost measures, management audits, and managerial reports.

Supply-price comparisons are intended to compare the price paid for an item against the price paid by other buyers. While many factors can affect price (e.g., purchase volume and delivery costs), comparisons can indicate the effectiveness of past practices and can help set goals for future buying.

The materials cost per patient day can be used in making comparisons with similar organizations. The ratio of all materials management–related costs (including labor, overhead, and all supply costs) to patient days (or some other common measure of volume) is a helpful benchmark.

Management audits are designed to monitor all aspects of the department's activities—inventory control, organization, personnel, procedures, pricing, and other operational parameters. Audits can be designed to focus on almost any aspect of the materials management operation or answer questions such as the following[25]: Are personnel performance appraisals done on materials management employees on a regular basis? Is there an effective materials orientation program for all institutional employees? Is there true centralization of purchasing or is the process regularly bypassed?

Periodic and special management reports are helpful in monitoring managerial performance. Like any other department, the materials management department should be required to report regularly on its routine operational activities (e.g., revenues and expense compared to budget and staffing levels; inventory levels). In addition, a number of other reports that address various productivity measures should be prepared at least quarterly. Examples include reports on supply usage, linen inventory and usage, stock turnover, and supply cost escalation.

The materials management department should also be subject to regular review by top management. Routine and special reports can serve as the basis for such review.

THE FUTURE OF MATERIALS MANAGEMENT

The resources an institution devotes to materials management can be considerable, and proper measurement in the allocation of these resources presents a great challenge. Materials management plays a central role in ensuring that these resources are well used and is critical in supporting the activities of other departments, ensuring they have the supplies and equipment they need to perform their duties.

In the recently developed hospital materials management field, computer systems are being used not only in purchasing and receiving but also for inventory control, menu planning, food service management, preventive maintenance monitoring, energy management, and project scheduling and control, among other applications. It should be noted that there is little question that electronic data interchange will become the predominant method for handling business transactions. The primary reason for this is the universal acceptance of the ANSI X12 standards for the formats of the most common business transactions (e.g., purchase orders, confirmations, invoices, and remittances).

In the health care industry, proprietary order entry systems are becoming less prevalent, and the ANSI X12 formats and communication protocol have correspondingly received sincere support. This is good news for everyone, because use of the formats will lower the costs of doing business universally. No longer will hospitals have to invest in separate software to transmit purchase orders to their various suppliers.[26] Another major factor is the increased importance of prospective payment systems, not to mention the growing relationship of materials management to financial management and its interface role in coordinating the functions still decentralized by product line. Because purchasing of food, medical supplies, and equipment is secondary to the cost of personnel in a modern hospital, the emphasis will be on managing purchasing resources in a manner that is expedient, is economical, and ensures quality. Finally, the advent of AIDS highlights the increased need for safeguards in central supply, the emergency room, and the nursing floor, all areas of major materials management concern.

ADDITIONAL RESOURCES

Organizations

American Society for Hospital Materials Management, American Hospital Association, 840 N. Lakeshore Drive, Chicago, IL 60611.

Health Care Material Management Society, 13223 Black Mountain Road, San Diego, CA 92129.

Periodicals

Hospital Materiel Management Quarterly, Aspen Publishers, 200 Orchard Ridge Drive, Gaithersburg, MD 20878.

Hospital Purchasing News, McKnight Medical Communications Company, 1419 Lake Cook Road, Deerfield, IL 60015.

Hospital Materials Management, Business Word, 5350 S. Roslyn Street, Englewood, CO 80111-2125.

Journal of Healthcare Materials Management, Mayworm Associates, Inc., 507 N. Milwaukee Avenue, Libertyville, IL 60048.

Materials Management in Healthcare, American Hospital Publishing, Inc., 737 N. Michigan Avenue, Chicago, IL 60611-2615.

Books

Ammer, D.S. *Purchasing and materials management for health care institutions.* 2d ed. Lexington Mass.: Lexington Books, 1983.

Aspen Reference Group. *Hospital material management forms, checklists and guidelines.* Gaithersburg, Md.: Aspen Publishers, 1991.

Holmgren, J.H., and W.J. Wentz. *Material management and purchasing for the health care facility.* Ann Arbor, Mich.: AUPHA Press, 1982.

Housley, C.E. *Controlling hospital supply inventories.* Gaithersburg, Md.: Aspen Publishers, 1983.

——*Product standardization and evaluation.* Gaithersburg, Md.: Aspen Publishers, 1985.

——*Strategies in hospital material management.* Gaithersburg Md.: Aspen Publishers, 1983.

Kowalski, J.C. *Materials management policy and procedure manual.* 2d ed. St. Louis: Catholic Health Association of the United States, 1990.

Sanderson, E. *Effective hospital material management.* Gaithersburg, Md.: Aspen Publishers, 1985.

Scheyer, W. *Handbook of health care material management.* Gaithersburg, Md.: Aspen Publishers, 1985.

NOTES

1. C.E. Housley, *Hospital Materiel Management* (Gaithersburg, Md.: Aspen Publishers, 1978).

2. J. P. Swindler, The Future of the Purchasing Agent: Material Management as a Professional, *Hospital Topics,* July-August 1978, pp. 22–26.

3. J.H. Holmgren, and W.J. Wentz, *Material Management and Purchasing for the Health Care Facility* (Ann Arbor, Mich.: AUPHA Press, 1982), 54.

4. Ibid., 54–55.

5. L. Lee, Jr., and D.W. Dobler, *Purchasing and Materials Management* (New York: McGraw-Hill, 1971).

6. Holmgren and Wentz, *Material Management and Purchasing,* p. 70.

7. Ibid., p. 216.

8. Ibid., p. 128.

9. J.R. Griffith, *The Well-Managed Community Hospital* (Ann Arbor, Mich.: Health Administration Press, 1987), 629.

10. D. Cobbs, How To Conduct a Physical Inventory, *Hospital Materiel Management Quarterly,* May 1981, pp. 92–96.

11. H.S. Rowland and B.L. Rowland, *Hospital Management: A Guide to Departments* (Gaithersburg, Md.: Aspen Publishers, 1984), 221.

12. D. Sapp, How We Use EOQ and RQL for Better Inventory Control, *Health Institution Purchasing,* October 1971, p. 25.

13. L. Adelung, The Materials Manager and Chief Financial Officer Succeeding as a Team, paper delivered at the 28th Annual Conference of the ASHMM of the American Hospital Association, Materials Management '90: The Age of Leadership, Washington, D.C., 1990.

14. L.F.Wolper and J.J. Pena, *Health Care Administration: Principles and Practices* (Gaithersburg, Md.: Aspen Publishers, 1987), 473.

15. J.H. Holmgren, Hospitals Need Disposables, *Nonwovens and Disposable Soft Goods,* June 1973, pp. 75–80.

16. J.J. Frommelt and J.L. Schanilec, The Integration of Central Services into Material Management, *Material Management and Purchasing.*

17. Ibid.

18. The American Society for Hospital Personnel Directors, *Health Care Occupations: A Comprehensive Job Description Manual,* vol. 2 (Chicago: American Hospital Association, 1985).

19. Henning, W.K. Application of the Prudent Buyer Principle to Purchasing Administration, *Hospital Materiel Management Quarterly,* November 1979, pp. 17–25.

20. Housley, *Hospital Materiel Management.*

21. Holmgren and Wentz, *Material Management and Purchasing,* 149.

22. Ibid., 74.

23. W. E. Deming, *Out of the Crisis* (Cambridge, Mass.: Massachusetts Institute of Technology, Center for Advanced Engineering Study, 1986).

24. C.B. Stearns, Getting Results from Your Materiel Manager, *Hospital Materiel Management Quarterly,* August 1979, pp. 35–44.

25. Rowland and Rowland, *Hospital Management,* pp. 250–252.

26. T. Pirelli, EDI in the 90's: New Developments for a New Decade, paper presented at the 28th Annual Conference of the ASHMM of the American Hospital Association, Materials Management '90: The Age of Leadership, Washington, D.C., 1990. (Pirelli updated remarks by phone to the authors, September 1991.)

William A. Gouveia

Pharmacy Services

20

Purpose: The purpose of pharmacy is to procure, distribute, control, and monitor the acquisition and use of drugs so that a patient's drug therapy is appropriate, safe, and cost-effective and meets the physicians', patients', and pharmacists' goals and expectations. Pharmacy is an information-, product-, and outcome-oriented profession charged by society with ensuring the safe and appropriate use of drugs. Pharmaceutical care involves responsibly providing drug therapy for the purpose of achieving definite outcomes that improve a patient's quality of life.

sponsibility comes at a time in which the complexity and cost of drug therapy is increasing and in which the concept of pharmaceutical care is gaining greater public attention. This chapter reviews the management principles that guide departments of pharmacy; reviews organizational roles and functions; and discusses the key functions of pharmacy departments in drug information, drug preparation and distribution, clinical pharmacy services, and teaching and research. Resource requirements are defined, as is the need for quality management.

INTRODUCTION

Pharmacy has a traditional role in providing, preparing, and distributing drugs throughout health care institutions. Pharmacists are playing an increasing role in ensuring that drugs provided to patients are selected appropriately and that their use is properly monitored. The concept of pharmaceutical care is based on the premise that pharmacists should assume greater responsibility for making certain that each patient's drug therapy achieves the proper outcomes.[1] This trend toward expanded re-

MANAGEMENT PRINCIPLES

The hospital medication system has traditionally encompassed the ordering of drug therapies by physicians; the preparation, dispensing, and distribution of drugs by pharmacists; and the administration of drugs by nurses.

Research on the medication system performed in the 1960s and 1970s identified problems within the existing individual prescription and floor stock system. These problems resulted in significant medication error rates.[2] The unit dose drug distribution system and intravenous admixture services were developed in response to concerns about medication safety.[3] Satellite pharmacy programs were developed to provide drugs in closer proximity to patients and served as a basis for clinical pharmacy programs.[4] Clinical pharmacy programs, developed largely in the 1970s and 1980s, were based on the use of pharmacists with special training and skills who practiced at patient care areas or bedside.[5]

Presently, the focus of pharmacy managers is to recruit and retain pharmacists who are specifically trained to manage drug therapies in collaboration with other health care providers. The pharmacy manager faces an escalating drug budget, and must balance clinical needs with economic reality. Finally, the pharmacy manager has a responsibility to ensure that medication "misadventures" are minimized in their institutions.

- Pharmacy practice is increasingly specialized to meet the unique needs of patients, physicians, nurses, and institutions. In pharmaceutical care, a primary care pharmacist might work with each patient, their physicians, and their nurses.

- Effective and appropriate drug surveillance requires a high degree of vigilance in order to meet the requirements of local and national guidelines and laws regulating the use of drugs, including controlled substances and investigational drugs.

- There is an appropriate balance between the roles of the various professional and technical personnel in pharmacy and an appropriate balance between labor costs and supply costs must be realized.

- Drug therapy is becoming increasingly precise, complex, and costly. Special procedures and protocols must be developed or employed to utilize new pharmaceutical products, including biotechnological products, properly.

- Pharmacists and technicians require a considerable investment for their personal and professional development and training as well as opportunities for career growth.

- There are environmental hazards associated with the preparation, use, and disposal of chemotherapeutic substances as well as other medications potentially harmful to individuals who handle them. The proper handling and disposal of these substances requires special training, careful application of techniques, and constant vigilance.

- Drug distribution systems must be tailored to each institution and often to each patient care area. Automation is just beginning to be applied to the drug preparation and dispensing process. The goals of automation are to decrease labor involvement and subsequent cost and ensure timely and accurate drug preparation and dispensing.

- Pharmacy departments have expanded their responsibilities to include outpatient dispensing, home care, and other practice innovations.

- The cost of drug therapy can be controlled in part through effective purchasing. However, the volume and mix and hence cost of pharmaceuticals is best related to patient volume and mix. The greatest reduction in drug cost can come from the concerted efforts of physicians, nurses, and pharmacists to reduce utilization of drugs and drug-related services, including, for example, drug serum level laboratory tests.

ORGANIZATIONAL ROLES AND FUNCTIONS

Pharmacy had its origins in the role of the house apothecary, who was usually a physician or student of medicine and surgery. Jonathan Roberts, the first hospital pharmacist in the United States, began practicing at Pennsylvania Hospital in 1752. The slow transition from the house apothecary to apprentice-trained pharmacist and finally to formally educated pharmacist took nearly two centuries to complete. The period 1920–1942 was especially important, because in these years a number of state and local hospital pharmacy associations were founded to support the needs of an increasing number of practitioners. In 1936, during the annual meeting of the American Pharmaceutical Association, hospital pharmacy was reorganized on a national level. The American Society of Hospital Pharmacists (ASHP) was founded in 1942, with 152 charter members, as an outgrowth of the hospital pharmacy section of the American Pharmaceutical Association.

Continuing education programs for hospital pharmacists were initiated in 1946 by the ASHP. An audit of pharmaceutical services in hospitals was published in the 1950s and provided the first comprehensive description of the pharmacy services offered by U.S. hospitals.[6] The *American Journal of Hospital Pharmacy* began as a monthly publication in 1958 and is the most important source of professional practice information. Hospital pharmacy residency programs began in the 1960s and continue to be an important means of training the prospective leaders of the profession. These programs, which are accredited by the ASHP and now number 250, are based on the application of rigorous practice standards for the institution, department of pharmacy, program director, and resident.[7] Pharmacy practice residencies with emphasis on pharmaceutical care have specific training requirements in acute patient care, ambulatory care, practice management, and drug information and policy development.

Today's pharmacist is involved with patients, physicians, and nurses in working prospectively to ensure that the drug therapy prescribed for each patient is optimal considering the therapeutic goals and cost, to monitor drug utilization for both proper effect and adverse reactions, and to analyze drug utilization retrospectively according to predetermined criteria. The pharmacist is responsible for drug distribution and control and for ensuring that legal and regulatory requirements are met.

Organizationally, the pharmacy is often placed within the professional or clinical services unit of the hospital. Through a variety of hospital and medical staff committees, including pharmacy and therapeutics, infection control, and the institutional review board, the pharmacy collaborates with the medical, nursing, and administrative staffs. Figure 20-1 is a typical organization chart for a pharmacy that provides comprehensive programs to meet patient and institutional needs. Smaller hospitals tailor their pharmacy services to meet their patients' needs and may combine some functions. For example, a pharmacy clinical coordinator may serve as a resource for drug information (including investigational drug data) and also provide patient-specific clinical pharmacy services (e.g., pharmacokinetic dosing for patients).

Increasingly, ethical considerations have developed that affect pharmacy operations. For instance, the issue regarding the conduct of drug research involving patients, or the issue of the influence that the pharmaceutical industry has in the marketing and sales of drugs within institutions must be resolved. The role of the clinical investigator and members of the pharmacy and therapeutics committees in decision making regarding the management of the hospital formulary must withstand consumer scrutiny. Institutions are developing codes of ethics that require disclosure of consultancies, stock ownership, and other potential sources of conflict of interest.[8]

DRUG INFORMATION AND EDUCATION

A drug information service provides unbiased, timely, and meaningful information on drug therapy to patients, physicians, nurses, and other health care professionals. Some of the functions of the typical hospital-based drug information service are described below.

The service provides answers to the questions from clinicians. Timely and carefully prepared and presented responses to questions require not only evaluation of the literature but critical interpretation of that literature in the context of specific variables that must be considered in tailoring drug therapy to benefit individual patients.

The pharmacy and therapeutics committee includes members of the medical staff and of the

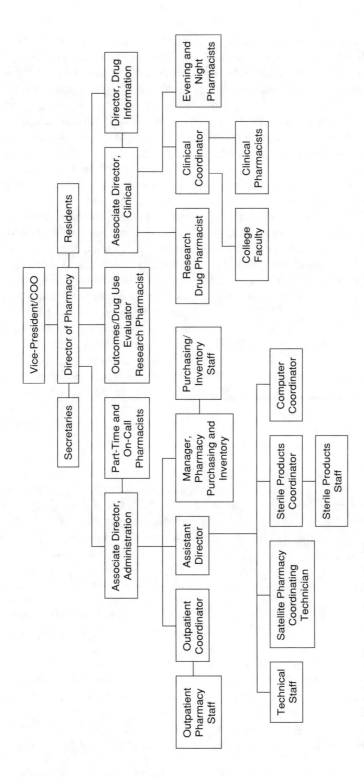

Figure 20-1 Sample Pharmacy Organization Chart

nursing and pharmacy departments and a representative of the administration. Its purpose is to develop and approve policies and procedures related to medication use in the institution, to develop and maintain the hospital formulary, and to identify and review all untoward drug reactions within the institution. Pharmacy and therapeutics functions are mandated by the Joint Commission on Accreditation of Healthcare Organizations.

The committee conducts drug evaluations, especially of new drugs requested for admission to the formulary. A comprehensive literature search is done, followed by the selection of specific comparative studies from the resultant bibliography. A critical evaluation of each study is performed by a drug information staff member trained in the evaluation of clinical literature. A thorough drug evaluation includes the following:

- the rationale for the formulary addition request
- the action(s) of the drug
- the drug's clinical pharmacology
- the drug's pharmacokinetics (the disposition of the drug in the body)
- dosage and administration
- drug interactions
- adverse reactions
- efficacy
- cost and cost comparison (drug versus similar drugs)
- concluding recommendations regarding formulary inclusion, need for drug use evaluation or other forms of monitoring, potential restriction of use within the hospital, and relationship to other drugs (e.g., deletion of an existing drug), along with pertinent references

Drug evaluations form the basis of the hospital formularly. The formulary reflects current clinical judgment regarding which drugs should be available in the institution for routine use. A highly restrictive formulary might have only one or two drugs available for each drug category. An unrestricted formulary allows a wide range of drugs to be used (a practice that may defeat the purpose of having a formulary). In a limited formulary, some drugs may be restricted to certain services, dosing regimens, or indications for use. Increasingly, new and high-cost drugs are added to the formulary only if the requesting physician provides an acceptable treatment regimen or service-specific protocol. Such protocols indicate conditions for patient selection, list laboratory and other parameters to be monitored, and provide specific instructions for administration.

A formulary consists of policies and procedures related to the prescribing, dispensing, and administering of drugs. In addition, it provides a list of the specific drugs selected by the pharmacy and therapeutics committee. It is recommended that a systematic review of each therapeutic category of the formulary be conducted annually and that the formulary be printed or available on-line so that relevant policies and procedures and an up-to-date drug list is available to all staff.

Drug use evaluations are conducted under the aegis of the pharmacy and therapeutics committee. Typically, the focus is on high-volume drugs, high-cost drugs, and drugs with a narrow therapeutic index (i.e., a narrow range between an effective dose and a potentially toxic dose). Current Joint Commission recommendations for drug use evaluations include the choice of drugs used for prophylactic, therapeutic, and empiric purposes. Criteria for the appropriate use of the drug are established by physicians and pharmacy clinicians based on the literature and their clinical judgment. Patient records (e.g., 50–100) are evaluated concurrently against the criteria. Discrepancies between the criteria and actual use are identified, and recommendations are made to the chief of service or to the prescribing physicians. It is expected that drug use evaluations will improve the prescribing practices within the institution.

The Joint Commission's flow diagram summarizing the issues related to the appropriate, safe, effective, and efficient use of medications is presented in Figure 20-2.[9] This diagram outlines the role of drug information, the drug use review process, and the reporting of adverse drug reactions.

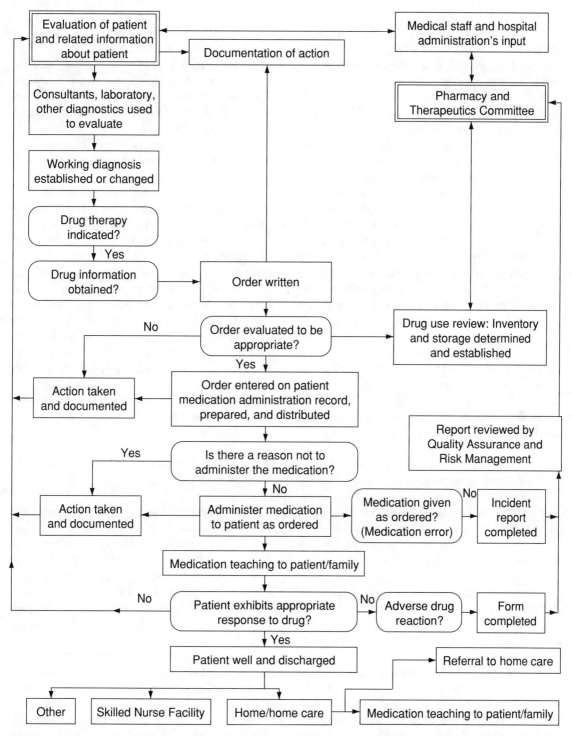

Figure 20-2 Medication Use Flow Chart. *Source:* Originally published in Nadzam, D.M. Development of medication use indicators by the Joint Commission on Accreditation of Healthcare Organizations. *American Journal of Hospital Pharmacy* 1991, 48: 1925–1930. Copyright 1991, American Society of Hospital Pharmacists, Inc. All rights reserved. Reprinted with permission.

The drug information service is also responsible for newsletters and bulletins targeted at specific professions (e.g., physicians and nurses). Typical contents may include brief therapeutic reviews (e.g., treatment of hypertension), specific drug evaluations, brief updates (e.g., new dosage forms of drugs), and newly reported adverse drug reactions.

The drug information service may serve as a catalyst for educational programs conducted by the hospital staff physicians or pharmacy clinicians. For example, in anticipation of the introduction of a new drug to the market, the drug information service may prepare a synopsis of its supporting published literature; plan a lecture series for physicians, nurses, and pharmacists; or prepare a full review of the drug for the pharmacy and therapeutics committee.

The drug information service frequently contributes to the proper control and recordkeeping associated with investigational drugs. (In some cases, this is a separate function independent of the drug information service.) The focus is on meeting the investigational drug requirements of various bodies that regulate the investigational drug process (e.g., the National Institutes of Health and the Food and Drug Administration). Investigational drug recordkeeping involves maintenance of current copies of investigational protocols and consent forms. The drug information service is ideally suited to prepare investigational drug monographs to be used by nursing, pharmacy, and physician personnel involved with the care of study subjects. Additional pharmacy services involved in the support of research include protocol development, patient randomization, preparation of special dosage forms, and related activities.

There are at least two reporting programs that typically are the responsibility of the drug information service: adverse drug reaction reporting and drug product defect reporting. Adverse drug reaction reporting is mandated by the Joint Commission. An effective drug information center can enhance both the quality and quantity of reporting by ensuring that the detailed steps in the reporting process are properly attended to and that reporting to the FDA, when indicated, is prompt. Drug product defect reporting involves reporting problems associated with commercially available drug products (problems related to drug manufacturing, packaging, labeling, and the like). These problems are usually discovered by nurses or pharmacists. Reports are submitted to the United States Pharmacopeia.

Some drug information centers also function as poison information centers. While the primary focus of the drug information service is the health care professional, poison centers receive a predominance of consumer calls. Although some databases and reference materials are common to drug information and poison information centers, the service requirements and staff training are somewhat different.

An effective drug information service uses a variety of computer databases, accessing them via CD ROM and on-line search systems, including MEDLINE and similar services. The typical center will maintain a library of current textbooks, journals, and other periodicals as well as a file for most drugs and/or disease states. Access to the primary literature is a must, and it is usually accomplished by establishing a close working relationship with a well-stocked medical library.

DRUG PROCUREMENT, RECEIVING, AND STORAGE

Computer-based systems are now commonplace for purchasing and inventory control. An effective drug procurement system should also involve active participation in group purchasing and the use of a prime vendor.[10] The use of electronic data interchange facilitates accurate and timely transmission of purchase orders to the vendor as well as immediate verification of the vendor's ability to supply each item. Such systems are available from drug wholesalers and medical supply companies. A computerized institution-wide materials management system may be used effectively by the pharmacy department to purchase and receive drugs, to provide current inventory information, and to facilitate vendor payments via the finance department. Such functions may also be a component of a dedicated pharmacy computer system package.

The decision of which purchasing group the institution supports is usually made by senior management. Input from affected departments, such as pharmacy, is strongly advised. Virtually all groups have a pharmacy purchasing program. Contract administration is usually the responsibility of a representative committee of pharmacists who award one-year to three-year contracts. Most purchasing groups require that the institution commit virtually all of its purchases to the group's contracts. In some cases, this might require that the pharmacy department staff work with nursing and medical staff to effect changes in the range of products offered by the purchasing group.

Many purchasing groups also provide additional services, such as educational programs for their members. Most pharmaceutical manufacturers mandate that an institution purchase only through a single group. Larger hospitals with significant purchasing power may find that individual contracting with drug manufacturers may better serve their needs and does not require the absolute commitment to a group's contract decisions.

A prime vendor is a single wholesaler that provides a large majority of an institution's purchases. Prime vendors operate on rather small margins (usually less than 5 percent of purchase costs), and each prime vendor expects a commitment by each client institution to purchase virtually all of its pharmaceuticals from that vendor. Most prime vendors provide electronic data interchange (which can produce a variety of reports analyzing drug purchases over time) and other services to attract and retain customers.

Receiving is a process that is usually conducted by pharmacy personnel, although in some cases materials management staff may perform some of the receiving tasks. Controlled substance receiving in all cases must be done by pharmacy personnel, since this responsibility rests with the pharmacy director for the institution.

Receiving can be done by exception—by identifying those products that have been ordered but not received. Alternatively, receiving can be done by indicating the quantity received in the receiving report. The method used is usually determined by the policies established by the finance and internal audit departments to maintain consistency with other hospital departments and audit requirements.

It is the responsibility of the pharmacy department, in conjunction with the security office and nursing, to set the standards for the storage of drugs throughout the institution. State and federal laws may dictate specific requirements for controlled substances control. Contemporary electronic security systems often allow for the recording of entry into each storage location and the establishment of passwords to limit access by location, time, and position. It is important that pharmacy staff develop a method for reviewing and documenting drug storage areas on a routine basis. Using a standard form, medication room inspections are performed monthly by a pharmacy staff member and a representative from each area. The medications are checked for expiration date, proper refrigeration, and the like. (See Chapter 19 for more on materials management.)

DRUG PREPARATION AND DISTRIBUTION

Drugs must be properly and safely prepared, labeled, and distributed according to legal and regulatory requirements, accreditation standards, and professional practice standards (as developed by the American Society of Hospital Pharmacists).[11] Figure 20-3 outlines the steps involved in the drug preparation and dispensing process for a typical hospital that utilizes the unit dose drug distribution system. Key components are the steps preceding the prescribing process and the actual writing of the medication order. The prescriber's knowledge of the patient (acquired through the diagnostic process) and of drug therapy is supplemented by the services of the clinical pharmacist and the drug information service when requested.

The prescriber should utilize the formulary to determine which drugs have been selected by the hospital's pharmacy and therapeutics committee

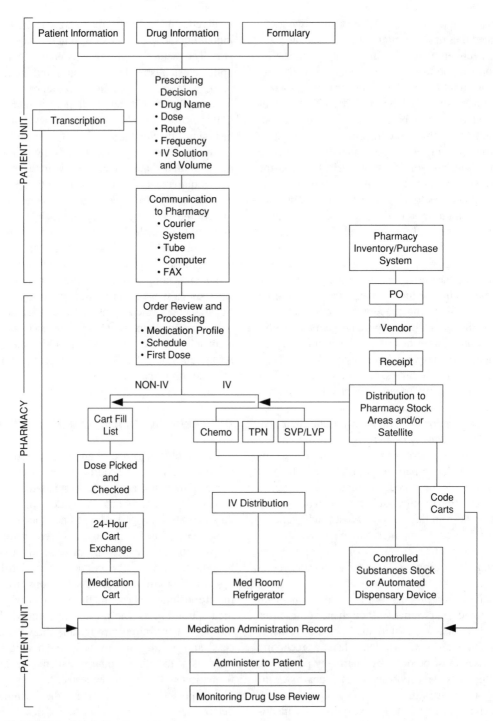

Figure 20-3 The Drug Distribution Process

and are available for prescribing within the hospital. Medication orders may be entered directly into a computer system by the prescriber or written on a form that allows a copy of the order to be transmitted to the pharmacy. If direct order entry by the physician is not possible, it is vital that the order, in the prescriber's original handwriting, be reviewed by the pharmacist so that transcription errors (e.g., those made by secretaries or nurses) are not transmitted to the pharmacist.

The review of the medication order by the pharmacist prior to drug administration is essential for ensuring safe and appropriate drug therapy. In addition to the clinical services detailed below, the pharmacist has a responsibility to recommend an appropriate dose and dose form, given the physician's therapeutic goals for a specific patient. In some cases the pharmacist will work with the medical staff to select a dose that can be accurately measured and still accomplish the intended clinical response. For example, a prescribed dose of gentamicin of 5.2 mg (calculated using the patient's body weight) is difficult to measure accurately, even using a syringe, and a dose of 5 mg may be appropriate in this case. In the case of an adult patient with a nasogastric tube, the physician's order for a sustained release dosage form of an antiarrhythmic drug to be administered twice a day may have to be adjusted so as to allow for more frequent administration.

The pharmacy, based on standard dosing schedules or on dialogue with the nurse, will prepare the number of doses required until the next medication cart is scheduled for delivery to the patient care unit. Nonintravenous drugs will then be dispensed according to the routine daily unit dose schedule. Carts are usually exchanged every 24 hours. During the exchange, the nursing medication administration record is compared with the pharmacy medication profile, and discrepancies are corrected. In the pharmacy, medication carts are often filled by the technician and checked by the pharmacist or another technician where permitted by law or regulation. Automated dispensing devices (similar in concept to automated teller machines) may be used to control and dispense controlled substances and other stock.

Preparing drugs for IV administration involves formulating chemotherapy solutions, total parenteral nutrition (TPN) solutions, small-volume parenterals (e.g., single doses of antibiotics), and large-volume parenterals (e.g., theophylline infusion). Because chemotherapy involves significant risk to the individuals preparing and administering these drugs, the Occupational Safety and Health Administration (OSHA) and the ASHP have developed guidelines for their preparation, disposal, and overall management.[12] Not only must the solutions be prepared in an aseptic manner, but their preparation must be done in a vertical laminar flow hood designed for this purpose, while the operator must protect him- or herself from the absorption of these hazardous drugs by the use of proper gowns, goggles, gloves, and other protective barriers.

The preparation of TPN solutions is increasingly accomplished through the use of automated mixing devices that allow the mixing of dextrose, amino acids, electrolytes, and other ingredients used in TPN. The preparation of these solutions and of small-volume and large-volume parenterals must be done in a laminar flow hood by well-trained operators. Rigorous policies and procedures as well as effective quality control and quality assurance measures are needed to ensure that these solutions are prepared aseptically and that all the proper drugs in the indicated volumes are included. Whether the solutions are prepared in decentralized areas (e.g., pharmacy satellites) or a central sterile products area, the same preparation and quality assurance policies should apply.

The administration of drugs and solutions by the intravenous route increasingly involves the use of infusion devices. The responsibility for their selection, distribution, and maintenance is shared by pharmacy and nursing as well as the patient care equipment department or the medical engineering department. Patient-controlled analgesia is increasing in utilization because of widespread patient satisfaction. It requires the use of narcotics (usually morphine or meperidine) and specially designed infusion devices. These devices are designed to allow the patient to select the dosing interval that the pump will infuse based on the program ordered by the physician.

The selection, purchase, receipt, storage, and distribution of intravenous solution and administration devices is usually within the province of nursing, materials management, and pharmacy, with each performing tasks commensurate with their responsibilities and resources. The purchase, receipt, inventory, and distribution of drugs rests legally with the pharmacy department. The distribution of drugs to clinics, to the emergency room, to operating rooms, and to code carts throughout the hospital involves both pharmacy and nursing. Drugs distributed within the hospital may be charged to the individual patients, or the cost can be distributed to the clinic, department, or area using the drug.

The revenue generated by the pharmacy from patient charges has been substantial in the past. Prospective payment in the DRG system for Medicare, fixed per diem or other charge systems for Medicaid, and capitated payments under HMO contracts have changed pharmacy's focus—from charges to costs. The application of cost-accounting systems in pharmacy is designed to define costs precisely and to relate pharmacy costs of labor, drugs, and supplies to patient utilization.[13]

The administration of drugs to patients is a time-honored responsibility of nursing. Although some pharmacy departments have developed pharmacy medication technician programs, their use has not expanded of late. They were developed to deal with a shortage of nurses and may emerge again as a means for controlling costs.

CLINICAL PHARMACY SERVICES AND PHARMACEUTICAL CARE

Clinical pharmacy services have evolved in response to needs and demands of patients, physicians, and nurses that have resulted from the complexity of new therapies. Indeed, these services are such a regular part of pharmacy practice today that the adjective *clinical* may not be necessary. The term *pharmaceutical care* has also been used to encompass the comprehensive provision of pharmacy services to ensure proper outcomes of drug therapy.[14] Clinical pharmacy services have been described in terms of the specialty involved (e.g., pharmacokinetics, oncology, nutrition), the type of patients serviced (e.g., pediatric or geriatric), or the location of the service (e.g., ambulatory or operating room or satellite). The role of the pharmacy has expanded to include clinical services, drug distribution, and teaching and research. Clinical pharmacists have begun to seek formal recognition as specialists credentialed by the Board of Pharmaceutical Specialties, a national credentialing body. Currently, the following specialties have been recognized or are in the process of trying to achieve recognition: nuclear pharmacy, pharmacotherapy, nutrition support, pharmacy practice, and psychopharmacy. As an example, a pharmacist with a specialization in oncology pharmacy practice should have the skills needed to

- conduct a patient medication interview
- monitor drug therapy for potential drug-drug, drug-test, drug-diet, and drug-disease interactions and make recommendations, when appropriate, to modify such therapy
- provide medication counseling for inpatients and outpatients.
- provide formal and informal education services to students and professional staff
- serve as a member of the oncology team
- evaluate drug studies reported in the oncology and medical literature
- communicate effectively with patients, physicians, nurses, professional peers, and students[15]

A pharmacist with this specialization should be knowledgeable about

- neoplastic disease, including the metastatic process and appropriate clinical management of hematological malignancy, solid tumors, and pediatric malignancies

- anticancer therapy, including antineoplastic agents, radiation therapy, and surgery
- supportive care, including nausea and vomiting care, pain control, mouth care, nutrition, transfusion therapy, and extravasation
- antineoplastic drug preparation and administration
- clinical research

TEACHING AND RESEARCH

Pharmacists have an important role to play in teaching individuals, especially students, who are in the profession and also other health care professionals. Teaching responsibilities within the profession include supervising clinical clerkships for baccalaureate and doctor of pharmacy students, residents, and interns and externs as well as pharmacy technician training. Pharmacists frequently help in the training of medical and nursing students and students in other health care professions.

Pharmacists' involvement in research has traditionally been focused on the proper control, inventorying, and monitoring of the use of drugs in research. Pharmacists who participate on institutional review boards utilize their expertise in drug information, therapeutics, pharmacokinetics, and pharmacy practice. Additionally, pharmacists have developed skills needed to conduct original research, usually building research programs in their specialty practice by integrating their training in study design, biostatistics, and clinical trials with their clinical practice.

RESOURCE REQUIREMENTS

Pharmacy managers are faced with the task of utilizing the resources entrusted to them in such a way as to ensure optimal, cost-effective drug therapy. Personnel needs are a reflection of the services the department offers as well as the amount of emphasis placed on the proper utilization and cost

control of increasingly expensive drug products. A number of studies have documented the positive impact of clinical pharmacy services on the quality of drug therapy and on costs.[16]

A variety of types of pharmacists and technical personnel are required in a contemporary pharmacy. The appropriate mix depends on the distributive, clinical, teaching, and research programs offered. Most pharmacists interested in hospital practice have a doctor of pharmacy degree, many have participated in residencies (twelve-month general and specialty postgraduate training programs accredited by the ASHP), while a few have completed fellowships (one- or two-year training programs in research). Technicians are usually hospital trained in either structured or unstructured programs lasting from weeks to months.

Space requirements include the need for satellite pharmacies in patient care areas so that pharmacists will be accessible to patients, physicians, and nurses. Sufficient space is also needed for the purchasing, receiving, and storage of drugs as well as for the production and distribution functions. Specific space requirements include the following:

- office and conference space
- drug information center space
- purchasing and receiving area
- alcohol and controlled substances vaults
- inventory storage area, including freezers and refrigerators
- sterile products preparation area
- outpatient pharmacy dispensing area
- unit-dose cart filling area
- satellite pharmacies, including one in the operating suite

The arrangement and location of pharmacies, offices, and so on, is partly dependent on the logistical requirements and physical features of the institution, such as the location of elevators, pneumatic tube systems, automatic conveyors, and the like.

The equipment needed in hospital pharmacies includes

- personal and departmental computer systems and associated software
- bar code readers
- FAX machines
- photocopy machines
- laminar flow hoods
- freezers and refrigerators

Some departments require unit-dose packaging machines, others use automated compounding devices for IV admixture, while those with outpatient pharmacies may use automated tablet counters as well.

Given the volume and complexity of transactions, computerization is essential to support dispensing and billing operations. Patient medication profiles are maintained for prospective review of clinical parameters and concomitant drug and intravenous fluid therapy. Many departments have special purpose microcomputer systems to support single-function applications (e.g., a pharmacokinetics dosing service). Automation of the drug dispensing or distribution process is somewhat limited, with only some initial efforts being made at this time.

QUALITY MANAGEMENT

As regards pharmacy, there are two principal foci for quality management: the services that pharmacy provides and the drug therapies prescribed for patients.

The hospital medication system has been under scrutiny because of the increasing public perception that prescribing errors by physicians, dispensing errors by pharmacists, and medication errors (usually committed by nurses) are increasing in frequency and gravity.[17] The negative consequences of drug therapy have been referred to as "medication misadventures." For example, adverse drug reactions result in as many as five percent of hospital admissions. Pharmaceutical care involves a more proactive roll for the pharmacist in reducing the problems associated with the use of drugs. Although medication error studies using controlled methodologies have been published, few hospitals collect data for use in trend analysis or for comparison with other institutions. Underreporting of medication incidents is common, and typically only the most trivial or the most serious errors are reported. The increased toxicity of current medications has heightened the need to continuously improve the quality of performance of the medication system. The development of a methodology for the assessment of the frequency and severity of medication errors is of paramount importance.

The Joint Commission, in its agenda for change, is in the process of developing outcome indicators to replace structure and process measures of service quality.[18] A number of these quality indicators include measures of the outcomes of medication treatment.

Even more complex is the issue of how to evaluate the quality of drug therapy decisions made in a given hospital. The drug usage evaluation process is intended to detect problems in the use of specific drugs or categories of drugs. Because the process can only encompass a few drugs in a given time period, it is important that hospitals develop comprehensive programs for the evaluation of drug therapy, including adverse drug reaction reporting, the reporting of the usage frequency of nonformulary drugs, and the reporting of medication errors. In time, as comprehensive outcome measures and management programs are developed and implemented, a definitive methodology for the assessment of the impact of drug therapies may be possible.

PERFORMANCE INDICATORS

Performance indicators have been used to measure cost, resource utilization, and workload for both drug utilization and the pharmacy department as a whole. Most health care managers operate on the premise that physicians, in their role as case managers, are responsible for the selection and volume of utilization of intermediate products, including pharmaceuticals. The department manager (the pharmacy manager, in this case) is responsible for the costs of production (ingredient and labor costs) of the intermediate products, which are components of the case costs.[19] For example, the cost of treating community-acquired pneumonia in hospitals comprises separate component costs for laboratory tests, radiology exams, and pharmaceuticals. It is the physician who determines the number and type of intermediate products, and it is the pharmacy manager who is responsible for ensuring that the drug and labor costs are reasonable.

Drug cost measures include drug cost per admission, per patient day, and per dose (see Table 20-1). Drug cost per admission varies based on the type of cases admitted, the acuity of those cases, and how the drug therapy is managed by physicians, pharmacists, and nurses. Drug cost per patient day depends on the length of stay, the intensity of drug therapy, and the choice of specific drugs. Drug cost per dose reflects how well the pharmacy purchases drugs (using purchasing groups, prime vendors, and effective contract negotiations) as well as the use of generic drugs, the presence of a therapeutic interchange policy, and the decisions of the pharmacy and therapeutics committee.

The use of generic drugs in hospital formularies has long been common and is encouraged and monitored by most pharmacy and therapeutic committees. Therapeutic interchange—substituting a drug with the same therapeutic use as, but a slightly different chemical structure than the one the physician originally prescribed—has also been effective in lowering drug therapy costs.

Increasingly, the literature has documented the effectiveness of clinical interventions by pharmacists.[20] Some of these initiatives are quality focused

Table 20-1 Resource Requirements

	ASHP*	Lilly†	UAB‡
Inventory			
Patient Day	$ 4.23	$ 3.27	$ 6.13
Occupied Bed		$ 1,195.00	$1,749.00
Admission		$ 22.66	
Turnover Rate	9.30	10.40	13.90
Expenses			
Drug Cost/Occupied Bed	$11,672.00	$12,373.00	
Total Expenses/Occupied Bed	$18,719.00		
Utilization			
Drug Cost/Dose		$	3.82
Doses/Patient Day			16.20
Drug Cost/Patient Day	$ 31.98	$ 33.90	$ 61.87
Doses/Admission			114.00
Drug Cost/Admission		$ 234.65	$ 434.64
Staffing			
Pharmacists/100 Beds			10.33
Support Staff/100 Beds			10.23
Total			20.56

*The ASHP National survey on hospital-based pharmaceutical services. Conducted every two or three years, it is a national mail survey of selected hospital pharmacies.

†The Lilly Hospital Pharmacy Survey, conducted annually by the Eli Lilly Company, uses questionnaires sent to hospital pharmacies throughout the United States.

‡The University of Alabama at Birmingham annual survey of selected teaching hospital pharmacies is conducted by Herman L. Lazarus, Director of Pharmacy.

(intended to reduce or eliminate problems associated with drug therapy), whereas others are cost focused. The drug use evaluation process has been an effective means of evaluating, both prospectively and retrospectively, the prescribing of drugs within institutions. Dialogue with the medical staff through the pharmacy and therapeutics committee has proven to be effective in decreasing the cost and increasing the quality of drug therapy.

Labor and productivity measures are also useful for evaluating the effectiveness of pharmacy services. Comparison of pharmacy full-time equivalents per 100 beds is usually not productive, since this simple measure does not reflect patient intensity or acuity, the scope and quality of services, or the impact of initiatives to improve quality or reduce the cost of drug therapy.

Pharmacy labor cost per dose, per patient day, and per admission are measures of variables controlled in large part by the pharmacy manager. They also reflect the availability of labor as well as salary and benefits offered by the institution. They may be added to drug cost per dose, per patient day, and per admission to more completely represent the cost of drug therapy. The number of occupied beds per pharmacist and per technician and the number of pharmacists and technicians in total are broad comparative measures that do not reflect the scope, quality, or impact of pharmacy staff involvement.

Intensity measures that reflect the pharmacy workload include the number and type of doses per patient day and per admission. The cost per dose reflects patient acuity and purchasing effectiveness. The number of doses per pharmacy full-time equivalent reflects productivity, yet it should be evaluated in the context of the scope and quality of services offered.

Finally, measures of fiscal performance such as inventory turns over and the dollar value of inventory per patient day, per occupied bed, and per admission have been used to assess pharmacy's purchasing and inventory control performance.

Comparing the institution's drug cost per admission with those of other institutions, even on a controlled basis (i.e., for specific DRGs or case types),

is not always fruitful. Physician prescribing and patient management have a major influence on drug cost per admission. The other factors mentioned above also affect this measure, including the extent and type of clinical pharmacy services, the use of generic drugs and therapeutic interchange, and the use of prudent purchasing techniques. Interinstitutional comparisons are mainly helpful in identifying potential problems that require further institutional study.

Quality measures must be used with caution. The number of adverse drug reactions or medication errors reported per unit of time might reflect the aggressiveness and effectiveness of reporting programs more than the prevalence of therapeutic misadventures.

THE FUTURE OF PHARMACY SERVICES

Recruitment, Retention, and Development of Professional Staff

As hospital pharmacy services have expanded and competition with other types of pharmaceutical services and organizations has become more intense, the recruitment of pharmacists has become increasingly challenging.

Salary levels have increased, as has the sophistication of the techniques for recruitment (which now often require the active involvement of human resource departments and sometimes even recruitment firms).

Similarly, because the roles and responsibilities of pharmacists have increased, skill training and professional development are even more important for maintaining effective pharmacy services.[21] Many programs can be developed within the institution. For example, pharmacokinetic services, which must be provided by trained specialists, could be offered throughout the institution and at all hours the department is open if an in-house program is developed to train staff. (An ongoing validation and certification process may be needed as well.)

Technicians require a wide range of skills. Computer order entry, medication cart filling, and the admixture of intravenous solutions are a few. An organized training program designed to meet the specific requirements of the institution is usually developed by the pharmacy staff. Such programs range from two weeks to months of full-time or part-time training. A certification process may be developed for each technician. The ASHP now accredits technician training programs based on specific criteria.

Expansion of the Roles of the Technical Staff

The expansion of the roles of the technical staff should keep pace with the increase in complexity of pharmacy department programs.[22] Within the proper legal and regulatory limits, the technicians' role in preparing, manipulating, and distributing drugs should be as highly developed as is feasible. Not only is this cost-effective, but it also increases the job satisfaction of pharmacists and technicians alike. Training programs, comprehensive policies and procedures, and attentive supervision by licensed pharmacists are essential.

Automation of the Drug-Dispensing Process

Although still in its infancy, dispensing automation can be used to fill unit dose carts and to prepare IV admixtures more inexpensively and with fewer errors than manual dispensing.[23] The use of automation also allows pharmacy services to expand without increasing labor requirements. Technology will play an ever-greater role in the manipulation and preparation of drugs, allowing pharmacists to concentrate on meeting the needs of patients. Benefits can accrue, for example, by having a device to prepare chemotherapy solutions, thereby reducing operator risk.

Development of Integrated Medication Systems

Current medication systems are insular and do not require nor facilitate communication between professionals on behalf of patients.[24] The implementation of management strategies and new information systems will help in the creation of a comprehensive medication system, as will the application of continuous improvement techniques and contemporary information technology.

Technology may facilitate the integration of the medication system by allowing medication ordering by physicians at the bedside and the use of bar code recorders by nurses to verify the appropriateness of medications. Patient physical parameters or the use of infusion devices can also be recorded in a technologically enhanced, comprehensive information system.

Development of Integrated Drug Therapy Databases

In order to properly manage resource utilization, clinicians must have access to information on the cost of therapies they initiate. For example, the presentation of cost information on both therapeutic regimens that use drugs requiring laboratory utilization and those that do not can assist the clinician in making effective resource decisions. As another example, a thorough analysis of the utilization of drugs for a specific diagnosis can assist the manager and clinician in discussions about the cost-effectiveness of drug therapies.

Development of Treatment Protocols

Increasingly, the management of certain disease states has been systematized (e.g., cancer, AIDS, and transplant surgery). Systematization can increase the efficiency of the clinical staff and also enhance their skills by giving them experience with specific patient care methodologies. Although a great deal of patient care must be individualized, treatment protocols can be facilitated by the use of information systems.

Development of Outcome Measures

Although the science of measuring patient care outcomes is still in its infancy, growing evidence suggests that it is feasible to measure the impact of drug therapy on a patient's quality of life, functional status, and satisfaction with the medical care process.

The development of the concept of pharmaceutical care reflects the development of comprehensive patient-centered outcome-driven pharmaceutical services.[25] Pharmaceutical care increases the pharmacist's responsibility for ensuring that drug therapy benefits patients. Pharmaceutical care involves all aspects of the use of drugs including responsibilities held by physicians, nurses, and pharmacists. Pharmacists are expected to take a leadership role in ensuring that the outcomes achieved are those that the physician and patient anticipated. Pharmacists are likely to have greater direct contact with patients as a result of pharmaceutical care. Some of the issues a department of pharmacy faces as it seeks to implement pharmaceutical care are listed below.

Biotechnological Drugs

Biotechnology poses enormous challenges to the health care system. Drug therapies are emerging that can treat diseases for which no therapy existed (e.g., Gaucher's disease), replace surgery (e.g., drugs that treat benign prostatic hypertrophy), and save lives that might otherwise have been lost (e.g., drugs that treat septic shock). Such drugs are extraordinarily costly, and their appropriate and safe use must be ensured. Treatment protocols, careful selection of patients, and careful monitoring of drug use are essential elements of any program that utilizes biotechnological products in institutional settings.[26] Reimbursement issues have also arisen, especially in regard to non-FDA-approved indications for use. Some third-party payers have refused payments for nonlabeled uses of biotechnological drugs. Hospitals must develop a strategy for dealing with this problem (e.g., researching the literature to build a case for nonapproved uses). As a result of these issues, hospitals must develop a comprehensive strategic plan for the management of high-cost drugs, including bio-

technological drugs. Planning for new patient care and research programs, as well as the recruitment of new physicians to the institution, should involve consideration for the use and cost of these new agents.

Drug Delivery Systems

Devices are being developed that involve the placement of sensors capable of measuring physical parameters of patients (e.g., devices that measure blood glucose and infuse insulin based on the patient's blood glucose level). Pharmacy management must accept the responsibility of ensuring that such devices are accomplishing what they are supposed to. Clinical pharmacists must be able to assess the efficacy of the devices and to counsel patients regarding their use. Clinical monitoring must occur to ensure that the devices are safe from failure.

Changes in Organizational Structure

Hospitals have been examining the relationship of pharmacy to other departments. Modifications will undoubtedly occur that reflect the change in focus from drug distribution and materials management to a more patient-centered set of programs and responsibilities.

ADDITIONAL RESOURCES

Organizations

American College of Clinical Pharmacy, 3101 Broadway, Suite 350, Kansas City, MO 64111.

American Foundation for Pharmaceutical Education, 618 Somerset Street, P.O. Box 7126, North Plainfield, NJ 07060.

American Pharmaceutical Association, 2215 Constitution Avenue, NW, Washington, DC 20037.

American Society of Consultant Pharmacists, 2300 Ninth Street South, Suite 515, Arlington, VA 22204.

American Society of Hospital Pharmacists, 7272 Wisconsin Avenue, Bethesda, MD 20814.

National Association of Boards of Pharmacy, O'Hare Corporate Center, 1300 Higgins Road, Suite 103, Park Ridge, IL 60068.

Periodicals

American Journal of Hospital Pharmacy, American Society of Hospital Pharmacists, 7272 Wisconsin Avenue, Bethesda, MD 20814.

The Annals of Pharmacotherapy (formerly *DICP*), P.O. Box 42696, Cincinnati, OH 45242.

Clinical Pharmacy, American Society of Hospital Pharmacists, 7272 Wisconsin Avenue, Bethesda, MD 20814.

Hospital Pharmacy, 1143 Wright Drive, Huntington Valley, PA 19006.

P&T (formerly *Hospital Formulary*), 105 Raider Boulevard, Belle Mead, NJ 08502.

Pharmacotherapy, New England Medical Center, 750 Washington Street, #236, Boston, MA 02111.

Topics in Hospital Pharmacy Management, Aspen Publishers, Inc., 200 Orchard Ridge Drive, Gaithersburg, MD 20878.

Books and Articles

American Society of Hospital Pharmacists. *Harvey A.K. Whitney award lectures.* Bethesda, Md.: American Society of Hospital Pharmacists, 1992.

American Society of Hospital Pharmacists. Directions for clinical practice in pharmacy. *American Journal of Hospital Pharmacy* 42 (1985): 1287–1342.

Bezold, C., ed. *Pharmaceuticals in the year 2000.* Alexandria, Va.: Institute for Alternative Futures, 1983.

Black, B.L. *Resource book on progressive pharmaceutical services.* Bethesda, Md.: American Society of Hospital Pharmacists, 1986.

Brown, T.R., and M.C. Smith. *Handbook of institutional pharmacy practice.* 2d ed. Baltimore, Md.: Williams & Wilkins, 1986.

Gouveia, W.A., et al. *1990 report: Hospital pharmacy computer systems.* Bethesda, Md.: American Society of Hospital Pharmacists, 1990.

Raehl, C.L., et al. Pharmaceutical services in U.S. hospitals in 1989. *American Journal of Hospital Pharmacy* 49 (1989): 323–346.

NOTES

1. C.D. Hepler and L.M. Strand, Opportunities and Responsibilities in Pharmaceutical Care, *American Journal of Hospital Pharmacy* 47 (1990): 533–543; R.P. Penna, Pharmaceutical Care: Pharmacy's Mission for the 1990s, *American Journal of Hospital Pharmacy* 49 (1990): 543–549; W.A. Gouveia, Caring for the Patient: Implications of Assuming Responsibility for Patient Outcomes, *American Journal of Hospital Pharmacy,* in press; J.C. McAlister, Opportunities for Fostering Pharmaceutical Care, *American Journal of Hospital Pharmacy,* in press.

2. E.L. Allan and K.N. Barker, Fundamentals of Medication Error Research, *American Journal of Hospital Pharmacy* 47 (1990): 555–571; T.S. Lesar et al., Medication Prescribing Errors in a Teaching Hospital, *Journal of the American Medical Association* 263 (1990): 2329–2334.

3. H.J. Black and W.W. Tester, Decentralized Pharmacy Operations Utilizing the Unit-Dose Concept, *American Journal of Hospital Pharmacy* 21 (1964): 344–350; K.N. Barker and W.M. Heller, The Development of a Centralized Unit-Dose Dispensing System, Part 1: Description of the UAMC Experimental System, *American Journal of Hospital Pharmacy* 20 (1963): 568–579; W.J. Durant and J.D. Herrick, A Unit-Dose Drug Distribution System in a Children's Hospital, *American Journal of Hospital Pharmacy* 27 (1970): 121–131; K.L. Rascati, Brief Review of the Literature on Decentralized Drug Distribution in Hospitals, *American Journal of Hospital Pharmacy* 45 (1988): 639–641; C.C. Pulliam and J.H. Upton, A Pharmacy Coordinated Intravenous Admixture and Administration Service, *American Journal of Hospital Pharmacy* 28 (1971): 92–101; N.W. Schwartau et al., A Comprehensive Intravenous Admixture System, *American Journal of Hospital Pharmacy* 30 (1973): 607–609.

4. Black and Tester, Decentralized Pharmacy Operations; A.G. Lipman et al., Decentralization of Pharmaceutical Services without Satellite Pharmacies, *American Journal of Hospital Pharmacy* 36 (1979): 1513–1519.

5. H.N. Godwin, Developing a Clinical Role for the Hospital Pharmacist, *Drug Intelligence* 2 (1968): 152–157; W.A. Miller, Selection, Training and Evaluation of Clinical Pharmacists, *American Journal of Hospital Pharmacy* 31 (1974): 448–455; J.E. Bell et al., A New Approach to Delivering Drug Information to the Physician through a Pharmacy Consultation Program, Part 4: Evaluation Results, *American Journal of Hospital Pharmacy* 30 (1973): 300–310; E. Owyang et al., The Pharmacist's New Role in Institutional Patient Care, *American Journal of Hospital Pharmacy* 25 (1968): 624–630.

6. D.E. Francke et al., *Mirror to Hospital Pharmacy* (Bethesda, Md.: American Society of Hospital Pharmacists, 1964).

7. *American Society of Hospital Pharmacists Residency Directory* (Bethesda, Md: American Society of Hospital Pharmacists, 1992); American Society of Hospital Pharmacists Accreditation Standard for Residency in Pharmacy Practice (with an emphasis on pharmaceutical care), *American Journal of Hospital Pharmacy* 49 (1992): 146–153.

8. American Society of Hospital Pharmacists Guidelines on Pharmacists' Relationships with Industry, *American Journal of Hospital Pharmacy* 49 (1992): 154.

9. D.M. Nadzam, Development of Medication Use Indicators by the Joint Commission on Accreditation of Healthcare Organizations, *American Journal of Hospital Pharmacy* 48 (1991): 1925–1930.

10. E.C. Buchanan, Planning and Coordinating Pharmaceutical Purchasing, *American Journal of Hospital Pharmacy* 41 (1984): 1829–1834.

11. *Practice Standards of the American Society of Hospital Pharmacists, 1991–1992* (Bethesda, Md.: American Society of Hospital Pharmacists, 1991).

12. American Society of Hospital Pharmacists, Technical Assistance Bulletin on Handling of Cytotoxic and Hazardous Drugs, *American Journal of Hospital Pharmacy* 47 (1990): 1003–1049.

13. W.A. Gouveia et al., Design and Implementation of a Cost Accounting System in Hospital Pharmacy, *American Journal of Hospital Pharmacy* 45 (1988): 613–620.

14. Hepler and Strand, Opportunities and Responsibilities in Pharmaceutical Care.

15. American Society of Hospital Pharmacists, Supplemental Standard and Learning Objectives for Residency Training in Oncology Pharmacy Practice, *American Journal of Hospital Pharmacy* 39 (1982): 1214–1215.

16. M.S. Willett et al., Prospectus on the Economic Value of Clinical Pharmacy Services, *Pharmacotherapy* 9 (1989): 45–56; H.T. Hatoum et al., Evaluation of the Contribution of Clinical Pharmacists: Inpatient Care and Cost Reduction, *Drug Intelligencer* 22 (1988): 252–259.

17. W. Bogdanich, *The Great White Lie* (New York: Simon and Schuster, 1992); H.R. Manasee, Medication Use in an Imperfect World: Drug Misadventuring as an Issue of Public Policy, Part 1, *American Journal of Hospital Pharmacy* 46 (1989): 929–944; H.R. Manasee, Medication Use in an Imperfect World: Drug Misadventuring as an Issue of Public Policy, Part 2, *American Journal of Hospital Pharmacy* 46 (1989): 1141–1152.

18. W.A. Gouveia et al., Paradigm for the Management of Patient Outcomes, *American Journal of Hospital Pharmacy* 48 (1991): 1912–1916; W.A. Gouveia, Measuring and Managing Patient Outcomes, *American Journal of Hospital Pharmacy* 50 (1992): 2157–2158.

19. R.B. Siegrist and C.S. Blish, Cost Accounting, Management Control and Planning in Health Care, *American Journal of Hospital Pharmacy* 45 (1988): 372–379.

20. Willett et al., Prospectus on the Economic Value of Clinical Pharmacy Services; Hatoum et al., Evaluation of the Contribution of Clinical Pharmacists.

21. J.E. Smith, Integrating Human Resources and Program Planning Strategies, *American Journal of Hospital Pharmacy* 46 (1989): 1153–1161; J.E. Smith and R. Shane, Clinical Career Ladders: Application to Hospital Pharmacy Practice, *American Journal of Hospital Pharmacy* 46 (1989): 2259–2262; P.A. Chase, Human Resources Management for a Hospital Pharmacy Department, *American Journal of Hospital Pharmacy* 48 (1989): 1162–1169.

22. Final Report of the American Society of Hospital Pharmacists Task Force on Technical Personnel in Pharmacy, *American Journal of Hospital Pharmacy* 46 (1989): 1420–1429; R.W. Anderson, Technicians and the Future of Pharmacy, *American Journal of Hospital Pharmacy* 44 (1987): 1593–1597.

23. S.M. Somani and T.W. Woller, Automating the Drug Distribution System, *Topics in Hospital Pharmacy Management* 9 (1989): 19–34; K.N. Barker et al., Effects of Technological Changes in Information Transfer on the Delivery of Pharmacy Services, *American Journal of Pharmacy Education* 53, suppl. (1989) 27S–40S.

24. W.A. Gouveia, Turbulence and Tranquility in the New Decade: Pharmacy Leader-Managers in Patient Care, *American Journal of Hospital Pharmacy* 47 (1990): 311–319.

25. Hepler and Strand, Opportunities and Responsibilities in Pharmaceutical Care.

26. E.T. Herfindal, Formulary Management of Biotechnical Drugs, *American Journal of Hospital Pharmacy* 46 (1989): 2516–2520; J.P. Santell, Projecting Future Drug Expenditures, *American Journal of Hospital Pharmacy* 50 (1993): 72–77; S. Huber, Strategic Planning for Colony Stimulating Factors, *Pharmacotherapy* 12 (1992): 399–435.

M. Rosita Schiller
Kay N. Wolf
Judy L. Miller

Food and Nutritional Services

21

Purpose: The purpose of food and nutrition services is to provide high-quality meals within budgetary guidelines, to meet the nutritional needs of patients, staff, and the public; to offer cost-effective clinical nutrition services to institutionalized, ambulatory, or homebound patients; to provide nutrition education and counseling to patients and the public; to provide professional education opportunities and conduct research for improved dietetic practice; and to maximize revenue for the institution.

INTRODUCTION

High-quality food and nutrition services are essential for optimal health care, high patient satisfaction, and sound fiscal administration. Well-managed food services, accompanied by first-rate clinical nutrition services and tasty meals served in a pleasant atmosphere, make a significant contribution to positive attitudes among patients, physicians, personnel, and visitors. Also, because a major portion of operating expenses, space, and equipment are allocated for dietary services, it is essential that administrators recognize the inherent

value of these services and carefully monitor the structures, processes, and outcomes of food and nutrition operations.

This chapter provides an introduction to the basic concepts, presents general information for communication and decision making, and discusses key issues facing the industry. Departmental functions are summarized, and general management principles are delineated. Major aspects of departmental organization are described, such as organizational models; food production and distribution systems; food services for patients, staff, employees, and the public; nutritional care services, including dietary counseling and nutrition education; professional education and research; and revenue generation. To facilitate informed decision making, resource requirements are summarized, including personnel, space, equipment, and meal costs. Quality control issues are discussed as they relate to food and food services, patient care, departmental management, and clinical nutrition services. And finally, some key issues are presented, such as marketing food and nutrition services, environmental consciousness, cost-benefit analyses of nutrition services, use of contract food services, productivity, new technologies, staff recruitment and retention, and public relations. Sources of additional information are also provided.

MAJOR FUNCTIONS

Key responsibilities of the department usually include

- menu planning for patients on regular and modified diets, institutional cafeterias and dining rooms, and catered events both on and off the premises
- food purchasing, according to specification and within budgetary limitations, as determined by established menus
- food storage at the point of both delivery and service, under safe and sanitary conditions, and with the desired degree of security and control
- food preparation that meets menu requirements and standards for nutrient retention, safety, sanitation, productivity, and food quality
- distribution of raw ingredients, menu items, supplies, and assembled trays as needed for distribution to patients, staff, and the public
- maintaining and merchandising quality food service to maximize use of institutional facilities and to promote patient and customer satisfaction
- disposal of plate waste and other garbage and dumping or recycling of nonfood trash, including paper and plastic packaging and supplies, glass and metal containers, and worn-out fabric, such as uniforms or table linens
- sanitation and cleanliness in both food service areas and food-handling procedures
- patient nutritional care services, including nutritional assessment, care planning, intervention, documentation, and evaluation
- dietary counseling and education for hospitalized, ambulatory, or homebound patients; staff members; and the public

- professional education of dietetic students, nurses, physicians, and other staff members

MANAGEMENT PRINCIPLES

The following principles should be kept in mind when planning, organizing, and directing food and nutrition services:

- A philosophy, goals, organizational structures, policies and procedures, and standards of practice are needed to guide food and nutrition services, and these must be delineated in writing and used as the basis for daily operations and communication.
- Food should be both safe and palatable, and food choices should be offered when appropriate so that individuals may select meals in harmony with personal preferences while conforming to dietary prescriptions and nutritional guidelines.
- Food and nutrition services and professional education programs must be in keeping with laws and standards established by regulatory agencies.
- Food service systems and subsystems (procurement, storage, preparation, distribution, and service) should be secured against theft, tightly controlled, and periodically evaluated.
- The nutritional status of all patients should be assessed, and patients at nutritional risk must be placed under the care of a registered dietitian for appropriate dietary intervention, monitoring, follow-up, and evaluation.
- Nutritional care must be documented in the medical record, and outcomes must be monitored through a comprehensive quality management program.
- Diet counseling and nutrition education should be provided for both hospitalized and free-living patients.
- Educational programs for physicians and other health care professionals, as well as in-service

training for all food service staff, should be provided on a regular basis.

- Effective operations require close collaboration between food and nutrition service personnel and physicians; between the food and nutrition services department and other departments such as nursing, pharmacy, medical records, clinical chemistry, maintenance, purchasing, and systems engineering; and between patients, clients, staff members, and the public.

ORGANIZATIONAL STRUCTURE

Historical Background

Through improved professional education, changing professional roles, and the emergence of support personnel, dietetics gained importance and prestige in the management and delivery of food and nutrition services. In the earliest hospitals, food services were supervised by the chef, the housekeeper, or the nursing department. Soon after dietitians were first employed in 1901, it became common practice for them to be put in charge of dietary departments and given responsibility for all food services, instruction of nurses, and nutritional therapy for metabolic diseases.[1] Key concerns of these early hospital dietitians related to budgets, organization, personnel management, quality food service, effective communication with physicians, and planning dietaries to meet special needs. Nutrition was widely recognized as an important aspect of medicine. Food prescriptions were handled somewhat like apothecary compounds, creating a demand for special diet kitchens.[2] The dietitian, recognized as the nutritional expert,[3] was responsible to the executive officer of the institution and had a status equal to that of the superintendent of nurses.[4]

Organizational Overview

Good nutrition plays a vital role in optimal health. Those who exercise, maintain a healthy weight, and consume a balanced diet glow with vitality and reduce their risk of developing chronic diseases. Alternatively, those who fail to meet their nutritional needs are more susceptible to infection and disease and are less capable of healing. Many persons, such as those with diabetes, coronary heart disease, Crohn's disease, and hypertension, must follow modified diets to control their disorders and maintain a normal life style. Because diet plays such an important role in health status, nutritional assessment services, appropriate dietary products, nutritional therapy, and education are necessary components of comprehensive health care services.

The process of producing and delivering food (Figure 21-1) begins with the menu, which is designed to meet the needs and preferences of the patient population. Planning the menu requires that consideration be given to the type of food service system and the labor pool as well as the food available in the marketplace. The menu determines the recipes, the foods to be procured and stored, and the food production schedule. A production manager must forecast the number of servings needed, determine the portion size of each serving, and assign staff to prepare menu items. Foods may be served immediately after cooking or stored for future use; either way, they must be transported to the point of service, then dished and served. Finally, soiled permanent ware is retrieved, sanitized, and stored, and other wastes are discarded or recycled.

The typical organization of clinical nutrition services is shown in Figure 21-2. Clinical dietitians work in conjunction with the medical staff and nursing personnel to provide clinical dietetic services, including

- patient nutritional status assessment
- development of appropriate nutritional care plans
- confirmation of physician diet orders
- dietary intervention as deemed necessary by the patient's condition
- supervision of patient meal services
- collaboration with other health professionals to provide specialized nutrition support such as tube feedings or parenteral nutrition

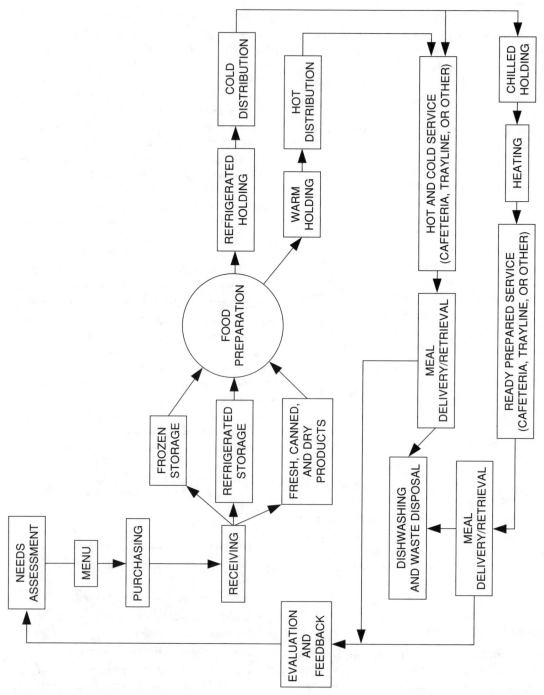

Figure 21-1 Overview of Food Services

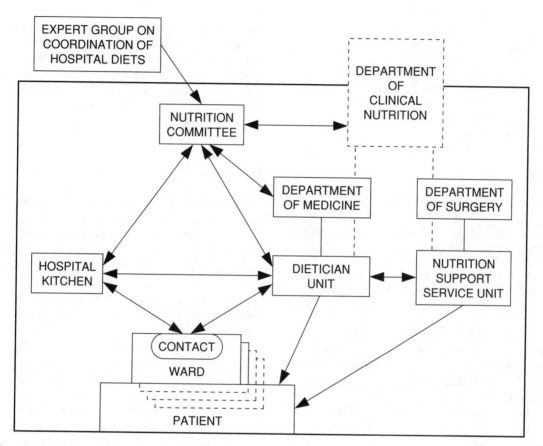

Figure 21-2 Organization of Hospital Nutrition Care. *Source:* Reprinted from B.I. Isaksson, Management and Organization of Modern Hospital Nutrition Care, in *Principal Aspects of Clinical Nutrition,* J.C. Somogyi and R. Wenger (eds.), p. 100, with permission of S. Karger AG, © 1983.

- observation of food acceptance and patient responses to evaluate achievement of nutritional goals and make changes where necessary

The organization of food and nutrition services varies with the size of facility and the services offered. Small hospitals often have one administrative dietitian acting as the director and one to two clinical dietitians providing clinical services; supervisors may oversee both food production and patient services (Figure 21-3). As the size of the institution increases, both the number and diversity of tasks increase. Many large hospitals will have one

dietitian or manager for each of the following areas: procurement, production, cafeteria services, catering, patient services, and training and development (Figure 21-4). The patient nutrition services area usually will have a clinical nutrition manager or chief clinical dietitian, several clinical dietitians specialized in diet therapy, and approximately the same number of dietetic technicians. Senior dietitians or clinical nutrition specialists may coordinate several clinical dietitians in large medical centers.

In recent years, other organizational designs have appeared. In some hospitals, food and nutrition services are separated, with each service hav-

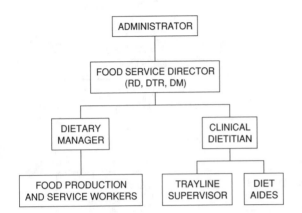

Note: RD = registered dietitian; DTR = dietetic technician, registered; DM = dietary manager

Figure 21-3 Typical Organization of Food and Nutrition Services in Small Hospitals and Nursing Homes

ing a department head. This separation fosters a stronger relationship between clinical dietitians and the medical staff but has the disadvantage of fragmenting responsibility for dietary services. Some hospitals position clinical dietetics within pharmacy, and in a few hospitals dietetic services come under the department of surgery. These unique configurations may affect only a few specialized dietitians who are members of a nutrition support service, research protocol team, or federally funded project.

Some extended care facilities operate like small hospitals. The food service director is frequently a dietetic technician or certified dietary manager. A recent trend is to hire a registered dietitian to be the director, and be given responsibility for both food management and clinical duties. A dietitian consultant reports directly to the administrator of the facility; he or she acts as a liaison with the food service manager but is responsible for all clinical nutrition services.

Free-standing community organizations that offer nutrition services are on the rise. Dietitians offer nutrition counseling at medical and women's health clinics; health clubs; government programs; weight reduction, renal dialysis, and wellness centers; and specialty agencies, such as local diabetes or heart associations. In these organizations, the dietitian is generally a staff member who collaborates in service delivery with other health professionals. Dietitians also oversee food service operations in nonacute settings, such as patients' homes and congregate feeding sites.

Food Production and Distribution Systems

Meal preparation and service are at the heart of a dietary department. Throughout the day, foods of numerous types are cooked, portioned, and delivered to a wide assortment of consumers, including patients, staff, and visitors. High-quality edibles, served with finesse, are essential to establish and maintain an untarnished reputation for food throughout the institution. The food service system is in part determined by the nature of the menus and the types of meal service offered by the facility.

The four principal types of food service systems used for food production and distribution are the conventional, commissary, ready-prepared, and assembly-serve (see Table 21-1). The conventional system remains the most common choice, although the ready-prepared system, also known as the cook-chill-freeze system, is gaining in popularity. In a ready-prepared system, food is prepared, then chilled or frozen prior to service. Items can be stored as individual servings or in bulk. Foods are reheated at the point of service.

The potential for savings from selecting one system rather than another remains controversial. A conceptual analysis shows a financial savings should accrue when changing from a conventional to a ready-prepared system.[5] One reason for savings is that the ready-prepared system allows for the purchase of convenience foods and the preparation of foods well in advance of service, eliminating productivity peaks and valleys. Also, cost reductions ought to result because less equipment and fewer staff members are needed, especially cooks and other skilled workers. Ready-prepared systems may also save time and cut waste by eliminating the long

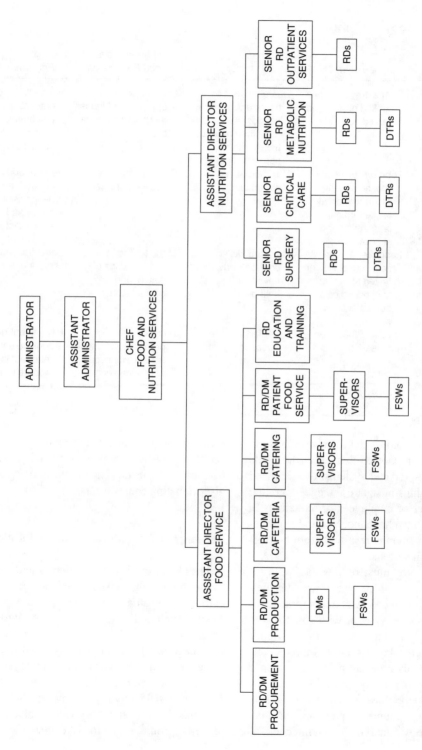

Note: RD = registered dietitian; DTR = dietetic technician, registered; DM = dietary manager; FSW = food service worker.

Figure 21-4 Typical Organization of Food and Nutrition Services in Large Hospitals

Table 21-1 Food Service System Types

Type	Characteristics	Labor	Implications for Food Preparation	Equipment Needs
Conventional (cook-serve)	Central tray line; food cooked on-site and served hot.	Operates 13–14 hours a day; peak periods at mealtime; requires highly trained cooks and bakers.	Use of mostly unprocessed foods; few preprepared or convenience items.	Need full line of food production equipment and system for keeping foods hot.
Commissary (satellite)	Food procured and cooked at central site; transported offsite for final preparation and service.	Maximum use of skilled labor.	Potential for large-scale purchasing.	Delivery equipment needed; each site needs service space and equipment.
Ready-Prepared (cook-chill; cook-freeze)	Food prepared in advance, chilled or frozen for future use; plated cold; heated at service site.	Reduced skilled labor costs; steady work flow; one 8-hour shift per day.	Menu limited by heating times of plated food combinations.	Decentralized heating system required.
Assembly-Serve	Procured foods ready for service.	Unskilled labor adequate for most positions.	All foods are prepackaged; must have ready supply of convenience items.	Heating but no cooking equipment required; large storage space needed.

process of cooking from scratch. However, a study by Greathouse et al. showed that, when hospitals switched to ready-prepared systems, they realized no significant savings in square footage, operating hours, and number of employees or reductions in absenteeism.[6] On the other hand, Vaz and Holm reported significant savings resulting from conversion to a cook-chill system.[7]

Each administrator must review available resources and determine which system would be best in the given circumstances. A common practice is to have a combination system, with some ready-prepared foods and some conventional items. Those with a limited labor supply, unpredictable food delivery, outmoded equipment, and cramped space may find a total ready-prepared system appealing. Alternatively, those with an abundant supply of labor, food, equipment, and space and a desire to maximixe the market for "homecooked" meals will favor a conventional system. Some health care institutions go all the way, offering gastronomic delights that cater to the culinary tastes of discriminating connoisseurs.

Feeding Staff, Employees, and the Public

The ability to feed staff members and the public first-rate meals in a fast, convenient, and economical manner is an asset for any health care facility. Meals purchased at the site translate into shorter breaks for staff and less time away from the bedside of a loved one for visitors. Discounted food prices can also be featured as a valuable employee benefit.

A host of methods are available for on-premise feeding of staff, employees, and the public. Most facilities, large or small, provide a cafeteria where all three groups may dine. At times the cafeteria may be closed to the public due to limited seating, but this is not usually a good marketing strategy. If a facility is too small to provide a cafeteria, arrangements may be made for visitors and employees to purchase patient meals.

In most facilities, employees and visitors dine together, but many American hospitals have either a separate dining room or special food service for physicians. The cafeteria menu can be used but many offer upscale menus and table service to enhance the dining atmosphere for both physicians and others.

Large hospitals may provide other dining services, such as a coffee shop or restaurant. These may or may not be managed by the dietary department. Vending machines, food courts, delicatessens, and takeout meals offer patients, employees, and guests alternative eateries when the main dining areas are closed. Another nice touch is to have a coffee cart accompany patient meal service so visitors can enjoy a beverage while the patients eat.

Feeding night shift employees can be a problem. Keeping the cafeteria open 24 hours a day is not cost-effective in most instances. Options include a limited cafeteria service for short periods of time (e.g., from 2:00 to 4:00 AM, vending machines, a 24-hour coffee shop service, a vending truck, or no service at all (staff are required to provide their own food).

Health care institutions can enhance their images by offering food services that foster positive health habits among staff and visitors. Good nutritional practices can be advanced by consistently offering healthy food choices that meet high standards of quality, attractiveness, taste, and economy and by providing information on written menus, the cafeteria line, or table tents regarding nutrient composition and the characteristics of a healthy diet.

Feeding Patients

Meals are a highlight of the day for many patients. Most patients recognize the importance of nutrition to well-being, but results of one study showed that only two-thirds of patients felt their hospital food was of good quality—tasted, smelled, and looked good and was fresh and nutritious.[8] Patient satisfaction may be improved through more appealing menu choices, greater attentiveness to individual patient preferences, upgraded table or tray appointments, better service, and marketing (all of which may require increased food prices).

Patient feeding may vary by type of menu (selective, restaurant, nonselective) and type of service provided (tray, cafeteria, dining room, hotel service). Selective menus allow patients to choose from a list of two or more entrees, starches, vegetables, salads, and desserts. Sometimes an extensive restaurantlike menu is used. Nonselective menus, used for patients unable to make balanced meal selections, tend to have lower food costs than selective menus but are not as popular with clients and may result in greater plate waste.

The most common meal service is the delivery of trays to patients' rooms for the standard three meals per day. Another alternative is the five-meal plan featuring early morning rolls and coffee, a mid-morning brunch, a full late afternoon dinner, and snacks in the afternoon and evening. Facilities serving ambulatory clients may provide meals in congregate dining areas. This can both stimulate client socialization and reduce labor costs. Discretion should be used because some clients resist eating with persons who are less alert than themselves.

In a highly competitive environment, hospitals often attempt to attract patients by offering upscale, private, luxury dining. Gourmet meals, flexible meal hours, and impeccable service add costs but also create a more favorable image. For example, elegant meals for new parents are often offered in maternity suites, and many hospitals set aside one or more units where all meals are served with fine china, linens, silverware, and fresh flowers.

Vending machines can be used for late admissions. Each nursing station is provided money to buy food for the patient. This procedure assists in the documentation of expenditures for food and allows the kitchen to be locked after dining hours, decreasing the chance for theft.

A large percentage of patients receive some type of between-meal nourishment or refreshment.

Foods available for all patients normally include juice, crackers, and carbonated beverages. These can be distributed from a cart by nursing or dietary aides. Nourishments, on the other hand, are considered an important part of individualized diet therapy and may include nutritional supplements, between-meal feedings for patients with diabetes or ulcers, and food with high nutrient density for patients who require additional calories or protein. It is common practice for the dietary department to leave nourishments for personnel in each unit to distribute as prescribed. Since hungry staff members may help themselves to nourishments, the system needs to be closely controlled by careful planning and documentation and strict monitoring.

Highly specialized needs may increase the cost of food production. For example, hospices or cancer hospitals take extreme measures to prevent microbial contamination and protect immunocompromised clients. Religious rituals and practices that require special foods, equipment, or storage should be taken into account when organizing a department and planning the annual budget.

Nutrition Services

Nutrition services encompass the full range of duties associated with patient care, such as screening for nutritional risk; nutritional status assessment; development of care plans and documentation in the medical record; provision of modified diets, tube feedings, or parenteral nutrition, as appropriate; continuous quality improvement programs; and diet counseling and nutrition education. These functions are provided directly by registered or licensed dietitians or by dietetic technicians or other qualified personnel under the supervision of a dietitian. In states that license dietitians or nutritionists, only authorized dietetic professionals may conduct nutrition assessment and counseling services. Dietetic technicians are usually employed full time, whereas the dietitian may be full or part time or retained as a consultant, as needed by the organization. Figure 21-5 presents major facets of the nutritional care process.

Nutrition Assessment and Care Planning

Studies indicate that about a third of patients admitted to hospitals and more than 75 percent of those admitted to nursing homes show signs of malnutrition.[9] Thus, every admission should be screened to ensure that such patients are identified and designated for appropriate levels of care.[10] Screening protocols require collection of pertinent information; screening is fast and can be completed by dietetic technicians or by admitting personnel. Using guidelines established by registered dietitians, technicians can determine which patients are likely to have nutritional problems.[11] They turn screening data over to a dietitian who then conducts a thorough nutritional assessment and develops a plan for each patient, including caloric and metabolic requirements, nutrient and fluid restrictions, diet patterns, supplemental feedings, and counseling needs. The physician's diet order must be confirmed and the care plan written in the medical record.

Nutritional Intervention and Evaluation

The institutional diet manual serves as a guide for specific diet modifications. Patients on special diets are encouraged to make food choices from a limited selective menu. Intakes are monitored to ensure understanding of the diet, compliance with dietary prescriptions, and adequacy of intakes.

Enteral (tube) feedings may be prescribed for patients who have an intact, functioning gastrointestinal tract but whose nutritional needs cannot be met by oral intakes. Ready-to-use tube feedings may be purchased, or the formulas can be prepared from such items as pureed foods, milk, and pasteurized eggs. Purchased formulas have the advantage of being free of contamination and having a free-flowing consistency that prevents clogged tubes. There is also a range of special products available to meet unique dietary needs, such as increased density, absence of lactose, controlled nutrient composition, and ease of administration. Typically, a tertiary care hospital uses 10–15 different commercial formulas (placed on bid according to established

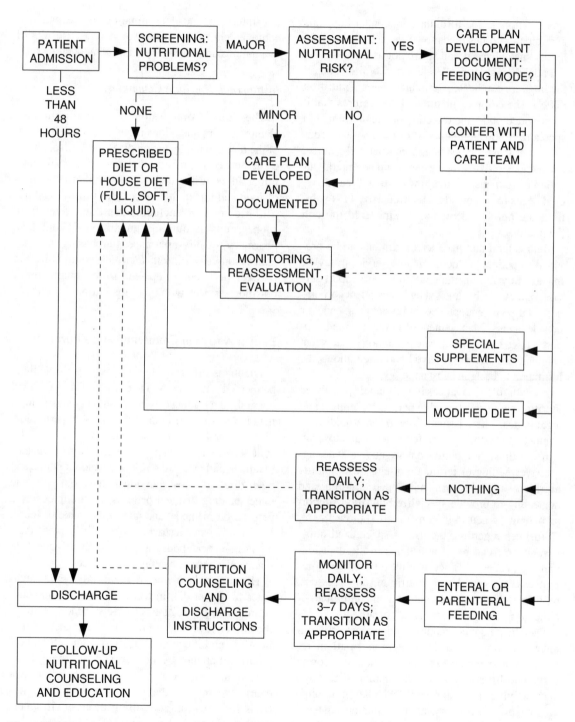

Figure 21-5 Major Facets of the Nutritional Care Process

specifications). The formulary in smaller hospitals and nursing homes tends to be more limited, since highly specialized products are not used.

Patients unable to tolerate either oral or enteral feedings are candidates for total parenteral nutrition (TPN). The complex nature of TPN requires that it be provided under the direction of a team trained in specialized nutrition support; often this team consists of at least a physician, a pharmacist, a nurse, and a registered dietitian. Enteral and parenteral nutrition are expensive, and how costs will be recovered needs to be considered. Ordinarily, TPN solutions are purchased by and administered through the pharmacy.

Both enteral and parenteral nutrition can be provided to patients at home. Home services may be managed by the institutional nutrition support service, or they can be directed by independent corporations staffed by entrepreneurial hospital personnel or outside agents. Management of home nutrition support service by the health care institution ensures that continuity of care is preserved and often allows the institution to bring in substantial revenue.

As with many advances in medicine, specialized nutrition support is linked to perplexing ethical and legal issues. These issues relate to force-feeding of competent patients, enteral feeding of comatose patients or those in a permanent vegetative state, aggressive feeding of terminal patients, withholding nutrition support from handicapped children, and neglecting to provide specialized nutrition support to patients when it is considered standard care. Guidelines regarding the use of specialized nutrition support can be of assistance in the decision-making process.[12] Since institutional ethics committees often grapple with nutrition support issues, registered dietitians are vital to such committees—either as regular members or as consultants.[13]

Dietetic personnel monitor and evaluate compliance with prescribed diet orders and patient response to nutritional intervention. Their monitoring responsibilities are ordinarily managed through such activities as meal rounds, calculation of nutrient intakes, observation and discussion during ward rounds, reassessment of nutritional status at 3- to 7-day intervals, and determination of the patients' achievement of nutritional objectives. Results of evaluations are documented in the medical record.

Institutional Nutrition Committees

The Joint Commission on accreditation of Healthcare Organizations requires annual approval of the diet manual by the medical staff. Also, physicians and other institutional personnel can make important contributions to the overall effectiveness of food and nutrition services. An institutional nutrition committee including representatives from such groups as nursing, nutrition and dietetics, pharmacy, quality assurance, purchasing, and human resources can both facilitate communication between pertinent groups and foster integration of nutrition services with other institutional services.

Patient Nutrition Counseling and Education

Dietitians offer nutrition counseling to facilitate patient self-sufficiency. Diet is associated with six out of the ten leading causes of death in industrialized nations (coronary heart disease, cancer, hypertension, diabetes mellitus, cirrhosis, and obesity), and lifestyle and dietary changes are necessary to enhance treatment and reduce the risk of developing these and other diseases. Most individuals have only a vague understanding of meal patterns, food composition, preparation methods, and nutritional value of foods. Particularly when a strict modified diet is prescribed, a nutritionist can both teach and motivate patients to make independent, healthy food choices.

Hospitalized patients are not usually good candidates for either diet instructions or nutrition counseling (see Table 21-2). Anxiety, time pressures, the influence of medications, and frequent interruptions all inhibit patient education.[14] Therefore, hospitalized patients are best served by giving them only rudimentary details of their diets before discharge and inviting them to return on an outpatient basis for nutrition counseling in an environment more conducive to learning.

Table 21-2 Diet Counseling and Nutrition Education

	Description	Setting	Time Requirements
Diet Instruction	Provision of basic information on a specific diet modification.	Prior to hospital discharge; at physician's office or nutrition clinic.	10–30 minutes.
Individualized Nutrition Counseling	Development of individualized diet plan to meet life-style preferences of the client; plan offers sufficient information and guidance so that the patient can make independent food choices.	Outpatient setting; nutrition clinics and private offices.	2–12 hours, depending on complexity of diet and lifestyle modifications; at least 4 sessions of 20–60 minutes recommended.
Group Nutrition Counseling	Informational sessions for individuals on similar diet plans, such as weight reduction, cholesterol and fat controlled, and sodium restricted or diabetic plans.	Hospital classroom or outpatient setting; nutrition clinic.	4–12 sessions each lasting 30–60 minutes.
Nutrition Education	Dissemination of general information to promote good nutritional habits.	Lecture hall, classroom, nutrition clinic, or private office.	Varies from 1-minute TV spot to regularly scheduled programs over an extended period of time.

Patients may benefit from sharing their experiences with others in similar situations. Thus, group nutrition counseling sessions are often held for patients who require modified diets to control conditions such as diabetes mellitus, elevated serum cholesterol, hyperlipidemia, obesity, hypertension, inborn errors of metabolism, and renal insufficiency.

Dietitians with well-honed counseling skills are often employed to provide nutrition services for ambulatory patients. Diet counseling may be organized as part of the outpatient department at the hospital or within a free-standing nutrition clinic sponsored by the institution. Many physician groups also employ one or more dietitians within group practices; these may compete with counseling services offered by the institution.

Nutrition education programs may be presented to foster better health among personnel at the institution. Examples of worksite nutrition education programs include posting nutrient composition of foods on the cafeteria line, featuring a nutrition col-umn in the company newsletter, and promoting dietary goals on table tents or bulletin boards. Some hospitals sponsor employee weight reduction classes or invite employees to spend "an hour with the chef" learning about low-fat or vegetarian cooking. Individual nutrition counseling services may also be offered to employees and covered by the employee health insurance policy. Coverage is especially common for employees who suffer from chronic health problems such as diabetes, obesity, hypertension, and coronary heart disease. The booklet *Worksite Nutrition: A Decision-Maker's Guide* contains several suggestions for planning and implementing employee nutrition programs.[15]

Nutrition education can be the basis for an outreach initiative to promote wellness and maximize institutional visibility and public relations in the community.[16] Classes at local libraries can successfully feature topics such as school lunches, eating out on a diet, popular food myths, and food secrets your mother never taught you. Other effective strategies for enhancing participation in outreach programs include computerized nutrient analysis of intakes, nutrition counseling at cholesterol screenings, body fat analysis at health fairs, modified diet cooking classes, and guided grocery store tours.

Packaged nutrition education programs and franchises are available, particularly for weight reduction. These programs are profitable and easy to use, but patients rarely retain the weight loss.[17] The decision to adopt structured programs should take into consideration professional guidelines, personnel skills, and the availability of other nutrition education resources.

Education and Research

Education and research work hand in hand to improve workers' knowledge base, ensure high performance, and advance levels of practice. Those who participate in continuing education programs develop the skills necessary for independent decision making, increasing their value to the institution. Registered dietitians and food service managers should provide educational programs designed to meet the specific needs of department employees, professional staff members, students and interns, physicians and other health care practitioners, and personnel at the worksite.

Many unskilled personnel are employed in food service departments. Because jobs in the department are diverse and there tends to be high turnover, the need for in-service education of dietary workers is particularly acute. Departmental policies ought to provide for regular training during working hours, attendance should be required, and space as well as other teaching resources should be provided.

Professional staff must have continuing education to remain current in their fields and to facilitate advancement of the department. Techniques for providing in-house continuing education include journal clubs, nutrition and medical rounds, circulation of scientific journals, use of loaned or purchased audiovisual programs, independent-study kits, and self-assessment programs. Frequently it is desirable for professional staff to attend local, state, regional, or national conferences, courses, symposia, and workshops. Institutional or departmental policies should be in place that provide for paid time off and payment of registration fees and travel expenses. On the other hand, staff who attend meetings at institutional expense should be expected to report back, spearhead projects, and apply learned information at the institution.

Departments may collaborate with educational institutions to provide supervised professional practice for students enrolled in dietary manager, dietetic technician, coordinated undergraduate, postbaccalaureate, and graduate programs. In such cases, professional staff members must help plan high-quality learning experiences, direct student activities, and evaluate student performance. Care should be taken to ensure that students engage in activities designed to meet defined learning objectives, do not replace regular employees, and are not paid for the time devoted to educational experiences. Collaboration between the health care facility and the academic institution should be formalized by a memorandum of agreement signed by the chief executive officers of both institutions.

It is also popular to offer summer practicums for undergraduate and graduate students especially interested in food service management or clinical nutrition or for faculty members who wish to update their practical knowledge of the field. One staff member should be assigned to coordinate such programs, which may vary in length from one to ten weeks. Trainees may work on special projects or shadow designated employees in various units to gain a broad perspective of the department. These training programs are sometimes supported by industry, and the department usually does not pay a stipend.

Hospitals may sponsor an accredited dietetic internship or an approved preprofessional practice program that meets standards established by the American Dietetic Association, Canadian Dietetic Association, or a similar professional group. The costs of these educational programs are offset by the benefits, which include

- ready access to a pool of qualified candidates from which to draw professional employees
- continual stimulation motivating the dietetic staff to remain current in both knowledge and practice
- contributions of interns or trainees to productivity in the department
- greater departmental prestige and recognition as a result of student assignments related to special meals in the cafeteria, bulletin board displays, miniresearch projects, patient nutritional care, and so on

Dietitians need to provide nutrition education programs for health professionals at the facility, including physicians as well as medical students, interns, and residents.[18] These programs usually involve one or more presentations at regular weekly conferences. Topics might include the institutional diet manual, procedures for ordering special diets or products, the role of the dietitian in health care delivery, and the range of nutritional services offered by the department. Some institutions hold medical conferences over lunch—a typical lunch for someone on a low-sodium, diabetic, weight reduction, or protein-restricted diet.

Dietitians may participate in clinical research projects either independently or in collaboration with physicians, educators, or other professionals.[19] At major health care institutions, clinical research is often written into the job description; this should be taken into account when setting departmental standards of practice, performance, and productivity. Research projects should be submitted for departmental and institutional approval according to defined procedures, and any outside funding should be strictly controlled to ensure compliance with monetary guidelines.

Generating Revenue

The wave of fiscal constraints affecting health care institutions triggered new methods for generating revenue. Some of these are outlined below.

Catering

Catering to outside groups is one option for generating additional revenue. The most common strategy is to use the kitchen during nonpeak times, such as evenings and weekends. Catering can bring in revenue, but it can also create hard feelings among nearby businesses who lose customers as a result.[20] Catering cannot be started without proper serviceware, serving utensils, delivery and heating equipment, and adequate personnel. Furthermore, pricing systems must be established to ensure sufficient profit.

Income-Producing Food Operations

Some successful expanded food service programs described by Super include

- takeout meals for customers
- frozen modified entrees (low-sodium, low-fat) for purchase by staff members or the public
- delicatessens
- baked goods sold to staff, guests, and local businesses
- hot dog stands in business or college sections of towns
- bulk food service to day-care and senior centers, small nursing homes, and private schools
- vending machine service
- individual food service to homebound senior citizens[21]

The department must be careful not to stretch profit-making enterprises to the point where the quality of food service provided to patients and staff declines.

Nutrition Services

Inpatient nutrition services are an important source of revenue for both the institution and the department. The institution benefits when improved patient nutritional status contributes to reduced lengths of stay.[22] Such improvement has been observed in both surgical and medical patients; lengths of stay were reduced up to five days, with average cost savings from $1,738 to $3,557 per patient stay.[23] Also, when malnutrition is documented in the medical record and listed as a comorbidity factor on the attestation sheet, revenues are increased over that usually allowed for the specific diagnostic related group (DRG).[24] Clinical dietitians play a major role in identifying and reversing poor nutritional status, thus optimizing revenue from treatment of malnutrition.

Revenues can also be increased by direct charges for clinical nutrition services. Many departments have separate cost centers for clinical nutrition; hospitalized patients are charged for any service not included in the per diem rate, including special diets, diet instructions, nutritional status assessments, nutrient intake evaluation, nutritional supplements, and tube feedings.[25]

RESOURCE REQUIREMENTS

Considerable resources are allotted to the department, including budgeted expenses for labor, food and supplies, furnishings, and equipment, as well as extensive floor space for the kitchen, offices, cafeteria, dining rooms, and storage. Judicious use of these resources hinges on creative budgeting and strict controls.

Dietetic Personnel

Dietary services are labor intensive. Table 21-3 summarizes the role functions and qualifications of personnel needed within the department.

The recruitment and retention of qualified professional personnel is a laborious process. This is particularly true when there is a disparity between competencies expected by health care operators and skills taught in educational programs. For example, Yates et al. found educators placed greater value on skills related to nutritional services, whereas executives desired greater emphasis on financial competencies, technical operations, and personnel man-

agement skills.[26] Educational programs, especially at the graduate level, now place greater emphasis on quantitative management techniques.

Recruiting unskilled employees also presents a challenge. The diminishing number of persons under 30 and the escalating wages offered by competitive for-profit operations intensifies the competition for unskilled laborers. Many new employees have no previous food service experience, increasing the need for extensive on-the-job training and education. Cross-training and career counseling are ways to boost job satisfaction and employee retention and facilitate growth toward full potential.[27] For example, diet aides may be trained to work on the tray line, assist with food preparation, serve food in the cafeteria, and wait on tables in the coffee shop, making their job more interesting and enhancing their value to the organization.

Staffing and scheduling of staff are highly variable in food service operations. Factors that affect staffing include facility size, physical plant, hours of operation, meal presentation, type of meal plan, nature of menu selections, variety and number of modified diets, amount of convenience food used, design of food service delivery systems, and use of disposables. Output is also influenced by the skill and longevity of personnel and the rate of labor turnover. Revenue-generating programs and the level of clinical nutrition services also affect staffing requirements.

Several indices have been used to estimate the labor hours needed per meal. A guideline of 10–17 minutes per meal or 3.5–5 meals per labor hour may be used as a staffing standard for a conventional food service system.[28] Exhibit 21-1 shows how to calculate staffing needs for a specific institution. These figures should be used with caution because a minimum number of people will be needed, no matter how many meals are served. The number will also vary according to the functions performed by the food service staff, such as tray distribution, food preparation, and catering. Table 21-4 presents estimates of staffing needs by facility size.

The current norm is one clinical dietitian for each 50 to 60 patients, although reported averages range

Table 21-3 Job Titles, Roles, and Qualifications

Job Title	Credentialing	Qualifications	Responsibilities
Director	Registered dietitian; Commission on Dietetic Registration of the American Dietetic Association	Baccalaureate or master's degree plus specified practicum experiences	Coordinates food service and clinical nutrition systems; administers personnel; designs and implements employee training programs; directs and evaluates food systems; controls departmental budgets.
	Dietetic technician, registered; Commission on Dietetic Registration of the American Dietetic Association	Associate degree	As above, under direction of a dietitian; helps dietitian to perform routine nutritional screenings, counseling, and patient menu coordination.
	Dietary manager, certified; Dietary Managers Association	One-year training program, correspondence course, or 90-hour course	Coordinates food service systems, hires staff, and conducts in-service training; all tasks performed under the supervision of a dietitian.
Clinical Dietitian	Registered by the American Dietetic Association	Baccalaureate or master's degree plus specified practicum experiences	Manages nutritional therapy and assessment; integral member of the health care team; as a consultant, serves as a liaison to the dietary manager or dietetic technician and the medical staff and administrator.
Diet Clerk	None	In-house training	Menu-processing and clerical duties.
Food Service Supervisor	May be certified dietary manager	In-house or dietary manager training	Directs personnel in a given area, such as food production.
Chef	Culinary arts school	May have associate degree	Prepares food items and special meals; assists with staff supervision.
Baker	None	Experience	Prepares desserts and baked goods.
Cook	None	Experience	Prepares hot food items.
Diet Aide or Food Service Worker	None	In-house training	Assists in all areas, including sanitation.
Storeroom Clerk	None	Honesty	Receives and distributes products according to specifications and requisitions.
Secretary	None	Secretarial school	Performs clerical duties.

Exhibit 21-1 Method for Estimating Staffing Needs

Considering each eight hours of employee time as a full-time equivalent (FTE), it takes at least 1.4 FTEs to fill each position on a daily basis. A department would need 8.4 FTEs to cover 6 full-time positions that need to be staffed seven days a week. This does not take into account sick time or vacation coverage.

To calculate staffing needs based on number of labor minutes required to serve one meal to one person (standard = 10–14 minutes), perform the following operations:

1. Determine total meals per week (number of residents × 21 + guest/employee meals/week).
2. Determine number of labor minutes needed to serve total meals per week (total meals/week × 12 labor minutes/meal).
3. Convert labor minutes to hours (labor minutes/week ÷ 60).
4. Divide labor hours per week by full-time work-week (total hours ÷ 40).
5. Convert workweeks into FTEs (workweeks × 1.4).

from 50 to 100 or more patients per dietitian.[29] Professional staffing requirements are chiefly dependent on patient mix, professional roles, and availability of trained support personnel.[30] The demand for clinical dietitians is expected to increase over the next few years.[31]

Table 21-4 Suggested Numbers of Food Service Personnel in Hospitals and Nursing Homes

	Number of Beds				
	25	50	100	200	500
Hospitals					
Number of FTEs	4	6–7	11–12	22–24	55–60
Extended Care Facilities, Nursing Homes, and Sheltered Care					
Number of FTEs	3	4–5	9–10		

Source: Adapted with permission of Macmillan Publishing Co. from *Food Service Organizations: A Managerial and Systems Approach* by Marian C. Spears, p. 401. Copyright © 1991 by Macmillan Publishing Co.

Space and Equipment Needs

Each food service area has its own unique space and equipment needs, as outlined in Table 21-5. The layout and design of the kitchen should evolve from a specific operational plan. The flow of products must be in a forward direction from raw ingredients to production to the service area. A rule of thumb for kitchen space allocation is 12–15 square feet per meal. This is a rough estimate, as a minimum amount of space will be needed regardless of the number of meals served.

The decision to use disposable dishes and serviceware in place of china and silver has a major impact on space and equipment. The use of more permanent ware means greater client satisfaction, but it is attended by frequent breakage and theft, higher water use, more labor hours, and greater investment in dishwashing and sanitizing equipment. Not only do paper and plastic products require more storage space, but they also have a negative impact on the environment and there is a greater need for refuge control.

Budgetary Considerations

Food and nutrition services consume about 5–8 percent of the direct expenses of the average hospital. The budget is affected by labor intensity; type of menu; type of services provided (e.g., table service); fluctuating costs of raw food, supplies, and materials; and equipment needs. Appropriate scheduling and limited use of overtime can assist in controlling labor costs. The use of part-time employees during peak production and service times can also help cut costs. Menus and types of diets can be altered to be less labor intensive, but the large number of complex modified diets now in use dictates even higher labor usage than was previously the case.[32] Dietetic technicians may be employed to do many routine tasks formerly done by clinical dietitians, whose salaries are higher. Optimal professional staffing is still required, however, to maintain high-quality patient food and nutrition services.

Table 21-5 Food Service Equipment and Space Needs

Area	Functions	Considerations	Equipment/Space Needs
Receiving	Ensures that products delivered were ordered and are of the quality, quantity, size, and price specified.	Storage areas should be convenient to receiving area.	Forklift or handtruck; an accurate scale; tools such as can opener, thermometer, crowbar, and short-bladed knife.
Storage	Stores and secures products.	Only authorized personnel should be allowed access to storage. Dry food and chemical storage must be separate. Storerooms should be locked and have only one door.	Storage space needed depends on type of food service system. Plan 42" between shelves for mobile equipment. Most shelves are 14" to 21" deep. Estimate storage by multiplying the number of meals served by ½ square foot. Walk-in refrigerators needed for 300–400 meals per day.
Production	Produces high-quality and safe food.	Nature of production varies with type and size of operation. Equipment controls types of items that can be on menu. Storage space is needed for raw ingredients and finished products.	Deck oven, convection oven, steam-jacketed kettle, steamer, fryer, tilting braising pans, grill, microwave, or specialized equipment for cook-freeze or cook-chill systems. An estimate of kitchen space requirements is 12' to 15' per meal. A person's work zone is 42" by 30". Aisles must be 42" for one person, 48" to 54" for two persons, and 5' for main traffic.
Distribution and Service	Assembles trays or bulk food and distributes to dining or patient areas.	Varies with type of system (centralized or decentralized). Trays assembled hot in a centralized area must be delivered within 30–45 minutes for maximum quality. Decentralized system food is delivered hot or cold and must be plated or heated at the distribution site. Distribution of trays may be by nursing or food service personnel.	Equipment to retain temperatures during tray delivery includes insulated trays and dishes, pellets, covers, and temperature support carts. Storage space for these items must be allocated. Insulated trays need special china or paper goods for the compartments. Cold tray assembly requires reheating equipment, which may cost $15,000 to $30,000. Space requirements at the serving site are estimated to be 120 square feet for 20 persons.

continues

Table 21-5 continued

Area	Functions	Considerations	Equipment/Space Needs
Dishwashing and Waste Disposal	Retrieves and sanitizes permanent ware and dispose of waste.	Type of machine based on amount of permanent ware to be sanitized in a set period of time. Reduction of waste options can be costly.	Dishwashing area must have space for soiled tableware, scraping, prerinsing and stacking, dishwashing machine, removal of dishes, and storage.
Cafeteria	Provides food service to staff and guests.	Hours of operation, number served (usually between 4 and 8 per minute), turnover, and types of service (self-serve, served, grilled items).	Serving area can be a single line, parallel lines, L-shaped, U-shaped, or double-U-shaped, or a scramble or wheel system. 32 square feet needed to seat 4 people; 20–60 minutes per meal.
Offices	Space for administrative personnel, the diet office, and clinical dietitians.	Administrative personnel should have offices within kitchen and should have windows to see the operation. Clinical dietitians should have offices on or near patient wards.	Office space depends on the size of operation and the number of personnel.
Classrooms	Rooms for personnel training, group instructions, and classes.	Instructional materials and audiovisual equipment must be available for teaching purposes.	Classrooms vary in size and may be used by other departments.

Raw food costs usually go up every year, as do expenses for materials and supplies. Average raw food costs depend on the types of services provided and the philosophy of the organization. For example, the more convenience items used, the higher the costs of food but the lower the labor costs. Also, using paper goods for the tray service will increase supply costs but may decrease water and electricity usage.

Capital budget expenditures are required to improve, expand, or replace equipment. Equipment life expectancy can be extended through a meticulous preventive maintenance program based on recommendations by the manufacturers. Good preventive maintenance and detailed repair records are essential for cost control and purchasing decisions. A food service operation cannot close, so budgetary allowance should be available for emergency purchase or repairs.

QUALITY CONTROLS

Quality is perhaps *the* word of the decade. Total quality management and its derivatives permeate discussions in the board room, at the bedside, and in the dishroom. Every health care manager must be held accountable for establishing standards of quality and ensuring that subordinates comply with maintaining these standards. Within dietetics, quality controls must be defined and maintained for food and food services, patient nutritional care, and general management of the department.

Food and Food Services

Quality standards have been established for specific food products.[33] These standards must be taken into account during the development of specifications for the purchase of fresh produce, frozen entrees, dairy products, meats, dry food items, canned fruits and vegetables, and specialty items. Constant vigilance is required to ensure that all purchased items meet quality standards upon delivery. Because quality may deteriorate rapidly during storage, foods should be used within the suggested shelf life. Both temperature and humidity must be carefully regulated in refrigerated and dry storage areas.

Dietitians, food service managers, and kitchen supervisors must give a high priority to providing high-quality food and impeccable service. Concern for superiority should be incorporated into job descriptions; recipes; and methods and procedures for food handling, preparation, and service. It is the practice in many institutions to conduct and document a food quality check of all items prior to serving each meal, or at least periodically.

Quality assurance probes can be used to assess such food service factors as tray appearance, food temperatures, tray accuracy, and the like.[34] Also, patient and customer surveys are often used to evaluate satisfaction with institutional food services. When performance in any of these areas deviates from established standards, care should be taken to identify and solve underlying problems, such as improper food handling, poorly maintained equipment, inadequate training, or poorly motivated employees. Improvement can often be achieved through the effective use of quality circles and other participative management strategies.[35]

Patient Nutritional Care

Regulatory agencies require an ongoing program of quality improvement of clinical nutrition in both hospitals and extended care facilities. Standards of performance can be established and monitored to ensure high-quality services related to the general aspects of nutritional care, such as screening, nutrition care planning, documentation, and evaluation. Also, quality assurance can be extended to encompass the nutritional value of patient menus, the adequacy of liquid diets, and compliance with standards for enteral and parenteral feeding, for example. Furthermore, standards of practice should be specified for patients with specific conditions, such as renal disease, cancer, burns, diabetes, or liver disease. Ordinarily, nutrition-related quality management programs are under the jurisdiction of clinical dietitians, whose job description includes responsibility for quality assurance. Time should be allocated for the tasks required by this role.

Food Service and Clinical Nutrition Management Audits

In the kitchen area, quality factors include sanitation, layout and equipment, personnel management, and policies and procedures. The American Society for Hospital Food Service Administrators of the American Hospital Association offers a comprehensive outline to assess all management aspects of the food service operation.[36] In addition, Schiller et al. developed an instrument that can be used to assess the overall quality of clinical nutrition services.[37]

THE FUTURE OF FOOD SERVICE MANAGEMENT

During the next several decades, health care administrators will face marketing, environmental, cost-benefit, contract food service, productivity, technology, and specialization issues.

Marketing Food and Nutrition Services

The dietary department can play an important role in marketing key services, increasing revenue, enhancing job satisfaction, and promoting a positive image for the department and the institution. Commonly used techniques include merchandising, public relations, and word-of-mouth communication. Both hospitals and nursing homes can market dietetic excellence, nutritious or gourmet meals, reshaped pureed food, ethnic meals, festive celebrations, luxury dining, and educational materials.[38] Numerous publications are available to help dietitians market, the most notable being *The Competetive Edge: Marketing Strategies for the Registered Dietitian.*[39]

Recycling and Environmental Concerns

Food and nutrition services can play a major role in preserving resources and protecting the environment. Operators sensitive to environmental concerns employ a variety of strategies for waste disposal and recycling. Waste can be minimized by purchasing fewer packaged, nonbiodegradable products. For example, bulk entrees create less refuse than individually packaged portions, and sliced or unsliced cheese in a single package generates much less waste than individually wrapped slices. Products made with recycled materials should be purchased whenever possible. The institution can also participate in municipal recycling and composting programs.[40]

When shifting from one environmentally sensitive practice to another, all ramifications need to be considered. What were thought to be solutions may cause other problems. For example, decreasing polystyrene products in favor of paper products may increase costs by two to three times.[41] Use of durable serviceware eliminates waste (i.e., discarded disposable plates, cups, bowls, and flatware) but increases breakage and the need for adequate dishwashing facilities.

Cost Benefits of Nutrition Services

The economic value of nutrition services is under investigation for both ambulatory and institutionalized patients. Early results support the economic benefits of nutritional care, but data are insufficient and too fragmented to make definitive statements. The anticipated outcome of these studies is third-party reimbursement for most nutrition services delivered by qualified dietitians. Increased revenues also accrue to hospitals when malnutrition is cited as a comorbidity factor resulting in extended hospital stays for patients. *Business Success in Dietetics: Generating Revenue and Saving Costs*[42] offers detailed guidelines on how to conduct a cost-benefit study.

Self-Operated versus Contract Food and Nutrition Services

During the next decade administrators will be faced with questions such as the following.

Should a commercial group be contracted with to manage food service operations? The pros and cons of both self-operated and contract services are outlined in Table 21-6. Although the final decision depends on individual circumstances, many health care institutions are attracted to contract arrangements because they offer cost savings; availability of qualified management personnel; standardized menus; and well-defined goals, policies, and procedures. Nutrition services are usually retained under hospital jurisdiction even when food services are rendered by an outside company.

Should contract services be negotiated between institutions in the same system or those geographically located near each other? For an established fee, a large hospital may provide a full range of services to smaller institutions, such as management systems, menus, purchasing, and prepared menu items. Benefits include maximum utilization of resources at the large institution and reduced staffing, especially at the management level, at the affiliated organizations. In one case, a hospital prepares foods in bulk and transports it to a retirement center, where the food is plated and served. Another model is for the hospital to prepare the trays prior to delivery. Dietitians and food service managers from the parent institution also provide a full range of professional services to the satellites.

Table 21-6 Pros and Cons of Facility-Operated and Contract Food Services

	Advantages	*Disadvantages*
Facility-Operated Services	Greater concern for and sensitivity to facility objectives Better maintenance of established standards Access to records and ability to monitor incurred costs Total accountability to facility administration Lower operating cost	Less flexibility; must work within institutional bureaucracy; expertise may be lacking for highly complex activities and decision making Continuation of past operational procedures Need for greater administrative input Higher operating costs because of inefficiencies and possibly poor management
Contracted Services	Access to wide array of organizational resources, including a variety of professional staff Group buying allows products otherwise not available to small facilities Increased operating efficiencies with lower cost Reduced direction required by internal administrators	Loss of internal control Attitudinal concerns Unavailability of facility support services in some cases, such as concurrent peak demand by several facilities Miscellaneous operational problems, such as unsatisfactory menus, poor quality food, communication problems

Source: Information from *Cost Effective Contract Food Service: An Institutional Guide* by B.H. Zaccarelli and J.D. Ninemeier, Aspen Publishers, Inc., © 1982.

Should clinical dietetic services be contracted for? Small institutions may not need the full-time services of a registered dietitian; these services can be obtained by employing a part-time dietitian or by contracting with an individual, institution, or agency. When professional services are covered by contract, the written agreement should be sufficiently detailed to address both procedural and legal dimensions of the arrangement. Consultant Dietitians in Health Care Facilities offers model contracts to guide decision making in this regard.[43]

Should an institution hold a fast-food or other franchise? Many institutions are pressured by consumer demand to install a McDonald's, Burger King, Wendy's, or other popular alternative to hospital food.[44] Such companies owe their success to tight quality controls, dependability, prompt service, strict standards of sanitation, and economy. Sometimes an institution is unable to match these characteristics; it may be better to retain some revenue from an in-house franchise than see employees stream to a nearby restaurant for meals and beverages.

Productivity

In dietary departments, labor accounts for 60–70 percent of total operating costs.[45] Concern for cost containment has intensified efforts to both accurately measure and increase labor output in the department. Exhibit 21-2 contains various formulas for calculating productivity in food and nutrition services. Labor minutes per meal equivalent is the most common measure of productivity. For a more accurate accounting, Brown and Hoover recommend a total-factor productivity model that relates food service output to all input resources.[46]

Productivity in clinical areas can be standardized through the use of time studies or an analysis of departmental charges. For example, a study of 283

Exhibit 21-2 Formulas for Calculating Productivity

1. Meals per labor hour $= \dfrac{\text{Total meals served per day}}{\text{Labor hours per day}}$

2. Minutes per meal $= \dfrac{\text{Labor minutes per day}}{\text{Total meals served per day}}$

3. Payroll cost per day = sum of hourly rate of each employee × hours worked for all employees

4. Payroll cost per meal served $= \dfrac{\text{Total daily payroll cost}}{\text{Meals served per day}}$

5. Labor cost per day = total payroll cost per day + total of all other direct labor costs (fringe benefits) per day

6. Labor cost per meal served $= \dfrac{\text{Total labor cost per day}}{\text{Meals served per day}}$

Source: Reprinted with permission of Macmillan Publishing Co. from *Food Service Organizations: A Managerial and Systems Approach* by Marian C. Spears, p. 409. Copyright © 1991 by Macmillan Publishing Co.

clinical dietitians showed a 41.3-hour average workweek, with 20.4 hours spent in direct patient care, 13.6 hours in indirect patient care, and 7.3 hours in non-patient-care activities.[47] For the most part, only direct patient care time is considered as "productive" because clinical output is often measured by reimbursable activities such as nutritional assessments, indirect calorimetry, nutrient analyses, diet counseling, and group classes. Any gain in productivity requires an upturn in the number or amount of patient charges; this means spending more time in direct patient care. When productivity is a concern, time should be carefully monitored to ensure maximum benefit from attending meetings, writing reports, coordinating nutritional services, and communicating with other members of the health care team. Time wasted in traversing from one unit to another and waiting on others should be kept to a minimum.

Monitrend (Hospital Administrative Services, American Hospital Association) offers a national productivity reporting system for dietetics. The standardized reports are based on paid hours per 100 meal equivalents and do not address clinical productivity. When comparing a specific facility to reported norms, individual circumstances must be considered. For example, some hospitals serve a higher percentage of labor-intensive patient meals than the average. Other facilities may sell more cafeteria meals, causing the product mix to be less labor intensive. The number of beds, turnover rate, number of part-time workers, and operating philosophies each affect calculated outcomes.

Productivity within a system can be augmented by using systematic analysis and application of systems engineering principles.[48] These four steps will lead to a more favorable outcome:

1. Show administrative commitment to productivity by making available a system in which each employee can efficiently perform designated tasks.

2. Focus on the personnel skills and capabilities needed to perform the tasks. Careful screening of job applicants, good communication, flexible schedules, and intensive on-the-job training can help.

3. Reinforce efficient work habits; watch for duplicative work efforts or wasted steps. Analysis of workflow processing and careful attention to principles of time and motion economy can enhance efficiency.

4. Use industrial engineering techniques to evaluate the necessity of an activity and the degree of compliance with the desired workflow and methods. Pilot projects can provide supportive data and evaluation documentation.[49]

Technological Advances

Computers

Computers are essential for the effective management of food operations, clinical dietetic services,[50] and evaluation activities.[51] Integrated systems offer the greatest assistance in master menu coordination, forecasting, food purchasing, requisition and inventory control, recipe and production control, pricing, generation of individualized patient menus, menu scanning, nutrient analysis of patient menus, and cost control. Despite the many applications of computers in food and nutrition services, this technology is not yet fully utilized in daily operations. Administrators need to foster the use of computers in food service management educational programs.[52]

Food Service Equipment

Advances in construction materials and electronics account for major advancements in this area. The advent of high-density plastics portends the availability of lightweight, durable equipment for food storage, transport, and service. Electronic controls mastermind such things as

- the speed of tray assembly belts to control productivity levels
- the mechanical delivery of tray carts to decrease dependence on labor
- point-of-service heating of patient trays to optimize food temperatures and decrease complaints about cold food and beverages
- the flow rate of tube feeding pumps to control formula usage

Nutrition Assessment Devices

Dietitian involvement in patient nutritional status assessment requires the availability of assessment devices. Three of the most popular devices include the following:

- Equipment for body composition analysis. For example, RJL Laboratories (Detroit) offers a Bioelectrical Impedance Analyzer (BIA) that rapidly and accurately measures body fat, water, and muscle mass. Health care facilities use this device to track fluctuations in body fluid, measure fat losses during weight reduction, and monitor changes in muscle mass resulting from exercise and body-building routines.

- Metabolic carts. Nutrition support dietitians or other personnel use metabolic carts to measure metabolic rates and determine patient energy needs.
- Anthropometric measuring devices. These tools include skin-fold calipers, knee-height calipers, scales, and tapes for determining head size and girth.

Specialization

Many dietitians are recognized as management specialists.[53] They may administer food service or clinical nutrition services operations or function in general management positions within the organization. Often these management specialists pursue advanced degrees in business administration, personnel management, law, or finance.

Dietitians who work in clinical dietetics may be generalists or they can obtain credentials for practice in a specialized area (e.g., some are certified diabetes educators and others are certified nutrition support dietitians). When specialty skills are desirable, the job specification should designate the need for certification.

In 1990, the American Dietetic Association recognized three areas of clinical specialization and delineated roles associated with specialty practice in renal dietetics, pediatric nutrition, or metabolic nutrition support. Training programs and certification exams are offered for these and in the future other areas of specialty practice may be developed.

It is common for major medical centers to have career ladders for staff dietitians, with clinical nutrition specialists at the highest level. These dietitians generally have several years experience and an advanced degree.[54] They may consult on complex cases or serve as supervisors for staff dietitians.

CONCLUSION

Food and nutrition services—and the work of both food service managers and registered dietitians—are crucial to health care organizations. Not only do food and dietetic personnel costs represent a significant portion of the institutional budget, but dietetic services play a key role in marketing and public relations. Through careful planning, innovative services, creative problem solving, and tight quality controls, food and nutrition services can enhance a hospital's reputation for excellent meals, high patient satisfaction, judicious use of resources, environmental sensitivity, attentiveness to nutrition as an important component of optimal health care, responsiveness to professional education needs, and participation in community efforts to improve the quality of life.

ADDITIONAL RESOURCES

Organizations

American Dietetic Association, 216 West Jackson Boulevard, Chicago, IL 60606-6995. 312\899-0040; FAX 312\899-1979.

American Society for Hospital Food Service Administrators, 840 N. Lake Shore Drive, Chicago, IL 60611. 312\280-6147.

Dietary Managers Association, 4410 West Roosevelt Road, Hillside, IL 60162-2077.

Periodicals

Food Management, published monthly by Edgell Communications, Inc., 1 East First Street, Duluth, MN 55802.

Food Service Director, published by Bill Communications, Inc., 633 Third Avenue, New York, NY 10017. 212/986-4800.

Restaurants and Institutions, published monthly by Cahners Plaza, 1350 E. Tough Avenue, PO Box 5080, Des Plaines, IL 60017-5080. 312\635-8800.

Books

American Dietetic Association. *Productivity management for nutrition care systems.* Chicago: American Dietetic Association, 1986.

American Dietetic Association. *Accreditation/approval manual for dietetic programs.* Chicago: American Dietetic Association, 1987.

Huyck, N.I., and M.M. Rowe. *Managing clinical nutrition services.* Gaithersburg, Md.: Aspen Publishers, 1990.

Jernigan, A.K. *Nutrition in long-term care facilities.* Chicago: American Dietetic Association, 1987.

Puckett, R.P., and B.B. Miller. *Food service manual for health care institutions.* Chicago: American Hospital Publishers, 1988.

Rinke, W.J. *The winning foodservice manager: Strategies for doing more with less.* Gaithersburg, Md.: Aspen Publishers, 1989.

Rose, J.C. *Handbook for health care food service management.* Gaithersburg, Md.: Aspen Publishers, 1984.

Schiller, M.R., et al. *Handbook for managing clinical nutrition services.* Gaithersburg, Md.:Aspen Publishers, 1991.

Schiller, M.R., et al. *Total quality management for hospital nutrition services.* Gaithersburg, Md.: Aspen Publishers, 1993 (in press).

Sneed, J., and K.H. Dresse. *Understanding foodservice financial management.* Gaithersburg, Md.: Aspen Publishers, 1989.

Spears, M.C. *Foodservice Organizations: A managerial and systems approach.* New York: Macmillan, 1990.

West, B.B., and L. Wood. *Foodservice in institutions.* 6th ed. revised by V.F. Harger, et. al. New York: Macmillan, 1988.

Zaccarelli, H., and J.D. Ninemeier. *Cost effective contract food service: An institutional guide.* Gaithersburg, Md.: Aspen Publishers, 1982.

NOTES

1. L. Graves, Dietetics Developing Rapidly, *Hospital Management* 10, no. 8 (1920): 51, 74–76.

2. J.B. Howland, The Function of the Hospital Dietitian, *Journal of the American Dietetic Association* 1 (October, 1925): 81–83.

3. R.M. Wilder, The Hospital Nutrition Expert, *Journal of the American Dietetic Association* 1, no. 3 (1925): 118–127.

4. W.H. Walsh, The Professional Standing of the Dietitian in the Hospital, *Journal of the American Dietetic Association* 1, no. 3 (1925): 103–105.

5. J.F. Freshwater, *Least-Cost Hospital Food Service Systems,* U.S. Department of Agriculture Marketing Research Report No. 1116 (Washington D.C.: U.S. Government Printing Office, 1980).

6. K.R. Greathouse et al., Comparison of Conventional, Cook-Chill, and Cook-Freeze Foodservice Systems, *Journal of the American Dietetic Association* 89 (1989): 1606–1611.

7. J. Vaz and S. Holm, Assessment Shows That Cook/Chill/Freeze Saves, *Health Care* 27, no. 4 (1985): 18–20.

8. D. DeLuco and M. Cremer, Consumers' Perceptions of Hospital Food and Dietary Services, *Journal of the American Dietetic Association* 90 (1990): 1711–1715.

9. S.K. Kamath et al., Hospital Malnutrition: A 33-Hospital Screening Study, *Journal of the American Dietetic Association* 86 (1986): 203–206.

10. D.A. Ford and M.M. Fairchild, Managing Inpatient Clinical Nutrition Services: A Comprehensive Program Assures Accountability and Success, *Journal of the American Dietetic Association* 90 (1990): 695–702.

11. A.M. Hedberg et al., Nutritional Risk Screening: Development of a Standardized Protocol Using Dietetic Technicians, *Journal of the American Dietetic Association* 88 (1988): 1553–1556. See also J.V. White et al., Nutrition Screening Initiative: Development and Implementation of the Public Awareness Checklist and Screening Tools, *Journal of the American Dietetic Association* 93 (1993): 163–167.

12. American Dietetic Association, Issues in Feeding the Terminally Ill Adult, *Journal of the American Dietetic Association* 92 (1992): 996–1005.

13. H. Brody and M.B. Noel, Dietitian's Role in Decisions to Withhold Nutrition and Hydration, *Journal of the American Dietetic Association* 91 (1991): 580–585.

14. S.S. Picus, Evaluation of the Nutrition Counseling Environment of Hospitalized Patients, *Journal of the American Dietetic Association* 89 (1989): 403–405.

15. American Dietetic Association; Society for Nutrition Education; U.S. Department of Health and Human Services, Public Health Service, Office of Disease Prevention and Health Promotion, *Worksite Nutrition: A Decision-Maker's Guide* (Chicago: American Dietetic Association, 1986).

16. E.M. Zallen, Dietitians' Participation in Nutrition Education Activities for the Public, *Journal of the American Dietetic Association* 90 (1990): 852–854.

17. M.J. Neely, Weight Management Programs Gain Profit, Image for Hospitals, *Clinical Management* 5 (April 1989): 13–16.

18. American Dietetic Association, Nutrition: Essential Component of Medical Education, *Journal of the American Dietetic Association* 87 (1987): 642–647. American Dietetic Association, Nutrition Education of Health Professionals, *Journal of the American Dietetic Association* 91 (1991): 611–613.

19. W.J. Rinke and M.W. Berry, Integrating Research into Clinical Practice: A Model and Call for Action, *Journal of the American Dietetic Association* 87 (1987): 159–161.

20. E. Faulkner, Institutional Operators Get Entrepreneurial Itch; Stretched Limits Strain Relations with Neighbors, *Restaurants and Institutions,* January 21, 1987, pp. 24–29, 36, 38.

21. K.E. Super, Hospitals Expanding Food Service Programs To Generate Added Revenue, *Modern Healthcare,* August 14, 1987, p. 56.

22. P.M. McMurray, Cost Savings through Nutrition Intervention: Implementing a System for Analysis, *Clinical Management* 5, no. 9 (1989): 32–35.

23. J.J. Reilly et al., Economic Impact of Malnutrition: A Model System for Hospitalized Patients, *Journal of Parenteral Enteral Nutrition* 12 (1988): 371–376.

24. K.G. Coats et al., Hospital-Associated Malnutrition: A Re-evaluation 12 Years Later, *Journal of the American Dietetic Association* 93 (1993): 27–33.

25. M. Smith, Dietitians Deliver Results with Fee-for-Nutrition Services, *Clinical Management* 4, no. 10 (1988): 33–36.

26. S.C. Yates et al., Competencies of Foodservice Directors/Managers Required in Health Care Operations, *Journal of the American Dietetic Association* 87 (1987): 1636–1643.

27. J. Sneed and C. Herman, Influence of Job Characteristics and Organizational Commitment on Job Satisfaction of Hospital Foodservice Employees, *Journal of the American Dietetic Association* 90 (1990): 1072–1076.

28. J.C. Rose, Containing the Labor Costs of Food Service, *Hospitals,* March 16, 1980, pp. 93–98.

29. S. Calvert et al., Clinical Dietetics: Forces Shaping Its Future, *Journal of the American Dietetic Association* 80 (1982): 350–354.

30. S. DeHoog, Identifying Patients at Nutritional Risk and Determining Clinical Productivity: Essentials for an Effective Nutrition Program, *Journal of the American Dietetic Association* 85 (1985): 1620–1622.

31. A.S. Ryan et al., The Role of the Clinical Dietitian, Part 2, Staffing Patterns and Job Functions, *Journal of the American Dietetic Association* (1988): 679–683.

32. K.W. McClusky et al., Nutrition Priority System: A Model for Patient Care, *Journal of the American Dietetic Association* 87 (1987): 200–203.

33. M.C. Spears, *Foodservice organizations: A Managerial and Systems Approach* (New York: Macmillan, 1990).

34. J. Renner-McCaffrey and A.H. Leyshon, *Quality Assurance in Hospital Nutrition Services* (Gaithersburg, Md.: Aspen Publishers, 1989). See also M.R. Schiller et al., *Total Quality Management for Hospital Nutrition Services* (Gaithersburg, Md.: Aspen Publishers, 1993).

35. D.D. Treadwell and J.A. Pfennig-Klein, Quality Circles in a Department of Dietetics, *Journal of the American Dietetic Association* 84 (1984): 682–684.

36. American Hospital Association, American Society for Hospital Food Service Administrators, *Hospital Food Service Management Review* (Chicago: American Hospital Association, 1988).

37. M.R. Schiller et al., *Handbook on Managing Clinical Nutrition Services* (Gaithersburg Md.: Aspen Publishers, 1991).

38. D.B. Molis, Innovations in Food Service, *Provider* 19 (April 1993): 19–28.

39. American Dietetic Association, *The Competitive Edge: Marketing Strategies for the Registered Dietitian* (Chicago: American Dietetic Association, 1986). See also S.C. Parks and D.L. Moody, A Marketing Model: Applications for Di-

etetic Professionals, *Journal of the American Dietetic Association* 86 (1986): 37–43.

40. C.W. Shanklin, Solid Waste Management: How Will You Respond to the Challenge? *Journal of the American Dietetic Association* 91 (1991): 663–664.

41. P. King and M. Pennacchia, The High Cost of Garbage Wars: Foodservice Fight for the 90's, *Food Management* 25, no. 1 (1990): 96–106, 110–115.

42. *Business Success in Dietetics: Generating Revenue and Saving Costs* (Columbus, Ohio: Ross Laboratories, 1990).

43. American Dietetic Association, Consultant Dietitians in Health Care Facilities, *The Consultant Dietitian: How To Consult—A Guide to Success* (Chicago: Consultant Dietitians in Health Care Facilities, 1988).

44. Wendy's Opens in Dayton Hospital, *Food Management* 20, no. 8 (1985): 29–30.

45. Rose, Containing the Labor Costs of Food Service.

46. D.M. Brown and L.W. Hoover, Total Factor Productivity Modeling in Hospital Foodservice Operations, *Journal of the American Dietetic Association* 91 (1991): 1088–1092.

47. M.K. Meyer, Productivity of the Clinical Dietitian: Measurement by a Regression Model, *Journal of the American Dietetic Association* 89 (1989): 490–493.

48. R.P. Puckett et al., Management Engineering Principles Applied to Foodservice Operation, *Journal of the American Dietetic Association* 87 (1987): 770–774.

49. E.K. Brendel et al., Strategies for Increasing Productivity, *Journal of the American Dietetic Association* 85 (1985): 966–969.

50. K.M. Duffy et al., A Computer-assisted Management Information System for Nutrition Services, *Journal of the American Dietetic Association* 89 (1989): 1296–1300.

51. D. Soergel et al., A Network Model for Improving Access to Food and Nutrition Data, *Journal of the American Dietetic Association* 92 (1992): 78–82.

52. J.L. Miller, Survey of Computer Technology in Foodservice Management Education, *Journal of the American Dietetic Association* 89 (1989): 1279–1281.

53. R.A. Dowling et al., Credentials and Skills Required for Hospital Food and Nutrition Department Directors, *Journal of the American Dietetic Association* 90 (1990): 1535–1540.

54. M.L. Bogel et al., Achieving Excellence in Dietetics Practice: Certification of Specialists and Advanced-Level Practitioners, *Journal of the American Dietetic Association* 93 (1993): 149–150.

Robert Douglass

Facilities Planning and Construction

22

Purpose: The purpose of facilities planning and construction is to define, plan, design, construct, and evaluate facilities that meet the programmatic needs of the health care organization, finish on time and within budget, and are financially feasible and operate efficiently. The necessity of bringing existing facilities into compliance with the Americans with Disabilities Act of 1990 will, by itself, guarantee years of facility evaluation and retro-fitting work for designers and contractors. Adapting existing facilities to changing priorities of health care access and to re-engineered patterns of patient service will likely dominate health facility construction in the coming decade.

INTRODUCTION*

The physical plant either facilitates or limits an organization's objectives. It imposes constraints on

*This section is adapted from Robert Douglass, Planning, Design and Building for Health Facilities, *Journal of Health Administration Education*, Vol. 6, No. 4, pp. 665–674, with permission of the Association of University Programs in Health Administration, © 1988.

movement and mandates many aspects of personnel utilization; equipment acquisition, use, and maintenance; technological innovation; and building maintenance. Therefore, the process of planning and design presents an important opportunity to shape the life of the organization for years.

A Sequential Process

Building development is a sequential process. Just as a building must rise from firm foundations, project planning and design must build upon clear and conscious commitments of the health care institution. Each step in the development process should provide a secure base for the next necessary step. The steps are facility master planning, functional and space programming, design, construction documentation, contracting and construction, commissioning and startup, and postoccupancy evaluation.

Although it is convenient to illustrate the building development process in a linear fashion, in practice the process involves many simultaneous, overlapping, and interactive activities. Intentional redundancy helps cope with complexity and seemingly infinite detail. The "final step" in the sequence, postoccupancy evaluation, really just starts a new cycle—the cycle of renewal necessary to protect and enhance the value of the project. Each subsequent project benefits from the accumulated experience, knowledge, and data.

Surviving Excellence

The chief executive's visible commitment to leadership is a hallmark of excellence in the management of projects. Such qualities as vision and leadership are difficult to define or describe, but building projects manifest their effects in tangible and highly visible ways. Executive leadership should create a working climate that fosters creativity and quality.

Achieving success requires avoiding failure, but achieving excellence entails risk. Psychologist Abraham Maslow used a pyramid to illustrate his suggested hierarchy of human goals. He placed survival needs at the lowest level and "actualization"—achievement that reaches beyond the limits of individual needs or appetites in order to benefit society—at the highest level. Similarly, in facility project development, there is a choice to be made between merely surviving and attaining excellence.

Buildings and built environments that reach beyond their functional tasks to empower their users and enrich their communities do not cost more dollars. They do, however, require a greater commitment from executive leadership. This leadership can provide the entire project team with the license and encouragement to reach beyond the normal limits of effort and imagination.

MANAGEMENT PRINCIPLES*

The following are management principles for executives who seek to attain excellence while improving their chances of success:

- Get personally involved. If things really go wrong, it will be your responsibility anyway.

Through involvement, you will be in a position to act decisively.
- Make sure your institution has a strategy for development before you start a project.
- Have complete and current information on the facility's utilization and productivity.
- Select design team members who are proven professionals. Look for proof of quality, as well as competence and experience, and for good chemistry.
- Delegate fully, but be aware of the key success factors. Computer printouts and spreadsheets often obscure individual responsibilities. Set up a feedback system that provides you with evidence of your team's personal engagement.
- Require a formal management framework for the project. The team needs to know clearly who is in charge of what and when it will occur. Users particularly need to know the authority structure of a project and the allocation of resources.
- Practice "creative clienting." Train yourself to think through rather than at the proposals of your design team. Try to think ". . . and if . . ., then . . ." more often than "Yes, but. . . ."
- Be a team builder with regard to your own staff as well as your consultants. Communicate your expectations and your appreciation of their best efforts. Encourage them to work hard for the pleasure of doing well rather than from fear of falling short.
- Be a role model and show enthusiasm and pride in the work of your team (both insiders and outsiders).
- Be a visible leader—but remember, you can accomplish more if you do not care who gets the credit.

---

*This section is adapted from Robert Douglass, Planning, Design and Building for Health Facilities, *Journal of Health Administration Education,* Vol. 6, No. 4, pp. 665–674, with permission of the Association of University Programs in Health Administration, © 1988.

THE ROLE OF MANAGEMENT*

In a health care executive's career, the project having the greatest financial risk will probably be a new building, but many administrators enter practice with only a superficial exposure to physical plant development. Some are fortunate enough to have gained prior experience in organizations that had building projects. Many, however, will arrive in senior management positions without any direct experience in facility development and no academic exposure to the process. Construction programs of some scale are a constant in most hospitals, with major projects typically occurring at less than ten-year intervals. This chapter identifies and explains the knowledge and skills administrators require for successful direction of facilities development. Three principles are key:

1. In order to manage the process of facility development, it is essential to understand what it is and how it works.
2. The complexity of the undertaking cannot be denied, but the process can be organized and controlled.
3. Failures occur when details overwhelm; it is important to focus on what really matters and to encourage simplicity.

Ten Key Success Factors

Strategic thinking and judicious application of both incentives and controls are keys to executive success in any venture. Administrators need to concentrate management resources on the following key factors in facility development.

Project Organization. Organize the project so it works for you, not you for it. This requires effective

---

*This section is adapted from Robert Douglass, Planning, Design and Building for Health Facilities, *Journal of Health Administration Education,* Vol. 6, No. 4, pp. 665–674, with permission of the Association of University Programs in Health Administration.

formal delegation and a clearly delineated decision process. For example, make your administrative team clearly responsible for defending the budget, controlling project costs, and securing user acceptance in their own departments. Do not allow yourself to become the arbiter of every debate over square feet.

The Project Team. The project team should mirror the organization of the institution. To act effectively, each member must have the benefit of appropriate authority.

Service Volume. Tie space and equipment needs directly to objective projections of service volumes. For example, a straightforward equation using volume and mix of patients for surgery can balance the numbers of operating rooms, recovery beds, surgical ICU beds, and general surgical beds.

Practices and Policies. Examine operational practices and policies to see if brick-and-mortar solutions are really necessary.

User Involvement. Give users a significant part in the process. Even if there were standard solutions to complex problems, your users would want to believe that their facility proposal is the best achievable.

People and Staffing. People and their activities create space needs. Staffing is a key check and balance to control space requests. For example, when radiology shocks you with requested space, look at the staffing instead of arguing about square feet. See if you really intend to have all those technicians and managers in your operating budget.

Space, Equipment, and Furnishings. Do not allow space to become equated with empire or esteem. For example, make use of standard square footage allocations for "generic" rooms in order to depersonalize and defuse potentially emotional issues such as office size.

Cash Flow Requirements. Do not just ask, "Can we afford to build it?" A financial model of a project may show a profit but require such large cash flows unrelated to income (e.g., interest and principal payments on debt) that the institution loses needed financial flexibility.

Operational Consequences. Model the operational consequences of any major capital project in both financial and nonfinancial terms and in relation to your institution's other operations. Test the model for sensitivity to variable factors. Develop contingency plans. For example, a new free-standing surgery center may attract new business, but how will it affect volumes and revenues in the main operating room? In the surgical intensive care unit? How will it affect surgical patient days? What about the feelings of the surgeons who may need to work in two locations?

Timing and Scheduling. Time is money, and a sense of urgency can help the decision process. Seek a demanding but achievable schedule. The feasibility of the project may hinge on getting to the market before competitors.

The Planning Framework

For more than a decade we have heard that hospital beds are oversupplied and health care costs out of control. Contraction rather than construction seems to be indicated. Health care construction, however, has increased during this time at an average rate of roughly 15 percent annually. Competitive pressures and market demand for more convenient and responsive health care require hospitals to build in order to survive in a shrinking market. One may be tempted to say, "Programs, not facilities, really matter." But buildings shape and limit activities and often must be adapted to the needs of new or evolving programs. Change is constant; construction and reconfiguration are always occurring in a responsive health care organization.

Health care construction grew steadily during the real estate crash of the late 1980s and peaked in 1990. It declined in 1991 and 1992 despite modest signs of recovery in the national economy. This may reflect the uncertainty of the 1992 presidential election campaign and subsequent promise of

health care reform by the Clinton administration. Figure 22-1 illustrates the annual volumes of health care construction reported for the years 1984 through 1992 by *Modern Healthcare Magazine.*[1] It seems likely that any comprehensive national health care reform will require adapting and redistributing facility resources–a process that could accelerate construction activity in both existing and new facilities.

Although the number of U.S. hospitals (currently over 6,000) is predicted to decline by one-third by the year 2000, the *Modern Healthcare* survey for 1991 reported 8,000 significant health care construction projects, 6,100 of which were hospital based. Given this persistent level of activity year in, year out, it is safe to say most health care administrators will have a construction project on their desks most of the time.

The construction projects reported in the *Modern Healthcare* surveys have included hospitals, ambulatory care centers, medical office buildings, and various specialty facilities. The overwhelming majority, however, are hospital based, and in recent years the trend has been toward facilities housing ambulatory services. Other types of projects falling to health care executives include research labs, parking structures, power plants, dormitories, elder-care centers, and other residential facilities.

Every change in hospital market, service mix, function, or technology affects facilities. The problem of obsolescence intensifies in today's environment of rapid change. Attractive facilities provide a competitive edge in attracting patients and medical staff. Every CEO is responsible for protecting a huge investment in physical plant and equipment.

In the 1980s, facility planning emphasized provider conveniences over customer preference. We listened more to ourselves than to our customers. We listened to our competitors and tried to "keep up with the Joneses" by means of facility expansions and ever bolder redecorating schemes.

The industry and the markets are changing. We must also change to achieve better competitive market position through new types and designs of facilities—facilities that are cheaper to build and operate

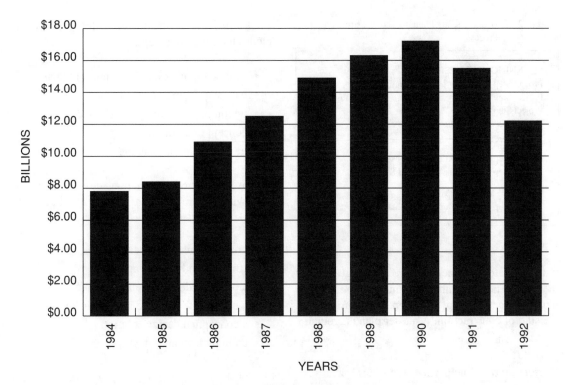

Figure 22-1 Health Care Construction (dollar value as reported by survey respondents). *Source:* Data from *Modern Healthcare Magazine,* annual, *Design and Construction Surveys,* 1984 through 1992, Crain Communications, Inc.

and are more appealing to customers. And as part of this whole process of change, we must adapt our approach to facilities planning and development.

Administrators are seldom called upon to create a hospital from scratch. In this era of health care reassessment and reform, they will be required to use existing space more efficiently, to remodel to enhance their hospital's image, or to build new facilities to house spinoff services. The trend has been toward systematic planning built upon comprehensive market research and the construction of facilities designed to improve cost-effectiveness.

The following three main sections present a seven-step model of the planning and construction process for a health facility project. Exhibit 22-1 contains an outline of the process.

PLANNING AND DESIGN

The initial phases of a construction project, planning and programming, establish the size, scope, budget, and basic structure of the project. Decisions made during this period are very important. Not only do these decisions affect every subsequent phase, but changes made later will alter project cost and completion time. In the health care environment, both of these issues are extremely important.

Every major project should include a market analysis; utilization studies of the service to be provided; an assessment of how the project relates to the institution's strategic plan; selection of the internal team; determination of essential support services and manpower requirements; involvement

Exhibit 22-1 Health Facility Planning and Construction Process

PLANNING AND DESIGN
Project Step 1: Facility Master Planning
Project Step 2: Functional and Space Programming
Project Step 3: Design
Project Step 4: Construction Documentation

CONSTRUCTION
Project Step 5: Contracting and Construction
Project Step 6: Commissioning and Startup

QUALITY MANAGEMENT
Project Step 7: Postoccupancy Evaluation

with regulatory agencies; and financing arrangements. It is not uncommon for one or more years to lapse between conceptualization of the project and the start of construction. A master plan is crucial.

Project Step 1: Facility Master Planning

*Development Process**

Master plan development must blend effective process management and creative product development to be successful. It requires a structured yet sensitive and responsive approach to selecting the players and establishing the framework of the process. This blend of process and product results in planning that will have the greatest opportunity for acceptance and implementation.

Characteristics of Master Planning. Master plan development is not a linear process. We must be willing to recycle the input of many participants in order to create a continuum of re-evaluation, process modification, and product modification.

---

*This section is adapted from David Ginsberg, Master Plan Development, *Journal of Health Administration Education,* Vol. 6, No. 4, pp. 723–732, with permission of the Association of University Programs in Health Administration, © 1988.

The *process* of master plan development includes the following steps:

- evaluation of external and internal factors
- data acquisition and analysis
- option or opportunity development
- concept or solution testing
- implementation planning

The *product* of master plan development will vary widely from setting to setting, but it generally includes

- goal and mission statements
- strategic and marketing plans
- a program development narrative
- a master site plan and a relationship plan
- a conceptual design solution
- an implementation plan

The Master Planning Organization. Asking people to participate in a process that competes with their daily responsibilities and looks creatively at the future is very difficult. Therefore, it is wise to precede or parallel master planning with a temporary set of actions intended to meet the highest priority needs. By demonstrating the tangible result of initial improvement, the subsequent master planning process is given credibility as a tool for response and change.

Balance must be maintained; people must not feel they have to get "all they can get" in this process. Priority and long-range needs should not be attempted simultaneously—the demands on time and attention will be too great. Ideally, as a result of this preliminary phase, the master plan development process can be carried out in a responsive environment.

Essential components of the master planning process are the *structure* and the *schedule.* The structure determines the manner in which the players are brought together in a series of regular and special events. The schedule provides a framework for these events and the discipline to sustain the process. Busy people appreciate a set of dates established well ahead of time and adhered to as closely as possible.

A key step in master plan development is the selection of *internal* and *external players*. No matter how talented any one individual may be, a group setting is essential. Be sure to include participants who are part of the institutional decision-making process and have special knowledge and/or creativity.

The best approach for involving internal players is to create a master planning or long-range planning committee. It should include the key individuals responsible for the principal elements of the institution, including its clinical, academic, administrative, and operational components.

The number of regular members of the committee will vary, depending upon the nature, structure, and complexity of the institution. A group of approximately 20 is ideal, 30 is possible, 10 is likely too few. If the executive committee meets frequently to make decisions, the master planning committee can afford to be somewhat larger.

The number of outside players, such as consultants and architects, also varies with the nature, structure, and capabilities of the institution. The number will increase as the process moves from concept to implementation.

Leadership of the master planning committee must make sense given the structure of the organization. For example, it is usually desirable for the CEO to chair the committee. It is possible to delegate the chair to the chief operating officer, but such delegation should not preclude the CEO's participation, nor should it be interpreted as an indication that the master planning effort is not of the highest priority.

It is important to set an appropriate series of guideposts to determine just how far to take the master plan process. In broad terms, the planning effort should concentrate on the principles of "what to do and why to do it." The specifics of exactly how to do it should be left to those directly responsible for management and operations. The master plan should define concepts and parameters but not contain detailed conclusions.

Developing the Master Plan. The first step is to establish the structure by determining leadership, selecting inside and outside players, and setting the schedule. It is important to have sufficient funds to accomplish the necessary tasks, but preconceptions regarding the costs of plan implementation should be avoided. Developing resources should be a part of the planning effort and not an initial constraint upon it.

External Factors. A series of factors external to the institution will shape the master planning process and its ultimate product. The following are examples of external factors:

- location
- transportation
- quality of life
- population demographics
- ethnic and sociocultural environment
- politics (local, state, federal, and institutional)
- regulations and reimbursement policies
- consumerism
- physician supply and practice patterns
- health professionals and labor availability
- institutional competition
- multi-institutional systems
- for-profit enterprises
- bed supply and average stay
- alternative delivery modes
- community needs

Internal Factors. Internal factors can bring the planning process into focus, providing guidance for organizing the subject-oriented subcommittees or task forces. The following are examples of internally generated factors to be considered:

- affiliations and interactions with other institutions
- clinical program development
- educational programs

- facility resources (financial and human)
- marketing
- physician development
- research development and application

Master plan development in the increasingly complex health industry is a demanding process and shows every indication of becoming still more rigorous. The new directions that can be seen in the external environment, as well as the new opportunities offered by the tools and techniques for planning, ensure the existence of this trend.

Accordingly, it is important to set realistic expectations for management of the process. In broad terms, the role of the "planning process manager" is becoming more complex. The planning process manager is increasingly a planning generalist who is able to help structure the approach and assist in selecting the individual specialists who will be responsible for the detailed work.

Reduce Risk, Improve Results . . . Combine Planning for Facilities and Finance*

Once planning has begun, administrators and the board (especially the planning and finance committees) can balance facility and financial aspects of a construction project by planning for each concurrently. This process starts with formal strategic plans. Facility and capital plans can then be advanced interactively, maintaining flexibility to ensure that the institution's objectives are met within manageable financial limits. The project thus planned will be the most effective and efficient project possible within defined constraints and will be ready for immediate implementation.

The need for a new, more adaptable planning process for hospital capital expenditures has been growing in the United States since the federal government changed its method of payment for hospital services in 1983. New reimbursement methodologies will continue to emphasize cost reductions in support of competitive pricing policies. Reimbursement of hospitals' capital costs may be severely limited.

The purpose of a facility master plan is to determine the most practical and effective use for the institution's physical resources while preserving future options. Anticipating implementation (i.e., building design and construction), the master plan includes schedules, phasing plans, and recommended budgets. Unfortunately, however, facility master plans often stop dead at the final report. Frequently, the cost of a recommended project is found to greatly exceed the institution's financial capabilities, and fallback options have not been thought through.

How a project may be affected by inflation, the cost of money (e.g., bond underwriting fees and interest on borrowings), cash flow requirements, and changes in revenues and expenses is often evaluated only after lofty building expectations have been generated. Dismay and disappointment are frequent consequences. In addition to costing dollars, these false starts result in lost opportunities and disillusioned users.

Planning is a continuous management activity. Consequently, effective planning models must be adaptable to constant change and provide for decisions based on incomplete, approximate, or evolving information. Figure 22-2 shows some of the forces affecting the planning continuum. It also shows that facility and capital considerations are interactive, not sequential, and are influenced by forces outside and inside the institution. Figures 22-3 and 22-4 compare the traditional sequential approach and the proposed concurrent and interactive approach to facility and capital planning.

The Team. Interactive facility-financial planning may be performed by in-house staff, outside consultants, or a combination. The facility planning team may consist of health care consultants, architects, engineers, and construction managers. The fi-

---

*This section is adapted from Robert Douglass and Scott Hoffman, Merging Facility and Financial Planning: A New Approach, *Journal of Health Administration Education*, Vol. 6, No. 4, pp. 703–715, with permission of the Association of University Programs in Health Administration, © 1988.

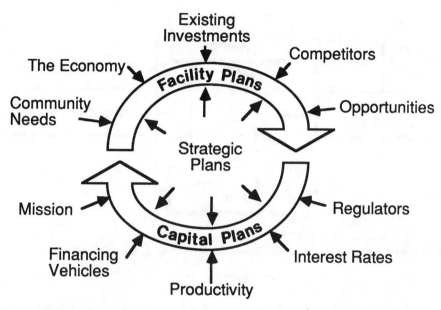

Figure 22-2 Forces Affecting the Facility Planning Process. *Source:* Reprinted from *Journal of Health Administration Education,* Vol. 6, No. 4, p. 706, with permission of the Association of University Programs in Health Administration, © 1988.

nancial planning team may include the hospital's finance group, financial consultants, investment bankers, legal counsel, and, increasingly, real estate development professionals.

Getting Started. One of the most difficult aspects of health care facility planning is getting started. The architect asks the CEO, "How much can we spend?" The CEO looks questioningly at the CFO, who shrugs and counters, "You tell me what you want to build, then I'll tell you if we can afford it."

The CEO senses that the real question is, "How much should we spend . . . over what time frame . . . and for what results?"

It makes sense to start the facility master planning process with the owner's wish list. This list typically includes more projects than the hospital can afford. Among planning professionals, the term *wish list* has come to suggest a set of extravagant and unrealistic ideas. In fact, the perceptions of owners and users are the only logical place to begin—they should not be lightly dismissed.

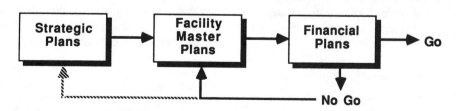

Figure 22-3 The Traditional Project Master Planning Process. *Source:* Reprinted from *Journal of Health Administration Education,* Vol. 6, No. 4, p. 704, with permission of the Association of University Programs in Health Administration, © 1988.

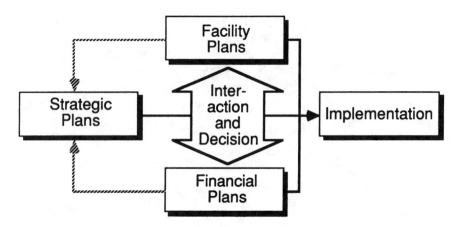

Figure 22-4 The Proposed Facility/Capital Master Planning Model. *Source:* Reprinted from *Journal of Health Administration Education,* Vol. 6, No. 4, p. 704, with permission of the Association of University Programs in Health Administration, © 1988.

The purpose of responsible planning is to objectively research and refine the wish list, balancing wants, needs, and resources. Developing facility and financial criteria simultaneously and interactively achieves this essential balance. Each perspective tempers the other, and issues of need and financial capability are reconciled.

The Facility and Capital Master Plan Model

Figure 22-5 displays the "two-track" facility and capital planning process in five phases. Facility and financial findings of each phase are integrated into interim reports so "go/no go" decisions are possible. The depth and detail of analysis in each phase increase as the process advances and approaches larger dollar commitments. Board planning and finance committees have clear milestones and explicit evidence on which to base their judgments.

Project Step 2: Functional and Space Programming*

Programming is the process of developing a statement of the requirements for a facility—the "pro-gram." Programs may be functional, describing the "what, who, how many" parameters of an individual space, a department, or a large group of spaces. They may also be physical, describing the need for space and equipment in terms of size, proximity (adjacencies), and quality in order to optimize the relationship between function and facility.

Typically, programs are developed by specialized consultants or architects, although they may be developed by qualified in-house health care managers and staff. Whether it makes sense to employ out-of-house consultants or architects depends on the time frame and the availability of skilled executives. The key is to begin the programming process as early as possible in the development of a facility project. Programming should be done before the commencement of feasibility studies and architectural planning and design.

A functional program must precede the development of a space program (see Figure 22-6). First, the programmers must identify and select the spe-

---

*This section is based on Merlin Lickhalter, How To Be a Good Consumer (Both Buyer and Manager) of Programming Services, *Journal of Health Administration Education,* Vol. 6, No. 4, pp. 741–749, with permission of the Association of University Programs in Health Administration, © 1988.

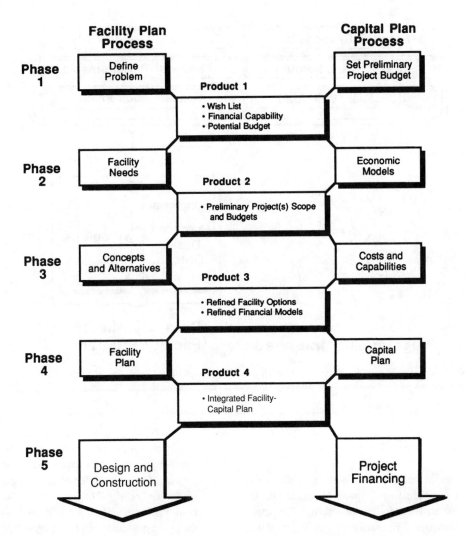

Figure 22-5 Combining Facility and Capital Planning for More Controlled and Efficient Results. *Source:* Reprinted from *Journal of Health Administration Education,* Vol. 6, No. 4, p. 707, with permission of the Association of University Programs in Health Administration, © 1988.

cific individuals within the institution who will provide input. It is important that these individuals adopt a global outlook when answering the "what, who, how many" questions.

In today's market-oriented environment, it may be difficult to make quantitative projections about future market shares of new product lines; an outside consultant may offer helpful guidance in this regard. In addition, consultants can often provide creative approaches to functional and organizational issues that influence space requirements (e.g., sharing waiting areas and clerical functions).

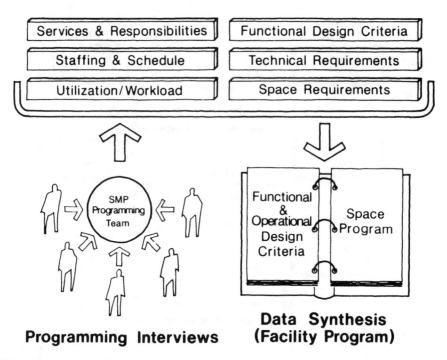

Figure 22-6 Development of a Facility Program. *Source:* Reprinted from *Journal of Health Administration Education,* Vol. 6, No. 4, p. 742, with permission of the Association of University Programs in Health Administration, © 1988.

How Is Programming Done?

There should be a smooth transition from the functional program to the space program (sometimes called an architectural program). The space program provides a quantitative statement of the following parameters:

- Quantity of space (by room) needed for each function (usually expressed in square feet, with any minimum required dimension noted). Since many individuals have difficulty understanding abstract concepts of space, there is often no substitute for defining space quantities, together with associated major equipment, in easily understood graphic terms (see Exhibit 22-2).
- Relationships of spaces to one another are defined. Depending upon the level of detail de-

sired, these may be relationships between departments or between rooms. They are usually expressed using such terms as "immediately adjacent" or "nearby." Often for ease of computerization, numerical equivalents are assigned to the desired adjacencies (see Figure 22-7).

- Major floor space–consuming equipment is identified (on a room-by-room basis). This often helps future users visualize and understand difficult abstract space concepts.
- Desired qualities or characteristics of environments are identified (e.g., "high tech" or "high touch").

It is best to avoid rules of thumb, published guidelines, and other prescriptive approaches when developing space programs. The emphasis should be on an approach that encompasses workload analyses and personnel/occupancy and scheduling analyses.

Exhibit 22-2 Sample Departmental Space Program: Acute Care Nursing Unit

Room Space	Qty	Unit Area	Net Area	Comments
12-BED CLUSTER NO. 1				
Private room	4	200	800	w/lav, toilet, shower
Semiprivate room	4	270	1,080	w/lav, toilet, shower
Support				
Nurse station	1	160	160	Includes unit clerk
Medication alcove	1	20	20	w/unit dose cart, casework, & sink
Doctors charting/dictation	2	30	60	
Clean supplies/linen	1	120	120	
12-BED CLUSTER NO. 2				
Private room	4	200	800	w/lav, toilet, shower
Semiprivate room	4	270	1,080	w/lav, toilet, shower
Support				
Nurse station	1	120	120	
Medications	1	20	20	w/unit dose cart & refrigerator
Doctors charting/dictation	2	30	60	
Clean supplies/linen	1	120	120	
SHARED SUPPORT (for 24 beds)				
Head nurse	1	100	100	
Social worker	1	100	100	
Crash cart	1	20	20	
Nourishments	1	80	80	w/refrigerator and ice machine
Equipment storage	1	200	200	
Soiled utility	1	120	120	w/trash compactor and linen chute
Staff locker lounge	1	200	200	
Staff toilet	1	30	30	
Stretcher/wheelchair alcove	1	60	60	
Patient tub/shower	1	80	80	Wheelchair and gurney access
Janitor closet	1	40	40	
Conference/teaching	—	—	—	Shared, see Dept. 213
TOTAL NET SQUARE FEET			5,470	NSF
NET TO GROSS CONVERSION FACTOR			1.5	
TOTAL GROSS SQUARE FEET			8,205	DGSF

Source: Reprinted from *Journal of Health Administration Education,* Vol. 6, no. 4, p. 744, with permission of the Association of University Programs in Health Administration, © 1988.

Documentation of the decision-making trail is essential. It is usually not sufficient to provide the functional and space program without accompanying material, perhaps including records of the programming discussions (e.g., assumptions, criteria, rationale, and special circumstances) that support the program. In the absence of this support, it is all too easy to "shoot down" elements of the program or, worse, eliminate certain elements during the design phase (typically, to reduce project costs) without a total understanding of the programmatic and operational consequences.

How Is the Process Managed?

The institution's corporate culture can have an impact on even the most rigorous analytic approach; this should not be overlooked by programmers. The key

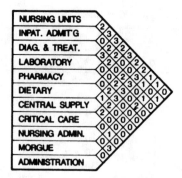

External Relationships (Adjacency Matrix)

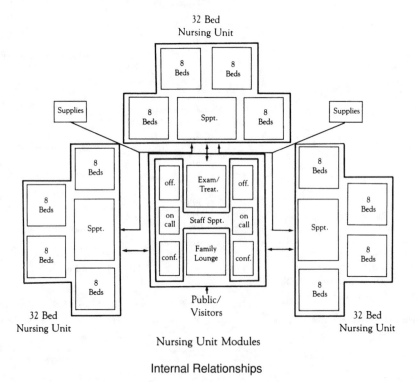

Internal Relationships

Figure 22-7 Departmental Functional Relationships. *Source:* Reprinted from *Journal of Health Administration Education,* Vol. 6, No. 4, p. 745, with permission of the Association of University Programs in Health Administration, © 1988.

to successfully employing analytic programming techniques is to use care in selecting the in-house individuals with whom the consultant or architect will be working. For example, consider programming for a proposed new ambulatory care center. Who are the key individuals the administrator wants on the programming team? What specific roles are envisioned? Will they acknowledge the authority of others on the team if the hierarchy of authority differs from the institution's normal organizational hierarchy? Exhibit 22-3 presents one model for dividing up programming roles among team members.

The programming process must be managed at a high level. Since a good program is a prerequisite for constructing a functional building, managing the programming must have a high priority. Continuity of leadership through the entire programming phase is ideal. The individual selected to manage must allocate sufficient time and resources. Generally, this means that this individual or his or her representative should be given provisional authority to approve or disapprove programming and must participate in all programming meetings.

Moreover, this individual must act as a catalyst to stimulate discussion, must often integrate the needs of two or more functions or departments, and must mediate internal conflicts involving function and space.

The opportunities for conflict seem greater at the programming stage than at any other phase in a project's development. This is probably because programming deals with fundamental internal and external issues. It strips away the usual camouflage provided by existing facilities when it asks questions like, "What is really needed—without regard to present facility constraints?" Great care must be exercised to avoid placing the consultant in the position of having to resolve organizational issues. It is a no-win trap and will lead to frustration and undermine project team effectiveness. A former CEO of a large university medical center once likened the programmer's role to that of a "cat scratching post."

Finally, when the program is in its final form, ready for institutional (or board) approval, the indi-

Exhibit 22-3 Sample Allocation of Programming Roles

	Roles		
	Determining Workload	Determining Adjacencies	Determining Extent of Shared Space
Administrator	○	●	●
Director of Planning	○	○	●
Chief of Staff	✓	✓	✓
Head Nursing	✓	○	●
Chief of Medicine	✗	✓	✓
Chief of Surgery	✗	✓	✓
Heads of Departments	●	○	●
Senior Nurses	✗	✓	✗

○ Approval Role   ● Leadership Role   ✓ Review Role   ✗ No Role

Source: Reprinted from *Journal of Health Administration Education,* Vol. 6, No. 4, p. 747, with permission of the Association of University Programs in Health Administration, © 1988.

vidual who has managed the programming process should assist the CEO and the consultant in making the necessary presentations and recommendations.

What Will the Program Accomplish?

Well-prepared functional and space programs offer several benefits. First, the discipline of the programming process itself provides an opportunity for analysis and reflection by the users. They will have much greater insight into the complex interrelationships of function and physical space. Space will no longer be an abstract concept to users. Further, by having worked together, the users will be in a much better position to make subsequent planning and design decisions as a team.

Second, good functional and space programs enable the users to later evaluate the quality and efficacy of the architect's plans. Too often, users evaluate and critique the architect's conceptual and schematic plans ineffectively, expressing vague and sometimes conflicting objections to certain aspects, with consequent delays, extra design costs, and loss of credibility. Conversely, if the plans are critiqued using the functional and quantitative parameters in the program—number of people occupying spaces, major equipment, relationships among spaces—the evolution and refinement of the plans is expedited and there is a higher probability of success.

However, the most sophisticated, analytic, and rigorous programs will not guarantee a good architectural and engineering outcome. A highly skilled architect must make the translation from program to design under the supervision of the administration.

Project Step 3: Design*

The Design Process, or How Not To Be Afraid of Building

One of the most challenging experiences in a hospital administrator's career is the building process. At its worst, it can be divisive, alienate the hospital board, cause controversy within the institution, and wreak havoc with the budget. At its best, it can be a positive, satisfying experience that fosters improved interdepartmental relationships, yields an improved facility, increases operational efficiency, and upgrades the hospital's image.

The design phase includes three important tasks: master zoning, schematic design, and design development. For many administrators, the tools used in communication during this phase are unfamiliar. They are excited about creating something new, but they do not know how to read plans; they do not know how to be part of the process; and they do not know how to relate to this whole new team of other professionals they have hired (architects, engineers, medical equipment specialists, and interior designers), all of whom speak a different language. The institution may have developed written documents outlining a strategic plan, a capital investment plan, and functional and space programs, but "blueprints" and "specifications" represent new and potentially intimidating graphic and codified communications.

The health client has the responsibility of establishing the criteria for a proposed facility project that is difficult to visualize and purchase as a single unit. When the process changes from a set of written documents that the client can control (the program) to one where architectural sketches, technical drawings, three-dimensional models, and other unfamiliar instruments are used to create a solution, a bridge is needed. The design process that works properly becomes the bridge between words and the resulting building.

Selecting the Architect

Architecture is not like buying a car—or even a building seen elsewhere. Each site is unique, each

---

*This section is adapted from James Falick, The Design Process, or How Not To Be Afraid of Building, *Journal of Health Administration Education*, Vol. 6, No. 4, pp. 761–770, with permission of the Association of University Programs in Health Administration, © 1988.

community and set of conditions is different, and buildings can rarely be ordered out of a catalogue.

In selecting an architectural firm, the client should ideally follow the guidelines of the American Hospital Association.[2] Unless the client has a history of working with a particular firm and is satisfied with the services provided, the design team of architects, engineers, interior designers, and medical equipment specialists should be selected after several qualified firms are contacted and invited to submit proposals. After proposals are screened and firms are invited for preliminary discussions, a short list is created to narrow the field to three or four firms, from which the finalist is selected. This exposure to a number of firms enables the client to learn about a variety of people and processes and how each proposes to provide services. Good chemistry counts.

Kickoff Retreat

The first part of any design process should include a retreat—for a day or a weekend—where all of the ideas and planning that have gone before are discussed openly and in the context of the resulting program. The administrator can facilitate these discussions by his or her personal leadership.

Master Zoning

With the architectural team brought up to date on early planning, it can begin work on the master zoning plan, which integrates internal function with overall site planning. A master zoning plan provides a diagram for growth that locates functional elements and delineates their three-dimensional relationship to one another on the site, including horizontal and vertical circulation patterns for various kinds of uses and users and preferred departmental locations.

Unlike an office building, a health care facility needs to change or grow regularly. If the circulation patterns of buildings and site are set properly, a variety of elements can be connected to the diagram at future dates, and the institution knows that at each phase it will operate as a whole. The existing, plus the new, plus the future can be designed to be one.

The master zoning plan is based on a block estimate of each department's gross square footage needs. Surgery in a master plan, for example, would be represented by a 10,000 departmental square feet (DGSF) block instead of detailing four operating rooms, recovery, and all the other individual spaces indicated in the functional and space programs. When departmental blocks are located and circulation is defined, the building gross square footage is calculated more accurately, because the circulation to hold the design together is included, as well as mechanical and service spaces.

A master zoning plan is important not only to test and develop the design options for the next phase and approximate schematic design but also for a first run at estimating total project construction costs. The team has a diagram for the project or can devise a workable pullback strategy in case cost reduction is necessary and is thus able to develop a project budget to which the board can commit.

Architectural Design

The American Institute of Architects Document B-141 provides a model for the standard agreement between owner and architect.[3] This document defines and codifies the basic and additional architectural services provided by the architectural team (see Figure 22-8). Two basic services, schematic design and design development, are included in the design phase.

Schematic Design

As master zoning sets the function diagram, schematic design sets the design parameters of a project. Depending on the project's scale and complexity, the master zoning plan may be part of the schematic design documents, and a portion of the fees will be credited to the schematic design effort. If master zoning is complex, schematic design will be an additional service, usually with a guaranteed maximum fee.

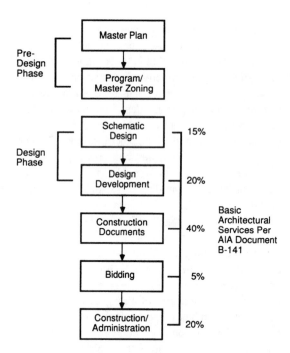

Figure 22-8 Phases of Architectural Services. *Source:* Reprinted from *Journal of Health Administration Education,* Vol. 6, No. 4, p. 765, with permission of the Association of University Programs in Health Administration, © 1988.

By contract, in the schematic design phase, the architect reviews the owner-provided program requirements and provides a preliminary architectural evaluation of program requirements, project schedule, and budget. Alternate design approaches and options are reviewed, and a project scope, budget, and schedule are agreed upon. The architect then prepares for the owner's approval a set of schematic design documents illustrating the size and relationships of the project components, drawn to a scale of ⅟₁₆" or ⅛" (i.e., one-sixteenth or one-eighth of an inch equals one foot). Schematic design represents 15 percent of the total architectural fee.

Design Development

During the second phase of basic services, design development, the approved schematic design is developed in greater detail. Drawings are usually at ⅛" or ¼" so the client can understand how the project will be described to the building contractor. The documents include architectural plans; structural, mechanical, and electrical systems drawings; and outline specifications. Selections of materials and building systems will be made as needed, and an estimate of the probable cost of construction will be delivered to the client for approval. Upon submission of the documents, an additional 20 percent of the total architectural fee is due.

Early Costing

What happens to the project if the dollars allocated for the building and the bids for the projects are not the same? This will not happen if the very first task of the design project is to use the space program to develop a sophisticated cost estimate. An estimate is possible at an early stage by making assumptions about building systems and materials. The design team must essentially develop and cost out a palette of building systems and materials that define the quality of the building: the type of heating, ventilating, and air conditioning; structural systems; landscaping; flooring; ceilings; hardware; and interior and exterior finishes.

The resulting budget should count the quantity of square feet per operational unit and include a cost estimate for equipment and furnishings. From the very beginning, and at each stage of the architectural process, probable cost assumptions must be brought up to date so that the client can know that the program and budget are in line.

Techniques and Tools To Improve Management and Communication

As architectural design continues through its various stages, a major concern for administrators is whether the process will be constructive or destructive for the institution. Good management of the process, including organization of the project team and the use of proven techniques to improve communication, can ensure quality input from all the team members, resulting in a better process and product.

Project Organization

The planning process requires an organization chart that clarifies the architect's role in the decision-making line so that the architect is not seen as making choices that properly belong to board, administration, or staff. The architect acts as staff to those groups by presenting options, instructing on the process, and providing technical advice.

Onsite Design

The best way to foster a climate of mutual respect and trust, as well as to share information, is for the administrators to encourage an interactive process that allows people to communicate easily. Onsite workshops can provide intense and fruitful exchanges between the architect and the hospital staff at intervals throughout the design process. (Such workshops are sometimes called squatters because the design team is virtually camping on the client's turf.)

Gaming

A technique called gaming is used to teach clients about physical planning. Gaming can help clients become familiar with reading blueprints and with understanding how money and design decisions relate in order to arrive at fair, functional trade-offs between their design needs and the money available to meet them.

The "game" employs a model in which each existing floor is a separate layer. The board is colored by function—blue for beds, red for diagnostic and treatment areas, and so on. Blocks of corresponding colors are cut out to represent the amount of space allocated for each department. Color-keyed tapes represent different kinds of movement—staff, patients, visitors, materials, information, and utilities.

Staff members who might have sat back if another process was used are delighted to pick up the blocks representing their space and work with the designer and other team members to find their best "zoning" or location. With existing colored areas plotted out for reference, hospital staff begin to understand how their plant is organized. They begin to feel a real sense of control over how new space can be arranged and develop a positive feeling about the design process.

Gaming gives everyone—administrators, physicians, nurses, architects, consultants—a solid basis for communication during the design phase. The architects thus become a trusted part of the team, not people with whom one communicates at a distance. There is an ease to peer review, since gaming allows everybody to pick up the "chips" and find out what the problems and opportunities are.

Computers as Communication

Computers now assist architects by providing greater visualization, suggesting economies, and detailing options for renovations and space fittings based on the program. As options are discussed, the computer makes the changes quickly and allows for immediate testing and review while saving all previous schemes. Each decision will have pluses and minuses. The computer allows the team to review all the options quickly and economically.

The computer-aided design and drafting system used by some architectural firms saves time and labor and increases quality control. It gives architects more time to review drawings and design solutions, while a machine actually draws the results and provides permanent storage and retrieval for drawings.

Finally, life cycle costing and rapid examination of alternative designs are virtually impossible without computers. An additional benefit is that telephone modems can be used to tie into outside time-sharing services of larger computer networks and commercial services and even into the hospital's computer if necessary, facilitating quick access to information.

Project Step 4: Construction Documents*

In the health facilities development process, the construction document phase follows the design

*This section is adapted from James Diaz, Construction Documents, *Journal of Health Administration Education*, Vol. 6, No. 4, pp. 771–775, with permission of the Association of University Programs in Health Administration, © 1988.

development phase and precedes the bidding and construction phases. If everything is going well, the construction document phase should proceed quickly, with less owner involvement than in previous phases. The owner, represented by the hospital administrator, has described the institution's needs during programming, participated closely in schematic design, and approved the documents for design input at the completion of design development. During the construction document phase, most of the action will be in the architect's court. It is the responsibility of the architect and the engineers to describe the project so that potential bidders will understand its parameters and submit responsive bids.

Construction Documents: The Tools for Building

Construction documents are tools for communication between builders and trades people. They are distinguished from design development phase drawings and outline specifications, which convey essentially the same information but in a language that can be understood by the owner for decision making and approvals. The construction documents consist of plans and specifications giving descriptive and technical information about the building design and materials, including how they are to be assembled.

When combined with the agreement between owner and contractor, the construction documents turn into contract documents and become legally enforceable. The contractor builds from these documents a building (or improvements) to be delivered to the owner by a specified date. The contractor is expected to subcontract for portions of work, and the subcontractors are also bound by the contract documents. Any addenda to the construction documents issued after execution of the owner-contractor agreement will also become part of the contract documents.

Owner and Architect Responsibilities: Facilitating the Construction Document Phase

Under a separate contract with the owner, the architect and his or her consultants work according to a predetermined schedule, with fees apportioned

out in percentages over the design and construction phases. Typically, 45 percent of the fee is allotted to construction documents and bidding, and 20 percent to construction administration (see Figure 22-8). The owner's specific responsibilities during the construction document phase are particularly important, since they affect the architect's ability to produce work on time and for the agreed budget. These responsibilities include reviewing and approving plans, finishes, and standards of construction in a timely manner; making decisions pertaining to the legal aspects and insurance requirements for the general, supplementary, and other "special" conditions; issuing bidding instructions; and sending information back and forth between the architect and the owner's many other agents, such as lenders, insurance brokers, and legal counsel.

A system of project management that identifies decision milestones and necessary owner input will help the construction document phase proceed smoothly. If unresolved planning and design issues exist, the design team's work during construction document preparation will suffer from needless interruptions, causing delays and perhaps additional fees. The owner bears responsibility if the architect shows that willful and unnecessary changes were made in areas previously approved by the owner, whether deliberately through a signed approval or tacitly by not commenting specifically on an issue assumed to be closed in earlier meetings.

Every effort should be made to negotiate additional fees and extensions before any additional service in question is undertaken. When a proposed change is out of sequence and countermands previous owner approvals and directions, the owner is obligated to pay any additional costs to the architect. The owner must also accept an appropriate delay in the completion of contract documents. Additionally, it is essential that the owner advise the architect of any impending change or untimely decision due to unexpected occurrences so that the project schedule and management system may be modified accordingly. When changes are anticipated, other avenues are open to minimize cost, delays, and the extent of change.

On the other hand, the architect is responsible for verbal and written communication with the owner to outline areas of general approval or uncertainty. The architect should alert the owner as to the impact of any change, including probable delays and additional fees that may be incurred. The architect should take action in any case where prompt review, responses, and decisions by the owner are not forthcoming. The intent is not to create a paper war but rather to use the management system to keep each party aware of the project's progress and anticipate stumbling blocks.

From Theory to Practice

No system is foolproof or sufficiently comprehensive. Therefore, the owner should identify a contingency allowance before project initiation. It is not uncommon for a new hospital staff member to be hired during the construction document phase and to demand changes in departmental design. Since hospital design and construction may take several years, the advent of a forceful new player is often not predicted or identified soon enough to allow his or her input to be timely or complete.

The owner and architect may mitigate the disruption by agreeing to select a special consultant to provide input on behalf of the department. Such a consultant should be on board as early as the programming and schematic design phases. The same is true for the selection of equipment, which may be postponed awaiting new technological developments or funds for purchase. An equipment consultant may be retained to review opinions and suggest alternatives. It always costs more to do it later.

Contracting for Success

Changes in the project's scope and design are inevitable during the construction document phase. They can be made smoothly if the responsibilities of the owner and architect are clear from the beginning of the project. The agreement between the owner and architect should fully and succinctly describe all responsibilities to minimize negotiations for additional fees and avoid time-consuming bickering. The pamphlet *Building Relationships: A Guide for Institutions*

on How to Work with an Architect, published by the American Institute of Architects, can help create understanding between the owner and architect.[4]

Owners should adhere as much as possible to standard forms of agreement, such as those published by the AIA, rather than attempt to prepare totally new documents. AIA contract formats have been used for decades, are recognized by the Associated General Contractors, and have been tested in court and arbitration proceedings. Nearly everyone in the construction industry accepts their nomenclature and definitions. Construction contracts are usually drafted in a form that parallels the AIA owner-architect agreements.

The hospital can allay fears that these basic contract forms favor architects by amending the documents slightly for its particular project needs. However, it is important to do so only by changing terms and conditions, preferably by adding, amending, or deleting articles on the standard AIA forms. This ensures that nothing vital to either party has been forgotten or eliminated during the process of negotiation. Nothing is more dangerous or costly to the interests of either side than a clean new contract draft invented from scratch by either party's attorney, and such a draft must be thoroughly reviewed for inadvertent deletions, omissions, and transpositions.

During contract negotiations, there is much room for inventiveness in the method of payment, description of project scope, and listing of items to be delivered by the architect. Any tendency toward changing key phrases or standard articles, however, may be detrimental to both owner and architect and should be discouraged. By straying from the general intent of the AIA documents and the recognized mutual responsibilities of each party (and of the general contractor later in construction), both the hospital and the architect may incur liabilities or responsibilities not covered by professional or owner's general liability insurance.

Enhancing the Process

If the hospital administrator recognizes the importance of a clearly understood contract and organizes the project so decisions are made in a timely fashion and costly changes are avoided, the construction document phase will be a positive experience. The architect will handle much of the work, while the administrator continues his or her invaluable role as communicator and coordinator of decision making during the health facilities development process.

CONSTRUCTION

Project Step 5: Contracting and Construction*

Despite misconceptions about the advantages of one method of contracting as compared with another, there are actually two basic approaches. The administrator must decide how much he or she can afford to spend and then endeavor to obtain the maximum benefit for that sum or must determine the mandatory needs and then attempt to meet them at the lowest reasonable cost. There are many variations on these basic approaches, but there is no magic method that results in a great bargain for the buyer.

A thousand bricks of a certain color, size, and type will cost almost the same amount to any contractor. The variation in final cost, when the bricks are built into a finished wall, results from the ability of the general contractor and subcontractor to manage the installation, finishing, and cleaning of those bricks to produce the desired results. The key is good management based on relevant experience.

Before deciding how to contract for construction, it is important to determine how the project will be managed. There is no substitute for putting individuals with demonstrated experience in charge of carrying out the project.

---

*This section is based on Thomas E. Batey, The Team Approach to Hospital Construction, *Journal of Health Administration Education,* Vol. 6, No. 4, pp. 777–784, with permission of the Association of University Programs in Health Administration, © 1988.

Methods of Contracting

There are several methods of contracting for construction, including lump sum bidding, cost plus fee (with and without a guaranteed maximum price), and construction management.

Lump Sum Bidding. Because of various legal, political, and other restrictions, lump sum bidding is probably the most frequently used method of contracting for construction. It generally requires a very complete and detailed set of bidding documents (architectural and engineering plans and specifications) so that bidders are able to clearly understand the basis for determining their cost of performing the work.

A lump sum bid for a total project is an accumulation by the general contractor of many lump sum bids for the various elements of the work, If the lower bidder is selected for each work element, each contractor, subcontractor, and material supplier is potentially in an adversarial relationship with everyone else; all the low bidders are seeking to perform their tasks at their low bid without delay or interference to make money on the project. Under this method, there can be difficulty in directing the efforts of several independent contractors and suppliers who may never have worked together and whose primary qualification for involvement is a low price.

There are ways of making the lump sum bidding process more effective. Bidders may be prequalified, with bidding limited only to those contractors and subcontractors who have demonstrated proficiency in hospital construction. It is essential to establish fair criteria and clearly state them in the bid documents.

Cost Plus Fee with Guaranteed Maximum Price. This method of contracting provides an owner with a degree of flexibility, since the project can begin before all plans are finalized and all decisions are made. The buyer of construction pays the actual cost of the various elements plus a reasonable fee to the contractor for his or her management of the work. In addition, the owner is guaranteed by the contractor that the cost will not exceed a specified amount. In effect, the owner buys "insurance" from the contractor that the project as it is initially defined will not exceed the guaranteed maximum price. Obviously the contractor, unless incompetent or willing to play games with the "costs," will not guarantee a price that is less than the estimated project cost. Therefore, the owner will eventually pay the contractor for the costs of the work, plus a fee that includes some profit, plus a "bonus" of some amount if the total is under the guaranteed maximum price.

Cost plus fee with a guaranteed maximum can be most expensive if the owner does not begin with a clearly defined plan. Changes in the project plan during construction will result in changes in the guaranteed maximum. An ill-defined project initiated under this method may not benefit at all from the original "guarantee" of cost. This method is appropriate when an owner is pushed for time and must have some handle on costs before beginning a project.

Cost Plus Fee without Guarantee. Cost plus fee without guarantee is an ideal contracting method—if all of the circumstances will permit. The owner pays exactly what the project costs plus an agreed fee for the builder—and no more or less than that. The contractor is not at risk, since all costs are covered, and the contractor's fee covers his or her overhead and profit. However, there are several mandatory elements that must exist if this method is to be used.

The critical element is mutual trust. The owner must have complete confidence in the contractor, since all costs are to be reimbursed. The contractor must be seen as an effective and efficient manager who will accurately present for payment only those charges required to complete the defined work.

A project handled by this method provides maximum flexibility. For example, the owner can speed up or slow down the project, change its scope, or make any other modifications (as long as he or she is prepared to pay the price).

In order to use this method of contracting effectively, an owner should employ an in-house project manager or engage a project management professional who can guide and facilitate the decision-making process. The absence of appropriate and timely decisions is the greatest contributor to excessive construction costs.

Construction Management. This method of contracting for construction involves just what the title implies: managing construction. In a typical arrangement, the construction manager is the owner's agent and contracts for the various components of construction in the owner's name. The management may be done by the owner's employed staff, or management services may be purchased from a broad range of professional groups. A construction manager, whether an individual or a large organization, may utilize any or all of the aforementioned contracting methods to develop a project. The key ingredient is the ability to control the project in all its aspects. Its adherents claim that what distinguishes construction management is that it is a service and that the construction manager represents the owner and acts for the owner's benefit.

The construction manager is a facilitator and decision "getter." Owners often require prompting in order to make necessary decisions. An effective construction manager must orchestrate contractors, subcontractors, suppliers, equipment vendors, and installers throughout the process if desired results are to be obtained.

Design-Build

With design-build, a single company can provide both design and construction.[5] Responsibility can be centralized, design and construction can be overlapped, and design can be improved through input from construction experts.

More projects would be design-build if it was easier to formulate an enforceable price before design. Most owners want to know what their building will cost before they hire a contractor. The paradox: It is hard to define the work to be done and arrive at an agreed price without a design, but if the design is done, then it is not design-build.

Some design-build companies work under an architectural engineering (AE) fee with a target price until the design is set. They then negotiate a final price. They agree that the owner may obtain prices from other contractors as well.

In this kind of arrangement, the design-build contractor begins in an agent role and switches to a vendor role. Although many contractors demonstrate integrity, it is potentially problematic to hire a contractor to represent your interests in defining a product that the contractor will then sell you.

There are a growing number of projects that have found a middle ground. Although the bid documentation consists of more than a simple written project definition package, it may stop short of a traditional full set of construction drawings (see below).

Bridging

Bridging is the name given to a hybrid process of project delivery that is gaining attention and advocates in the United States as this volume goes to print.[6] Bridging combines aspects of several traditional project delivery methods to "bridge" the expertise gap between architects and builders. It seeks to connect the architect's functional and aesthetic *design* solution to the builder's expertise in *construction*. Advocates of bridging say the owner wins with savings and improved building technology—better projects completed sooner and for less money. Bridging targets four problems of the traditional processes:

1. It takes too long and costs too much to deliver an enforceable fixed cost for construction. Often the budget is blown after much time and money have been spent.
2. Building technology is not adequately incorporated into design, so construction costs more than it should. There is little economic motivation for contractors to invest in R & D to improve building technology.
3. Everyone is exposed to more claims than necessary. Legal costs add to budget overruns for clients and destroy profits for architects, engineers, and contractors.

4. There is divided responsibility for the project during and after construction.

How to do it? Simply put, bridging separates the traditional design and construction process into three segments: project definition and final engineering and construction. See Figure 22-9 for a comparison of bridging and the traditional project delivery process. Project definition is carried out by the owner's designer or project manager (probably an architectural firm with planning, design, and project management skills, or a team possessing those skills) and is generally equivalent to the traditional process from planning and budgeting through completion of design development. At this point a contractor is selected (by competitive bidding, negotiation, etc.). In addition to construction, the contractor becomes responsible for production of the final architectural and engineering drawings and specifications—all subject to review by and approval of the owner and the "project definition" architect. Documents for this phase, equivalent to construction documents, are called final engineering documents.

Bridging is seen as an innovation in building construction in the United States, although similar methods are commonly used in heavy engineering projects and by many overseas contractors. Is it a fad or a trend? Will it reshape project delivery or quietly join the ranks of good ideas that did not quite make it? Time will tell, but today bridging seems worthy of serious consideration.

A Lawyer's Response: In Defense of the Conventional System

Professor Carl Sapers teaches design and construction law at Harvard University and from this vantage point has watched many innovations come and some go. He offers this perspective:

Your Board of Trustees has just authorized construction of a new facility. What they expect is commodity, durability, delight, and economy; and the greatest of these—it has been made clear to you—is economy. You have the sense and experience to

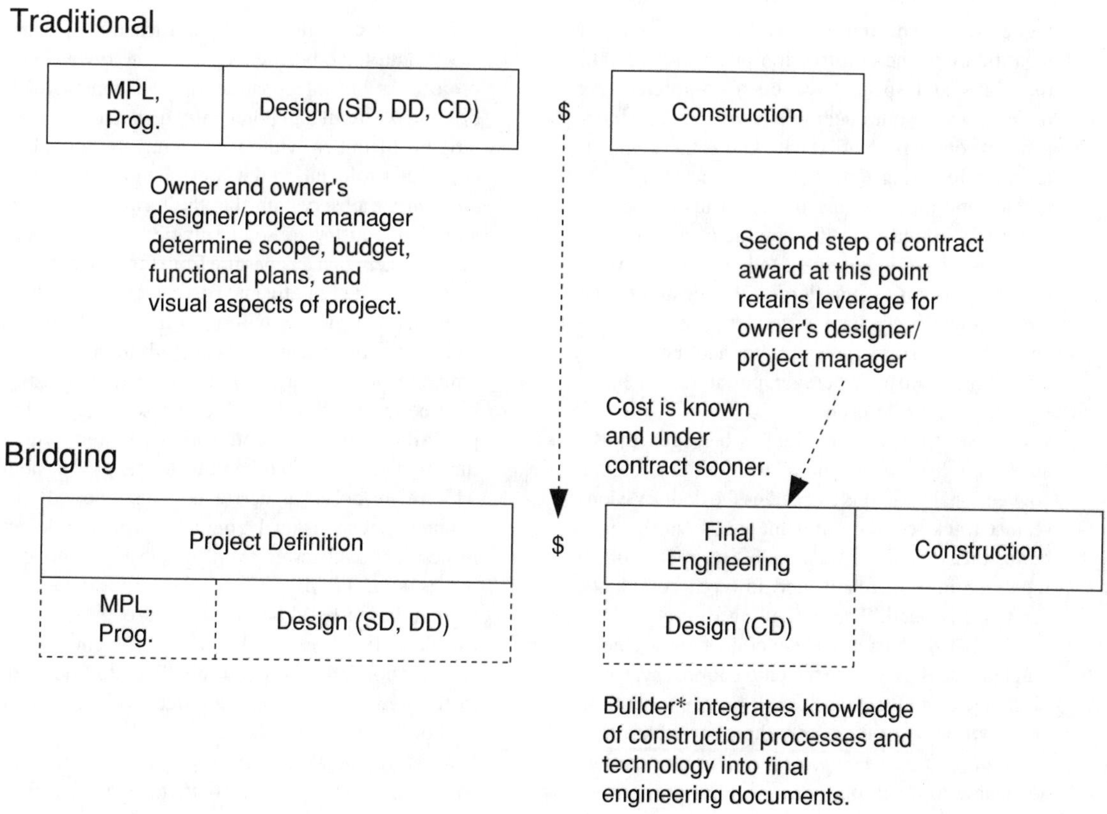

Traditional

MPL, Prog.	Design (SD, DD, CD)

$

Construction

Owner and owner's designer/project manager determine scope, budget, functional plans, and visual aspects of project.

Second step of contract award at this point retains leverage for owner's designer/ project manager

Cost is known and under contract sooner.

Bridging

Project Definition

$

Final Engineering	Construction

MPL, Prog.	Design (SD, DD)

Design (CD)

Builder* integrates knowledge of construction processes and technology into final engineering documents.

Key: MPL = Facility Master Plan
Prog = Functional and Space Programs
SD = Schematic Design
DD = Design Development
CD = Construction Documents
$ = Bidding, Negotiation of Construction Contract

*includes contractor and contractor's architects, engineers, and subcontractors

Figure 22-9 Comparison of Bridging and the Traditional Project Delivery Process

know that the highest construction bid may not produce the most expensive project. Conversely, the lowest bid may not produce the best bargain. Delays, cheap materials, shabby construction, serious disputes, unclear responsibility, unexpected extras; these hazards are seldom revealed at the time bids are received.

Wisely, you had best consider at the outset the basic form which your institution's construction will take. For a hundred years or more, the conventional form is to engage an architect/engineer, who prepares line drawings (plans) and prose descriptions of the various aspects of the building (specifications) (together referred to as "construction documents"), to solicit bids from contractors for doing what the construction documents require, and then to have the building built by the lowest bidding contractor under the watchful eye of the architect. The sequence of events implies that the contractor is not identified, nor the construction price known, until the plans and specs have been completed. As project owner, your client will have two quite independent contracts: the first with you as the architect/engineer requiring that you act as the client's inspector and agent during the construction period, while the second with the contractor admonishes him to do what the architect tells him to do. Built into the conventional system is the tension of the architect/engineer characteristically demanding a better product from the contractor and the contractor seeking to trim wherever possible to achieve greater profit for himself.

Almost at once your client is besieged by the apostles of "newfangledness" who tell him that the conventional system is as dead as the dodo. Visions of fast track, construction management, design-build, turnkey, fixed responsibility, reduction in time, certainty of result, and lowered cost dance through his head. The preceding discussion has catalogued the virtues of several of these "newfangled" ideas. But since the conventional system is disparaged on all sides, we will here extol the old gent's virtues by setting forth three principles.

There ain't no free lunch. . . . This proposition, applicable to much of a man's endeavor, has particular applicability in the construction industry. If you would have a fixed price commitment early, someone has built into that price a protective contingency factor. That is inevitably the case in the design-build or turnkey arrangement. In the conventional arrangement, the owner will calculate a contingency; but if the contingency is not used, the money remains in the owner's pocket. In the other two arrangements, the money belongs to the design-build team. Similarly, a reduction in the time it takes to construct the project inevitably bears with it the freight of additional risk on the promising party. That party, if he understands the economics of his endeavor, will include that risk cost as part of his price.

I want a girl just like the girl that married dear old Pa. . . . Much can be said for sticking with the conventional system, despite its defects, on the grounds that it has been around for a long time and the players understand it better. For example, there has yet to be published a careful contract document which separates out the respective responsibilities of an architect/engineer and a construction manager when both have been engaged by the owner on a project. As a result, construction management leads often to wasteful and potentially disputatious overlapping of duties without reducing the architect/engineer's role during the construction period. It is an accurate observation that the forms in the construction industry are so closely tied to the conventional system that a departure from the conventional system requires careful and costly legal work which many owners are not willing to finance. As if this were not enough, the courts and arbitration panels, which resolve disputes in the construction industry, may be expected to continue to resolve those disputes in terms of the conventional system which they understand rather than the newfangled system which they do not understand. Thus, one still encounters decisions analyzing a construction defect in conventional terms even though the court observes, almost in passing, that the parties in fact entered a design-build arrangement. If one is looking for clear, fixed responsibility for problems in the construction industry, one is not likely to find them in the new, innovative techniques unless a great deal of lawerying is involved.

Pending the perfection of mankind, a system of checks and balances is devoutly to be wished. . . . Owners who employ responsible and skilled architects and contractors may choose any form they wish without running any substantial risk on their construction project. The real concern is of course where one party or the other is less than adequate and is subject to the frailties which afflict mankind. The founding fathers decided that the way to deal with imperfections was to establish a constitutional system of checks and balances; the conventional system for constructing facilities is based on that same principle. The architect/engineer is not in the control of the contractor (as in the case of the design-build or turnkey arrangement) but is really the contractor's natural adversary. The architect/engineer's natural interest is durability, commodity, and delight, while the contractor's interest is economy. Each critical player, the owner, the contractor, and the architect/engineer, stands at the points of a triangle with the lines between representing lines of tension. Notwithstanding all of the problems that the construction industry has produced, and notwithstanding the fact that there are circumstances where some of the less conventional approaches may be most effective, it is the opinion of the author that this tension creates a better product than any other form or organization yet devised.[7]

Project Step 6: Commissioning and Startup*

Planning for occupancy parallels construction. The construction phase includes enforcement of contract specifications in the architect's walk-throughs and punch lists; enforcement of written warranties and guarantees of performance for all types of equipment, systems, and construction details; and time for the housekeeping staff to clean the facility to their standards. A shakedown period is recommended to test all systems in operation before moving in.

The process of commissioning the engineering systems and making the transition to occupancy begins as the construction phase is completed. There is a familiar and well-documented process for testing the plant before takeover. Essentially, commissioning is the process by which a statically complete installation is converted into an actuated, live, and integrated system that performs its functions in accordance with good engineering practice and the design intent manifested in the specifications and contract drawings.

It is helpful to look at a hospital as a set of three interactive systems (see also Figure 22-10):

1. the static system (the frame and envelope)
2. the energized system (the building services)
3. the human system (the patients and staff)

In developing a commissioning program, the hospital should conceptualize the task so that its strategy

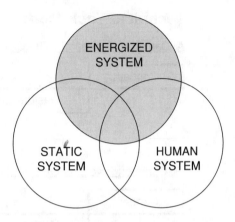

Figure 22-10 Interactive Hospital System. *Source:* Reprinted from *Journal of Health Administration Education,* Vol. 6, No. 4, p. 804, with permission of the Association of University Programs in Health Administration, © 1988.

is comprehensive, systematic, and timely. There are two acknowledged models for determining goals, time frames, components, and responsibility: the managerial process model and the technical task model. The latter model focuses specifically on the logistics involved in physically moving from the old to the new. Under this model, the time frame is short and basically spans the period from substantial completion of the facility to move day. The managerial process model is more comprehensive and longer range. This model is predicated on the idea that planning decisions are based upon knowledge of operating intentions and that the critical link between the two is the commissioning process.

In Figure 22-11, the managerial process model approach is integrated into an overall framework for planning. The figure compares the traditional and technical task models with the preferred managerial process model. The major steps in the process include these six:

1. The selection, purchase, receiving, and installation of all existing and new equipment that is not in the contract but is required for the operation of the facility.

*This section is adapted from B. Jon Jaeger and Louis E. Swanson, Facilities Planning: Opening and Activation, and from Iain F. Clayre and J. Gordon Pincock, Commissioning, *Journal of Health Services Administration Education,* Vol. 6, No. 4, pp. 795–818, with permission of the Association of University Programs in Health Administration, © 1988.

Technical Task Model

A. Common Illustration - Theory

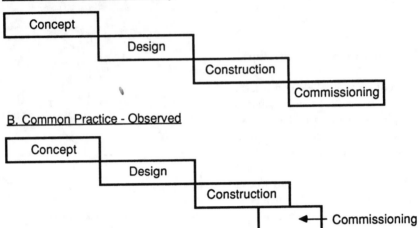

B. Common Practice - Observed

Managerial Process Model

C. Recommended Practice for Best Results

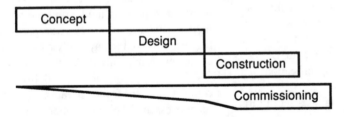

Figure 22-11 Steps in the Development of a Building. *Source:* Reprinted from *Journal of Health Administration Education,* Vol. 6, No. 4, p. 807, with permission of the Association of University Programs in Health Administration, © 1988.

2. Engineering commissioning to test and approve the facility's mechanical and electrical systems.

3. The orientation and training of existing personnel and the recruitment and training of any additional personnel.

4. Review of the nonpatient program, which includes supplies, furnishings, and equipment.

5. Development of a public relations program, which includes a dedication ceremony, public tours, and preparation of information for the media. Graphics included in the contract should be in place, and landscaping should be completed.

6. The actual move of patients to the facility. If the previous steps have been performed well, this last step is almost anticlimactic, but it is still important. It is likely to be the most dramatic step and thus of special interest to the media.

These steps are usually assigned to members of the operational staff. One person should be given the responsibility to plan and coordinate the overall occupancy process, especially the overlap with construction. This person must develop a schedule of events and activities, including established deadlines. The schedule must be realistic and provide adequate time for each activity. Implicitly or explicitly, a critical path method approach should be followed. The occupancy date, determined far in advance of the actual date, will change, and every change must be communicated promptly to everyone who needs to know.

Engineering commissioning does not just involve isolated pieces of machinery but the building systems themselves, such as the air conditioning and electrical distribution systems. Each system is made up of components that should be checked to make sure they are correct and in the correct place, able and ready to do the correct work.

Second, engineering commissioning has to be systematic. A rigorous commissioning program must be established and followed, and shortcuts or tempting compromise solutions based on charitable assumptions should not be permitted. Order, logic, discipline, and attention to detail are essential.

Third, commissioning has to be recorded. At each stage, the commissioning engineers will consult the records of design data—assumptions made where actual numbers were not known at the time, permitted tolerances, and changes in the original concepts. They will examine test certificates for the individual components and the sign-off sheets for the subassemblies prepared by the mechanical and electrical inspectors who supervised the installation. They themselves will be recording correct performance.

The commissioning and startup process is illustrated in Figure 22-12. The systems are divided into two main streams, mechanical and electrical. Within these divisions, the individual systems are set out in a logically dependent order: Transformers that regulate incoming power have to be proven before it makes sense to test the items of equipment that depend on that power. It also shows how tasks can be put into an efficiently planned program that harmonizes with the contractor's finishing schedule.

Experienced hospital commissioning engineers have, over the years, developed their own style of testing and documentation to keep them from overlooking any important program detail. There are also a number of well-established models, such as those of international engineering organizations like the American Society of Heating, Refrigeration and Air Conditioning Engineers. In Alberta, the first province in Canada to address the commissioning of hospitals in a formal and funded way, the Department of Hospitals and Medical Care has prepared its own guide to commissioning procedures.

Equipping the Project

The institution has the responsibility to acquire some items of fixed equipment and all the movable equipment and furnishings. There are consulting firms that can help to implement this step. Regardless of how the process is administered, the planning team must identify every piece of equipment and the furnishings that will occupy space or be part of a system in the design development stage. The team must also ensure that selected equipment meets departmental needs and institutional standards.

This process is long, tedious, and monotonous. The purchasing phase starts at least six to eight months in advance of the earliest scheduled occupancy date. On large projects, an equipment planner or consultant may be employed. Responsibility for furnishing and installing each piece of fixed equipment must be clearly established. The choice of who is responsible usually depends on which alternative will economically benefit the owner most, but other considerations—such as available manpower, the quality of the purchasing department, and the scope of the project—may come into play.

The institution wants equipment that will be as close to state of the art as possible when the project is activated. Some items have a long lead time for procurement and therefore must be ordered early. In the case of many items, market factors will determine whether it is more economical for the supplier

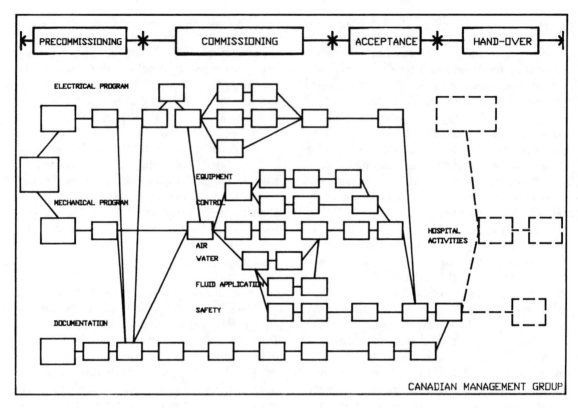

Figure 22-12 Activity Organization Chart. *Source:* Reprinted from *Journal of Health Administration Education,* Vol. 6, No. 4, p. 810, with permission of the Association of University Programs in Health Administration, © 1988.

to ship early and for the owner to provide (or pay for) local storage or whether the items should be held by the supplier for delivery on a specific date.

The supplier can usually best install complicated technical equipment, and the owner will pay a lower price and avoid a markup by the contractor if he or she buys it directly. The contractor still has to provide the installation requirements (such as for utilities) in specific locations and dimensions. In this event the contract should specify that equipment would be owner furnished and installed by the vendor (OF/VI), and the contract drawings should show where and in what quantities the utilities will be located. A second alternative is to have the contractor furnish and install equipment that is readily available (CF/CI). A third is for the owner to buy the item advantageously and have the staff install it (OF/OI). A fourth alternative is to have owner-furnished equipment installed by the contractor (OF/CI). Again, the rule for decision makers is to determine which approach provides the greatest benefit to the owner; this is usually determined through an item-by-item appraisal.

The project team and its designated leader are responsible for providing cost estimates for the equipment and installations that are not in the contract. Equipment and furnishings are grouped into bid packages, and preferred suppliers are selected. The chief engineer and his or her staff are key people in the selection and installation of complex equipment and systems. Suppliers of complicated equipment should be on duty during occupancy, along with the necessary operational manuals, to provide any needed services and a few spare parts to help ensure a smooth move.

Personnel Orientation and Training

In addition to commissioning the institution's equipment and engineering systems, the administrator may need to employ additional people to staff the new facility well in advance of occupancy. Smooth initial operations will depend on adequate planning sessions for all employees. They must be familiar with circulation patterns, standard locations for supplies and services on repetitive floors (such as nursing units), and new operating systems and equipment. This is a good time to initiate any desired changes in operating policies.

All employees, physicians, and volunteers must understand the operational concepts on which the design was based and the procedures that the facility supports. Some radical changes take months to assimilate. It is tragic and costly to abandon expensive mechanical systems simply because the staff has not learned to operate them properly.

Moving In

The move is broken into two parts, a nonpatient move and a patient move. Both follow the recommended shakedown period, when all systems are put into operation for a final testing. The nonpatient move can be done by professional movers to save the institution's staff for operational tasks.

In relocating staff and equipment, it may be necessary to double staff to maintain a minimum level of services at both ends of the move. Existing pieces of equipment that cannot be moved until the last minute must be tagged with their new room numbers and given top priority.

An adequate number of vehicles must be on hand to move existing furnishings and equipment. The telephone system and special communications must be "cut in" on schedule. Hardware and keying, key control, and distribution of keys are important. Security is essential, this is a time of confusion and unusual accessibility.

The census in the old area should be reduced in the days just prior to the actual move. Physicians should be asked to discharge as many inpatients as possible and reduce admissions to only those requiring hospitalization. Whenever possible, start admitting patients to the new facility only after the existing patients are moved.

All available staff, including physicians, nurses, and volunteers, must be mobilized. Most of the remaining patients will be critically ill or require longer stays than usual, and they will need special attention during the move. Patients' charts must accompany them, and the categories of staff attending the patients must be designated. There might be three teams: one to send the patients, another to accompany the patients, and the third to receive the patients in their new locations.

QUALITY MANAGEMENT

Project Step 7: Postoccupancy Evaluation*

Of all the steps involved in realizing a health care building program, evaluating the final product is the most often overlooked. The primary measure of success is user and client satisfaction. Evaluation is part of an ongoing process that looks back, but its benefits are in the future—for both the health care administrator and the architect.

An evaluation might be undertaken for many reasons:

- To justify actions and expenditures. Accountability is often demanded in the case of large buildings, especially if public funds are involved.

- To measure design quality. The quality level of the end product is a reflection on the entire institution.

*This section is based on Paul Kennon, Jay Bauer, and Steven Parshall, Evaluating Health Care Facilities, *Journal of Health Administration Education,* Vol. 6, No. 4, pp. 819–829, with permission of the Association of University Programs in Health Administration, © 1988.

- To fine-tune the systems in the new building.
- To prepare for a future building program, renovation, or expansion. The results of a post-occupancy evaluation are most useful when they contribute to improving the design of later projects.
- To adjust a repetitive program. A hospital may be built in phases, with additional wings constructed over time, or a free-standing clinic may build several facilities. An evaluation can help iron out snags encountered the first time around.
- To research human-environment relationships. A medical facility can be a stressful place for patients and staff. Information may be applied toward improving other facilities or the performance of the evaluated facility.
- To test the application of new ideas. Innovation involves risks, but new ideas are necessary to make advancements. These should be tested before further application is made.
- To educate past and future participants. Evaluation is helpful to both the client and the architect. New personnel arriving at any point in the program could benefit greatly from lessons learned from an evaluation and by participating in the evaluation process.

Method

Most new-facility evaluations occur after occupancy. By waiting until the facility is in use, the evaluation team can consider responses from facility users, who are the best source of information. The first major performance evaluation should occur between six months and two years after occupancy.

The evaluation team members should have different backgrounds and points of view; this makes the evaluation more objective. The size of the team varies between three and seven members, with one person as team leader. The team might include the administrator, the facilities manager, a user representative, a programmer, the designer, and the project manager.

The team may use different data-gathering techniques. Observation requires touring the facility. Interviews, whether formal or informal, allow a deeper investigation. Surveys reach a greater number of people than interviews and can be both comprehensive and specific.

Five Steps and Four Areas of Focus

Hospital facilities are very specific types of buildings that must fulfill certain atypical needs. However, they are easily evaluated using the postoccupancy evaluation process described below. This process is pragmatic and comprehensive, yet simplified enough for practical application. It consists of the following five main steps:

1. Establish the purpose.
2. Collect and analyze quantitative information.
3. Identify and examine qualitative information.
4. Make an assessment.
5. State the lessons learned.

The process also focuses on the following four areas (or considerations): (1) function, (2) form, (3) economy, and (4) time.

Evaluating, like programming, requires an organized, comprehensive process. The organization of the process should correspond to the framework used for programming. The similarity of the organization, content, and format will increase the usefulness of the evaluation results for programming and design in the future.

Purpose. It is essential that everyone involved has a clear understanding of why the evaluation is being undertaken. Successful evaluation depends on cooperation.

Quantitative Description. The second step includes collecting factual data on the building as constructed. Analyzing parameters provides a basis for comparing this facility with similar ones.

Functional adequacy is a measure of the amount of area per primary unit of capacity. The analysis might also compare the capacity for planned procedures with the actual operations performed.

Space adequacy checks the net assignable areas, including the sum of all spaces serving functional requirements. Unassigned areas include all other spaces in the building, specifically circulation areas, mechanical areas, public toilets, janitor closets, unassigned storage, and walls and partitions. The gross area of a building is the sum of the net assignable area and the unassigned area. The ratio of net assignable area to unassigned area indicates the building's efficiency.

Construction quality is the unit cost associated with the quality level of the building measured as the building cost per gross square feet. It is also helpful to note unique building systems that minimized cost and unusual constraints (e.g., codes or site location) that increased costs.

Technical adequacy measures the cost of fixed and special equipment (e.g., renal dialysis or laser surgery devices) represented as a percentage of the building cost, though it is also possible to represent it as a unit cost.

Energy performance is a measure of the amount of energy per gross square foot consumed for the standard operation of the building.

Assessing user satisfaction requires direct input from users as to how satisfied they are with the facility.

Qualitative Description. A qualitative description includes the following:

- Goals that convey the client's stated intention. Sometimes clients express great aspirations that are not fully achievable in the end because of budgetary or operational constraints.
- Concepts. Programming concepts represent abstract relationships and functional arrangements. Design concepts are physical responses that provide a unifying theme to the building solution.
- Problem statements. These demonstrate recognition of the critical project conditions and offer direction for the design effort.

- Changes since occupancy. These are indicators of new requirements or inadequacies.
- Issues that are unsettled and controversial decisions that are in dispute. These are posed by the occupants or owner of the facility during the evaluation or raised by the evaluation team.

Assessment. The evaluation is based on answers to standard questions that reflect important values (see Exhibit 22-4). Quality judgments vary with individuals. But although the judgments are ultimately subjective, rating does provide a mechanism for identifying the differences in the way the building is perceived by the various evaluators. Better understanding is possible when the evaluation team discusses these differences. Rating also allows explicit patterns to emerge that reflect how the parts contribute to the whole assessment. Clearer knowledge of the strengths and weaknesses of the building is possible when the evaluators compare these patterns and discuss them.

Lessons Learned. Lessons learned are conclusions about strengths or weaknesses. Rarely should an evaluation conclude with more than 12 statements. There should be at least 4 statements though—one for each of the major areas of focus:

1. Function. When evaluating functional performance, it is important to refer to the original goals and concepts that influenced the design.
2. Form. The evaluation must include aesthetic standards to determine the physical design excellence. This is the most difficult part of the evaluation, since aesthetic standards are ever changing.
3. Economy. It is important to consider the original quality goals in light of the initial budget. It is unrealistic to expect grand results if the budget allowed for no more than an economical level of quality.
4. Time. Because two or three years may elapse between programming and occupancy, the initial users may be different from those involved in the original planning. A certain amount of

Exhibit 22-4 Question Set for Health Care Facility Evaluations

Instructions
1. Use this form for rating a facility.
2. Review the criteria for each consideration and agree on the meaning for the particular type of health care facility being evaluated.
3. Enter score from one to ten for each criterion:

1 = Complete Failure	6 = Good
2 = Critically Bad	7 = Very Good
3 = Far Below Acceptable	8 = Excellent
4 = Poor	9 = Superior
5 = Acceptable	10 = Perfect

4. Add the scores and divide by six to get an average score for each major consideration.

FUNCTION   *Score*
A. THE OVERALL ORGANIZATIONAL IDEA
 (the big functional concept)   _____
B. EFFECTIVE ARRANGEMENT OF SPACES
 (activities and functional relationships) _____
C. WELL-PLANNED CIRCULATION
 (entry, orientation, flow)   _____
D. ADEQUATE SPACE ALLOCATION
 (net assignable/unassigned area, parking) _____
E. RESPONSE TO USER PHYSICAL NEEDS
 (comfort, safety, convenience) _____
F. RESPONSE TO USER SOCIAL NEEDS
 (privacy, interaction, sense of community) _____
SUBTOTAL   _____
DIVIDE BY SIX   ÷6
AVERAGE FUNCTION SCORE _____

FORM   *Score*
A. CREATIVITY AND EXCELLENCE IN DESIGN
 (imagination, innovation)   _____
B. PERFORMANCE OF BUILDING SYSTEMS
 (structural, mechanical, electric, signal) _____
C. RESPONSE TO SITE CONDITIONS
 (physical, climatic, aesthetic) _____
D. PROVISION FOR ENVIRONMENTAL CONTROLS
 (light, sound, temperature, ventilation) _____
E. RESPONSE TO USER PSYCHOLOGICAL NEEDS
 (order, color, variety, views) _____

F. APPROPRIATE SYMBOLISM
 (image, character, scale)   _____
SUBTOTAL   _____
DIVIDE BY SIX   ÷6
AVERAGE FORM SCORE   _____

ECONOMY
A. REALISTIC SOLUTION TO A BALANCED BUDGET
 (initial cost control)   _____
B. RETURN ON INVESTMENT
 (most for the money)   _____
C. MAXIMUM EFFECT WITH MINIMUM MEANS
 (elegance, multiple purpose) _____
D. EFFICIENT PLAN AND SHAPE
 (unassignable area, volume) _____
E. EASE OF BUILDING MAINTENANCE
 (materials and building systems) _____
F. COST-EFFECTIVE OPERATIONS
 (energy efficiency, minimum upkeep) _____
SUBTOTAL   _____
DIVIDE BY SIX   ÷6
AVERAGE ECONOMY SCORE _____

TIME   *Score*
A. CONVERTIBLE SPACES FOR CHANGES IN FUNCTION
 (dynamic activities, universality) _____
B. FIXED SPACES FOR SPECIFIC ACTIVITIES
 (major static activities)   _____
C. PROVISION FOR GROWTH
 (expansibility, shell space) _____
D. VITALITY AND VALIDITY OVER TIME
 (sustaining quality, holding power) _____
E. HISTORICAL AND CULTURAL VALUES
 (significance, continuity, familiarity) _____
F. USE OF MATERIAL AND TECHNOLOGY
 (expression of the times or advanced systems) _____
SUBTOTAL   _____
DIVIDE BY SIX   ÷6
AVERAGE TIME SCORE   _____

1. Use this graph for illustrating the pattern of scores.
2. Enter the average score for each consideration on the graph.
3. Mark the point on the graph representing the score.
4. Connect the points on the graph to form a quadrilateral.

continues

Exhibit 22-4 Continued

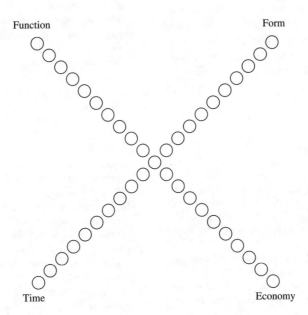

Source: Reprinted from *Journal of Health Administration Education,* Vol. 6, No. 4, pp. 828–831, with permission of the Association of University Programs in Health Administration, © 1988.

user satisfaction, therefore, depends on periodic interior design or on the degree to which partition and utility service changes are possible within the basic structure.

Evaluation Activities

The typical sequence of activities is as follows:

1. Initiation. The object is to establish the purpose of the evaluation and identify the background data requirements.

2. Preparation. Background research is used to prepare the quantitative and qualitative descriptions. User surveys should encompass description, satisfaction, and evaluation.

3. Tour. The evaluation team makes a visual inspection of the facility. Evaluators may undertake random interviews with users.

4. Discussion after the tour.

5. Assessment. Each evaluator makes a judgment as to the facility's success by assigning a score. The ratings are recorded on a special graph, which illustrates the pattern of each assessment.

6. Summation. The evaluation team reviews the quantitative and qualitative descriptions, along with the assessment ratings, and prepares a statement of the lessons learned.

7. Presentation. The team leader presents the conclusions.

8. Documentation. The team leader prepares a report of the evaluation process.

The five-step process described above (including the eight activities listed here) is practical enough for use in evaluating most health care facilities. As an aid to the programming process, it is appropriate to conduct an evaluation prior to initiating a new building program, remodeling a facility, or discontinuing the use of a facility. This allows the administrators of the institution to have greater confidence that they know what the problems are that need to be avoided or solved and what the goals of the program should be.

ADDITIONAL RESOURCES

Organizations

American Association of Healthcare Consultants, 11208 Waples Mill Road, Suite 109, Fairfax, VA 22030. 703\691-2242. The association puts out a directory of member firms, some specializing in prearchitectural programming and planning for health care facilities.

American College of Healthcare Executives, 840 North Lake Shore Drive, Chicago, IL 60611. 312\943-0544. This organization sponsors seminars on managing hospital and construction programs approximately three times per year (open to nonmembers).

American Hospital Association, American Society for Hospital Engineering, 840 North Lake Shore Drive, Chicago, IL 60611. 312\280-5223. The society sponsors two seminars on hospital design and construction (open to nonmembers).

American Hospital Association, Design and Construction, Douglas Erickson, Director, 840 North Lake Shore Drive, Chicago, IL 60611. 312\280-5223. Design and Construction functions as a clearinghouse. It will provide references to member institutions with related project experiences and problems and it cosponsors, with the Society for Hospital Engineering, health facility seminars, architectural exhibits, and trade shows.

American Institute of Architects, Committee on Architecture for Health, 1735 New York Avenue, N.W., Washington, DC 20006. 202\626-7366. The committee sponsors seminars on heath facility planning and design as well as tours of significant completed projects (open to nonmembers). It also sponsors research and publications by committee members.

American Institute of Architects, Library and Archives, 1735 New York Avenue, N.W., Washington, DC 20006. 202\626-7492. The library maintains book and periodical bibliographies on related topics, such as hospitals, health care facilities, ambulatory care facilities, medical offices, hospices, etc. The bibliographies are available to nonmembers.

Books and Directories

American Hospital Association. *Health care facility planning and construction.* New York: Van Nostrand Reinhold, 1989.

American Institute of Architects. *Building relationships: A guide for institutions on how to work with an architect.* American Institute of Architects, New York. Pamphlet.

American Society for Hospital Engineering. *Directory of planning and design professionals for health facilities.* Chicago: American Hospital Association, 1992.

Carpman, J.R., et al. *Design that cares: Planning health facilities for patients and visitors.* Chicago: American Hospital Publishing, 1986.

Covert, R., et al., eds. *Estimating space needs: A discussion of space planning for health facilities.* Chicago: American Hospital Association, 1984.

Cushman, R.F., and S.R. Perry. *Planning, financing and constructing health care facilities.* Gaithersburg, Md.: Aspen Publishers, 1983.

Elrod, J.L., and J.A. Wilkerson. *Hospital project financing and refinancing under prospective payment.* Chicago: American Hospital Association, 1985.

Guidelines for construction and equipment of hospital and medical facilities. Washington, D.C.: American Institute of Architects Press, 1992.

Hardy, O.B., and L.P. Lammers. *Hospitals: The planning and design process.* Gaithersburg, Md.: Aspen Publishers, 1986.

King, J., et al. *Preconstruction evaluation of hospital rooms.* Ann Arbor, Mich.: University of Michigan, Architectural Research Laboratory, 1982.

Klein, R. and A.J. Platt. *Health care facility planning and construction.* New York: Van Nostrand Reinhold, 1989.

Malkin, J. *Medical and dental space planning for the 1990s.* New York: Van Nostrand Reinhold, 1990.

Nackel, J., et al. *Working with health care consultants.* Chicago: American Hospital Association, Hospital Management Systems Society, 1986.

National Fire Protection Association. *NFPA health care facilities code 99-90,* Quincy, Mass.: National Fire Protection Association, 1990.

National Fire Protection Association. *NFPA life safety code 101–91,* Quincy, Mass.: National Fire Protection Association, 1991.

Porter, D.R. *Hospital architecture: Guidelines for design and renovation.* Melrose Park, Ill.: Health Administration Press, 1982.

Rea, J., et al. *Building a hospital: A primer for administrators.* Chicago: American Hospital Association, 1978.

Rohde, D.J., et al. *Planning and managing major construction projects: A guide for hospitals.* Ann Arbor, Mich.: Health Administration Press, 1985.

Rostenberg, B. *Design planning for freestanding ambulatory care facilities.* Chicago: American Hospital Association, 1987.

Setland, T., ed. *Health facilities research bibliography 1979–1986.* Washington, D.C.: Health Facilities Research Program, 1988.

Sloan, R., and B. Sloan. *A guide to health care facilities.* Ann Arbor, Mich.: Health Administration Press, 1991.

Thompson, J.D., and G. Goldin. *The hospital: A social and architectural history.* New Haven, Conn.: Yale University Press, 1975.

Toland, D., and S. Strong. *Hospital-based medical office buildings.* Chicago: American Hospital Association, 1986.

NOTES

1. *Modern Healthcare Magazine* annual Design and Construction Surveys from 1985 through 1992: K.E. Super, Healthcare Building Drops in '85, February 28, 1986, pp. 37–80; K.E. Super, Building Activity Jumps 16% in '86, February 27, 1987, pp. 37–80; K. Super-Palm, Construction and Architects Survey/Guide, February 26, 1988, p. 64; E. Gardner, Construction and Architects Survey, February 24, 1989, pp. 23–50; E. Gardner, More Hospitals Ready To Rebuild, February 19, 1990, pp. 20–44; E. Gardner, Healthcare Construction Survives Ailing Economy, March 11, 1991, pp. 25–40; L. Scott, Providers May See Lower Building Bills, March 23, 1992, pp. 25–46; L. Scott, Construction Key: Keep Options Open, March 15, 1993.

2. American Hospital Association, *Selection of Architects for Facility Projects* (Chicago: American Hospital Association, 1975).

3. AIA standard contract forms, available through the American Institute of Architects, 1735 New York Avenue, N.W., Washington, DC 20006 (202/626-7475) or local AIA chapter offices.

4. American Institute of Architects, Building Relationships: A Guide for Institutions on How to Work with an Architect. (American Institute of Architects, New York, pamphlet).

5. Courtesy of George T. Heery and Charles B. Thomsen, lecture materials presented at Harvard Graduate School of Design, May 27, 1992.

6. Ibid.

7. Adapted with permission of Carl Sapers from Legal Cases and Materials for the Construction Professional, vol. 2 (Harvard Graduate School of Design, privately published teaching case material), 516–520.

Thomas E. Skorup

Technology Assessment and Management

Purpose: The purpose of technology assessment and management is to optimize the effectiveness of existing and future technologies through the use of five principles: technology assessment, strategic technology planning, technology acquisitioning, technology management, and technology auditing programs.

INTRODUCTION

Physical assets in the health care arena can be separated into health care facilities, fixed, and ancillary equipment categories. Each category of equipment fulfills a specific, yet different, need within a health care institution. However, from an equipment management standpoint, all categories share a common life cycle. Whether we are discussing an advanced ultrasound unit or a common file cabinet, the management principles remain the same.

The concept of a life cycle and its cost is often neglected or misunderstood. Through a better understanding of the life cycle concept and its elements, management of physical assets becomes far more cost-effective. By better understanding the relationships between events such as needs assess-

ment, inventory control, and procurement, managers can implement more effectively the principal programs to control health care technology. These programs begin with *technology assessment* and *strategic technology planning,* before equipment procurement, followed by *technology acquisition, technology management,* and *technology audit* programs during physical equipment life. These techniques are interrelated and should be integrated for the most effective results.

Every health care administrator faces the dilemma of budget preparation with too many equipment requests chasing too few resources. Wish lists from departments must be scrutinized and, after internal negotiating and prioritization, be transformed into an overall capital equipment budget. This process will always prove challenging, but through improved asset management can be made more effective.

Many health care personnel think of technology as major medical equipment or medical devices in general, but the correct definition is much broader. As defined by the United States Congress, many international agencies, and academics, health care technology encompasses "drugs, devices, and procedures"—so that everything from pharmaceuticals, gene therapies, and biotechnologies employed

470

in health care to devices, equipment, and surgical and medical procedures are included. This chapter addresses strictly the medical device portion of health care technology.

Technology assessment and management responsibilities typically are located in several departments within a given health care facility. Clinical engineering, plant engineering, and purchasing departments maintain equipment records. The data from these departments is rarely integrated, however. Thus, the completeness and accuracy of each department's data typically suffers, and redundant files are often maintained for the same devices. Of these three areas, management of biomedical technologies offers the greatest challenge to a hospital. The Joint Commission of Accreditation of Healthcare Organizations (JCAHO) and the Food and Drug Administration (FDA) Safe Medical Device Act (SMDA) requirements mandate the collection and storage of equipment information in a specified format. Although this chapter emphasizes the management of biomedical equipment, the broad picture of consistent information throughout the hospital must always be maintained.

To optimize use of capital resources, hospitals require effective technology assessment, strategic technology planning, technology acquisition, effective technology management, and technology audits. The planning for and management of health care technology can be conceived as a series of building blocks. Each successive activity builds, in part, on the information gathered from the previous one, as shown in Figure 23-1.

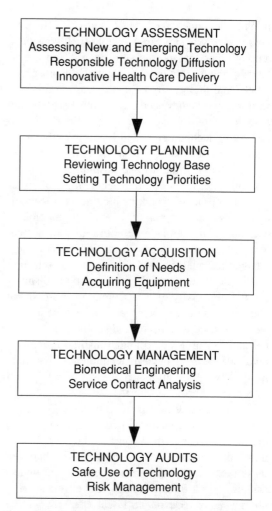

Figure 23-1 Technology Planning and Management Block Diagram. Courtesy of ECRI, Plymouth Meeting, Pennsylvania.

TECHNOLOGY ASSESSMENT

Technology assessment is defined as a rigorous analysis of a particular technology for its unique attributes of clinical efficacy and utility, safety, and relative cost-effectiveness compared to (1) alternative preventive, diagnostic, and therapeutic technologies intended to serve the same purpose and (2) its value and significance in relationship to other health care needs of a specific facility.

The original meaning and significance of the term technology assessment—as intended by the progenitor, the U.S. Congressional Office of Technology Assessment—has been distorted over the past few years by health care facilities, hospital groups, and commercial organizations, primarily in the United States, but, increasingly, in other nations.

Technology assessment, as first conceived and practiced, is a macroanalytical approach to determining the value, risk-benefit, and cost-effectiveness of a new health care technology. It considers, among other factors, the significance and prevalence of the disease to be prevented, diagnosed, or treated and the priority of that disease in relationship to other health needs. It examines safety and risk, costs, the value of a technology compared to competing technologies, and legal and ethical dilemmas or issues associated with a new technology.

Individual institutions and hospital groups, considering acquisition of a new technology, often refer to their process of making judgments as technology assessment. In reality, it is a combination of examining marketplace demographics in a local area (taking into account disease incidence), local competition analysis, and the equipment selection process. It lacks, generally, the economic disinterest and objectivity of true technology assessment and has far narrower perspectives, because it is intended to cope with needs and business opportunities at the local level. Still other institutions and individuals are using the term technology assessment to identify the traditional processes of equipment selection and procurement.

The net effect is that the term technology assessment means different things to different people, and the higher order term is, increasingly, applied to more mundane activities. To distinguish between these processes for the sake of clarity and understanding, refer to these higher order efforts as *technology macro-assessment*. Local efforts would be considered *technology micro-assessment,* and once a decision was made to acquire a technology, regardless of brand or model, the follow-up process would employ the traditional terms of equipment or technology selection and acquisition.

Technology Assessment Process

This section covers two technology assessment processes. The first process, macro-assessment, is intended primarily for use at teaching institutions and medical centers and is best suited to examine some justifiable and virtually all emerging and experimental technologies.

Technology macro-assessment at the medical center level has several purposes. One is to prevent premature adoption of technologies that are not yet proven to yield significant patient care benefits that are commensurate with their costs. Another purpose is to maintain a proper order of health care objectives and practices by comparing the significance of an emerging or future technology against other requirements for essential, advanced, and justifiable technologies, because no health care institution has unlimited resources to spend.

Whereas technology micro-assessment consists largely of organizing information that is usually readily available to support departmental decision making, macro-assessment has more uncertainties. This information is usually harder to find, less tangible, and less reliable; it has not been ripened by time. Macro-assessment is, in a sense, more theoretical, but failure to undertake it effectively often leads to wasted resources. It is, in a real sense, both an art and science of coming to judgment without sufficient information, despite which one is justified in having a high level of confidence that one's judgment is correct. It therefore requires a willingness to change one's mind based on available new information and the requirement that one accepts technology assessment as a continuing process until all questions are resolved about the validity of the information or related conclusions. Whereas micro-assessment demands more clinical knowledge, macro-assessments rely heavily on epidemiological and economic analysis, because they consider patients as a large scale statistical aggregate.

Decisions to adopt a new medical technology are a response to a perceived clinical problem or need. Individuals performing assessments of medical technology should keep the clinical need foremost in mind and not be influenced by high-tech appeal. This is equally important whether the desire is to (a) improve or replace an existing method or procedure or (b) introduce a technology that has not been available before.

Technology Macro-Assessment Methods

Macro-assessment of technology is a tool for reviewing the clinical, social, and economic consequences of a technology and provides a basis for making decisions. The primary value of technology assessment for decision making lies in determining the safety, efficacy, and cost-effectiveness of medical technologies and discrimination between appropriate and inappropriate indications for use.

Specific criteria should be adopted to screen new technologies and to order priorities for assessment purposes. These criteria include medical significance, potential benefit and clinical utility, proportion of population affected, ease of diffusion, economic incentives, impact on the health care delivery system, and important legal, ethical, and social considerations.

The following elements are part of a typical health care technology assessment:

1. Identify technology to be assessed, and prepare brief research protocol.
2. Establish a technical advisory panel made up of individuals who are familiar with the technology to provide assistance.
3. Contact appropriate professional organizations to provide input as needed.
4. Prepare a detailed research protocol, including background information on the technology, a list of sources of primary data, a brief description of the analysis plans, and a schedule for project activities.
5. Collect data.
6. Analyze data.
7. Prepare draft report.
8. Widespread critical review and comment.
9. Prepare final report.

The assessments should include these basic elements:

- a statement of clinical objective

- a projection of the need for the technology, and the potential for its wide application
- an estimate of the survival rates (if applicable) or improved quality of life of the recipients of the technology
- considerations of the availability of the technology and its stage of development
- a complete evaluation of the cost of the technology, including the cost of alternative treatments for the disease or condition in question
- a full assessment of the purported benefits of the technology including both objective and subjective parameters, and qualification of its reliability
- a review and evaluation of any legal concerns associated with the use of the technology, including patient selection, imposition of risk, distributional concerns, and conflicts with regulations and practices

Many innovations in health care technology rest on theoretical ideas held by the innovators. These ideas range in strength from well-informed to outright speculation. Beyond this, a few innovations are purely empirical, in that someone noticed that the technology seemed to work, even though no underlying mechanism was proposed or understood. If, in practice, the innovation is clearly better or clearly worse than existing technologies, then the innovation deserves either adoption or rejection. In considering medical technologies, no matter how strong or weak the theoretical justification, well-founded experience is the decisive factor, and technology assessment is the way to validate it.

Technology Micro-Assessment Methods

Micro-assessment of technology, the second process, is intended to evaluate a medical technology to be adopted and also to monitor the value of a technology once it has been integrated into a health care facility's operations. The process consists of six steps that answer key questions:

1. Clinical assessment to determine whether the technology is desirable from a clinical and epidemiological perspective.
2. Financial assessment to analyze the financial aspects of the planned acquisition (cost, not just price). Is it affordable? Where does it rank with other practices?
3. Facility assessment to explore practical considerations specific to the health care facility. Does the facility have the physical and human resources to assimilate the technology?
4. Vendor/equipment assessment to evaluate the vendor and specific items being considered for acquisition. Is it the right technology from the right source?
5. Integration of assessments to make a final decision based on information and conclusions drawn from previous assessments. Should it be adopted?
6. Reassessment to reevaluate the technologies and related processes adopted. Was it worth it?

It is not necessary to perform every step in the process each time an acquisition is being considered. For instance, issues considered in the facility assessment are not always specific to individual technologies and may need to be evaluated only superficially to bring the information up-to-date.

Persons performing the assessments should consider anticipated changes as well as present circumstances. Possible future obsolescence should be a major concern, and the assessors should obtain historical data in order to project trends as to future need, utilization, costs, and revenue.

Reassessment is important to determine if the recently adopted technology has fulfilled expectations and if the expected quality-of-care improvements have been achieved. Technologies should, at a minimum, be reassessed by the facility one year and three years after becoming operational. This follow-up information will be useful in future assessments.

The frequency of subsequent reassessments depends on the size and resources of the facility, but, at the very least, a medical technology should be reassessed whenever a replacement is being considered. Again, new technologies should always be compared to all possible alternatives, including those already in use in the facility, as well as other options that have emerged. Replacement equipment should be assessed in a similar manner.

The medical technology assessment process can be modified for reassessments performed one year later by addressing new or changed issues. Reevaluation is not a static process, and outside sources of information and data should be monitored for changes.

If this process is used for technology assessments appropriate to the technology under consideration, health care facilities should realize several major benefits:

- meeting the health care needs of the served population
- cost savings from enhanced productivity and from avoidance of unnecessary or obsolete technology
- improved quality of care and safety
- technology that is consistent with the facility's mission and level of service
- baseline information that can be used in reevaluations, planning, and examination of cost-effectiveness and cost-benefit

STRATEGIC TECHNOLOGY PLANNING

Under enormous pressures from its medical staff, hospitals frequently find themselves responding to physician requests that are not always feasible, are duplicative of existing services, and are not analyzed with regard to clinical need, risks, costs, or other hospital priorities. Hospital management spends much time responding to physician requests because there is no mechanism to allow for the rational deployment of technology in the support of services.[1] This scenario outlines a distinct lack of strategic technology planning.

A strategic technology plan provides a cohesive, coordinated, and prioritized strategy for a health care institution's short- and long-term goals. By identifying immediate and not so immediate technological needs, hospitals can project capital investments over a five- or seven-year period. This allows new or replaced technologies to be phased in at the most feasible and appropriate time. The most difficult step in technology planning is to determine which technologies warrant serious consideration and how they best fit into the hospital's strategic plan (see Figure 23-2). Health care organizations must provide a mechanism for the following tasks:

1. Monitor and analyze new and emerging technologies to provide the hospital with sufficient lead time to plan and develop new clinical services. This will require an in-depth understanding of what changes are occurring in diagnostic and therapeutic technologies in each specialty. What new technologies should the hospital be considering? What additional emerging technologies, which may not yet be approved by the FDA for general marketing, should be monitored? What technologies are not appropriate for acquisition because of insufficient proof of their effectiveness or safety, inadequate reimbursement, or inadequate utilization? What technologies support and can expand existing services such as peripheral vascular programs, cardiology services, and women's services?

   Without answers to such questions, it is difficult to determine when to invest in the tech-

nology—and timing may determine the success or failure of the acquisition and the related service. In fact, timing, more than the technology itself, may be the primary strategic factor.

Such knowledge also provides the hospital with a firm ground when it must withstand pressures from consumers and medical staff. Emerging technologies sometimes receive considerable media attention and generate interest among physicians and patients even before formal clinical trials have begun.

2. Assess the impact of new technologies on the hospital to ensure coordination with the organization's strategic plan, assimilation into the hospital's care, satisfaction among physicians and staff, and sufficient utilization of the equipment in light of medical staff preferences, internal and external competition, and service area demographics.

   Services should be enhanced using technology as a tool, and not be driven by technologies, which can result in short-sighted, costly errors in judgment. Support services cannot be neglected; proper tools must be available in the clinical laboratory, anesthesia, and other areas.

3. Consider how specific technologies will affect staffing, delivery of care, and facility design, including space planning, utilities, and physical and mechanical systems (structural, environmental, shielding).

4. Evaluate economic considerations such as the effects of reimbursement, the technology's life-cycle cost, cost and revenue shifting within the institution, the ability of the technology to be provided in a freestanding facility, and its potential to attract investors.

5. Analyze risks associated with new and replacement technologies including reuse, upgrades, complete or partial modification of equipment, and compatibility with the existing system.

6. Consider the impact of third-party payers on technology. Decisions by Medicare and oth-

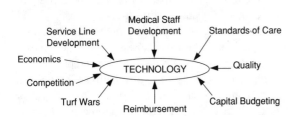

Figure 23-2 Strategic Technology Planning. Courtesy of ECRI, Plymouth Meeting, Pennsylvania.

ers about paying for new technologies will assume more importance than ever before as the broad trend away from cost-based payments continues.

With a decrease in Medicare reimbursement of capital-related costs, the amounts reimbursed are at least 12 to 15 percent below annual depreciation, interest, and leasing costs. Few other third parties now specifically reimburse capital costs, so, for most hospitals, future prospects for adequate capital-related income are likely to be no better than for operating income.

Further, hospitals are beginning to see reductions in outpatient revenue levels similar to those of inpatient revenues under prospective payment and HMO/PPO pressures. Under Public Law 100-203, clinical laboratory fee-for-service payments are further reduced, and, for the first time, Medicare revenue for other outpatient diagnostic services has been removed from a cost-reimbursed basis. This change became effective October 1, 1988 for diagnostic imaging modalities and October 1, 1989, for cardiology and all other diagnostic services.[2]

Few third parties will knowingly pay for the use of a technology before it has received FDA approval, and manufacturers sometimes prefer to sell, rather than lend, the devices that are to be used in clinical trials. This means that a few hospitals must make substantial expenditures just to conduct the trials necessary to obtain FDA and third-party approvals.

Thus, as hospitals develop strategic technology plans to chart a course and budget for their futures, an in-depth analysis should be made for each new technology, and a reevaluation of existing technologies.

TECHNOLOGY ACQUISITION

In the past, the decision to procure new equipment was often made by physicians and passed on to administration without adequate regard for patient need, equipment obsolescence, standards of care, or even awareness of product alternatives. Today, administrators must be acutely aware of these and other issues, before proceeding with an equipment acquisition.

Many hospitals have established multi-disciplinary committees to review equipment requests. These capital equipment committees are typically comprised of representatives from clinical departments, risk management, purchasing, biomedical engineering, and administration. By utilizing these diverse perspectives, more unbiased and effective procurement decisions can be gained.

In addition, opportunities such as purchase bundling, which may not have been realized, arise from the committee approach. Bundling of acquisitions often provides hospitals with special leverage at the negotiating table through the combining of acquisitions into a single package. (See Chapter 16 for more on financing capital expenditures.)

TECHNOLOGY MANAGEMENT

Technology management is an accountable, systematic approach to ensuring that cost-effective, safe, and appropriate equipment is available to meet the demands of quality patient care. Hospitals that have fully embraced technology management know it is worth the effort. Smarter technology decision making conserves resources, improves the quality of care, and reduces risks. Proving the truth of these assertions takes time, but that is true of all new concepts. The evidence from many hospitals is clear; technology management is worth doing. It has a financial, safety, and quality-of-care payback.

Indiscriminate use of equipment and operator error continue to be the weakest links in health care technology. Inappropriate selection and purchase of equipment often results in acquisition of equipment that is unnecessary, unsafe, overly expensive, or difficult to service. This, in turn, creates an excessive inspection, preventive maintenance, and service burden and leads, directly or indirectly, to dangerous, inadequately maintained, malfunctioning, or nonfunctioning equipment. Then, faced with insufficient reliable equipment to meet patient needs, hospitals, paradoxically, buy more of the same equipment.

Figure 23-3 illustrates the typical hospital's dilemma in employing and managing clinical equipment. It depicts broad relationships between management of equipment, risk to patients and staff, cost-effectiveness, compliance with regulations, and the quality of patient care.

For many hospitals, technology management will be the responsibility of an in-house biomedical engineering department; for others, materials management or, sometimes, administration will handle it. But who is assigned to implement technology management is less important than doing it, and doing it well.

In addition to an equipment control function, technology management entails greater attention to technology planning, acquisition, and replacement to equipment-related facilities planning, with intensive involvement of biomedical engineering, fiscal, and materials management. Technology management records and expertise will also improve the allocation of resources throughout the hospital. Identifying which items of equipment experience frequent repair requests may indicate overutilization, poor-quality equipment, or poor user training, and will aid in prioritizing capital budget requests. A general knowledge of current developments involving new and emerging technologies will also aid in allocating capital resources wisely among strategic planning options and capital budget requests.

Development of Clinical Engineering Departments in Hospitals

A number of diverse factors have influenced the development of clinical engineering departments and associated biomedical services in the past 20 years. The primary factor was a significant increase in the scope and complexity of the hospital's technology base and the use of this equipment for patient care (i.e., as opposed to basic or applied research). This resulted in clinical engineering departments assuming responsibility for the inspection, preventive maintenance, and repair of a portion (but not all) of the hospital's biomedical equipment.

An additional factor during this period was a major increase in codes and standards, their requirements, and their enforcement (particularly those of the Joint Commission and the National Fire Protection Association [NFPA]). These added significantly to the rationale for obtaining clinical engineering capabilities, particularly to perform required inspection and preventive maintenance and related documentation activities. Other factors included the increasing cost of purchasing repair services for biomedical equipment, the major growth of liability concerns regarding equipment-related incidents and malpractice claims, the need for more thorough, intensive training of equipment users, and educational needs related to the training of physicians, nurses, and allied health technologists.

Due to the economies of scale, clinical engineering departments in hospitals with more than 500 beds typically support the majority of the hospital's biomedical technology. Clinical engineering departments in hospitals of 200 to 350 beds typically consist of a clinical engineer or senior biomedical equipment technician (BMET) and two to four BMETs, depending on the type and number of devices to be supported by the department.

Clinical engineering departments now routinely report to administration (e.g., vice president of operations or support services), rather than to plant or facilities engineering due to this close connection between their responsibilities and patient care. In all hospitals, however, a successful technology management program is predicated on good communication between the clinical engineering and the plant engineering departments to ensure that all devices are appropriately managed. It is not expected that the director of plant engineering will be familiar with all biomedical engineering concepts, but he or she must understand that the tasks performed on biomedical equipment are distinct and

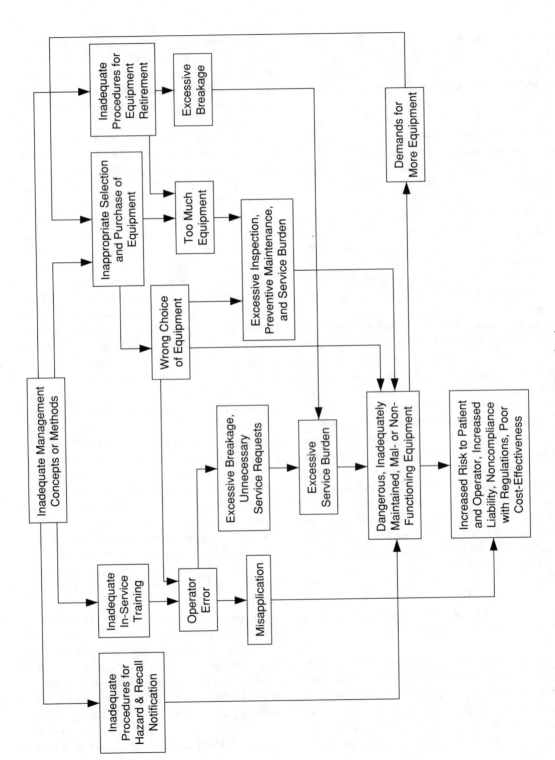

Figure 23-3 Ineffective Equipment Control. Courtesy of ECRI, Plymouth Meeting, Pennsylvania.

different from those performed on physical plant equipment because of the involvement of medical personnel who use the equipment and the interface with patients.

In addition to the inspection, preventive maintenance, and repair of equipment, the management of biomedical technology requires a commitment to other issues, such as acquisition and training. A clinical engineering department should be perceived, organized, and managed as a technical support service for the hospital, its medical staff, and clinicians. Its stated mission should be to provide guidance in the selection, acquisition, and application of biomedical equipment technology and to provide technical support through inspection, preventive maintenance, and repair of biomedical equipment, in addition to consultative and fiscal reviews of technology for administration.

Regardless of the size of the clinical engineering department and its responsibilities for in-house support of biomedical equipment, one group or person must be responsible for managing all biomedical technology, including those services provided by outside service vendors. In many institutions, uncontrolled service agreements are responsible for poorly maintained devices, costly repairs, and unnecessarily expensive contracts. Some institutions are using or considering maintenance insurance as a method to reduce expenditures and the number of service contracts. The devices placed on maintenance insurance are usually those with already high service costs (i.e., computed tomography scanners), and savings are often apparent within the first year. However, someone must still be responsible for managing the insurance company relationship and tracking any increased downtime or lost revenue due to the conditions of the maintenance insurance provider.

Also, clinical engineering departments now have yet another role in the hospital, because of the SMDA. Hospitals are now required to report all incidents of adverse outcomes or the possibility of adverse outcomes that involve *all* medical devices. As the regulations are written, everything from a mammography machine to a catheter is covered by SMDA. The clinical engineering departments and risk managers should collaborate in determining what happened in all medical device-related incidents that occur in the hospital.

Finally, the Joint Commission is placing greater emphasis on integrated technology management through its Plant, Technology, and Safety Management (PTSM) standards. For the first time, the Joint Commission is allowing individual hospitals to quantify and evaluate the risks associated with patient care equipment. These identified risks should then form the basis of each hospital's equipment management program. Clinical engineering must evaluate the equipment's function, clinical application, maintenance requirements, and incident history to have an effective management program. The equipment management program must include all capital equipment bought by the hospital, as well as all leased, loaned, borrowed, or rented equipment. With adequate staffing and experience, the clinical engineering departments can handle these responsibilities.

Equipment Control System and Documentation

All major medical equipment is tagged and placed on the department's computerized inventory/preventive maintenance (PM) scheduling/ maintenance history system.

There is a system to track in-house work orders and a history file for each inventoried device that contains data on work orders, PM calls, and repair costs. There is also a filing system for all technical and service data and manuals. A regular calibration schedule and documentation system have been instituted for clinical engineering (CE) test equipment.

Currently, the CE department only provides quarterly reports of PM calls accomplished and due to each cost center receiving services. The data captured in the equipment database are comprehensive enough to produce the following types of reports:

- a maintenance activity summary that lists the total number of PM calls by device type and includes the number of devices in service, number inspected, number failed, number not found, and comments, if any

- a serviced equipment maintenance history by device type that lists the inventory control number, model number, purchase price, remaining depreciated value, accumulated labor and parts cost (cost of ownership), last PM call date, total number of repairs, average repair time, and average time out of service
- an equipment service report (a printout of all BMET service reports from that time interval) that documents the details of each repair performed for that department or cost center
- the year-to-date charges to each cost center within a department, detailing total hours, parts costs, and total costs

The serviced equipment maintenance history could be made to flag certain instances, such as devices whose total or projected cost of ownership exceeds their remaining value or devices whose remaining depreciation has reached zero.

The current quarterly reports provided to department managers should be expanded in terms of the type of data presented. An executive summary that provides an overview of activities; recommendations for items requiring replacement or other managerial attention; current major issues or announcements of common interest, such as scheduled meetings or in-service training or new regulations pertaining to medical equipment; and a current calculation of mutually agreed upon quality/value indicators or progress toward specific mutual objectives would provide the department managers with a valuable tool to assist in their managerial functions. Data should include, in a convenient format, tracking and planning information such as: a summary of charges for that reporting interval, the total lifetime repair costs as a percentage of purchase price, the total lifetime out-of-service hours and repair hours, the projected replacement costs, the total user errors detected, and the number of repeat service calls or callbacks on particular devices. The use of graphics to represent data on the equipment databases is recommended, such as the number of PM calls performed versus the number scheduled, the total number of overtime hours charged, or other data requested by department managers, if available.

From the data currently available in the CE equipment databases, there are several possible quality and management indicators that could be calculated and reported on a regular basis to show trends, identify problem areas, or evaluate effectiveness. One or more such indicators should be included in regular management summaries to clinical department managers after the types of such indicators have been mutually agreed upon as being most useful in departmental and hospital management and planning functions. Possible indicators could include:

- Service Quality/Efficiency
  1. Percentage of downtime
  2. Percentage of callbacks
  3. Percentage of PM calls completed
  4. Average response time
  5. Average time to repair
  6. Hours of PM versus hours of repair
  7. Hours worked versus hours paid
- Economic Quality
  1. Total maintenance costs as a percentage of replacement costs on a hospital-wide, annual basis
  2. Maintenance cost as a percentage of replacement cost by device to date
  3. Cost savings of in-house CE versus third-party service organization or manufacturer
  4. Cost of downtime (also compare for in versus out)
- Other Quality Indicators
  1. Hours of training per year per BMET
  2. Equipment training received by users
  3. Number of outside calls for assistance
  4. User errors found per piece of equipment per area per month/quarter/year
  5. Equipment-related incidents

It is extremely important that a central equipment inventory be compiled, confirmed, and regularly updated. An accurate and complete inventory of all clinical devices is especially necessary for compliance with SMDA.

Equipment Acquisition and Standardization

A formalized, prepurchase screening program for medical device acquisitions should be included in written hospital policy to require review and sign-off by both CE and plant engineering departments. This policy should be formulated by a Product Evaluation and Standardization Committee comprised of representatives from the appropriate clinical departments, risk management, purchasing, clinical engineering, and other administrative departments. This committee's scope should include standardization and purchase approval for supplies, consumables, and clinical equipment. Since individual departments within a hospital often maintain autonomy in their purchasing, this committee serves as a hub for pulling together similar equipment requirements for standardization. Thus, specification, bidding, and negotiation should be handled with assistance from purchasing and clinical engineering departments.

All incoming medical equipment in a health care facility shall be routed to the CE department for safety inspections and performance tests and appropriate manuals should be included. This policy would assure that even leased or physician-owned equipment would be inspected for safety before commencing operation within the hospital.

Health care facilities should review all existing policies to ensure that there are complete, written policies governing the assessment, acquisition, and acceptance of all biomedical equipment. These policies should include procedures for assessing needs, financing acquisitions, and performing comparative equipment evaluations. They should address performance, safety, serviceability, and equipment/facility interfaces.

From initial screening to pre-use testing, the acquisition process should include the following steps as a minimum:

1. Assess needs
2. Evaluate effects on existing technology
3. Plan for service coverage
4. Ensure proper approvals
5. Develop qualified vendor lists
6. Request proposals/bids
7. Compare the request with other departments' needs for similar equipment
8. Analyze vendor responses
9. Evaluate sample devices
10. Investigate interfaces with other equipment and systems
11. Select vendor finalists
12. Negotiate purchase/acquisition
13. Review installation and user training plans
14. Make the award
15. Monitor delivery and installation
16. Review documentation and manuals provided
17. Verify acceptance testing and user training
18. Perform incoming tests/inspections, and place in the inventory

The following standard contractual terms and conditions for medical equipment acquisition should be required:

- installation and approval
- payment, assignment, cancellation
- obsolescence protection
- software requirements/updates
- documentation and manuals
- clinical and technical training
- acceptance testing (hospital and vendor)
- warranty, spare parts, and service
- price protection

Acquisition support should be one of the primary functions of a CE department acting as an in-house technology manager. This involvement must be supported by administration. The savings in dollars and time with a properly implemented system can be significant.

Equipment Inspection, PM, and Repair

The CE department should have complete responsibility for the management, inspection, PM, and repair of all hospital biomedical equipment. In some facilities, this responsibility is divided among the many clinical department managers, which dilutes the effectiveness of centralized equipment management.

Most of the equipment that is managed by the CE department is scheduled for PM two to three times a year, with documentation provided to the respective clinical departments. The procedures for performing this work should reference manufacturers' requirements, as well as other current applicable standards and codes.

Overall hospital biomedical equipment acquisition costs can be in the hundreds of millions of dollars for very large medical institutions. An acceptable ratio for calculating expected servicing costs, based on national averages, is in the range of 3 to 7 percent (per year) of the acquisition cost for nonimaging equipment and 7 to 11 percent of the acquisition cost for imaging systems, depending, of course, on sources of coverage and the age of equipment.

Many clinical engineering departments maintain intensive on-hand inventories of very specialized spare parts. However, because nearly all biomedical equipment repair parts can be obtained within 24 to 72 hours in North America and due to the rapid changes in equipment technology, such investments should be minimized. Inventories should be audited annually to identify any areas of surplus inventory.

In larger health care institutions, technology managers or chief technology officers (CTO) are being added to act as coordinator/managers of all equipment services. This person is responsible for all technology-related issues at the hospital and any satellite facilities and reports directly to upper-level hospital administration. Walk-throughs of clinical areas should be performed on a regular basis. The CTO should also have responsibility for the assessment of new technologies and should assist in determinations of appropriateness and eventual implementation, if appropriate.

The only current means of truly capping costs is through maintenance insurance or an agreement with an outside contractor who will guarantee all costs in advance. Although the latter would appear to be a cost-effective solution at first glance, such arrangements are always fraught with surprises, hidden costs, and other problems associated with the lack of full hospital control over the process. The problems of outside contractors should not become those of their clients, but that is sometimes unavoidable. The risk of being without in-house capabilities and being completely dependent on an outside vendor with its own agenda and priorities, with the chance of being left totally without service, is more than most hospitals exceeding 200 beds may reasonably care to assume.

Service Contracts

A single point of coordination and responsibility for the approval and monitoring of medical device service contracts should be established. Often individual departments have autonomy in making decisions pertaining to equipment maintenance coverage, with the department managers having responsibility for monitoring contractor performance and for maintaining service documentation on their own equipment. This approach leads to inconsistent tracking of service contractor performance, if at all, and provides no means of verifying what work is performed and what documentation is provided by outside service contractors.

Thus, responsibility for coordination of all biomedical technology service contracts should be centralized under a technology manager and/or the

CE department. The function should be responsible for evaluating the need for service contracts, their cost-effectiveness, and the actual performance of each vendor.

The first priority in monitoring service contracts is to list the inventory of outside service agreements by department. A central location or department should have all the service contracts, indicating the devices covered and the hours and other conditions of coverage. Full-service agreements should be listed separately from time-and-materials agreements. A listing of full-service contracts should indicate start and stop dates and cost per year, whereas time-and-materials agreements should include travel expense per service call, hourly rate, and a parts cost budget.

It is also necessary to determine whether a service contract covers adequate inspection and PM. If a device is covered by a time-and-materials agreement and no call for service is made during the year, will it be inspected and will preventive maintenance be performed? Also, if a full-service contract exists for a specific device, the service must include full PM and safety testing with proper documentation of same provided to the department at the time of service. All service contracts or extended warranties should be negotiated at the time of equipment purchase as part of the bargaining process. Copies of all present and future service contracts should be maintained in device-specific files and in a master file by the CE department. Department heads should receive a copy of all service contracts for their equipment, including complete costs and conditions of service. Without centralized coordination and approval of all outside service, there is no means to accumulate and track actual costs or even to confirm that basic documentation requirements for safety and quality assurance are being met.

Generally, manufacturer, third-party vendor, or insurance service should be used for equipment that requires very specialized training or prohibitively expensive spare-parts inventories or that is a one-of-a-kind item. The equipment is usually revenue producing, and extensive downtime for repair cannot be tolerated (e.g., CT systems).

As previously discussed, the technology management function should monitor the work of outside service vendors to ensure the timely and cost-effective performance of inspections, PM, and repairs. This function should be assigned responsibility for the coordination of all contracted repairs, including requesting service, quality control, monitoring of performance, and invoice approval. Contract terms should be standardized, and certificates of insurance should be requested and filed. If maintenance insurance is obtained, this function would also be responsible for submitting requests to and tracking reimbursements from the insurance carrier.

Close monitoring of service calls performed on a time and materials basis may allow CE department personnel to learn how to eliminate user error and routine service problems. CE department personnel can also better assess the level of effort, training, and test equipment required for in-house service. Responsibility of service should not be assumed by the CE department until its staff has been properly trained, however. Interim measures should include supervision of service calls, leading to the initial screening of service calls by the department. Once screening is begun, service contracts should be renegotiated with the vendors to increase savings.

Disposal of Obsolete Equipment

Most hospitals have a procedure for decommissioning or disposal of biomedical equipment and materials. However, criteria for identifying obsolete, ineffective, or nonrepairable equipment and designation of the authority for removing such equipment from service does not exist in most institutions. This policy should require a disclaimer that any equipment sold or donated to any other organization is taken "as is," without any implied or expressed warranties. Any identification material related to the seller's facility should be removed.

Hazards and Recalls

Responsibility for disseminating hazard and recall information and for monitoring action should be assumed by the CE department or risk manager, and supported by written hospital policies to this effect. Materials management and the purchasing department can be important resources in tracking disposable products. To facilitate dissemination of hazard and recall information, it should be routinely directed to the same individual (i.e., the department administrator or nurse manager) in each clinical area. In addition, to complete the loop, the information must be returned to the originating party.

In-service Training and Continuing Education

The CE department should establish and maintain a cooperative relationship with the nursing education department and participate in nursing in-service training for technical matters pertaining to medical equipment.

Because of the critical relationship between user error, patient injury, hospital liability, and technical support of biomedical equipment, the CE department should continue to be part of the training process in either a formal or a consultative role. As a minimum, a representative from CE should be included in any user training that the manufacturer provides for new equipment acquisitions. This will facilitate detecting user error and the need for re-training. Whatever role is established, a formal working relationship among the nursing service, CE, and all other allied health professionals must be maintained. This will go a long way toward mini-mizing equipment-related problems and injuries. Additionally, maintenance training should be included in most capital acquisitions.

The department director should evaluate the bio-medical knowledge of each technician with regard to the various devices being inspected and maintained. The director must ensure that the technical staff fully understands how and why devices are used. If weaknesses in biomedical knowledge are identified, the director should provide for appropriate training.

CE staff should demonstrate that they are keeping abreast of relevant standards, technical devel-

opments, and new biomedical applications. Education and training (e.g., manufacturers' training schools, professional conferences and seminars, professional journals and publications) should be encouraged and funded. Purchase conditions for new equipment that require the manufacturer to provide operator and service training at no additional cost can frequently be negotiated. CE technicians should also attend any local courses related to Association for the Advancement of Medical Instrumentation (AAMI) certification.

Equipment-related Incidents

Hospital incident reporting and investigation systems should be expanded to include the requirements of SMDA, which was to be effective in May 1992. However, the requirement for full compliance was delayed until September 1993. There should be a written, approved hospital policy to include requirements for impounding equipment, accessories, and disposables; criteria for independent investigation; and criteria for participation by equipment manufacturers and service contractors, as appropriate.

TECHNOLOGY AUDITS

Standards of care surrounding the safe use of health care technology are changing rapidly. In addition, each technology has a typical useful service life and a point at which it becomes clinically and technically obsolete.

Although most hospitals maintain equipment inventory records in their accounting and biomedical engineering departments, few systematically review this data for decision-making purposes. By reviewing equipment inventories, touring facilities, and interviewing key clinicians and department managers, hospitals can identify areas of risk and develop priorities for equipment replacement. These audits allow hospitals to identify and minimize liabilities associated with high-tech equipment, supplies, and supporting systems. Such audits identify defective, unsafe, and inappropriately used medical devices and staff. They help meet the need for hospital risk management that is evolving at the insurance company and state level. These have become even more important with recent Joint Commission requirements.

A technology auditing program provides a quality assurance system for health care institutions to measure the success of all technology management strategies. By identifying weaknesses in acquisitioning, assessment, or other programs, these audits help hospitals to more effectively manage technology.

THE FUTURE OF TECHNOLOGY ASSESSMENT AND MANAGEMENT

Many health care institutions have implemented programs to manage current and future technologies, but these programs rarely utilize or combine the advantages of all technology control techniques. Fragmented strategic technology planning, technology acquisition, management, and auditing programs are common in today's health care environment, and are rarely integrated to maximize their effectiveness. As the advantages of effective technology control become more evident, more health care institutions will invest in strengthening and integrating these programs.

Technology assessment programs should provide a new focus for health care institutions into the twenty-first century. As health care reforms, regulations, and competition drive medical facilities toward greater levels of efficiency and accountability, technology assessment programs will aid health care institutions in critiquing new technologies and their overall potentials. Since technology assessment programs are rare in the current health care market, this strategy should experience significant growth in the coming years.

Health care institutions should look for increased integration of all technologies using the concepts discussed. The future in overall technology management will provide departments other than clinical engineering departments access to accurate, current, and useful inventory data. Thus, wise management decisions will be possible for all levels of technology.

ADDITIONAL RESOURCES

Organizations

American Society of Hospital Engineering, c/o American Hospital Association, 840 North Lake Shore Drive, Chicago, IL 60611. 312-280-6180.

Association for the Advancement of Medical Instrumentation, 3330 Washington Boulevard, Suite 400, Arlington, VA 22201. 703-525-4890.

ECRI, 5200 Butler Pike, Plymouth Meeting, PA 19462. 215-825-6000.

Periodicals

Health Devices, ECRI, 5200 Butler Pike, Plymouth Meeting, PA 19462.

Health Devices Alerts, ECRI, 5200 Butler Pike, Plymouth Meeting, PA 19462.

Health Facilities Management, American Hospital Publishing, Chicago, IL.

Health Technology Trends, ECRI, 5200 Butler Pike, Plymouth Meeting, PA 19462.

Hospital Materiel Management Quarterly, Aspen Publishers, Inc., 200 Orchard Ridge Drive, Gaithersburg, MD 20878.

Journal of Clinical Engineering, Quest Publishing, Brea, CA.

Books and Articles

American Institute of Architects. *Guidelines for construction and equipment of hospital and medical facilities.* Washington: American Institute of Architects, 1993.

Cook, A.M., and J.G. Webster, eds. *Therapeutic medical devices: Application and design.* Englewood Cliffs, NJ: Prentice-Hall, 1982.

ECRI. *Health devices inspection and preventive maintenance system.* Plymouth Meeting, PA: ECRI, 1990.

ECRI. *Health devices sourcebook.* Plymouth Meeting, PA: ECRI, 1993.

ECRI. *Healthcare standards.* Plymouth Meeting, PA: ECRI, 1993.

ECRI. *Healthcare technology management.* Plymouth Meeting, PA: ECRI, 1990.

ECRI. *Universal medical device nomenclature system.* Plymouth Meeting, PA: ECRI, 1992.

Webster, J.G., ed. *Encyclopedia of medical devices and instrumentation.* New York: John Wiley, 1988.

NOTES

A portion of the material in this chapter originally appeared in a *Healthcare Forum* article entitled "Strategic technology management" (Vol. 32, No. 5, Sept/Oct 1989), by David A. Berkowitz. Other contributors for materials used in this chapter are Joel J. Nobel, M.D; David A. Berkowitz, MSE; and Peter R. Suydam, CCE, PE., and are provided courtesy of ECRI.

1. David A. Berkowitz, *Strategic technology management*, 5.
2. David A. Berkowitz, *Strategic technology management*, 6–9.

Paul A. Johnson

24

Housekeeping and Environmental Services

Purpose: The purpose of the housekeeping department is to maintain an orderly, clean, and aesthetically pleasing environment within the hospital and to ensure that all patient and nonpatient areas comply with internal and external standards and regulations regarding appearance, orderliness, sanitation, infection control, and environmental contamination.

INTRODUCTION

Planning, organizing, and maintaining a housekeeping department has been recognized as essential for the efficient operation of a health care facility. It is no longer a question of how clean a health care facility should be or whether it is willing to pay for what it expects. The major issue is whether the facility is receiving the quality of service it should be receiving given the amount of money it has allocated for housekeeping.

This chapter discusses various methodologies that can assist the housekeeping management and the administration in developing a successful housekeeping program.

A good housekeeping department can be the best customer relations tool a hospital has. First impres-

sions are lasting impressions! If family members step inside a health care facility and see a dirty, cluttered lobby or smell offensive odors, they will immediately have doubts about the ability of the staff to provide quality patient care to their loved one.[1]

The governing board of directors has the ultimate responsibility for establishing the standards of cleanliness for the hospital.[2] It is unlikely, however, that it will get involved in setting the various department standards. This will be the responsibility of the administration, the housekeeping management, and the specific departments. Tailoring the level of cleanliness and financial responsibility to an individual department's needs and expectations may not be an entirely new concept, but it is one that is taking hold in the industry. Third-party payers such as insurance companies and government agencies (Medicare and Medicaid) are demanding justification of all expenses.

Housekeeping department functions include

- establishing cleaning standards that will enable staff to determine whether levels of cleanliness are acceptable
- establishing cleaning tasks and frequencies in order to justify resources

- scheduling routine, special, and periodic cleaning assignments that are consistent with the cleaning standards and resources
- providing trash removal services to meet local, state, and federal standards
- providing trash removal schedules in order to keep the garbage and trash from accumulating in soiled utility areas
- assisting in the disposal of medical and hazardous waste
- maintaining interior finishes and furnishings by establishing a repair and replacement schedule

MANAGEMENT PRINCIPLES

- Management should ensure that the work is equally divided according to the cleaning standards for the given area.
- The housekeeping director should have the authority and responsibility to conduct the operations of the department within the scope of the department's mission.
- The department should have sufficient supervision to properly manage housekeeping activities.
- The housekeeping director should encourage esprit de corps in order to develop unity and good discipline within the department.

ORGANIZATIONAL ROLE AND FUNCTION

Background

When looking back through history, one can see that cleanliness has played an important role in well-organized societies. Its importance can be traced back to the fourth century B.C. when Hippocrates wrote his Hippocratic oath. He emphasized the value of hand cleaning, keeping soil excluded from wounds, and boiling water before cleansing wounds.[3] These prescriptions are still valid today.

According to Mildred Chase,

> Up until the 19th century, the history of medical work seems to indicate that nursing personnel—men and women—did not only nursing work, but housekeeping and cooking as well. The lack of proper housekeeping and good preparation caused Florence Nightingale to separate these three important phases of hospital operation. So while Florence Nightingale is considered the mother of Nursing, she can just as aptly be referred to as the mother of housekeeping and food service.[4]

Chase also points out that early in the twentieth century, housekeepers were accepted members of the staff in such institutions as colleges, clubs, hotels, and hospitals. During that time, the hospital head nurse or matron had direct control of the housekeeping function. A book written by Charlotte A. Aikens in 1910 was the first work to indicate that housekeeping should be a separate area, even if a head nurse was ultimately responsible.[5]

The actual title Executive Housekeeper was not utilized until 1930. At that time, a group of housekeepers in New York City formed the National Executive Housekeepers Association.

The housekeeping department is normally part of the support services division, which includes departments such as security, maintenance/engineering, dietary, materials management, and laundry (see Figure 24-1).

Infection Control

Joseph Lister, Ignaz Semmelweis, and Louis Pasteur were pioneers in battling cross-infection. The housekeepers of today assist in this important activity.[6]

Institutions accredited by the Joint Commission for Accreditation of Healthcare Organizations must have infection control committees that monitor and enforce infection control policies and procedures. Since proper housekeeping is crucial to infection

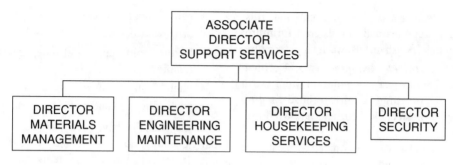

Figure 24-1 Organization Chart for Support Services Division

control, it is always a key item on the committee's agenda, and the director of housekeeping should be a member of this committee.

The manual *Infection Control in the Hospital* states,

> To the extent that nosocomial infection may be a consequence of exposure to contaminated air, dust, furnishings, equipment and other fomites, effective environmental sanitation is required to lessen such hazards. Frequent thorough cleaning of hospital interiors is necessary to reduce the number of pathogens. Environmental sanitation is not believed to have as its primary purpose a direct antibacterial effect by the cleaning agents themselves; its main purpose is to physically remove microorganisms from the various fomites that might transmit them to patients.[7]

Standards

The first step in organizing an efficient hospital housekeeping department is recognizing the importance of housekeeping. Once this has been recognized, then appropriate standards can be established in order to provide services.

The purpose of setting standards is to (1) equalize the workload of employees, (2) ensure that each employee knows what is expected in the time allowed, and (3) maintain high-quality service.

Edwin B. Feldman states that payroll amounts to 90 percent or more of the housekeeping budget.[8] This is the overall average for industry; in health care, 80–85 percent is devoted to labor, primarily because of the use of higher priced disinfectants and petroleum products such as plastic bags. Other items that affect the nonpayroll portion of the budget include

- exterior window cleaning
- pest control
- repair and maintenance
  —upholstered furniture
  —windows
  —wall coverings
  —floor coverings

As a labor-intensive department, housekeeping needs to give a great deal of attention to task standards. These are the specific standards for tasks expected to be completed when cleaning areas. The tasks are typically divided into routine, weekly, and periodic tasks:

- *Routine cleaning tasks.* Empty, wipe out, and reline wastebaskets; dust furniture; vacuum; spot-clean carpets, doors, and walls; clean restrooms and showers; replenish supplies; dust and wet mop hard or vinyl floors.

- *Weekly cleaning tasks.* Vacuum vents and grills; vacuum draperies and upholstered furniture; clean blinds; polish metals; wash vinyl furniture.
- *Periodic project cleaning tasks.* Refinish floors; shampoo carpeting and furniture; wash walls; clean ceiling; clean overhead lighting and vents; wash cubical curtains and windows.

Frequency standards are determined by the degree of cleanliness needed and the resources that are available. In other words, each area within a facility will have different requirements—patient rooms will require more cleaning than offices, and the operating room will require more than patient rooms. Other relevant factors include the amount of traffic, the type of dirt, and the function of the room or area.

Scheduling cleanings would be simple if there were sufficient resources available. Then every area could be cleaned every day, which would ensure consistently high levels of cleanliness. The availability of adequate resources is rare, and therefore priorities for cleaning must be determined.[9] Prioritization must be done conjointly by the administration, the manager of the department receiving the services, and the housekeeping director.

The following must be considered when establishing cleaning frequencies:

- expected standard of cleanliness (how clean it should be)
- available resources (manpower, equipment, money, and time)
- physical properties (ease of cleaning furniture and fixture surfaces)
- amount of room usage (heavy or light)
- kind of usage (whether subject to frequent spills or messy dirt)
- accessibility (number of people who use the area and whether occupied by incontinent, geriatric, or ambulatory patients)

Established frequencies might be as follows:

- patient room areas—daily

- patient treatment support areas—daily
- offices—weekly
- lecture, conference, and meeting rooms—as required
- public lounges and waiting areas—daily
- trash collection and restrooms—daily

In the areas that have been designated as needing daily cleaning, not all items must be cleaned every day. In patient rooms, those items that patients do not have direct contact with on a daily basis can be cleaned less frequently (see Exhibit 24-1).

In the case of restrooms and public areas such as lounges and waiting areas, daily cleaning is appropriate. These areas may also have to be policed several times a day to maintain neatness.

The housekeeping director must be familiar with cleaning tasks and allot sufficient time to properly clean a given area. It must be remembered that the time allotted for a specific task does not usually include setup time or personal, fatigue, and delay time. Setup time is the time spent getting ready to begin daily assignments or periodic project cleaning assignments. Personal, fatigue, and delay time includes restroom breaks, waiting for elevators, and waiting for access to patient areas. It also includes slowdown from fatigue due to working on one's feet, bending, stooping, reaching, and lifting during a shift. In most cases, personal, fatigue, and delay time adds 10–27 percent to the standard time for a task.

Cleaning the operating room, labor and delivery rooms, recovery areas, intensive care units, and nurseries involves special cleaning activities, but in some hospitals, housekeeping may provide only limited services to these areas, with cleaning responsibilities assumed by the appropriate department. In most hospitals, housekeeping does not provide services to mechanical areas, storerooms, and dietary or cafeteria areas. These areas are cleaned by employees in the appropriate departments. There may be some geographical and seasonal tasks, such as assisting in snow removal or dealing with flood plain problems. The department may contract out responsibility for the cleaning of windows, pest control, and solid waste management.

Exhibit 24-1 Cleaning Schedule

Clean Occupied Rooms
Patient Rooms:
( ) Empty, wipe out, & reline wastebasket at 7:15 a.m.
( ) Clean public restrooms at 7:30 a.m., police at 9:30 a.m., 12:00 p.m., & 2:30 p.m.
( ) Clean basin
( ) Clean tub & shower
( ) Clean toilet
( ) Clean overbed table
( ) Vacuum carpet
( ) Empty all wastebaskets at 2:30 p.m.
( ) Check & refill soap, toilet tissue, & paper towels
( ) Dust & damp mop bathroom floor
( ) Spot-clean carpet as needed
( ) Clean bedframe day of surgery

Clean Support Areas
Clean support areas, nurses stations, kitchen, utilities, & restrooms:
( ) Empty trash
( ) Clean basins, hoppers, & sinks
( ) Spot-clean and vacuum carpet
( ) Clean restrooms
( ) Clean counter tops
( ) Dust & damp mop floors
( ) Clean table tops

Patient Rooms:
Monday:
( ) Clean bedside table
( ) Clean foot stool
( ) Spot-clean walls, doors, & frames
( ) Clean telephones

Tuesday:
( ) High dust vents, lights, & bedframes
( ) Wash window inside
Wednesday:
( ) Clean telephone
( ) Clean television
( ) Clean wardrobe
Thursday:
( ) Dust & vacuum upholstered chairs
( ) Dust & clean vinyl chairs
Friday:
( ) Clean nurse call device
( ) Clean television control

Support Areas:
Monday:
( ) Spot-clean doors, frames, & walls
( ) Clean glass in doors
Tuesday:
( ) High dust vents & lights
Wednesday:
( ) Clean telephones
( ) Dust picture frames
( ) Dust bulletin board
( ) Dust wall clock
Thursday:
( ) Dust chairs
( ) Spot-clean doors, frames, & walls
Friday:
( ) Dust refrigerator
( ) Dust blinds
( ) Clean glass in doors & windows

Waste Management

Hospitals generate 15–20 pounds of discards (waste) per patient day. Disposing of this waste has become a major problem over the past several years. Regulating agencies such as the Environmental Protection Agency (EPA), the Occupational Safety and Health Administration (OSHA), and the Centers for Disease Control (CDC) as well as state, county, and local governments have become involved in the classification and disposition of medical waste. The housekeeping director must keep abreast of the ever-changing regulations in this area

to ensure proper compliance. The housekeeping director must also be aware of the volume of trash that is being generated.

Charles Miller points out that "all trash and waste are potentially dangerous."[10] Waste can cause contamination and can constitute a fire hazard, and it needs to be handled very carefully. The housekeeping director should review collection and disposal procedures to ensure that they are adequate for the location, type, and amount of disposal.

Miller makes the following suggestions pertaining to the collection and internal transportation procedures[11]:

- Sharp objects should be deposited in a proper container to prevent them from protruding or escaping. (It is recommended that all sharps be collected at the site of use.) Containers for sharps need to be impregnable and should have self-closing lids. When full, they are to be discarded.
- Waste containers in rooms, offices, and laboratories should contain a plastic liner. When full, the liner should be tied closed and discharged into a proper container for collection and removal.

Medical waste that is contaminated or considered infectious needs to be placed in double-lined containers that have distinct color (usually red) and are marked with identifying stickers. If the facility has an EPA-approved incinerator, then the waste can be handled onsite; otherwise, it must follow the local or state regulations that apply to medical regulated waste.

A great deal of the trash generated at any facility is recyclable. Paper, cardboard, plastic, glass, metal, aluminum, yard waste, and many other materials that were just thrown away now can be reused. Even though a profit may not be realized, recycling these items can reduce trash removal costs.

If trash cannot be disposed of at the facility, then the housekeeping director needs to make arrangements for trash disposal. The most practical way is to contract with an independent vendor. Miller suggests the following issues be dealt with in the contract[12]:

- frequency of pick ups
- periodic cleaning of containers
- leak proofing and maintenance of unit
- alternative service during failure or breakdown of mechanical unit
- monthly cost of contract to include hauling and tipping fees
- insurance to include liability (because the facility is responsible for its waste from "cradle to grave")

Maintaining Interior Finishes and Furnishings

The housekeeping director needs to be knowledgeable about the various types of finishes:

- flooring: carpet, vinyl composition tile, sheet vinyl, ceramic tile, quarry tile, terrazzo
- walls: vinyl wall covering, wall fabrics, painted surfaces
- ceilings: acoustical tile, plaster
- furnishings: drapery, blinds, furniture, mattresses, lighting

The housekeeping director should advise the administration on finishes and furnishings, because the housekeeping department will most likely be responsible for maintaining them. Proper selection will aid in reducing early replacement and will therefore decrease the probability of incurring additional expenses.

RESOURCE MANAGEMENT

A hospital normally spends about 50–60 percent of its budget on labor and benefits.[13] Housekeeping, however, is very labor intensive and spends 85–90 percent of its budget on labor and 10–15 percent on supplies and other expenses, not including capital equipment. Capital equipment consists of individual items that exceed a set cost, have a specified minimal useful life, and are budgeted separately from the department's operating budget.

Personnel

In terms of full-time equivalents, housekeeping is one of the largest departments in the hospital. Its total budget is usually 1.5–2.0 percent of the hospital's total budget.

Hospitals use various units of measure to calculate the cost of housekeeping services. The two most commonly used are cost per patient day and cost per 1,000 square feet. Whichever measure is used, when a comparison is made between hospitals, clarification is needed to ensure that the departments are providing equivalent services.

What size staff is necessary for cleaning a facility? That is difficult to determine. Later in this chapter is a discussion of the data required to do a staffing study.

The housekeeping department's organization depends upon the size of the hospital. In hospitals under 150 beds, if the director is only responsible for housekeeping, he or she will often serve as the day supervisor, with second-shift and weekend supervisors coordinating their activities with the director. Hospitals with less than 150 beds do not usually provide third-shift coverage.

In hospitals of 150–300 beds, the director usually coordinates activities through supervisors on each shift. Hospitals of 250–300 beds may also have an assistant director for the department. Hospitals over 300 beds will usually have a director, an assistant director, and a supervisor for all shifts.

Many housekeeping departments use "lead persons," who work with small groups of staff in coordinating activities such as project assignments or tasks within specific areas of the hospital (operating rooms, labor and delivery, combined nursing units). These individuals are not supervisors per se but rather facilitate work flow with work crews. In addition, some departments delegate responsibilities by designating some housekeepers as Level I and others as Level II housekeepers. Level II housekeepers typically have more experience, are trained to work in several areas of the hospital, and have a thorough knowledge of equipment and cleaning procedures.

Titles in housekeeping have changed over the years in order to eliminate any hint of discrimination. The terms *janitor* and *maid* are no longer used. Housekeepers are now referred to as *housekeeping assistants* or *environmental assistants* or *technicians*.

Over the years, housekeeping staffing methodologies have relied on square footage as the workload indicator. Square footage, however, is not an accurate indicator, nor does it reflect productivity changes as patient days or discharges fluctuate.

A better method is to calculate the amount of time spent on individual cleaning activities summarized by unit or service (e.g., nursing unit, radiology department, laboratory, physical therapy, and administration). The normal times for these activities are computed using accepted housekeeping industry standards. Sources that provide housekeeping time standards include the American Hospital Association, Chicago; the Minister of National Health and Welfare, Ottawa, Canada; and the International Sanitary Supply Association, Lincolnwood, Illinois.

As indicated previously, no two hospitals are alike. Therefore, a significant number of data are necessary to accurately assess the staffing needs of the department.

The data required to do a staffing study include but are not limited to the following:

- square footage cleaned by housekeeping (measured from blueprints)
- room type
  - —private and semiprivate rooms, wards
  - —each department (radiology, laboratory, administration)
  - —carpeted versus noncarpeted areas
  - —corridors, waiting or lobby areas
  - —restrooms, locker rooms
- patient data
  - —annual patient days
  - —annual discharges, transfers, and isolations
  - —annual operating room cases
  - —annual births
- annual hours
  - —vacation
  - —sick days
  - —holidays
  - —breaks

A review of cleaning, task, and frequency standards should be done when conducting the data collection outlined above. Revise the cleaning standards when appropriate (do not change the time standards utilized). Review the updated changes with the department director and obtain his or her approval of the revised standards. There should be cleaning standards for each of the following functional areas:

- patient rooms (daily)
- patient rooms (following discharge)
- nonpatient areas of the nursing unit
- offices
- lobbies and waiting rooms
- public restrooms
- treatment and exam rooms
- lounges and break rooms
- corridors
- labor and delivery rooms
- birthing suites
- operating rooms
- outpatient areas
- radiology
- laboratories
- physical therapy

Establish reasonable frequencies for project cleaning of the above areas (e.g., wall washing, ceiling cleaning, stripping and refinishing floors, shampooing carpets, and cleaning upholstery).

Data collected will be divided into three categories depending upon whether they concern variable workload standards, constant workload standards, or management supervisory standards:

- Variable workload standards pertain to the cleaning of patient rooms, isolation rooms, labor and delivery rooms, suites, and operating room suites.
- Constant workload standards pertain to the cleaning of nonpatient units, corridors, lobbies and waiting areas, public restrooms, offices, and project assignments.
- Management supervisory standards pertain to the management, supervisory, and clerical activities needed to manage the housekeeping department.

When all the workload volumes are collected and calculated, the total hours required to clean the hospital and manage the department are to be divided by annual paid hours less benefit hours to calculate a productivity percentage.

Equipment

Housekeeping personnel must be provided with sufficient labor-saving equipment to enable them to carry out their tasks efficiently.[14] The equipment selected will have a direct effect on the quality and the associated cost of the work performed.

Housekeeping equipment, if properly utilized, often pays for itself in a very short time. In addition to cost savings, there are other advantages:

1. Using properly selected equipment generally gets better results than manual techniques. Both a mop and a wet vacuum will dry a wet floor, but the vacuum will do it faster and leave the floor cleaner.
2. Housekeepers will become less fatigued using power equipment, raising their productivity.
3. State-of-the-art housekeeping equipment may be viewed as a status symbol and can boost morale. It enhances the prestige of the individual housekeepers and the department as a whole.
4. Housekeeping equipment promotes safety. Vacuums and automatic scrubbers clean and dry floors quicker, reducing the risk of falls. Vacuums equipped with wand extensions reduce the need for ladders and scaffolding.

Edwin Feldman describes what a program of housekeeping equipment would include[15]:

1. A survey of the needs based on an evaluation of the work to be done in the various areas.
2. Development of equipment specifications. Since equipment and supplies constitute only a small portion of the housekeeping budget, it

is poor economy to provide less than the best equipment available. Best, however, is not synonymous with the most expensive. Things to consider when writing specifications include appearance, size, weight, quality of manufacture, electrical characteristics, attachments, flexibility, safety features, noise level, horsepower, warranty, and filter capability.

3. Proper attention should be given to the supplier and the supplier's ability to furnish service and parts.

4. Equipment should be purchased under arrangements that best suit the hospital (e.g., outright purchase, lease, or rent).

5. The manufacturer or a representative should provide training and retraining in proper use and preventive maintenance.

Supplies and Other Expenses

Supplies and other expenses, which usually make up 15 percent of the operating budget, can amount to hundreds of thousands of dollars. Effective inventory control is critical in running an efficient housekeeping department. The department manager should routinely examine the inventory and expenses to ensure that they are within budget and that expenditures have been justified.

Depending on the hospital's accounting system, the department budget line items may include the following (in addition to wage and salary items):

- medical supplies (e.g., rubber gloves)
- office and administrative supplies (e.g., paper and pencils)
- cleaning supplies (e.g., disinfectants, all-purpose cleaners, and floor maintenance products)
- paper and plastic supplies (e.g., paper towels, toilet tissue, and plastic liners)
- minor equipment (e.g., mop buckets and waste cans)
- repair and maintenance (e.g., parts for equipment and furniture repairs)

- other purchased services (e.g., pest control and window washing)

Cleaning, paper, and plastic supplies will be the items that will require the most attention.

The questions that the director must ask are, "What do I need? How much do I need? When do I need it?" The department should have no more cases of a product on hand than it would normally use in a month. Overstocking ties up the hospital's cash and consumes valuable space that could serve other functions. In fact, if deliveries can be made more frequently than monthly, then that should be taken into consideration.

When a purchasing and inventory system is being set up, the director should do a value use analysis of all the products being considered. The same questions should be asked about each product, including these five[16]:

1. Is the product used as recommended by the manufacturer?

2. Is this the best product to use?

3. Does the product do the job?

4. Is there a less expensive product that will do the same job?

5. What is the end-use dilution cost for the product? (The end-use dilution cost is the actual cost of the product after it has been diluted. Products such as strippers, disinfectants, and all-purpose cleaners are sold in concentrates and are diluted before use. If, for example, a disinfectant costs $12.00 per gallon, but is diluted to a ratio of 1:128, the end-use dilution cost will be 9.375 cents per gallon.)

In most cases, 10 percent of the products will be responsible for 70–80 percent of the supply budget (typically, these products will include disinfectants, floor care materials, hand soaps, paper towels, and plastic liners). The best tactic for achieving immediate cost savings is to concentrate cost-reduction efforts on these products.[17]

Once the value use analysis has been completed and the products have been chosen, the next step is to develop an ordering cycle. It is helpful to first decide upon the working stock level for each product, which should be 50 percent of the amount that will be used over a predetermined period of time (weekly, biweekly, monthly).[18] For most items, the ordering cycle should be less than one month.

An effective inventory control system depends upon reliable suppliers who will deliver when expected. Getting such suppliers may require formal bidding of all supplies. If bidding is used, the expected delivery schedule should be included in the bid specifications. If the vendor cannot meet the specification schedule, then the contract can be terminated.

QUALITY MANAGEMENT

In the past, the Joint Commission's accreditation manual for hospitals stated, "In order to guide personnel in providing a hygienic environment for patients and staff, departmental procedures shall be developed for: the evaluation of cleaning effectiveness . . ."[19] Accordingly, a sound quality assurance program should include[20]

- identification of potential problems or related concerns in the care of patients
- an objective assessment of the cause and scope of problems or concerns
- implementation by appropriate individuals or through designated mechanisms of decisions or actions that are designed to eliminate, insofar as possible, identified problems
- monitoring activities designed to ensure that the desired results have been achieved and sustained
- documentation that reasonably substantiates the effectiveness of the overall program to enhance patient care and to ensure sound clinical performance

Today more than ever, the quality of health care services is the focus of national attention. Housekeeping departments are not excluded from public scrutiny.[21] Many people judge the quality of a hospital by its cleanliness and overall appearance. As hospitals compete for patients and physicians, their housekeeping departments must provide services that are cost-effective and of the highest quality. Studies have shown that when hospitals are recruiting physicians, cleanliness ranks among the physicians' top five priorities.

When developing a quality control program, the administration and the housekeeping management must have a firm grasp of what they want it to accomplish. The most common goal is to develop the ability to measure the relative quality of cleaning in a given area at a given time. Before quality can be improved, there must be a way of measuring it. Ten different people can inspect the same room and give ten entirely different opinions on the degree of cleanliness. To solve the problem of subjectivity, it is necessary to standardize scoring procedures.

Usually "satisfactory/unsatisfactory" ratings will suffice. This type of scoring will force the inspector to make a decision as to whether or not the item meets specified standards (see Exhibit 24-2).[22] Limiting the number of people involved in quality control inspections will also reduce the risk of varied opinions. In a large hospital, it is not uncommon to have only one person responsible for the quality control program. If only one person is involved, all areas will be evaluated by the same set of standards. The Joint Commission has no specific requirements for the quality control program; it can take whatever form is necessary to provide the manager with the information needed to assess the quality in the housekeeping department's areas of responsibility.[23]

To be effective, quality control must be ongoing, consistent, accurate, focused on system improvements, and have the absolute commitment of top management.[24]

THE FUTURE OF HOUSEKEEPING AND ENVIRONMENTAL SERVICES

Computers

In an article I wrote for *Executive Housekeeper Today*, I pointed out that the next decades are going

Exhibit 24-2 Hospital Cleanliness Standards

1. Ceilings: Clean, free of dust and spots, paint intact, vents clean and free of dust and lint, lights replaced.
2. Room Walls: Clean, no lint, paint intact, free of finger marks and stains.
3. Floors: Clean, free of dust, lint, and stains, no wax buildup or accumulation of soil in corners, free of heel and scuff marks, free of discolored wax.
4. Cove Bases: Clean and clear, no wax buildup, no mop marks, no accumulation of soil in corners, intact around room (firmly affixed to wall with no signs of being loose at junction with floor).
5. Doors: Clean, free of marks, finish intact, kickplate clean and shiny, top free of dust and lint, edges clean, handle or knob clean, hinge facing and doorframe clean, door vent clean and free of dust and lint, window and frame clean and free of dust and lint (inside and outside).
6. Windows: Clear and clean, not in need of immediate washing, frame clean, glazing intact, sill clean, paint in good condition.
7. Window Drapes: Free of lint, properly hung on tracks, not faded, no stains, yellowing, or tears, pulleys and pull cords intact and working, pins installed correctly in drapes and on carriers.
8. Cubicle Curtains: Clean and free of stains, not faded, pull freely in tracks, properly mounted, no tears, adequate length and width.
9. Beds: Headboards and footboards clean, metal upright and horizontal frame members clean, control unit and cord clean and working, linen clean and free of stains and tears, bed properly made, undercarriage free of lint and soil, wheels clean and free of lint.
10. Mattresses: Clean, free of stains and lint, in good repair without rips or tears, thoroughly deodorized, mattress turned on each discharge.
11. Overbed Tables: Clean and free of dust, elevation controls working properly, drawer and drawer mirror clean and free of dust, lint, and streaks, base, frames, and wheels clean and free of dust and lint.
12. Bedside Console Units: Counter top, shelves, and facings clean and free of dust and spots, no accumulation of soil in corners, stainless steel sink and plumbing fix-

tures clean and free of spots and streaks, clothes closet clean and free of dust and lint.
13. Chairs: Clean, free of lint and dust.
14. Television Sets: Clean, free of dust and lint, shelf clean, free of dust and lint.
15. Toilets: Toilet bowl clean inside and outside, no stains, streaks, or residue, toilet seat clean, free of spots, stains, or streaks and tightly fastened to toilet, plumbing fixtures clean, free of dust, spots, and streaks, plumbing connections to toilet free of alkali buildup and dirt, base of toilet free of soil buildup and stains.
16. Sinks: Clean, inside, outside, and underneath, free of spots and streaks, plumbing fixtures on top and underneath free of dirt, spots, and streaks, base of plumbing fixtures free of alkali buildup.
17. Mirrors: Clean, free of spots and streaks, frame top and edges free of dust and lint, shelf clean, free of spots and streaks.
18. Shower Stalls: Walls clean, free of soil buildup, caulking intact, fixtures free of spots and streaks, floor frame and glass free of dust, lint, spots, and streaks, horizontal crossbars above door free of dust, lint, spots, and streaks.
19. Dispensers: Soap, paper towel, and seat cover dispensers clean, free of dust and lint on top and underneath, free of spots and streaks, supplies replenished.
20. Refrigerators: Clean, free of dust, spots, and stains, shelves and facing clean and free of spots, spills, and stains, freezer clean and free of stains, motor vent clean and free of dust and lint.
21. Ovens: Stainless steel top, sides, and metal or glass door clean and free of spots and streaks, interior shelf, sides, and top free of stains, no accumulation of soiled food on surface of oven (interior).
22. Counter Tops: Clean, free of dust, stains, and finger marks.
23. Telephones: Clean, free of dust and lint, receiver, mouthpiece, and dial free of dust and lint.
24. Drinking Fountains: Stainless steel free of spots and streaks.

Source: Reprinted from *How To Organize and Maintain an Effective Hospital Housekeeping Department* by C. Miller, with permission of the American Hospital Association, © 1991.

to be an especially challenging period.[25] Hospitals are becoming more information oriented and more dependent on computers, and housekeeping will not be immune to this trend. Housekeeping directors will need to become computer literate.

In an age when computer software programs are being effectively utilized in all types of industries, it is time for housekeeping to benefit from this technology. The computer is the tool of choice for improving productivity and quality service.

Constant pressure to keep costs under control has become a way of life in the health care industry. With cutbacks in Medicare, Medicaid, and private insurance payments, the industry has become a financial battleground—and will most likely continue to be one. These cutbacks are going to have a direct effect on all support activities regardless of the size of the hospital. Housekeeping departments will be asked to hold the line and even cut back on expenses. At the same time, health care institutions will be attempting to be more competitive in the market and increase their revenues by offering more services to the community. The goal, in short, is to provide more with less and maintain quality service. Computerizing housekeeping operations will be of major assistance in meeting this challenge.

Revenue Production

Housekeeping could become a revenue-producing department by offering consultancy services or by contracting with other health care facilities, such as nursing homes, clinics, and physician's offices, to provide cleaning services.

New Services

The nursing shortage is still going to be a major problem in the decades ahead. Alternate methods of providing patient support services will have to be considered. Some hospitals have given housekeeping employees new duties or created a new job classification that encompasses housekeeping, food service, and nurse's aide responsibilities. Employees with this classification might

- clean patient rooms
- make the beds of ambulatory patients
- deliver patient meals, ice water, and snacks
- provide assistance to those patients who need help eating

- provide patient support supplies
- assist in orienting family members to the hospital

According to one hospital that has given housekeeping employees expanded responsibilities, the benefits include

- cleaner units
- increased patient satisfaction with all support services
- the development of matrix management relationships (housekeeping employees were treated as integral members of the nursing staff)
- increased job satisfaction for housekeeping employees, increased personal and professional esteem, and higher wages
- personalized, hotellike service for the patients

The hospital made the necessary changes without increasing the hospital budget.

Medical Waste

Medical waste is becoming more and more difficult to dispose of. Federal and state laws are becoming more restrictive and now require documentation of how waste material is handled.

Legislators at all levels are demanding waste reduction. They want less going into landfills and at the same time they want to allow less incineration. And although there is a general trend toward recycling, consumers of recycled material have concerns about items coming from hospitals because of possible contamination.

In most hospitals, the housekeeping department is responsible for the handling of waste, and therefore the director must be knowledgeable about the waste stream. Normally there are five definite types of hazardous waste that health care facilities must deal with: (1) chemical waste, (2) infectious waste, (3) chemotherapeutic waste, (4) radioactive waste, and (5) sharps.

Hospitals and other medical facilities must monitor and control the movement of these wastes, define the locations where they are produced, and use appropriate methods for disposal (as outlined in local and federal regulations).

Customer Relations

Service is not *a* competitive edge, it is *the* competitive edge.

In their book *Service America*, Karl Albrecht and Ron Zemke make the point about service strategies:

> Factors like cleanliness, attractive physical surroundings, and the flavor of food often do not qualify as elements of a service strategy. If the customer expects you to have a clean hospital, you get no bonus points for cleanliness; you only get demerits if it is not clean. In such a case, cleanliness is a minimum requirement to complete, not a strategy element. If all the other hospitals are dirty, then cleanliness might offer a competitive edge. If the other hospitals are clean, yours had better be clean, too.[26]

Hospitals are no longer the only providers of health services. During the eighties, outpatient clinics, ambulatory surgical centers, walk-in emergency centers, and home health services came into vogue, and all of them compete with hospitals. As a result, hospitals have begun to question their service ethics. Each hospital is now more concerned about perceptions of its services. What are the perceptions of the patients and of others who come in contact with the hospital? How do the employees of the hospitals behave toward the various clients? How do the employees treat each other?

If a hospital is going to improve its guest relations, it needs to know what the internal relations are. All departments including housekeeping must be involved in programs to enhance the manner in which services are provided. Housekeepers are very visible in the hospital, coming in contact with everyone who enters the hospital regardless of the time of day. Therefore, they are important members of the guest relations program. When dealing with patients, they must, for example, knock, state that they work in housekeeping, and introduce themselves when entering patients' rooms; use patients' names when speaking to them; refrain from making negative comments about the facility or staff members; offer assistance whenever they can provide it; and follow up on service requests or inform the requestors if there is to be any delay.

Education and Training

Housekeeping directors will be expected to complete a higher education. In most instances, the minimum requirement will be a bachelor's degree, coupled with 1–5 years of experience in a hospital setting, depending on the size of the recruiting hospital.

Housekeeping directors need to have good employee relations skills and be team builders. They will also have to be capable of training employees in basic housekeeping procedures and of educating them about right-to-know laws, hazardous waste, the American Disabilities Act, and other relevant topics.

Continuing education will also be needed so that the directors will be able to stay abreast of the ever-changing regulations and new developments in the science of management.

ADDITIONAL RESOURCES

Organizations

National Executive Housekeepers Association, Suite 301, 1001 Eastwind Drive, Westerville, OH 43081. 614\895-7166; FAX 614\895-1248.

Environmental Management Association, 4350 Dipalo Center, Suite C, Dearlove Road, Glenview, IL 60025. 708\699-6362.

American Society for Healthcare Environmental Services, American Hospital Association, 840 North Lake Shore Drive, Chicago, IL 60611. 312\280-6245.

Periodicals

Cleaning Times, International Sanitary Supply Association, 7373 North Lincoln Avenue, Lincolnwood, IL 60646.

Books

Albrecht, K., and R. Zemke, *Service America.* Homewood, Ill.: Dow Jones-Irwin, 1985.

Applebaum, S., and W.F. Rohns. *Time management for health care professionals.* Gaithersburg, Md.: Aspen Publishers, 1981.

Feldman, E.B. *Housekeeping handbook for institutions, business and industry.* Hollywood, Fla.: Frederick Fell, 1982.

Griffin, W.R. *The complete custodial handbook.* Englewood Cliffs, N.J.: Prentice-Hall, 1989.

Hazardous-infectious waste management for hospitals and health care facilities. Torrance, Calif.: American Environmental Systems, 1985.

Housekeeping procedure manual. Chicago: American Hospital Association, 1984.

Housekeeping staffing methodology. Ottawa, Ontario: Health Services Directorate, 1985.

Housekeeping workload measurement system. Ottawa, Ontario: Minister of Supply and Services, 1985.

Infection control in the hospital. Chicago: American Hospital Association, latest edition.

Miller, C.B. *How to organize and maintain an efficient hospital housekeeping department.* Chicago: American Hospital Association, 1991.

Safety guide for health care institutions. Chicago: American Hospital Association, 1988.

NOTES

1. C.B. Miller, *How To Organize and Maintain an Efficient Hospital Housekeeping Department* (Chicago: American Hospital Association, 1991),1.

2. Ibid., 1.

3. E.B. Feldman, *Housekeeping Handbook for Institutions, Business and Industry* (Hollywood, Fla.: Frederick Fell, 1982), 13.

4. M. Chase, *Housekeeping Management for Health Care Facilities,* rev. ed. (New York: Catholic Hospital Association, 1978), 17.

5. Ibid., 18.

6. Feldman, *Housekeeping Handbook,* 15.

7. American Hospital Association, *Infection Control in the Hospital,* 4th ed. (Chicago: American Hospital Association, 1989), 67.

8. Feldman, *Housekeeping Handbook for Institutions,* 363.

9. Miller, *How To Organize and Maintain an Efficient Hospital Housekeeping Department,* 6.

10. Ibid., 73.

11. Ibid., 73.

12. Ibid., 74.

13. V.K. Omochonu, *The Quality and Productivity Management in Health Care Organizations* (Milwaukee: American Society for Quality Control, Norcross, Ga.: Industrial Engineering and Management Press, 1991).

14. Feldman, *Housekeeping Handbook for Institutions,* 315.

15. Ibid., 315–316.

16. H. Kendrick, Effective Inventory Control, *Executive Housekeeper Today,* August 1990, pp.2–6.

17. Ibid., 2–6.

18. Ibid., 2–6.

19. Ibid., 4–5.

20. H. Kendrick, Quality Assurance—A Case in Point, *Executive Housekeeper Today,* May 1983, pp. 4–5.

21. C. Richards, What a Quality Assurance Program Will Do for Your Housekeeping Department, *Executive Housekeeper Today,* June 1988, p.5.

22. Ibid., 5.

23. R.J. Gibler, Improving Quality Control, *Executive Housekeeper Today,* May 1987, p. 5.

24. Ibid., 5.

25. P.A. Johnson, Improving Housekeeping Performance with Computers, *Executive Housekeeper Today,* August 1990, pp. 8, 10.

26. K. Albrecht and R. Zemke, *Service America* (Homewood, Ill.: Dow Jones-Irwin, 1985), 72.

Allan McLean
Fredrick G. Roll

Safety and Security

25

Purpose: The purpose of safety and security is to allow patients, visitors, physicians, associated health care workers, and others using the health care facility to deliver and receive quality services in an environment where unsafe conditions and practices are minimized and where they need not be unduly concerned about intrusive, threatening, or illegal acts directed toward their person or property.

INTRODUCTION

The terms *safety* and *security* are closely linked. Safety involves activities designed to minimize injury or harm resulting from hazardous practices or conditions. Security involves protection of people and property from the unlawful acts of others. Both are aimed at minimizing risks—either the risk of personal injury or the risk of losing or damaging property. While the nature and level of risks faced by health care institutions varies widely and are influenced by a host of factors, the following principles of safety and security management are widely applicable:

- Health care institutions have a special obligation to protect patients and others who, because of their illness, infirmity, age, or other factors, may be especially vulnerable to hazards or breaches of security.

- Risks are inherent in all areas of activity. Each department and service must be responsible for anticipating, identifying, and controlling risks in their own areas of work.

- Hazards are conditions that can lead to harm or loss. Hazards are predictable, can be identified, and can be minimized or eliminated. Health and environmental hazards, such as infectious or contaminated materials and waste, should be monitored and controlled.

- Training is required to help people identify risks and hazards and to alter behavior or conditions necessary to minimize personal injury or loss of property.

- Property is susceptible to damage, loss, theft, and misappropriation. These risks can be minimized through well designed systems of documentation, accountability, security, and verification.

- People and property are susceptible to the risks of accident, fire, and natural disaster. These risks should be anticipated and appropriate preparations and responses should be planned and rehearsed.
- All accidents and incidents should be reported and their cause and implications documented.
- The institution and its directors, agents, and employees should be protected from the financial implications of risk through an appropriately designed program of insurance. (See Chapter 26 for more on risk management and insurance.)

While safety and security activities are often managed together, the current trend in health care is toward separation, as both disciplines are becoming more specialized.

SAFETY

Safety management might well be founded on the same injunction given to physicians in the Hippocratic Oath—*Primum non jacere* (first, do no harm). As with medicine's growing stress on preventive and primary health care, safety management emphasizes prevention rather than cure.

Historical Development

Over time, the field of safety management has expanded its focus from a primary concern with the safety of buildings and equipment to a broader concern with the entire physical environment in which care and therapy take place.

Among the first regulations in health care were building safety and fire codes. Early life safety codes regulated the exiting from buildings and set standards for construction methods and building design for health care facilities.

Later regulation by government agencies and private regulatory agencies was limited to listing generally applicable "safety rules," usually based on well-publicized incidents or individual regulatory agency perspectives. These lists of rules and requirements grew longer over time until the regulatory burden became difficult to manage. In addition, many of the rules did not seem particularly effective.

Because of changes in the health care climate, including demands for more accountability and quality, the standards and regulations have had to change as well. There is a trend toward performance-oriented safety standards and monitoring the outcomes of the various safety program activities.

The role of groups such as the Joint Commission on Accreditation of Healthcare Organizations, the National Fire Protection Association, and other professional organizations and government agencies has increased, both in terms of the number of regulations and standards and the range of health care activities now regulated. Regulations and recommendations cover inpatient and outpatient operations, long-term care, psychiatric care, community mental health, home health care, hospices, and other areas.

Current Expectations

Safety management is now recognized as being as important as quality assurance and risk management in continuously improving the quality of the health care environment. Safety is an organization-wide responsibility that depends on constant evaluation of the overall environment in which health care and therapy take place.

Safety programs and activities are becoming performance based. It is now expected that institutions will set goals and measure progress toward those goals. Goals are generally based on regulatory expectations or an acceptable level of risk balanced by available resources. To ensure continuous incremental improvements, safety programs should be designed to ratchet up the standards or benchmarks as they are achieved. Goal setting should take into account the experience of the organization and not simply the number of accidents reported in the past. In many well-run organizations, especially smaller ones, there are no longer enough accidents to base predictions on. Evaluation of the effectiveness of the various elements requires specific data to be gathered.

External demands for greater safety are increasing. Government regulation of safety once had minimal impact on most hospitals, because the Occupational Safety and Health Administration (OSHA) standards were primarily industry based. However, bloodborne pathogens and laboratory standards are now a focus of attention by OSHA. Standards for handling biohazardous materials and wastes, standards for laboratory handling of hazardous chemicals, and guidelines for handling cytotoxic (antineoplastic) drugs also impact on internal hospital activities.

Enforcement of regulations is also increasing, and OSHA is looking more carefully at all areas of health care. Once considered not to need special attention, health care is being held to new and higher standards.

At the same time, the government and consumers want higher quality health care at lower cost to patients and insurers. The new expectation that quality will be measured has led to the creation of a number of methods to define and monitor quality. The same methods are being used by safety departments to measure their effectiveness.

Widespread publicity regarding medical wastes has caused concern and drawn regulatory attention, even though there has been little actual evidence of a public health hazard. Because of this publicity and OSHA's bloodborne pathogen standards, a new, expensive waste disposal industry has come into existence. Furthermore, given the increasingly tight standards for air quality, most hospital incinerators will be unable to handle infectious or biohazardous wastes, and waste disposal costs will increase.

In addition, more attention is being given to the sewage effluent from health care organizations, and some materials that have traditionally been treated as sewage may no longer be accepted, again pushing up disposal costs. While technological advances may assist in dealing with this problem, the result will still be an increase in the cost of patient care and research.

Finally, staff, visitors, and patients are now more intolerant of unsafe conditions. Traditionally, health care facilities have been considered safe-havens for the sick and injured and quiet, secure places to work. Recent litigation trends indicate that visitors and patients feel entitled to medical and environmental safety. Employees are also better educated about occupational hazards and more aware of the long-term effects. They are therefore demanding more (and more expensive) precautions and modifications to the work environment.

Future Expectations

Safety standards in the future will increasingly be performance based, and skillful monitoring of activities will be used to assess the effect of the safety program. Indicators, both internally developed and regulatorily mandated, will become the primary means of assessment by outside agencies and by the program itself. Assessments will be done more frequently, and the results will be reviewed by the top administrators and the governing body as well as by outside agencies. If expectations are not met, changes will need to be made quickly, not at multiyear intervals.

Monitoring will include more direct measurement of activities and effects, and there will be less reliance on paper-based documentation. Documentation will still be critical, but it will be less easy to fabricate and more dependent on the observation of actual activities. Attendance will no longer be a measure of performance. It will be replaced by methods that assess the benefits or behavior changes resulting from activities.

Training will become ever more important, and the documentation of such training will need to indicate the outcomes: the knowledge gained and the behavior changed. Testing and observation will be used to demonstrate the effectiveness of the training, and evaluation of the content and need for training will become more critical. The goal will be to ensure the best use of training resources, which often represent a substantial expense for a health care facility.

Employee health issues will continue to be a major concern, particularly occupational exposure to a variety of types of hazards. Chemical, radiation, infectious, and pathological materials; trace contamination in the air; ventilation and the quality of outside air brought in for ventilation—all of these issues will need to be addressed. Many current practices will be discontinued or modified to ensure the reduction of health hazards. The hazards themselves will become more subtle and difficult to measure, and thus it will be harder to ensure safe levels. As we learn more about cancer and similar diseases, some currently accepted practices and materials will become unacceptable, and more expensive substitutes will be required.

There will be related concern about the impact of health care facilities on their local environment. The casual assumption that hazardous materials can be safely injected into the atmosphere will be challenged, and use of some chemicals (such as ethylene oxide) may be challenged or complex chemical filters may be required to prevent their release.

The role of information management will expand. Measurement of all kinds of performance will occur more frequently, and by using electronic data collection and evaluation, surveys will be able to focus on organizational and industry-wide outcomes. The definition of indicators of performance will become more critical, and both straightforward and subtle indicators will be developed and mandated for all facilities. These indicators will drive the search for quality improvement, and fixed standards will become more flexible, meaning that the standards will become gradually more difficult to meet.

Elements of an Effective Safety Program

The functions of a safety program include performing activities to ensure safety, collecting data to measure the effectiveness of the activities, and translating the data into useful information for management decision making.

The Safety Officer

The safety officer is the individual responsible for executing the day-to-day tasks of the safety program and achieving the outcomes defined by regulatory intent. Although the position is not necessarily full time, the safety program generally requires more hours than are available because of the scope of the duties.

The safety officer is a staff officer and generally reports to the CEO and, through the CEO, to the governing body. The safety officer should already be trained or receive training in government regulations; national consensus and accreditation standards; safety inspection and survey methods; accident information collection and analysis; training methods; identification and control of recognized hazards and risks in the health care setting, including hazardous materials and hazardous wastes; emergency preparedness, life safety, and fire protection; and identification of operational risks, such as equipment and utility system risks.

Safety Department

The safety department carries out various activities to ensure that the organization has appropriate safety policies and procedures, methods for monitoring and assessing compliance with standards, and methods for reporting information to the appropriate managers.

The size and composition of the department is less critical than the use of effective methods. Some organizations use a safety committee to carry out safety-related activities in lieu of a safety department. Others use other departments to perform the necessary tasks.

Safety Committee

This committee plays a central role in the assurance of safety. To a great extent, it serves as the conscience of the organization. It is charged with reviewing the safety policies and procedures of the organization to determine if they are realistic and in the best interests of the organization, the employees, and the patients. Committee members come from a wide range of disciplines to ensure that key concerns are not overlooked.

All of the information about safety performance, safety problems, identified hazards, and the organization's response to problems and hazards should go through this committee, and its findings and recommendations should go to all levels of management. If any department or person comes between the committee and the CEO and governing body, the safety program may be weakened. Also, great harm can result from sugarcoating the problems and hazards identified by the safety committee. If there is not an effective method for the committee to communicate its concerns and suggestions to the appropriate managers, safety is likely to be jeopardized.

The responsibilities of the safety committee include annual review of the overall safety policies and procedures, the safety policies and procedures for each department, and all training programs (to ensure that they are effective and that the training is appropriate to the needs of the organization). The committee also receives reports of accidents and incidents of all kinds (including errors or failures in use of equipment or utility systems, security incidents, and hazardous material or waste problems) and critiques of drills of emergency preparedness plans.

The safety committee shares information with other organization-wide monitoring programs such as quality assurance, infection control, and risk management programs. It uses this information to evaluate the safety program, to prioritize the use of the organization's resources in order to correct the most critical problems and control the most serious risks, and to monitor the effectiveness of training and other corrective programs and various departmental activities.

Quarterly Report

In order to organize and share information, reports should be prepared for middle and upper man-

agement on a quarterly basis. This schedule allows the identification of useful trends, permits timely responses to identified problems, and provides opportunities to take corrective action if the responses are not sufficient.

The quarterly reports should be provided, at least in summary form, to the top administrators and the governing body so that they are aware of the most serious problems identified and the effectiveness of the safety program. The information is also critical for all levels of management, particularly where it might have an impact on operations and decisions. Ideally it should be presented in a format that allows managers to understand their problems and successes and to make the changes necessary for improvements in areas for which they are responsible.

The Safety Cycle

Any effective safety program can be defined by a basic conceptual model, sometimes called a safety cycle. (The concept of a cycle is incorporated in most management methods.) The cycle is ongoing, but, for purposes of understanding, we will assume it begins with information collection and problem identification. The second step is analysis and prioritization. The third step, corrective action, involves changing the work environment and the behavior of people. The final step involves monitoring and evaluating the results of the corrective changes to ensure they have solved the problem or to identify where they have failed. This information then becomes input for a new information collection and problem identification phase, and the cycle begins again. The prioritization of problems to be dealt with is particularly critical, since the resources of any organization (time, enthusiasm, money, and staff attention) are limited. Focusing on those problems that have the greatest negative impact is the best, most cost-effective strategy.

Information Collection

There are several basic sources of information for the identification of problems. The most traditional consists of accident and incident data. Although these data represent safety system failure, they are nonetheless important to collect and analyze. In effective systems, the trend is to collect more data about the less severe incidents. It has long been understood that accident data can be conceived of as points on a probability table, and the more points, the more accurate the predictions of the types and locations of future incidents.

The second traditional source of data is surveillance (safety inspections and surveys). Ideally, accident-producing situations can be identified and corrected prior to an injury or loss. Gathering information through surveillance is useful in two ways. First, the information can be used to predict accidents. Second, the process of data collection can be used to train managers how to discover unsafe conditions in their areas of responsibility.

A wide variety of other sources of data for accident prediction are currently available but underutilized, including such diverse sources as plant management records, infection control reports, security round reports, and inspections by outside agencies.

Prioritization and Analysis

The analysis phase is one place the safety committee can provide critical guidance. Prioritizing problems may not be simple, but identifying the most critical problems and focusing the energy and attention of the organization on them is one of the best ways to achieve quality improvement and increase the safety of the environment.

Prioritization and analysis should be based on criteria that reflect both safety and larger institutional interests. Criteria might be developed around the following issues: extent of potential injury or damage, probability of injury or damage, liability or financial exposure (risk), nature of corrective action, cost of corrective action, and other areas of concern.

Corrective Action

Corrective action involves changing the work environment or changing the behavior of people. Envi-

ronmental changes, such as installing guards or putting needle collection containers near use sites, have been the mainstay of safety management for decades, and they are often effective. Once done, they increase safety as long as they are not reversed.

Modifying behavior is also a workable tactic, but it is generally less reliable. Once persons are trained, they still have to be supervised to ensure they continue to do things the "right" way. However, because changing physical conditions is becoming more difficult (hazards are more subtle and difficult to guard against), training will take on a greater importance. It has long been recognized that most accidents are partly due to unsafe conditions and partly due to an unsafe act. Traditional safety techniques attempt to identify unsafe conditions and acts and to correct them both. Recently, the focus has narrowed, and the emphasis is on preventing unsafe acts. Training is the general method, but training requires a major investment in resources, especially if it is to be effective.

Monitoring and Evaluation

The key to safety program effectiveness is the monitoring of outcomes. Feedback is needed for an activity to ensure that the activity is on track. One traditional feedback measure has been the number of accidents that occur. However, this measure has several shortcomings. First, it depends on the injury of people, rather like the destructive testing of a piece of chain. The weak link is identified, but the chain is useless. Breaking chains may be acceptable, but allowing people to be injured is not. Second, gathering accident data is a slow process, since accidents usually do not occur with great frequency. This means problems will take a long time to identify.

More effective methods for monitoring safety activities include the use of available information from other sources, such as safety rounds, focused surveys, questionnaires and interviews, infection control reports, and plant maintenance reports.

One technique used in quality assurance—identifying specific indicators and establishing baseline

benchmarks or thresholds for acceptable performance—is very effective for evaluating the safety
program.

Employee Health

Because of the increased interest in the long-term
effects of occupational exposures and because of a
number of mandated safety regulations, employee
health is receiving greater attention. Once seen as
first-aid units, employee health departments are
now branching out into monitoring for exposures to
occupational health hazards and chemical contami-
nants in the workplace, exposures to radiation
(nonionizing as well as x-ray and radioactive materials), ergonomics (repetitive trauma disorders such
as carpal tunnel syndrome), substance abuse, and a
wide range of other health-related areas.

It has become well accepted that in the next decade occupational health will become as important
as more traditional safety concerns were during the
seventies and eighties. Many organizations are hiring industrial hygienists to complement their safety
staff and have begun aggressive programs to investigate occupational exposure to commonly used
chemicals. In addition, government regulatory
agencies (such as OSHA) regularly add chemicals
to their warning lists and reduce permissible exposure levels of known hazardous materials. More
sensitive monitoring methods, new technology, and
wider employee education have expanded awareness of hazardous materials from the few traditional, well-recognized chemicals.

Some regulations require medical surveillance or
preassignment physicals. For example, staff members who need to wear respiratory equipment (res-
pirators, gas masks, self-contained breathing equipment) must undergo a medical examination prior to
starting the assignment even if the equipment will
be rarely used (e.g., only in emergencies). Staff
members exposed to specific chemical hazards,
such as ethylene oxide or formaldehyde, will have
to be subjected to medical surveillance if overex-
posed on the job or exposed to unknown levels during an emergency. Staff members exposed to asbes-

tos also need to be included in specific, mandated
medical surveillance programs. As regulations become tighter, more and more employees will fall
into the exposed or potentially exposed categories.

Hazardous Materials and Waste

Hazardous materials programs are structured to
meet regulatory requirements of "right to know" and
"hazard communications" standards set by government agencies. There are several elements that need
to be in any such program. It should also be noted that
hazardous materials programs and hazardous waste
programs are inherently different, and most health
care organizations must have both types of programs.

Hazardous Materials Programs

The first task of a hazardous materials program is
to identify all hazardous chemical materials in the facility and all that are being ordered. The end result of
this investigation is an inventory list of materials categorized by department or physical area. This inventory list becomes the cornerstone of the program.

Once the materials are known, the next step is to
ensure that a materials safety data sheet (MSDS) or
the equivalent is available for each material on the
inventory list. If an MSDS is not in the facility, it
must be requested from the supplier or vendor.
Copies of the MSDSs should be readily available to
employees, either in the department or in an always
accessible location well known to all employees.

Materials must be labeled to ensure that users
know the contents and can consult the appropriate
MSDSs if they have further questions. In general, the
labels materials arrive with are adequate, but if materials are transferred into other containers for use or
ease of handling, those containers must be labeled.
Excepted from this rule are containers used and emp-
tied within a single shift by the same person, such as
mop buckets, graduates, and similar containers.

All employees should receive some training in
the use of hazardous materials, and employees who
typically use these materials should receive special-

ized training. The basic training should be included in the orientation for new employees, and refresher training should be included in an annual safety in-service. The basic training should give orientees some understanding of the hazardous materials program and should inform them who is responsible for maintaining the program and how to get copies of the MSDSs. The programs for users need to include specifics about the hazards of the chemicals they will use or come into contact with.

These programs should be monitored for effectiveness. Such monitoring can be done through inspections, review of records, and observation of staff in action. For example, it might be worthwhile to review the inventory process to make sure all materials are included and an MSDS exists for each of them, to observe staff to make sure they are using proper personal protection, and to inspect chemical materials to make sure they are adequately labeled.

Hazardous Waste Programs

Hazardous waste programs are related to hazardous materials programs but are concerned with different regulations and cover a wider variety of materials. In general, hazardous waste must be separated from ordinary waste, and each type must be segregated and handled in a way that reflects its hazards. Specific disposal protocols often must be followed, and the methods of handling and the locations must be documented for legal purposes.

There are several categories of hazardous waste that must be considered:

- Infectious (medical) waste. This category includes materials that contain or may contain bloodborne pathogens and other infectious materials (as defined by infection control specialists).
- Sharps. These are a special subset of infectious waste and are handled similarly, except that they should be collected in special puncture-resistant containers and handled in such a way as to minimize the chance of a puncture or laceration injury.

- Chemotherapeutic waste. Chemotherapeutic (antineoplastic or cytotoxic) waste can cause cancer and thus must be separated and destroyed using specific protocols defined by OSHA.
- Chemical waste. Chemical waste (as defined by the EPA) must be collected and usually removed by a licensed chemical disposal contractor.
- Radioactive waste. Radioactive waste is among the most regulated of hazardous materials, and its handling and disposal are explicitly determined by the license for use. In general, low-level radioactive materials are handled according to the regulations of the state in which they are licensed.

Policies and procedures for the collection, transport, storage prior to disposal, and disposal of each type of hazardous material present in the health care facility must be devised and followed. These should be reviewed annually by the safety committee to verify they remain appropriate, and the actual handling and disposal should be monitored at least quarterly to ensure that materials are being dealt with in accordance with the approved procedures.

Documentation of the handling of hazardous materials is critical. The facility must be able to establish that legal requirements are being met and that all handling is being done in a manner that protects both the employees and the community. Licenses and manifest documents are often required, and these must be maintained to provide legal protection and to prevent harmful public disclosures and bad publicity.

Monitoring and Evaluating Safety Programs

Monitoring and evaluating all areas of a safety program is critical for ensuring effectiveness. Feedback allows the safety manager to check that the message has gotten through and that everyone is doing what needs to be done. Formal methods of monitoring and evaluating programs are being mandated by more and more regulatory bodies.

Developing specific items to be monitored and objective performance levels will make understanding the role of safety management easier for all managers and will assist in defining what middle managers must do to meet upper management's expectations.

In general, monitoring is done by selecting specific objective, quantifiable features or aspects that reflect the overall quality of the program being evaluated. The next step is to define where the data are to come from and how they can be collected. The data may already exist as a subset of previously collected information, or they may have to be gathered during routine inspections and surveys or by observing staff behavior.

Once the data are collected, the evaluation phase begins. Generally, data are collected over a predetermined period of time, such as a month, a quarter, or a year. The data are then reviewed, ranked, sorted, and processed to determine the performance level. That level is compared to predetermined thresholds or benchmarks set by the organization or outside agencies. If the performance level is acceptable, no further action may be needed. If it is less than acceptable, some programmatic changes will probably need to be made. Continuous quality improvement efforts may also indicate that threshold levels could reasonably be raised to provide motivation for improvements in service.

All areas of the safety program should be examined. However, some areas have historically been of special concern and should receive special attention. These include the following:

- Hazardous materials and waste. Special attention should be paid to training, MSDSs, and labeling so that staff know what to do and have the necessary information available in an emergency.
- Emergency preparedness. An evaluation of the disaster plan should be done after each incident or drill and should include all areas of the plan, not just those involved in the incident or drill.
- Fire safety preparedness. Staff members' knowledge of their proper role in a fire emergency has proved to be one of the critical factors contributing to patient survival. Making certain that medical and service staff know what to do and where to go is very important.
- Fire response. Measurement of staff knowledge and behavior during fire drills and actual fire incidents is related to fire safety preparedness and is equally important.
- Management of patient care equipment. Patient care equipment must be tested regularly and kept in working order.
- Operation of utilities and emergency power. Methods are needed to ensure that errors and failures are effectively responded to.

Information gathered from evaluating these areas needs to be shared with department and service managers, senior management, the governing body, and other organization-wide monitoring programs, such as the quality assurance program.

Resource Requirements

The perception of safety as one of the engineer's responsibilities was due to the early emphasis on fire and life safety and on the safety of buildings and grounds. Recent changes in expectations make it clear that safety is a primary management responsibility. Among other things, this means new safety management methods and techniques are required.

Top Management Support and Participation

Safety has only recently been recognized as an organization-wide responsibility. The entire obligation to manage safety was often shifted to staff safety officers, but experience has shown that any safety program is more effective if senior management and the chief executive officer take a personal interest in it.

Safety Staff Requirements

In this era of lean management and cost consciousness, most safety programs are understaffed. The traditional ratio of safety staff to other employees (one safety staff member for every 300–500 employees) is rarely found in health care. Although in organizations in which managers really do have responsibility for safety performance, somewhat fewer staff resources are needed, and increased government requirements mean that staffing cannot be ignored. Understaffing has its own costs. An old truism in safety is that "you pay for the program whether you have it or not" (if not, you pay in preventable accidents and injuries and their attendant costs). Inadequate staff support means that some safety responsibilities are not met (which generally shows up during surveys and inspections by outside agencies) or some of the other responsibilities of those doing the safety tasks are not met. With safety responsibilities and expectations expanding, the costs of understaffing will increase.

Computer Support

Given the emphasis placed on collection, processing, and distribution of data, the most critical tool in most safety operations is the computer. Although the computers need not be the most expensive or fanciest available, they are, along with database management and word processing software, among the most cost-effective investments a safety department can make (see Chapter 13 for further discussion of information management).

SECURITY*

The aim of security management in health care is to protect persons and property from undesired and threatening intrusions and losses. Unlike law enforcement, which primarily responds to unlawful acts, security management emphasizes prevention. While security officers must understand the extent of their authorities to enforce rules, regulations, and laws, the bulk of their time is typically devoted to anticipating and limiting potential security problems.

Source: The section on Security is excerpted from *Healthcare Security Management Handbook* with permission of Fredrick G. Roll, © 1992.

In most health care institutions, security services are nonrevenue-producing activities and their value to the organization may be challenged. Security managers must be able to identify the services they provide, their contribution to other departments and services, and their role in helping the institution fulfill its overall mission.

Security's Organizational Role

The history of hospital security is covered in *Hospital Security* by Russell L. Colling.[1] Colling traces the lineage of hospitals back to twelfth-century England. The first designated managerial position in security was the "office of the porter," and the "beadles" acted as stationary guards.

Security management in the United States has developed in several stages. In the period 1900–1950, protective duties (e.g., watch rounds and fire watch) were performed by maintenance personnel. There is little mention of designated security personnel. In the 1950s, there was a shift from fire watch to law enforcement, and police officers began to work in hospitals in larger communities. The 1960s saw the beginning of the security management era, and the range of protective duties expanded beyond dealing only with illegal activities.

In the late 1970s, security and safety management began to join together, and managers became more recognized. Finally, in the decade just past, security began to have an even more expanded role in the hospital environment. There was a greater emphasis on the protection of assets and greater demand for flexibility and interaction with other team players.[2] During the 1990s, the trend toward the application of professional management concepts and team interventions is expected to continue.

The overall role of security is to provide a secure and safe environment. Public law enforcement is deemed responsible for the enforcement of laws enacted to protect the general public. Because this is a very broad responsibility, law enforcement usually devotes its resources to responding to criminal activities that have already occurred. Security services, on the other hand, are usually specific to a single organization, and their primary function is to prevent incidents from occurring. They are concerned not only with the breaking of laws but also with breaches of the organization's rules, regulations, and policies. Laws may be enforced, but under the same authority vested in any private citizen. Police officers should still be called upon to deal with public law violations.

Table 25-1 lists some of the differences between security and law enforcement. Table 25-2 compares the two in terms of the total number of personnel and dollars expended annually. The trend is toward a greater role for private security programs, and thus law enforcement personnel will rely on institutions such as hospitals to assume more responsibility for their own security and the protection of their staff and clientele.

Hospital security must first focus on the protection of persons, then on the protection of property. Its safeguarding responsibilities encompass patients, physicians, staff, visitors, and others as well as their personal property and the assets of the hospital. In some larger and more sophisticated hospital security departments, security staff may also be involved in in-depth investigations of computer fraud or loss of financial assets. For the most part, however, hospital security is oriented toward prevention. This orientation requires the security department to identify incidents that might have an adverse financial impact upon the hospital, including injuries or deaths on hospital property as well as theft of or damage to personal or hospital property.

Prevention is usually accomplished through the use of "preventive patrols." These patrols allow

Table 25-1 Comparison of Security and Law Enforcement

Security	Law Enforcement
Loss prevention	Loss recovery
Protection of specific clients	Protection of the general public
Enforcement of rules and regulations	Enforcement of laws
Prevention of crimes	Apprehension of criminals
Proactive	Reactive

uniformed security officers to maintain high visibility and to verify that conditions are as they should be. The intent is that the high visibility of the officers will deter someone contemplating the commission of a criminal act. The patrols also give the officers the opportunity to discover such things as a stuck door that might allow unauthorized access or a cracked water pipe that might eventually cause serious damage. No matter how sophisticated electronic security systems become, there will always be a need for security officers to go on patrol and respond to problem situations.

Vulnerability in Health Care Institutions

For the past several years, the International Association for Healthcare Security and Safety has been conducting crime surveys on hospital-related crimes. It is evident from the surveys that hospitals are not the sanctuaries they once were. Patients are usually in a

Table 25-2 Summary of Private Security and Law Enforcement Employment and Expenditures, 1980–2000

Year	Private Security Employment (millions)	Law Enforcement Employment (millions)	Total Protective Services Employment (millions)	Private Security Expenditures (billions)	Law Enforcement Expenditures (billions)	Total Expenditures (billions)
1980	1.0	0.6	1.6	$20	$14	$34
1990	1.5	0.6	2.1	$52	$30	$82
2000	1.9	0.7	2.6	$103	$44	$147

Source: Reprinted from *The Hallcrest Report II* by Cunningham, Strauchs, and Van Meter, p. 229, with permission of Hallcrest Systems Inc., © 1990.

vulnerable condition; hospitals have large supplies of items useful to the general public, including food, clothing, computers, and drugs; and the large number of female employees working various hours creates opportunities for sexual assault.

The surveys indicate that all types of crime do in fact occur in hospitals, including homicide, rape, arson, kidnapping, armed robbery, assault, and theft. In one highly publicized homicide, a female physician was brutally raped and murdered by a homeless vagrant while working in her research laboratory at Bellevue Hospital in New York in 1989. The offender was discovered to have actually lived in a machinery area of the hospital for over a month prior to the murder. Infant kidnappings are also on the increase. From 1983 to January 1992 there were 116 successful or attempted abductions from U.S. health care facilities.

Although the numbers and percentages of the crimes vary, hospitals in all geographical settings, from inner city to rural, reported criminal incidents. Furthermore, the perpetrators ranged from employees to patients to persons off the street. Obviously, security management and administrative personnel need to analyze the security risk at their facilities and take appropriate action.

It is difficult to identify in terms of dollars how much property is stolen or misappropriated in hospitals, since many thefts and incidents go undetected or unreported. Hospital-owned property loss is estimated to be between $2,000 and $3,000 per bed per year on average. Assuming the average is $2,500 per year, a 300-bed hospital would lose $750,000 annually. The theft of patient property, in addition to the dollar loss, has a tremendous impact on patient relations, and the theft of employee property negatively affects employee morale.

Assaults, thefts, kidnappings, and other crimes have led to an epidemic of legal actions against hospitals based on charges of inadequate security, including lack of security, insufficient numbers of security personnel, untrained security personnel, poor security management practices, failure to meet perceived national or community standards, and failure to foresee criminal activity. Hospitals must meet the

public's expectation that they offer a caring and protected environment. The difficulty of meeting this expectation is complicated by the fact that health care dollars are becoming increasingly tighter and security services are becoming more costly to maintain.

In fairness, however, most security problems in health care institutions are not as dramatic or as devastating as kidnapping, murder, rape, or armed robbery. A security service is likely to devote most of its time and resources to tasks such as assessing security risks, conducting security patrols, controlling traffic, assessing and addressing the risks of theft and pilferage, and advising on methods to control internal fraud and pilferage.

Security Programs and Structure

Security programs differ in size and complexity depending on the type of health care institution. The Joint Commission for Accreditation of Healthcare Organizations states that each hospital must provide a security management program that meets its specific needs. In other words, in a small rural hospital, the program might consist of maintenance personnel who lock and unlock doors at certain hours; small problems are handled by staff members and larger ones by the local law enforcement agency. So long as the program meets the needs of the facility and there is documentation that the program has been reviewed and is viable, it will be deemed an adequate security program. Some small hospitals will supplement such a minimal program with onsite security personnel for after-hour coverage. Figures 25-1, 25-2, and 25-3 present organizational security models for organizations of different sizes.

The organizational reporting level of formal hospital security programs also varies. In some large multifacility organizations, a vice-president for security operations heads the program, and there are individual managers at each facility. In most medium to large hospitals, there is a director or manager of security who usually reports to an assistant administrator responsible for several ancillary departments. In most cases, the manager of security is

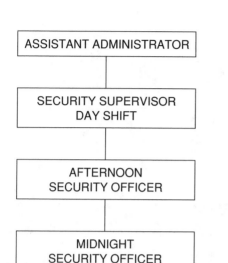

Figure 25-1 Sample Organization Chart for a Small Security Department

large hospital, especially if it is located in an urban area, security is a major responsibility requiring the manager's full attention.

At one time, security was thought of as a responsibility of the physical plant department, and security personnel reported to the plant manager. As security problems have become more complex and the responsibilities have become greater, this type of minimal program exists only in relatively small facilities.

The important point to remember is that security operations are intended to enforce rules, regulations, policies, and laws and to safeguard the institution from financial loss. Rule enforcement and protection from loss are basically administrative duties, and the security department acts as the administration's agent. Therefore, the security department should, when possible, report to someone in the administrative hierarchy who understands the importance of security and can take appropriate administrative actions as needed.

The interdepartmental relationships of the security program are also very important. As previously

considered to be at the department head level. The manager might have other areas of responsibility, such as parking, safety, and transportation, but in a

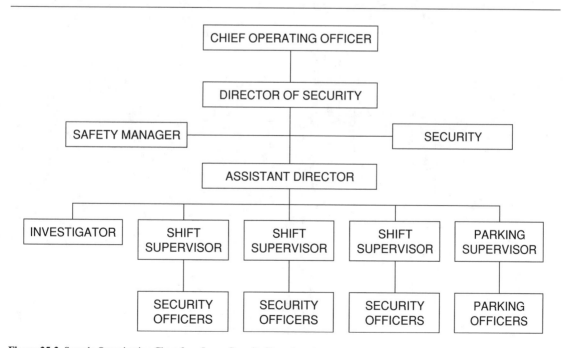

Figure 25-2 Sample Organization Chart for a Large Security Department

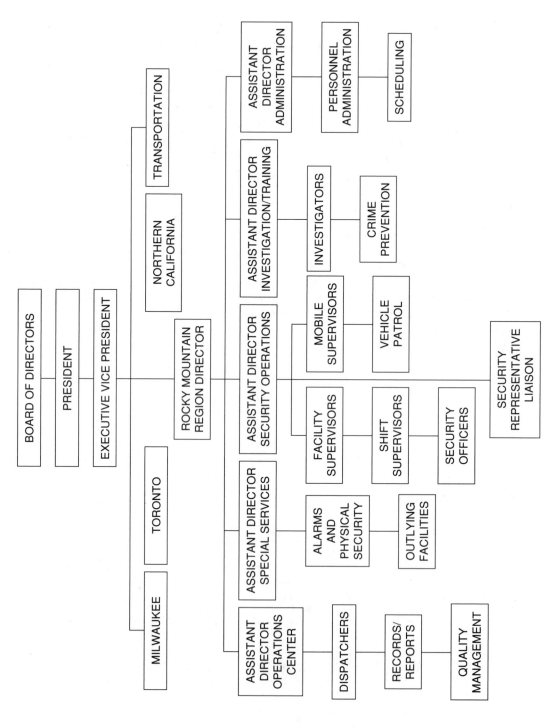

Figure 25-3 HSSC Organization Chart

mentioned, security is the responsibility of every unit within a hospital. Staff members must take an active role in protecting persons and property within their work area. At a minimum, this might involve contacting a security officer when a suspicious person is seen and securing personal and hospital property to avoid theft.

The security program must establish close relationships with the safety, risk management, and quality assurance programs. These latter programs are all involved in loss prevention. In some hospitals, the security program is responsible for dealing with general liability issues, whereas the risk management program focuses on insurance issues and, in conjunction with the quality assurance program, medical malpractice issues. Many security programs also work closely with human resources and employee health departments on such issues as background screening, employee assistance, and substance abuse.

Although a few security departments use sworn law enforcement personnel, most have individuals who possess the same authority as any private citizen. Using such individuals allows for greater flexibility when dealing with interdepartmental issues, since they can be handled administratively and not necessarily legally. There are, however, some advantages associated with law enforcement authority, and these will be discussed later.

Persons who are hospitalized expect that, besides being provided with high-quality services, they will be safe and secure. When incidents such as physical and sexual assault, theft of valuables, infant kidnappings, or even the loss of eyeglasses or dentures occur, there is major disappointment on the part of the patients and the community. The astronomical awards issued in medical malpractice and inadequate security cases indicate the public's view on this matter.

Staff members and physicians also expect a crime-free environment in which they can concentrate on their primary function, patient care. Criminal activity or the sense of a lack of security has a major impact on the productivity and morale of staff members.

On the other hand, security officers are often called upon to perform security-related functions that might offend staff members. These include inspection of packages or lockers, parking enforcement, and enforcement of specific rules, regulations, and policies. In other words, security officers are expected to be helpful public relations representatives on the one hand and private police officers on the other, which does not make their job an easy one.

Security Resources

In the area of human resources, flexibility is probably the most important attribute a security officer or security manager can possess. Hospitals are extremely complex institutions whose activities range from performing high-tech procedures to giving a helping hand. Security personnel must keep in mind public relations while performing enforcement functions. The key is to handle each new situation in an appropriate manner. For example, an officer might be on an exterior patrol at 3:00 A.M. without seeing anything but parked vehicles and locked doors for a long period of time and then be called to the emergency room to confront an uncontrollable patient. The two situations demand substantially different ways of behaving.

Whether the security officers are male or female, young or old, they must give the impression that they can in fact fulfill a security function. Persons in a health care setting will not feel secure if the security officers do not seem competent and self-assured. One factor that can help or hinder is their visual image. Uniforms, whether blazers or traditional uniforms, are a visible sign of authority. Of course, if security personnel wear uniforms, they will frequently be asked for information and directions as well as for help. By answering questions politely and demonstrating concern for people, they can help engender a sense of security and confidence in their ability.

Security managers must also be flexible. They will usually be asked to participate on a number of committees and must be able to communicate the security point of view. Basic management and human relations skills are needed in addition to the ability to enforce policies.

In order to assist security officers, supervisors, and managers, the International Association for Healthcare Security and Safety has developed training guidelines and certification programs. At the present time, the certification standards are the only recognized standards in the health care security field. Exhibit 25-1 contains an outline of the 40-hour security officer's training program. An advanced program is available for security supervisors, leading to the designation of Certified Healthcare Protection Administrator (CHPA). Another prominent general security organization, the American Society for Industrial Security, also offers a management certification program. A manager who completes this program is designated a Certified Protection Professional (CPP). Hospital security managers should be encouraged to attempt certification and should be rewarded if they succeed. Both credentials indicate a high level of professional accomplishment. Since the CHPA and CPP require initial testing and periodic recertification, they also demonstrate continued commitment to the field.

The appropriate number of security personnel for providing security is an important issue in litigation claiming inadequate security. Many people have attempted to devise a method for determining the number based upon bed size, square footage, acreage, number of employees, number of patient days, location of the hospital, and so on. The best way to determine it is to use the results of risk assessment and a review of services rendered by security personnel. The assessment must include such factors as the location of the hospital, the surrounding crime rate, the frequency and severity of past incidents in or near the hospital, the local and community standards, the functions and responsibilities assigned to the security department, as well as the size and complexity of the hospital. The development of a program necessitates a full review of these factors and also periodic reviews to determine if there have been changes that call for an increase or decrease in the number of personnel. More is not necessarily better. The number of personnel might need to be adjusted upward to handle the opening of a new facility or downward if electronic devices are installed that can perform specific tasks. In some cases, security personnel have been assigned numerous ancillary service duties because few serious security incidents have occurred. This may mean that the original security functions are no longer being performed. Periodic reviews will allow for checks on the adequacy of security staffing.

An outside security consultant can assist in conducting such an assessment. An outside consultant will likely have the same orientation as the expert witnesses who would review the security program if litigation were to occur. The consultant's objectivity will be helpful in determining the risk potential under the current staffing plan, and the consultant can make appropriate recommendations to the hospital.

In most proprietary security programs, the security personnel earn wages somewhat above entry-level employees. Contract security agencies often pay their security officers at or slightly above minimum wage. In some institutions this may be appropriate, but in others, unacceptable.

Proprietary versus Contractual Programs

There are several types of security programs, including proprietary, contractual, off-duty law enforcement, and shared service programs. Following is a brief discussion of each.

Proprietary Programs. A proprietary program, a program operated by the institution, offers the institution the ability to directly select and supervise the security employees. Consequently, there is usually adequate training, adequate supervision, and quality control, and the program is more likely to become an integral part of the hospital. On the negative side, high and escalating costs for wages and benefits often result. It is also difficult to terminate substandard officers, and officers may have a harder time enforcing rules against fellow employees. Finally, a proprietary program can make it

Exhibit 25-1 International Association for Healthcare Security and Safety Basic Training Program Curriculum

	No. Hours		No. Hours
Note: Courses marked with an asterisk are elective. Mandatory training of 34 hours must be completed with an additional 6 elective hours required to complete the 40 hour program.			
Introduction to Hospital Security		Physical Security Controls	1*
Hospital Organization	1	Alarms	1*
Security as a Service Organization	1	Equipment Usage/Maintenance	1*
Public and Community Relations	1		
Labor Relations	1	**Hospital Safety and Emergency Preparedness**	
		Functional Safety	2
Developing Communication and Investigative Skills		Fire Prevention	2
Investigations and Interviews	2+1	Fire Control	2
Report Writing	3+2	Bomb Threats	1
Patrol Procedures/Techniques	3	Disaster Control	2
Handling the Disturbed Patient, Visitor, Employee	1	Civil Disturbance	1
Courtroom Procedures	1		
		Security and the Law	
Security's Role in Hospital Operations		Laws of Arrest/Search/Seizure	2
Nursing Units	1	Narcotics and Dangerous Drugs	2
Business Office	1	Law Enforcement Liaison	1*
Pharmacy	1		
Dietary Service	1	**Specialized Skills**	
Ancillary Services	1	Career and Professional Development	1*
		Self-Defense	2*
Protective Measures		Weapons: Use and Handling	2*
Hospital Vulnerabilities	1	Emergency First Aid/Life Saving Techniques	1*
Lock and Key Systems/Access Control	1*		

Source: Courtesy of the Training Committee, International Association For Healthcare Security & Safety, Lombard, Illinois.

more difficult for the hospital to find out about security problems occurring at surrounding hospitals and to be fully prepared to deal with them.

Contractual Programs. Contract security programs are less expensive, since the contractor is responsible for all wages, benefits, insurance, and overhead and the wages and benefits are usually not based upon a hospital scale. The hospital can calculate a fixed annual budget for the program. Also, the personnel burden remains with the contractor, meaning that the hospital can demand replacements for marginal or inadequate officers.

On the downside, contract agencies often pay low wages and benefits and may attract low-quality personnel. There is often inadequate supervision, and the officers may suffer from low morale and confusion about whom they really work for. There is often high turnover, which can result in a lack of proper hospital training. The officers may rotate from hospitals to businesses and have less of a commitment or desire to work in the hospital environment.

Some organizations have found that supplementing proprietary supervisors and key personnel with contract personnel can be effective in providing security. This approach, however, still has some of the difficulties associated with totally contracted programs.

Using Law Enforcement Officers. The number of off-duty police officers providing hospital security functions continues to decline except for some specific applications. The presence of a law enforcement officer was once considered a plus by many hospital administrators. For one thing, these officers have had excellent police training and create a strong security presence. They are also vested with the authority to make certain arrests that a security officer could not make.

Using law enforcement officers does, however, have several negatives. In many cases, law enforcement officers are not willing to perform the vast variety of security functions necessary for full-service security operations. Second, despite being off-duty, they still have an obligation to their oath of office to act in their sworn capacity when they observe certain violations of the law. The actions they take may not always be in the best interest of the hospital. In some instances, however, it may be necessary to use sworn law officers for specific functions, such as directing traffic on a city street, which may not be done by non-law-enforcement personnel.

Shared Services Programs. Another security staffing model gaining popularity is the shared service or hybrid model. In this model, more than one hospital or group of hospitals share the various components of a hospital security program that they could not afford independently. The costs of a quality hospital security manager, supervisors, investigators, communication center, high-tech equipment, and so on, are funded based upon the size, scope, and use of each member hospital. Since the program is restricted to hospitals, the security personnel can develop expertise in hospital security. Because the hospitals (usually through representatives or board members) govern the program, they have a direct method of quality control—similar to the control they would have over an in-house program but without the higher costs.

On the downside, each hospital must give up a certain amount of autonomy for the overall good of the program. (If developed properly, this program operates in the same manner as shared purchasing programs.)

No matter what the type of program, consideration should be given to the use of part-time personnel. By developing a mix of full-time and part-time personnel, adequate and flexible coverage can be maintained while minimizing the use of overtime. The mix would vary, of course, based upon the size and complexity of the security program.

In some hospitals, the security personnel are so-called commissioned law enforcement officers or special police officers. These types of officers generally have the authority to enforce parking regulations under a municipal ordinance but lack full police powers. Some hospitals, however, do have full police authority, which allows the security personnel to enforce laws with the same authority as the local law enforcement officers. This can make it difficult to determine what is an administrative action as opposed to a legal action, and there may also be a problem deciding who holds the final authority in some situations, the chief of police or the chief executive of the hospital.

Security Equipment

There are numerous equipment systems and components available to enhance a hospital security program. It is important to remember that there needs to be a balance between security devices and personnel.

Uniforms. Uniforms allow the security personnel to project a certain image. Traditional police-style uniforms continue to be the most popular, although many facilities are switching to the blazer look. Larger institutions often use a combination: Outside personnel wear a full uniform to create a deterrent effect, whereas inside officers wear blazers to provide a "softer image." The best uniform is one that meets the mission of the security department and the aims of the facility.

Nonprotective Equipment. A two-way radio is often referred to as the most valuable piece of equipment a security officer can have. Two-way radios allow officers to maintain continuous communication while moving about their patrol areas and to summon each other as necessary. The sophistication of radio systems varies tremendously. Features include paging, alarm and telephone interface, and multiple frequency capabilities. Units also come in various sizes. Once the specific purposes are defined, manufacturer representatives can submit proposals to the hospital.

Protective Equipment. There is also the question of the type of protective equipment that should be issued to security personnel. Protective equipment includes nightsticks or batons, handcuffs, chemical gases, electronic stunning devices, and firearms.

The administration of the hospital must evaluate the security risk level and decide if weapons should be issued (and if so, what type). In some institutions, the security personnel were unarmed until there was a significant problem, then armed until there was a problem involving a weapon, then disarmed, and so on.

At this time, there is a national trend toward disarming the majority of security personnel (including security personnel in health care institutions). The general opinion seems to be that carrying firearms can be a greater liability than not carrying them in most settings. However, in some facilities weapons may be essential.

At Hospital Shared Services of Colorado, which provides security coverage for over 50 health care–related facilities in Colorado and Wyoming alone, the percentage of armed personnel is declining. In some facilities where all of the security personnel were once armed, the revised model calls for only one officer to carry a firearm. This allows for better control yet quick response if an armed officer is required.

In any event, the use of firearms, electric stunning devices, chemical gases, handcuffs, batons, and so on, requires complete and documented initial and continued training. The improper use of any weapon will immediately result in the potential of litigation. The training course, the instructor, and the proficiency of users need to be closely scrutinized. Proper documentation of all training is essential.

Security Devices

There are some basic security components that almost any health care facility should consider purchasing, including proper lighting, fences and barriers, and locking devices. These components must be assessed regularly to ensure they are providing the basis for a sound physical security program.

Electronic security components are becoming an integral part of many health care security programs. These components include closed-circuit television, video recorders, electric locks, card control access systems, alarm identification systems, computer systems, and robotics. These components can be used independently or integrated into security packages. For example, if a computer-based physical access system was being used, the system not only could decide if an attempted access was valid but could also activate a closed-circuit camera and time-lapse video recorder to visually document the occurrence. It could also set off an alarm if the access was in fact invalid.

The best use of electronic security systems is to augment the overall security program. This program must consist of sound physical security (i.e., locks, fences, lighting) and adequate security personnel (in quantity and quality). When properly blended, electronic security systems can allow a single security officer at a stationary position to monitor and control a number of access points and vulnerable areas. Combined with alarm monitoring and telephone and radio communications, such systems can increase the cost-effectiveness of the security program.

Some caution, however, is warranted in the area of electronic security. Use of dummy or simulation closed-circuit cameras has led to successful litigation because victims established there were expectations of security that were not fulfilled. Similar types of litigation have also been successful when live cameras were not monitored or had become inoperative. The use of electronic security measures requires careful initial financial consideration, a regular review of the purpose of the installation, and a sound maintenance program.

Quality Management in Safety and Security

Quality management depends on having a quantifiable method of determining the effectiveness of the safety and security program. Different institutions use different methods, but most develop indicators for evaluating specific aspects of service. These indicators would usually be expected to fall within certain thresholds.

In order to identify and analyze aspects of service, safety and security managers should use this six-step process.

1. Identify areas of concern or problems the safety and security department is held accountable for.

2. Analyze each area of concern or problem as it relates to safety and security department services and expectations of performance.

3. Examine all potential methods for dealing with the area of concern or problem.

4. Select the best possible method for addressing the concern.

5. Implement the chosen method.

6. Monitor the implementation and take corrective action as necessary.

By using a format like the one shown in Exhibit 25-2, the safety and security manager will be able to quantify and evaluate departmental actions. Identifying an aspect of service allows the manager to describe intended actions. The manager can then state the objective or rationale, which addresses why the aspect was picked out. The manager then chooses indicators for evaluating the intended actions and lists the indicator thresholds, which set the acceptable parameters for the actions. These should be realistic, achievable goals. The methodology establishes how the evaluation is to be done. Finally, the manager lists sources—documents or sources of information to be consulted for evidence that the goals are being met.

The format in Exhibit 25-2 was used in the quality management program for security services at Baptist Medical Center in Jacksonville, Florida. The same basic format was also used by other departments to identify areas of concern. The reports were given to the Medical Center Quality Assur-

Exhibit 25-2 Monitoring and Evaluation Summary

DEPARTMENT: Safety, Security, and Parking

DATE: August, September, October

ASPECT OF CARE/SERVICE: The Safety, Security, and Parking Department will respond to various emergency situations within two minutes.

OBJECTIVE OR RATIONALE: To insure a prompt response to emergency situations.

INDICATOR(S):	Thresholds for Evaluation
1. Fire responses	95%
2. Intrusion/robbery alarms responses	95%
3. STAT/emergency responses	95%
4. Patient restraint assistance responses	95%

METHODOLOGY (time frame, sample size, staff, how?): Because of the new computerized reporting system, 100% of the incident reports and fire reports are being reviewed on a monthly basis by the Security Supervisor.

DATA SOURCES:
1. Daily activity reports
2. Incident reports

Source: Courtesy of Baptist Medical Center Quality Management Department, Jacksonville, Florida.

ance Committee for consideration. Each major department was required to submit reports on a quarterly basis.

Quality management should not be viewed as extra paper work or filling out forms or pure statistics. It should be utilized to track and monitor ongoing activities within the safety and security department. This will allow the manager and administration to determine the effectiveness of the department as well as pertinent trends. These trends can then be used to help identify corrective actions and strengthen the safety and security program. For example, if security personnel are not responding to emergency calls within the appropriate time and within the thresholds for evaluation, this might be a signal to administration that more personnel are required.

THE FUTURE OF SAFETY AND SECURITY MANAGEMENT

As health care continues to become more sophisticated, it will be essential that each hospital department keep pace, including the safety and security department. The education and integration of the various departments and employees with regard to safety and security issues will become even more essential.

The trend toward increased litigation will continue, and safety and security incidents that occur at hospitals will be closely examined. The competency of security managers and officers will be reviewed by expert witnesses, and the education, experience, training, and certification of managers and officers will be scrutinized.

The following trends (derived from the professional literature, national and regional seminars, and Hospital Shared Services consulting projects) are offered as an indication of what safety and security programs can expect in the future[3]:

- Increased training for all levels of hospital safety and security personnel.

- Increasing involvement of hospital employees, including non-security supervisory personnel, in contributing to the maintenance of safe and secure premises.

- Epidemic levels of litigation concerning safety and security programs.

- More security personnel working in an unarmed capacity.

- A shift from safety and security by providing non-security–related services to a greater emphasis on the basis of "pro-active protection activities."

- A trend toward separating safety and security management as the safety function becomes better defined. Security personnel to continue as being ancillary to the safety function.

- A decrease in the overall use of centralized closed circuit television and a shift to departmental systems.

- Increased use of alarms, computerized card access controls, and integrated security systems.

- A greater awareness by the hospital administrative staff of the need for more loss prevention safeguards to enhance the bottom line.

- Violence in emergency rooms remaining at the high level experienced during the past several years.

- Increasing security budgets despite attempts to supplement security manpower with physical security systems.

- Greater organizational demands on security as law enforcement services continue to diminish.

A specific responsibility of the safety and security manager will be to perform regular and documented risk assessments of the facility. It will become more popular to utilize outside consultants to give objective views of the safety and security risks and make recommendations to be considered by the safety and security manager and hospital administration. Litigation increasingly will be a problem because of reductions in personnel, improper or inadequate training, lack of documentation, not addressing foreseeable crimes or incidents either on hospital premises or surrounding area, not attaining local or national standards for safety and security services, lack of or malfunctioning equipment, lack of policies, and lack of administrative support for the safety and security program.

In the years ahead, a continued emphasis will be placed upon safety and security managers to provide a high-profile enhanced public relations image for the facility. Uniformed security personnel are perceived by the public as administrative agents of the hospital. It will be necessary for the administration and the various departments of a hospital to realize and accept this elevated role within the organization.

Effective liaison with law enforcement agencies will become critical. As the number of law enforcement personnel becomes fewer per capita, security organizations will take on a greater responsibility to provide protective services within their respective organizations. Increased security emphasis will be placed on high-risk areas in health care facilities such as emergency departments, nurseries, psychiatric units, drug and alcohol units, and pharmacies. This will require the security personnel to have a greater understanding of how to deal with people under stress or with those displaying aggressive and assaultive behavior.

A continued and greater emphasis will also be placed on crime prevention efforts. This includes crime prevention materials, handouts, flyers, and posters. Security fairs allowing the security staff to interface with other hospital personnel to gain understanding and support for the security program will become more popular.

Quality management will continue to be a driving force in ensuring that proper documentation is maintained. This facilitates trend analysis and corrective action in problem areas. Along the same line, risk management will ensure that incident forecasting is maintained to avoid unnecessary losses.

With the continued financial strain in health care, loss prevention will become a more important issue in the next decade. Security, safety, risk management, and quality assurance departments must strive together to identify, prevent, and deal with incidents that might result in financial loss.

Colling, H.L. *Hospital Security.* Stoneham, Mass.: Butterworth Publications, 1982.

Cunningham, et al. *The Hallcrest report: Private security trends, 1970–2000.* Stoneham, Mass.: Butterworth-Heinemann, 1990.

Faitz, S., ed. *The healthcare security crisis handbook.* Port Washington, N.Y.: Rusting Publications, 1987.

Hospital safety handbook. Boca Raton, Fla.: CRC Press.

National Fire Protection Association. *Healthcare facilities handbook.* Current ed. Quincy, Mass.: National Fire Protection Association.

National Fire Protection Association. *Life safety code handbook.* Current ed. Quincy, Mass.: National Fire Protection Association.

Purpura, P. *Security and loss prevention.* Stoneham, Mass.: Butterworth Publications, 1984.

Turner, J.T. *Handbook of hospital security and safety.* Gaithersburg, Md.: Aspen Publishers, 1983.

Periodicals

Health Facilities Management, American Hospital Association.

Hospital Security and Safety Management, Rusting Publications, 430 Main Street, Port Washington, NY 11050.

Journal of Healthcare Protection Management, International Association of Healthcare Security and Safety, P.O. Box 637, Lombard, Ill. 60148.

Professional Safety, American Society of Safety Engineers, 1800 East Oakton Boulevard, Des Plaines, Ill. 60018.

ADDITIONAL RESOURCES

Organizations

American Society for Industrial Security.

International Association for Healthcare Security and Safety, P.O. Box 637, Lombard, Ill. 60148.

Books

Cherry, D. *Total facility control.* Stoneham, Mass.: Butterworth Publications, 1986.

NOTES

1. R.L. Colling, *Hospital Security,* 3d ed. (Stoneham, Mass.: Butterworth Publications, 1992), 58–60.

2. J. Richards III and P. Rathbum, *Medical Risk Management* (Gaithersburg, Md.: Aspen Publishers, 1983), 4–5.

3. Colling, *Hospital Security.*

Aaron Liberman

Risk and Insurance Management

26

Purpose: The purpose of risk management is to create and maintain a safe, secure, and properly insured health services environment and to contain the cost of insurance.

INTRODUCTION

In developing the subject of risk management and its capacity to reduce loss due to litigation, one is immediately impressed with the complexity of problems confronting health care organizations and the multiplicity of approaches to control specific risk-producing situations.

With the emergence of modern medical technology, the public has raised its level of expectation so far as the availability of health care services is con-

cerned. Medical care is increasingly viewed as a right rather than a privilege. This new perspective is exerting significant economic and clinical service pressure on health care providers. The public now rightly expects quality care. They similarly expect to receive treatment that parallels the goods and services promised by this society's scientific and technological advancements.

It was not long ago that hospitals were viewed as eleemosynary institutions, and because of the prevailing doctrine of charitable immunity, accountability for quality of care was rarely an issue. In a 1965 landmark case, *Darling vs. Charleston Memorial Hospital,* the court ruled that hospitals, like other corporations, have responsibilities toward their clients.[1] The public sector began to expect more from care providers, and in recent years the public's expectations have impacted the economics of operating health care institutions.

Additionally, patients have come to view health care as a product rather than as a service. This has encouraged many recipients of care to use product liability as a rationale for seeking court relief for actions considered wrongful or injurious.[2] The emphasis on consumer rights and a concomitant move

Portions of this work are based on a previously prepared document authored by Aaron Liberman and published by the Center for Research in Ambulatory Health Care Administration of the Medical Group Management Association, Englewood, Colorado. The original publication was directed toward meeting the needs of individual organizations in establishing risk management programs for medical group practices.

523

toward the normalization of compensatory reimbursement for injuries also encourage litigation.

Although malpractice claims originally constituted a small part of this trend, a cyclical pattern has developed as the number of cases and resulting awards have grown. Moreover, the legal profession now treats health care malpractice and liability as a specialty field, which has increased the number of medical and legal experts versed in this area of the law. It is now much easier for patients to seek judicial relief. Thus, the attendant risks health care organizations would normally experience have been multiplied by favorable court decisions on behalf of litigants. In turn, this has affected the ability of health care organizations to operate as free-standing and independent entities.

To further understand why professional liability claims are occurring, one need only consider this additional fact: Often a liability claim is filed not because of incompetence on the part of a health care provider but because of negative perceptions of the process or personnel who support that health care provider.

The term *risk* can be used to refer to

1. the possibility of loss or injury
2. a dangerous element occurring in a given situation
3. the chance of loss in an insurance contract
4. the degree of probability of such loss
5. the presentation of a person or object that represents a specified hazard to an insurer
6. an insurance hazard from specified cause or source[3]

For purposes of this discussion, the term *risk* shall be considered to refer to the possibility of financial loss due to an unexpected contingency.

Risk management programs have been available for many years in the business world. Industry-wide use of risk management began during the 1950s, although it was not referred to as risk management in the early days.[4] The health field, until recently, only adopted individual components of risk management. The current approach to dealing with risk is much more comprehensive. Indeed, the containment of insurance costs is vital for a hospital's continuing existence as an effective provider of care.

The object of risk management is to reduce or eliminate the potential for financial loss resulting from occurrences of a fortuitous nature. It involves more than the management of malpractice claims, because financial loss due to litigation can result from other aspects of a health care organization's operations.

In the ensuing discussion, legal liability in the health care setting is the primary focus. This chapter also contains practical suggestions for minimizing and in some cases even eliminating the probability of a claim occurring. There is no guarantee, however, that the suggestions will provide solutions for any particular organization. There is and probably always will be great differences among organizations and between their philosophies of treatment and service.

MANAGEMENT PRINCIPLES

The following are key principles in establishing an appropriate program of risk and insurance management:

- Management should establish a risk and insurance management program that emphasizes the safety and security of patients, staff, and visitors.
- Management should develop a comprehensive and integrated system to reduce and control the incidence of loss-producing situations.
- Management's expectations regarding the risk and insurance management program should be clearly presented as measurable outcomes.
- Management should provide a loss control component of the program that encourages the active involvement of all staff members.
- Management should publish clear safety rules and regulations.
- Management should include patient quality assurance and clinical record maintenance as integral parts of the risk management program.

- Management should provide follow-up assessments to staff as feedback regarding the success or shortcomings of the risk management program.
- Management should make available objective information regarding benefits and savings realized from the program.
- Management should be prepared to redefine efforts to minimize the incidence of liability claims.

The success of a risk management program depends on following these principles and on manipulating the professional disciplines through which the incidence of risk is controlled.

HEALTH SERVICES ORGANIZATIONS AND LITIGATION

In the years since World War II, the legal liability exposure of all health care providers has expanded at an alarming pace (see also Chapter 27).

As noted previously, the landmark *Darling* case opened the doors to litigation. As a result of this case, the court granted payment of $110,000 in damages to a patient because of the negligence of the hospital staff. The doctor referred to in this case admitted his liability and settled with the patient, thus leaving the path clear for abrogation of the doctrine of charitable immunity as it pertained to health care organizations. Upon appeal and subsequent review of the case by the Illinois Supreme Court, the following remarks were made for the record:

> The conception that the hospital does not undertake to treat the patient, does not undertake to act through its doctors and nurses, but undertakes instead simply to procure them to act upon their own responsibility, no longer reflects the fact. Present day hospitals, as their manner of operation plainly demonstrates, do far more than furnish facilities for treatment. They regularly employ on a salary basis a large staff of physicians, nurses, and interns, as well as administrative and manual workers, and they charge patients for medical care and treatment,

collecting for such services, if necessary, by legal action. Certainly, the person who avails himself of hospital facilities expects that the hospital will attempt to cure him, not that its nurses or other employees will act on their own responsibility.[5]

The decision not only removed charitable immunity as a means of defense; it also placed a greater burden of responsibility upon boards of trustees to ensure that the quality of care satisfies basic standards, that its own rules and regulations are obeyed by the medical staff, and that general practitioners actively seek specialist consultation in the care and cure process. These determinations placed health care organizations in a more exposed position with respect to malpractice and legal liability.

Litigation against health care organizations has come of age. To succeed in a malpractice claim, a plaintiff must prove a case that stands on four distinct premises, which are referred to as elements of professional liability. They are as follows:

1. A professional relationship has been established between the organization or provider and the patient. At this point, the organization or provider incurs a legal duty for the provision of quality care.
2. There is a demonstrable standard of care and the organization or the practitioner has breached that standard. In other words, the organization or practitioner is said to have practiced below the standard of care.
3. The patient suffered discernible injury or harm. This must clearly be established and demonstrated in the patient's case.
4. The organization or practitioner breach of duty to practice within the standard of care was the proximate cause of the patient's injury. This means that the injury was a reasonably foreseeable consequence of that breach of duty.[6]

In theory, the plaintiff always bears the burden of establishing the existence of each element for a successful professional liability claim. If more than one cause of action is cited during the course of litigation, the plaintiff is required to prove each of the elements for each occurrence. In practice, however, juries often find for a plaintiff even though the proof of a particular case element is incomplete.

One basis for claims of negligence is the notion of strict liability. Health care organizations are generally charged with providing a reasonable standard of care. If, for example, defective equipment is involved, the organization must offer evidence of a standard of care by which ultimately it will be judged. Conversely, proof must be shown by the plaintiff that the defendant has failed to meet a defined standard of care, thereby causing proximate injury to the plaintiff. When a court asserts strict liability, the determination that a defect was present and that it resulted in the plaintiff's injury is all that is required. Under such circumstances, no proof of fault becomes necessary.

Another basis for litigation is the doctrine of informed consent. Litigants almost always contend that it is a hospital's and a provider's obligation to inform a patient fully of all details pertinent to the care that is to be rendered. If subsequent treatment proves less than satisfactory, a patient can reasonably claim that had he or she known all of the risks involved, he or she would not have granted permission for the procedure to be performed.

Health care organizations and providers also have been found liable based upon the locality rule. For many years, a finding of negligence depended on the manner in which care was provided in the particular community. In other words, health care organizations and providers in a small rural community were not expected to provide the same level of care as those in a larger urban area. The case that effectively abolished the locality rule involved a woman who was brought to a radiology department for diagnostic tests. Although it was stated in the patient's chart that she could faint if placed under any stress, no one provided the information to the consulting radiologist . Consequently, when the patient was placed on the x-ray table, she fainted, and as the table was being tilted, she rolled off, suffering a serious head injury. The organization defended itself against an assertion of negligence on the grounds that no other hospital in the area took a history in the x-ray room and therefore this accident should not result in a judgment against the organization. The court stated that there are some situations in which an entire community or an entire profession had erred, and this was one of those occasions. The court thereupon held the hospital liable.[7]

IMPLICATIONS FOR THE DELIVERY OF HEALTH SERVICES

Although the cases involving health care organizations represent a small fraction of the total number of liability claims filed each year, it should be obvious that courts and litigants increasingly believe it is the joint responsibility of the governing body, administration, and clinical staff to provide the best possible care and treatment for a patient. As previously noted, a health care organization can be held liable for the negligent conduct of any person in its employ; in addition, the organization is likely to be held accountable for the acts of any provider who has not personally been engaged by a patient to provide a service. Even in instances when the provider who acts negligently is not on salary and enters into a direct contractual arrangement with the patient, the organization and its trustees may be held liable if they fail to exercise due diligence in granting privileges to the provider or in supervising his or her performance.

As to the possible implications of the burden of liability, a single large judgment against a hospital involving capital assets can impair or even destroy the hospital's ability to render a high level of care.[8] Consequently, it is the duty of a health care organization's administrators to become informed about the best methods of minimizing or eliminating their liability risk. Much of the responsibility for the care of patients falls upon the administrators even though they are not directly involved in delivering treatment. The board of trustees similarly is being held more accountable, and the trustees, through their administrators, are now expected to ensure that the clinical staff develops standards to prevent the occurrence of problems. One requisite for achieving this is adequate communication with the clinical staff, and another is the exercise of proper authority over the clinical staff to enforce appropriate standards of practice and rules of conduct. Health care administrators, therefore, must be effective managers and be aware of those standards of practice that will ensure the quality of care and limit the damage caused by a service problem.

The foregoing discussion has emphasized the extent to which liability claims have become a major problem throughout the health field. There are few health care institutions in America today that can realistically state that this crisis has not in some way affected their operation and management. Indeed, the cost of liability coverage represents one of the major expenses incurred by hospitals and other health services providers.

In recent years, many different approaches to the problem have been tried. However, it is generally agreed by people knowledgeable in the field that anything short of a complete risk management program simply will not be sufficient to meet the challenges at hand.

MANAGEMENT OF RISK

In *Health Care Risk Management,* Gary P. Kraus identified risk management as a process comprising a complex set of tasks, functions, and decisions carried out with the objective of reducing unexpected financial loss to an organization.[9] It is recognized that prevention, although not always possible, is the best means of managing risk. Unless there is an aggressive and ongoing program of prevention, the risk management program will not be able to achieve its goals.

Identification of Risk

It is seldom easy to discover situations capable of producing an incident that might result in a financial loss. Identifying the chance of loss requires regularly scheduled reviews of all physical assets belonging to the organization. Conducting inventories of cash, securities, patient property, and physical assets is essential for identifying risk. Inviting

an insurer to participate and, in some instances, to provide leadership when undertaking risk detection can enhance the process. The use of fact finders, which are provided by most insurance companies that offer professional and general liability coverage, can also be quite helpful. Another possible tool is the organization's incident report form. Traditionally, this form has been used to help establish an organization's defense during the course of litigation, but it can also provide assistance in preventing claims from ever being filed in the first place. These documents should be reviewed periodically so that the organization can uncover any developing negative trends.

Risk Evaluation

The evaluation of risk can be accomplished by reviewing and categorizing all available incident reports for a time period of at least six months. Comparing data on incidents involving other organizations can also be of benefit. Using the incident reports, the severity and frequency of incidents should be assessed. Medication errors are among the most important types of incidents to look at. The success of the evaluation process depends on the application of reason and judgment and on the collection of comprehensive information from internal accounting records.

Elimination of Risk

Once a risk has been determined to exist and has been evaluated, it does not usually pose an invincible threat. It is not possible, of course, to eliminate all of the incidents that could produce losses. However, if identified early enough, a risk can be corrected. A sound loss control program (one that emphasizes and unifies the medical and nursing services review processes) can substantially minimize the chances of a loss occurring. Risk managers and working hospital committees must be made aware of the potential consequences of needless and dangerous procedures being performed under the aegis of the health care organization.

Risk Reduction

All of those risks that cannot be eliminated should be reduced. A risk is reduced or controlled when losses can be predicted more accurately.[10] Risk reduction should also minimize both the probability (frequency) and the severity of negative incidents. For example, exposure to loss from a fall on a stairway cannot be completely eliminated, but the addition of a handrail and nonskid tread strips can reduce both the probability and the resulting seriousness of such falls.

Managerial controls also tend to reduce incidents. These include material control systems, accounting controls and audits, and product inspections. If it has been found that incidents can be reduced sufficiently, the health care organization may benefit more than by insuring against risk. Also, insuring against risk may best be accomplished through the use of an internally funded insurance mechanism. However, whether to use such a mechanism depends on the extent to which the organization is willing to assume responsibility for losses.

Risk Transfer

There will be some risks an organization is unable to eliminate or reduce and cannot afford to assume responsibility for. The strategy for these risks is to transfer them through service contracts or the purchase of insurance. For example, purchasing or leasing equipment, acquiring supplies or products on a daily basis, and utilizing needed services of outside agencies can in effect transfer the risk of loss away from the health care organization.

If outside providers are brought in on a contractual or admission basis to provide services to patients or the organization, hold-harmless and additional insured agreements become legitimate tools for transferring a portion of the risk. It is important to remember that once the organization establishes a contract, that contract is binding. Therefore, it is critical to insist that the contractor furnish evidence of having secured proper insurance coverage.

If a health care organization finds the insurance marketplace unresponsive or too costly, there are at least three other methods of securing liability insurance: pooling, joining a captive plan, and self-insuring.

Carriers may voluntarily underwrite assigned risk or pooling plans. If a particular geographic area lacked malpractice insurance, a voluntary pool of carriers could provide adequate coverage. In such circumstances, premiums may be higher than before, but the availability of insurance would be ensured.

A captive insurance plan is a company formed by a group solely to insure the members of that group. Captives have been employed, with varying degrees of success, to provide more predictable premium structures for organizations susceptible to marketplace fluctuations. If not professionally managed, captives have been known to fail and create even greater market instability.

Self-insurance involves setting up an internal fund for insurance purposes. The organization establishes the limit to which it will self-insure any risks. The problem is that the money set aside is often insufficient or is used for emergency purposes.

PREVENTIVE MEASURES

Before any prevention program can be successful, a system for the prompt recording of incidents must exist. The records of an incident can play an important legal role if the incident becomes cause for a lawsuit. It can also help determine whether litigation is resorted to.

Attention to records management should not be restricted to the maintenance of clinical records. All recordkeeping systems of the health care organization can be scrutinized in the event a claim in filed.

The degree of safety in a health care facility depends on the characteristics of people who frequent the facility and on the physical features of the buildings.[11] The responsibility for ensuring safety rests at all levels of management and staff. One essential task is to collect and collate information for the purpose of assessing safety performance. If performance is poor, corrective actions must be instituted by management through its span of control. A fully integrated safety program will draw on the resources of all departments and will include input from management and staff alike. The integration of functions is essential to developing a cohesive program in which all employees strive for the resolution of problems.

Risk is inherent in all activities and should be identified and controlled. Each department or service is responsible for the prevention of hazards and the control of risk within its sphere of responsibility.

The use of written policies and procedures contributes to safety and security. For example, food service personnel are responsible for the preparation of meals and for maintaining a high standard of cleanliness. If a hospital kitchen is unclean and careless practices are allowed to persist, it will be only a matter of time until the lack of quality is reflected in a series of food-related problems. The use of written policies and procedures affords a viable mechanism for staff training and also establishes parameters of accountability for food service employees.

As a second example, hospital reception personnel, including volunteers, are ideally situated to identify and report persons who appear to present a threat to security. Appropriate policies and procedures will allow such personnel to help maintain an effective security net.

A safety and security committee should be established and charged with oversight responsibilities. The committee should meet regularly, and its evaluations and recommendations should be shared with department and service heads alike. Safety and security programs should include methods of monitoring and measuring health and environmental hazards, including air contamination, biological hazards, hazardous materials, hazardous waste, and the potential for infection. There should be programs that regularly evaluate and disseminate information about accidents and incidents that occur in the organization. Areas of special focus should include the management of hazardous waste and hazardous materials and the management of fire and building safety. (For more on safety and security see Chapter 25.)

THE INSURANCE MARKETPLACE

In this section, several fundamental concepts will be presented as well as summary descriptions of several types of business insurance typically purchased by health care organizations. The types include fire insurance, liability insurance, boiler and machinery insurance, special multiperil insurance, workers' compensation insurance, crime insurance, fidelity bonds, and fiduciary insurance.

There are two distinct categories of business insurance: essential and attractive. Essential insurance, as the name implies, must be purchased to protect the business and its officers against catastrophic occurrences. In choosing among essential insurance policies, cost is not the only factor to be considered. At the same time, it makes sense to comparison shop and purchase the least expensive of comparable policies. Attractive insurance policies may be purchased or ignored without exposing the organization to unmanageable forfeitures. The lesser losses insured against may be absorbed by the organization, though not necessarily without financial stress. Examples of attractive insurance include plate glass insurance and rent insurance.

The focus of the following discussion is on essential insurance coverage, which, if not prudently purchased, can affect the financial integrity of the hospital.

Fire Insurance

An uncontrolled fire is without question one of the more devastating events an organization can face. A standard fire policy is one that a state insurance department has accepted as standard for purposes of effecting coverage within that state. When a policy is considered to be standard, it is designated as such.

A standard fire policy contains the following elements: an insurance clause; stipulations and conditions that govern the basic contract; any additional coverage provided in the contract; the forms that list the property coverage. The building and contents form is generally used for business and public building coverage. Excluding endorsements, a standard fire policy protects against direct loss from three perils: fire, lightning, and the temporary removal of goods from the premises due to fire. The decision as to whether a fire is a just cause for remuneration is based upon state statutes and court decisions that determine the exact definition of the term *fire*.

All other perils (generally referred to as "AOP" in the policy) must be added to the basic policy by attaching one or more forms. It is generally smart to assume that unless a fire policy mentions a specific peril, the organization is not insured against that peril. Conversely, if the declarations page of a policy has "AOP" or "All Risk" written on its face, it may be assumed that the policy covers all such perils unless otherwise noted. Smoke or water damage during a fire is not covered by a standard policy unless specified in the insurance clause.

The extended coverage endorsement covers each of the following perils: windstorms, hail, explosions, riots and civil commotions, damage by aircraft or vehicles, and smoke damage. There are three general exclusions: war, nuclear hazards, and water damage.

The coinsurance clause in a fire policy is frequently misunderstood. This clause requires the policyholder, if accepting 80 percent coinsurance on a building, for instance, to insure to 80 percent of the value; otherwise the payment in the event of loss will be reduced by the proportion to which the policyholder failed to insure. For example, if the building has a value of $100,000, with an 80 percent clause it must be insured for $80,000 or more. If not, then a loss could mean that less than the actual amount of damage would be recovered. In essence, the coinsurance clause is both a penalty and

an incentive clause encouraging the policyholder to purchase adequate coverage.

There are forms that may be added to the fire policy to cover additional losses (generally referred to as indirect or consequential losses). For example, business interruption insurance is designed to offset the expense of salaries, taxes, interest payments, and other related items during the rebuilding or repairing of a facility. The period for which the policy will continue to indemnify depends on the length of time required to complete repairs with due diligence and dispatch—and of course on the face value of the policy.

The payment for gross earnings losses is payable in a single amount and is based upon lost income less costs. Generally, a coinsurance clause is required for gross earnings insurance.

As previously mentioned, all-risk coverage (AOP endorsement) is designed to fill the gaps left by an extended coverage endorsement. The all-risk endorsement typically excludes floods, wars, nuclear hazards, earthquakes, boiler and machinery exposures, and electrical equipment failures.

The valuation of lost property may be based upon the actual cash value (the insurance company calculates the original purchase price less depreciation) or the replacement cost value (the original purchase price plus any appreciation due to escalation of replacement costs). The policyholder may select either alternative at the time the policy is purchased.

Liability Insurance

Professional liability insurance protects an organization against charges of negligence or incompetence in the provision of professional services. The selection of a professional liability insurance program that meets the organization's needs is essential. Too often an insured organization may find that its management has misunderstood the requirements for participation in the program or the policy's limitations or exclusions.

There are some basic criteria that should be used for selecting a professional liability insurance program. Cost is one criterion, but inevitably not the most important, as an organization will come to understand once it has been sued.

The single most important factor for the purchaser of professional liability insurance to consider is the policy form under which the coverage has been written. There are two specific forms of coverage available today to health care organizations: claims made coverage and occurrence coverage.

A claims made policy states that the policyholder is covered for those claims filed while the policy is in force. A claims made policy does not cover the policyholder after the policy has expired or been cancelled unless "tail coverage" is purchased. Tail coverage protects against claims filed for incidents alleged to have taken place during the policy period. An organization that has purchased a claims made policy may find, much to its chagrin, that it must pay more than twice the final year's premium to purchase tail coverage, which may only extend for three months to one year. A claims made policy may ultimately prove to be an excellent purchase, but it is important that the insured organization understands the implications of that purchase at such time as the policy expires, is retired, or is replaced due to economic or coverage considerations.

Occurrence coverage provides that the insured organization is covered for incidents that have occurred during the policy period, even though the filing of claims is actually done after the policy expires. Under this form of coverage, there is no necessity to purchase a tail, because coverage is valid at any time a claim is filed even though the policy may not be in force. In the long run, occurrence coverage offers the most viable and broadest form of protection that can be purchased.

Still another factor to consider in evaluating claims made versus occurrence coverage is the carry over of policy limits from one year to the next. With claims made coverage, it is as though the insured organization moves from one room of a building to the next, permanently closing a door. In other words, a claims made policy form carries all of the potential exposures from the retiring year and places them in the new policy year. As a result, after three or more years of coverage, there can be so many potential exposure units that the limits of liability of the original policy may not be sufficient to cover the accumulated exposure. Hence, it may be necessary for the insured to increase the policy limits and thereby significantly increase the premium.

With occurrence coverage, the policy limits remain in force for each of the years that have passed. If claims are filed for incidents occurring during the past year of coverage, those limits apply only to the incidents that are alleged to have occurred during that year. The result is a flattening of exposure units and, although the cost of coverage may be higher during the initial years, there is a tendency for that cost to remain at a more predictable level during subsequent years.

Figures 26-1 and 26-2 depict what could happen in the event multiple claims are filed under a claims made policy versus an occurrence type of policy.

In Figure 26-1, there have been three claims filed in year 4 for alleged incidents that took place in years 1, 2, and 3. Because the policy is a claims made type, all three claims and the resultant legal costs and awards are credited to year 4 liability, which has a one-million-dollar limit.

One additional aspect of claims made coverage not indicated in Figure 26-1 is that a claims made policy normally has a five-year period of maturation. During this period, the premium levels are adjusted to reflect the frequency and severity of claims and losses. However, if losses persist beyond that period, there is no guarantee that the premium will stabilize. In other words, an insured sacrifices the period of time in which the carrier will accept responsibility for a loss and gains few material concessions in return. Hence, the effects of multiple claims being filed during a single policy year could be significant and financially damaging to the organization.

In Figure 26-2, the organization also has had three claims filed during year 4. But because the policy is an occurrence type policy, the claims and resulting judgments and legal expenses are credited against the years in which the incidents are alleged to have occurred. Figures 26-1 and 26-2 together highlight a primary benefit of occurrence coverage (both while the policy is in force and beyond).

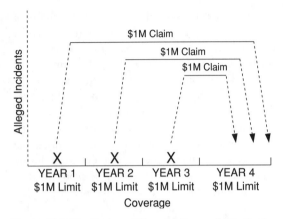

Figure 26-1 Distribution of Financial Responsibility for the Payment of Judgments with Claims Made Coverage

Directors and officers liability insurance provides protection for individual trustees in their capacity as policy makers of an organization. It is important to note that there are two specific types of policies. One insures the organization and governing board as a whole through limits that apply in the aggregate to all participants of that board. The other type provides protection for the insured organization as well as individual directors and officers. For organizations that have wealthy individuals as

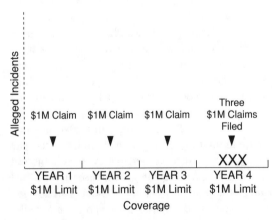

Figure 26-2 Distribution of Financial Responsibility for the Payment of Judgments with Occurrence Coverage

board members, an enhanced form of coverage that extends protection to the assets of each governing board member is a far more desirable type of coverage than a policy that only provides blanket coverage for the organization as a whole.

General liability insurance covers two contingencies: property damage and bodily injury. In the case of most business liability policies, the property and bodily injury coverage varies from one jurisdiction to another. In general, however, an accident may be defined as a sudden and unanticipated occurrence at a definite time and place.

It is important to note that general liability and professional liability coverage responsibilities sometimes become blurred because of the nature of an alleged injury. Blurring is especially common in the case of mental health patients who are given advice that results in an injury on or in proximity to the premises of the organization. In these instances, there is some uncertainty as to whether the claim will be litigated as a professional liability claim or as a general liability claim.

A general liability policy normally contains the following elements:

- The name of the insured. The policy normally includes the corporate entity and in some instances will add the chief executive officer or administrator as an additional named insured.
- The area covered. The physical area covered encompasses the designated premises and the area immediately adjoining the premises, including sidewalks and parking lots.
- The hazards covered. Building and operational hazards are the main hazards covered. Product liability and contractual liability coverage may also be deemed necessary and can be added by endorsement.
- The perils covered. A lawsuit charging negligence resulting in bodily injury or property damage is a primary example of the type of peril covered. The policy also may provide coverage for losses from the payment of dollar awards made by the court or by out-of-court settlements. The cost of investigation, legal

defense, and negotiation and all other reasonable expenses similarly must be covered by the policy.

It is generally considered advisable for a health care organization to purchase its general and professional liability insurance from the same insurance company. This will avoid jurisdictional disputes as to which insurance company bears responsibility for the defense of a particular claim.

Umbrella liability insurance increases the protection and liability limits of general liability, professional liability, and automobile liability insurance. Some policies also will extend coverage of the employer's liability section of a workers' compensation policy. If the additional coverage provided is for only one element of coverage (such as auto liability), it is commonly referred to as excess coverage. Coordination of underlying and umbrella or excess coverage through the same insurance company will in most instances minimize potential conflicts in the event a loss occurs.

Automobile liability insurance and auto loss coverage are generally handled together and together constitute the standard auto policy. This policy provides basic protection from liability claims for bodily injury or property damage arising out of the ownership, operation, or use of an insured vehicle. The coverage extends to employees and any person operating a vehicle with permission from the named insured. It is important to note that automobile insurance covers the vehicle being operated. The driver receives protection as an extension of that coverage.

Uninsured motorist coverage in effect makes the insurance carrier responsible up to the policy limits for any uninsured or hit and run motorist who injures the operator or a passenger of an insured vehicle. Similarly, *underinsured motorist coverage* provides protection in the event an insured vehicle is struck by another vehicle not having sufficient insurance to cover the monetary loss resulting from that incident.

Medical payments coverage provides for payment of reasonable medical expenses or funeral expenses and a death benefit because of an injury incurred by any individual upon entering or alighting from an insured vehicle.

Collision coverage applies to direct accidental damage to the insured vehicle resulting from a collision or upset. It usually includes a deductible.

Comprehensive coverage addresses direct accidental loss of or damage to an insured vehicle other than through the incidence of collision.

Representative losses are those occasioned by fire, theft, glass breakage, flying objects, explosions, windstorms, floods, and vandalism.

Towing and labor coverage pays for emergency repairs to a stalled or damaged vehicle or the towing of such vehicle.

Boiler and Machinery Insurance

This is a highly specialized type of insurance offered by some of the oldest insurance companies in existence. Generally speaking, it protects against losses caused by explosions of furnaces, steam boilers, and engines and damage to electrical equipment. The policy specifically lists coverage for the loss of a boiler or other insured machinery, expenditures required to resume operations, property damage, and bodily injury. Losses are paid up to an aggregate limit, which represents the maximum payable per accident.

Special Multiperil Insurance

Special multiperil policies provide fire and extended coverage insurance on all buildings and their contents, plus premises and operations liability. Simply stated, this type of policy is similar to a homeowner policy. Because it bundles an array of types of coverage in a package, it is usually offered at a discount.

Workers' Compensation Insurance

Workers' compensation insurance provides coverage for occupation-related diseases and injuries. Premiums are paid by the employer to the workers' compensation carrier (Part A coverage). The statutes governing workers' compensation are compulsory and guided by federal regulation. The workers' compensation program covers loss of pay, medical expenses, rehabilitation or retraining expenses, and payment of a death benefit to the survivors of an individual who dies as the result of a work-related incident.

Part B of workers' compensation coverage includes what is called employer's liability insurance. This insurance protects an employer in the event an employee is awarded damages because the workplace environment was unsafe or inhospitable.

There are two major determinants of workers' compensation premiums: the frequency of claims and the severity of claims. These factors modify premium amounts. Organizations with positive claims experience customarily will see their premiums reduced, whereas organizations with poor claims experience will be assessed a penalty.

Crime Insurance

Following are the most common types of crime insurance policies.

A *storekeeper, burglary, and robbery policy* provides coverage for each of the following:

- robbery inside the premises
- robbery outside the premises
- kidnapping
- forcible entry into the premises and theft of merchandise or equipment
- damage to property due to any of the above types of occurrences

An *office burglary and robbery policy* is useful in covering office equipment, such as calculators, typewriters, and other items that have a marketable street value.

A *paymaster robbery policy* covers loss of payroll money and checks by robbery occurring either inside or outside of the office. The policy may also cover damage occurring to office furniture and fixtures during a robbery.

A *mercantile safe burglary policy* covers loss of money, securities, and other property due to burglary of safes or vaults after they have been properly locked.

An *interior robbery policy* covers loss of or damage to money, securities, and other property inside the premises. The policy covers losses due to the following types of events:

- A robber enters an office open for business and forcibly takes property that is in the care of a custodian.
- A custodian or messenger is kidnapped while off the premises and compelled by threat of violence to admit a person to the building after it is closed.
- Property is stolen from within a display window by a person who has broken glass from the outside while the office is open for business.

A *messenger robbery policy* covers loss of or damage to money, securities, or other property in the custody of a messenger while off the premises. The money must be forcibly taken from the messenger by violence or the threat of violence.

Fidelity Bonds

Fidelity bonds represent a contract designed to provide protection against losses resulting from employee dishonesty. There must be a commitment to prosecute if a bonded employee is discovered to have perpetrated a theft. There are several types of fidelity bonds.

A *named scheduled bond* is used by many organizations. Here the organization simply lists the names of the specific individuals it wishes to bond and the amount of the bond it chooses to carry on each person.

A *position bond* lists specific positions rather than individuals. One benefit is that it does not have to be changed each time a person leaves the employ of the organization.

A *blanket bond* covers all employees regardless of position and regardless of turnover. The advantage of this alternative lies in its simplicity. Such a bond may also provide protection for the following loss exposures:

- safe burglaries
- safety deposit box theft
- forged or altered checks

A *commercial blanket bond* indemnifies up to the limit of the bond on each loss.

A *forgery bond* covers losses resulting from forged or altered checks. The principal type is called a depositor's forgery bond, which protects the organization and its bank against such losses while the bond is in force.

A *surety bond* guarantees that the principal bonded party will carry out the work that the obligee has hired him or her to perform. It serves as insurance that the principal is honest and has the necessary ability and financial capacity to fulfill the obligations for which the bond has been issued. The most common use of surety bonds is to guarantee construction contracts. Surety bonds are commonly referred to as three-party contracts or agreements.

Fiduciary Liability Insurance

This policy covers the duties of trustees in the dispatch of their responsibilities on behalf of a group of designated persons. A specific type of fiduciary liability is that which pertains to the prudent management of a pension trust or a vacation trust. The Employee Retirement Income Security Act of 1974 has greatly increased the responsibilities of fiduciaries or trustees of employee benefit or retirement plans. A number of insurance carriers now are providing insurance policies to protect both the plans and the individuals acting as trustees or fiduciaries from lawsuits alleging wrongful acts (e.g., errors and omissions in the handling of investment funds).

There are no standardized forms, and the plan of an individual carrier should be referenced. The Pension Reform Act allows for such insurance, but if the premiums are paid for by the retirement plan's

funds, then a policy may permit action by the insurer against any negligent fiduciary. Some fiduciary liability policies permit the inclusion of a "no recourse endorsement," which protects the individual trustees. A policy may be written with a minimum deductible of $1,000. Companies may issue policies with the basic limits, including a $1,000,000 aggregate or more, but some companies will issue policies to fiduciaries with limits as low as $250,000.

QUALITY MANAGEMENT OF RISK

Each hospital should have an ongoing and active risk management program designed to objectively evaluate the quality and appropriateness of clinical care as it relates to the chances of loss to the organization. The risk management program should be supported by a risk and insurance management committee, which provides input into the process of developing and maintaining the program.

There are five generally accepted phases of a risk management process[12]:

1. identifying loss exposures
2. examining the feasibility of alternative risk management techniques
3. selecting the best technique for problem resolution
4. implementing the chosen technique
5. monitoring and improving the risk management program

Prior to the establishment of a risk management program, there should be a clear understanding of the goals of the program. This will help to maximize the involvement and commitment of various key hospital participants.

Second, spheres of authority should be defined, and the reporting relationships of a risk manager or risk management committee should be clearly delineated. In addition, it is essential that the flow of information to and from the risk management office be clearly defined so that realistic expectations can be established among the various participating departments.

Third, it is important that the internal organization of the risk management program be clearly articulated to those responsible for managing the process. This will provide further support for proper information flow. Clear standards of performance are also necessary, and monitoring whether the standards are being met will assist in strengthening the program.

Finally, the publication of a clear policy statement from the office of the chief executive officer of the hospital will help in legitimizing the program and its relationship to other key players in the hospital organization.

Quality assurance is mainly responsible for monitoring and evaluating the quality and the appropriateness of clinical care. It is normally supported by a clinical services and pharmaceutical committee, which monitors and evaluates clinical practices and reviews and modifies clinical policies.

In almost all hospitals, there is a written quality assurance plan that describes in brief but precise terms the mechanisms utilized to sustain effective monitoring, evaluation, and problem-solving efforts. The scope of the quality assurance program includes the following:

- the quality and appropriateness of diagnostic and treatment procedures
- the completeness of clinical record entries
- the administering of clinical care
- the prescription and use of medications as part of treatment
- patient satisfaction with the care provided
- the quality and appropriateness of emergency services

The role of risk management in the hospital is to review and evaluate the quality assurance process. This is critical, because a flawed quality assurance program can heighten the organization's exposure to liability loss. Assessing the program requires the sharing of information gleaned from quality assurance efforts. If problems are discovered, corrective measures must be instituted to ensure that the mechanisms being utilized are appropriate and in line with the expectations of all parties. Furthermore, the effectiveness of the corrective measures must be assessed, and if they are found not to solve the problems, new measures must be substituted.

To facilitate the quality assurance process, there should be ongoing collection and evaluation of information regarding significant aspects of patient care. The focus should be on identifying opportunities to improve care and problems that may impede the improvement of care. If problems are identified, written protocols should be developed and published that articulate expectations for patient care improvement. Although it is essential that the clinical services review committee oversee the process, the risk management department should be available to ascertain the time required to improve or resolve given situations.

In addition, information should be communicated between the appropriate departments when opportunities to improve patient care involve more than one department or service. The evaluation of the effectiveness of the quality assurance program requires that there be an ongoing assessment of the patterns of communication between the departments and clinical services of the hospital. This assessment can also help ameliorate conflicts over turf.

It is important that the hospital publish principles of professional practice that reflect an ongoing concern for the acceptability, accessibility, and availability of clinical services. There should be a description of the system for providing emergency and routine patient services both during and after peak hours of operation, and there should be specific information about gaining access to emergency treatment as well as documentation of the use of appropriate diagnostic procedures, including laboratory and radiologic studies. It is equally essential that informed consent procedures be established and followed throughout the organization.

The main object of having an active risk management program is to assess on a regular basis the effectiveness of the hospital and its departments in maintaining a fail-safe system of care and treatment. The risk management department, besides ensuring that the program is appropriate and in the best interests of the hospital and its staff, also plays an important communication role, providing both empirical and descriptive information to the staff regarding the effectiveness of the program.

It is important to make sure that utilization review and precertification programs are not merely paper-and-pencil exercises performed for accreditation purposes. When untimely or inappropriate use of services is identified or new needs are recognized, corrective actions or new services should be developed and implemented. The risk management program can help prevent the political structure of the hospital from becoming an impediment to the effectiveness of the precertification, utilization review, and quality assurance programs.

In summation, it is obvious that there should not be duplicate or unnecessary diagnostic or treatment procedures. Case management and individual treatment plans should be employed to ensure appropriate use of services, and treatment plans should encompass both the inpatient and the outpatient components of the hospital. The risk management department is in an excellent position to provide an independent evaluation of costs and benefits to determine which procedures are necessary and appropriate and will in the long run raise the quality of care while simultaneously demonstrating cost consciousness. Hence, cost-effectiveness studies should be included in the risk management program, and there should be regularly scheduled meetings with quality assurance staff participants to discuss such studies.

RISK MANAGEMENT INVOLVEMENT IN EVALUATING CLINICAL RECORDS

Each organization should maintain a clinical records system that permits the prompt retrieval of needed information. Clinical data should be documented accurately and promptly and should be readily accessible to both administrators and clinical practitioners. Without a comprehensive clinical records system, it is impossible to implement a viable quality assurance process. The collection, processing, maintenance, storage, and retrieval of clinical records information is essential to the timely study and follow-up of those situations in which problems are likely to occur. Clinical information pertinent to the care of a particular patient should be available to the practitioner providing care as well as to support staff and others who may be evaluating that care. Records should be protected from loss, destruction, and unauthorized access or removal (see Chapter 14).

The role of the risk management department is to ensure that there are written policies and procedures concerning the use, maintenance, and retention of clinical records. In addition, the risk management department should be involved in evaluating the quality of clinical records, including the consistency of information that is being retained. Through its involvement in this process and through working with the hospital's legal counsel in defending any claims that may have been filed, the risk management department can substantially lessen the chances of a major liability judgment being levied against the organization.

The risk management department should be involved in the following activities:

- the maintenance of confidentiality of information
- the mechanisms for safeguarding clinical records from loss
- the entry of data into the clinical records
- the release of information contained in the records
- the use of informed consent procedures
- the retention of active clinical records
- the retirement and storage of inactive clinical records

The involvement of the risk management department in the assessment process will enhance the quality of the clinical records program and will consequently lessen the likelihood of a successful malpractice claim being filed against the organization.

THE ROLE OF THE RISK MANAGER IN ESTABLISHING CONTRACTUAL RELATIONSHIPS

Although it is the responsibility of the hospital's legal department to negotiate and implement contracts, the risk manager can contribute significantly to the development of legal relationships, especially contractual relationships with professionals who are not directly employed by the hospital. Through appropriate wording to gain additional insured endorsements from the coverage of a consultant, physician, or paramedic, the hospital can become secondary to any litigation that may be filed against that individual. Furthermore, the requirement that such coverage be in force prior to finalizing a contract will protect the organization in the event a claim should arise.

THE ROLE OF THE CEO IN ESTABLISHING A RISK MANAGEMENT PROGRAM

The tone set by the chief executive officer in developing and implementing a risk management program determines whether the program becomes fully legitimized. If the purpose of the program is simply to satisfy the accreditation requirements of the Joint Commission on the Accreditation of Healthcare Organizations, the program will probably not enhance the quality of patient care, nor will it demonstrate a commitment to cost-effectiveness. Moreover, the lack of an appropriate risk management program may ultimately encourage legal actions against the organization. This can defeat the ultimate purposes of such a program and, in the extreme, can contribute to its demise.

In short, a risk management program can be viewed either as a bureaucratic necessity or as a significant contributor to the quality of the hospital's care and cure process. The effectiveness of the pro-

gram ultimately depends on the administration and its willingness to present the program as an essential component of care provision.

THE FUTURE OF RISK AND INSURANCE MANAGEMENT

Risk and insurance management has slowly been gaining acceptance during the last decade and a half. The use of computers has increased enormously the ability of organizations to evaluate their risk and loss exposures and to provide baseline information for the development of prevention programs. Their use also facilitates a more comprehensive approach to management and decision making. During the next decade, the most prominent risk management issues will center around prevention as an integrated function throughout the hospital and its departments. There is also an emerging realization of the need for a better understanding of the potential for liability losses.

At least one state, Florida, requires the presence of a risk manager or a risk management consultant at each hospital. With the state now mandating certification of risk management in all licensed facilities, hospitals are reviewing more comprehensively their loss exposures on a timely basis.[13] It is anticipated that the continuing need for risk management consultation and a better understanding of its benefits will increase the prominence of risk managers in health care organizations of the nineties.

ADDITIONAL RESOURCES

Organizations

Risk and Insurance Management Society, 205 E. 42nd Street, New York, NY 10017. 212\286-9292.

Books

Bennett, B. et al. *Professional liability and risk management.* Washington, D.C.: American Psychological Association, 1990.

Bjorn, J., and H. Cross. *Problem oriented practice.* Chicago: McGraw-Hill, 1975.

Gordis, P. *Property and casualty insurance.* Indianapolis, Ind.: The Rough Notes Company, 1986.

Hassard, H. *Medical malpractice: Risks, protection, prevention.* Oradell, N.J.: Medical Economics Books, 1966.

Head, G.L. *Essentials of risk control.* Vols. 1, 2. Malvern, Pa.: Insurance Institute of America, 1989.

Head, G.L., and S. Horn. *Essentials of risk management.* Vol. 1. Malvern, Pa.: Insurance Institute of America, 1992.

Kraus, G.P. *Health care risk management.* Owings Mills, Md.: National Health Publishing, 1986.

Liberman, A. *A risk and insurance management guide for medical group organizations.* Englewood, Co.: Center for Research in Ambulatory Health Care Administration, 1988.

Vickery, D., and J. Fries. *Take care of yourself: A consumer's guide to medical care.* Reading, Mass.: Addison-Wesley, 1981.

NOTES

1. H.L. Hirsh, Risk Management—The Physician's Role, *Legal Aspects of Medical Practice,* January 1979, p. 1.

2. S.L. Salman, A Systems Approach Can Ensure High Quality Care and Low Costs, *Hospitals,* September 16, 1980, pp. 48–50.

3. E.J. Vaughan, *Fundamentals of Risk and Insurance Management* (New York: Wiley, 1986), 3.

4. T. Dankmyer and J. Groves, Taking Steps for Safety's Sake, *Hospitals,* May 16, 1977, p. 62.

5. J.M. George, When Is a Hospital Liable for Negligence to Its Patients, *Canadian Hospital,* October 1970, pp. 26–27.

6. B.E. Bennett et al. *Professional Liability and Risk Management* (Washington, D.C.: American Psychological Association, 1990), 35.

7. N.L. Chayet, Corporate Responsibility for Medical Care, *Hospital Progress,* January 1972, pp. 32–37.

8. D.M. Holcomb, Risk Management Techniques in Short Term General Hospitals in Iowa (unpublished master's thesis, 1967), 49.

9. G.P. Kraus, *Health Care Risk Management* (Owings Mills, Md.: National Health Publishing, 1986), 16.

10. R.I. Mehr and B. A. Hedges, *Risk Management in the Business Enterprise* (Homewood, Ill.: Richard D. Irwin, 1963), 89.

11. G.L. Head, Maintaining Security, in *Essentials of Risk Control* (Malvern, Pa.: Insurance Institute of America, 1989), 71.

12. G.L. Head and S. Horn, *Essentials of Risk Management* (Malvern, Pa: Insurance Institute of America, 1992), 165.

13. Edward N. Willey, personal communication, May 15, 1992.

David Warren
Douglas Hastings

Legal Services

27

Purpose: The purpose of legal counsel is to help ensure that the institution (1) is organized and operated in a manner that conforms with relevant laws, regulations, and legal standards; (2) avoids unnecessary legal exposure to liability affecting its financial resources, employees, reputation, and legal status; (3) respects the rights of patients and other users of the institution's services; and (4) has procedures for recognizing and resolving legal issues fairly and economically.

INTRODUCTION

This chapter provides health care executives with a management perspective for dealing with legal issues and using legal resources. It explores the relationship between law and management in health care organizations by looking at the legal and regulatory environment of the health care industry and the application of key management principles for the effective use of legal services. The role of legal counsel is often crucial in avoiding unnecessary legal liability, in making decisions that are more likely to be legally viable in the long run, and in minimizing internal and external disputes and regulatory difficulties.

Legal matters permeate nearly every aspect of management of a health care organization. Law is a crucial factor in making management decisions. It requires health care executives to be aware of the legal and ethical implications that may arise in situations ranging from providing patient care to paying vendors. It involves patients' rights, since health care is inherently a personal service that affects an individual's ability to function and his or her sensibilities and dignity. It involves employees and contractors and others who do business with the organization, since contractual rights and responsibilities attach to these relationships. It involves obligations to other health care organizations who are affiliates or competitors, since none are exempt from the rules of the marketplace. Ultimately, law imposes upon health care executives the responsibility to operate within the regulatory parameters of the various levels of government and the framework of applicable statutes and judicial rulings.

MANAGEMENT PRINCIPLES

- Health care executives should be well informed on legal issues and procedures so that

540

they understand the legal and ethical implications of operational decisions affecting the organization.

- Health care executives should know when and how to involve legal counsel in obtaining advice on a timely basis and helping the organization prepare for and respond to changes in the legal and regulatory climate.
- The organization should plan and carry out its activities in a manner that proactively avoids consequences that invite legal difficulties and litigation.
- Procedural mechanisms should be established that manage risks as effectively as possible and address conflicts internally and externally in an effort to resolve them as expeditiously as possible.

A health care executive who does not pay close attention to legal issues or procedures or does not seek legal advice when indicated risks both personal and institutional liability as well as the unraveling of plans and programs. Even if a legally careless or improper management decision does not result in litigation, it may still be costly in terms of time and resources. For example, if a radiology technician is unnecessarily exposed to more radiation than permitted under current standards and makes a claim for subsequent disabilities, the hos-

pital loses both the worker and the workers' compensation payments. Or if a hospital gives a monetary reward to a physician for patient referrals, both may be penalized under antikickback regulations. Or if a contract between an HMO and a particular provider contains no provisions for evaluation of the work performed and no cancellation procedure, the health care executive may spend considerable time attempting to negotiate out of an unsatisfactory arrangement and may even end up in court.

It is clear that the legal consequences of poor planning, inappropriate policies, or below-standard performance in a health care organization can be serious (see Table 27-1). Of course, the most severe results could be bankruptcy for the organization and jail terms for its directors and officers.

THE ROLE OF LAWYERS AND LEGAL SERVICES IN HEALTH SERVICES MANAGEMENT

A health care executive should be able to comprehend and apply many of the relevant legal principles and government regulations by staying current with legal and management literature and complying with existing institutional policies and procedures. Increasingly, however, it is necessary for managers as well as board members and professional staff to con-

Table 27-1 Implications of Inattention to Legal Issues

Group	Potential Liability
Patients	Malpractice, breach of confidentiality
Other Users of Services (cafeteria, labs, shops)	Negligence, breach of contract
Employees	Workers' compensation, collective bargaining, discrimination
Medical Staff	Antitrust, due process, defamation
Contractors and Vendors	Breach of contract, liens
Other Health Care Organizations	Antitrust, breach of contract
Insurers	Breach of contract, utilization review
Local Government	Zoning, property taxes, employment regulations
State Government	Incorporation, licenses, taxes, Medicaid, certificate of need
Federal Government	Antitrust, taxes, fraud and abuse, reimbursement, Medicare compliance

sult regularly with legal counsel. Many larger health care institutions are creating legal services departments to provide internal advice and to assist in obtaining specialized outside legal services. This trend may be attributed to a recognition of the complexity of applicable law and regulations and a concern about liability. Deciding when and how to use legal services is a critically important task of management.

Evolution of Health Care Law

Health care law has evolved rapidly in the last 25 years (see Table 27-2). The passage of the Medicare and Medicaid legislation in 1965 was the beginning of an era of increasing government regulation of the accessibility and availability of health care services. Numerous extensions of this legislation have been passed to cover more patients and services while at the same time imposing more procedural restrictions for purposes of cost containment. Health planning legislation in many states has created a web of controls over facility and equipment acquisition. In some states, rate regulation has been implemented. All institutions are subject to a wide variety of laws affecting employer-employee relations. Tax laws at every level of government directly affect the activities of health care organizations whether for-profit or nonprofit.

Judicial Influence on Health Care Law

In addition to new legislation, health care law has developed rapidly in the courts during this same period. The landmark 1965 ruling in an Illinois case (*Darling v. Charleston Memorial Hospital,* 211 N.E. 2nd 253 [Ill. 1965], *cert. denied,* 383 U.S. 946 [1966]) created the concept of "corporate liability," which was adopted and expanded in other state court decisions, heightening the necessity for risk management and risk financing. Other cases have developed clearer concepts about patients' rights, employee relationships, governing board conflicts of interest, medical staff responsibilities, and contract obligations.

Table 27-2 Highlights in the Evolution of Health Care Law

Date	Event	Impact
1948	Hill-Burton Act	Community service obligation
1965	Medicare and Medicaid	Reimbursement rules and conditions
1966	*Darling v. Charleston Hospital*	Corporate liability doctrine
1972	*Canterbury v. Spence*	Informed consent doctrine
1973	Labor law amendments	National Labor Relations Act jurisdiction over nonprofit institutions
1973	Rehabilitation law	Nondiscrimination of handicapped
1975	Health planning legislation	Certificate of need
1976	*Hospital Building Co. v. Rex Hospital*	Antitrust laws apply to hospitals
1977	Anti-fraud-and-abuse amendments	Sanctions for kickbacks
1983	Professional review organization law	Utilization review
1985	*Utah County v. Intermountain Health Care*	Tax exemption challenge
1986	Emergency Medical Treatment Act	Sanctions for patient dumping
1986	Health Care Quality Improvement Act	Promotes peer review
1990	National Practitioner Data Bank	Reporting physician disciplinary actions
1991	Safe Harbor Regulations	Restriction on joint ventures
1991	Patient Self-Determination Act	Promotes advance directives

Trends in Health Law

Health care executives need to be aware of the continuing development of the legislation, regulations, and court decisions that constitute health care law. The following areas are particularly important, and managers should know when to seek legal advice when decisions involve these matters.

- corporate law
  - incorporation as a for-profit or nonprofit organization
  - limitations on corporate powers
  - governance principles
  - joint ventures
  - affiliations, mergers, and consolidations
  - bankruptcy
  - securities law issues
- tax law
  - filing and reporting requirements
  - criteria for obtaining and retaining tax-exempt status
  - private inurement and unrelated business income issues
  - tax issues related to joint ventures, mergers, and acquisitions
- labor and employment law
  - organization and recognition of collective bargaining units
  - restrictions on strikes
  - federal conciliation and mediation services
  - employment discrimination issues
  - negligent hiring and firing
  - HIV and drug testing in the workplace
  - substance abuse policies
- medical staff issues
  - granting, restricting, and denying admitting privileges
  - peer review activities
  - due process in disciplinary proceedings
  - exclusive contracts

  - reporting disciplinary actions to the National Health Practitioner Data Bank
- antitrust laws: Sherman Act combinations and conspiracies in restraint of trade
  - joint activities affecting price
  - horizontal mergers and joint ventures
  - downstream referrals
  - medical staff antitrust issues
  - Federal Trade Commission unfair trade and advertising practices
- patient care issues
  - admission, transfer, and discharge
  - consent and refusal of treatment
  - confidentiality
  - AIDS-related issues
  - special problems related to mental health and substance abuse
  - emergency room cases and the antidumping laws
- liability issues
  - professional liability
  - expanding liability concerns in managed care
  - tort reform initiatives
- third-party payers
  - changing hospital and physician reimbursement rules under Medicare and Medicaid
  - professional review organizations
  - utilization review issues
- fraud and abuse concerns
  - impact on joint ventures and business contracts
  - antikickback law and safe harbor rules
  - the Stark legislation
  - civil and criminal sanctions
- managed care
  - point-of-service products and other new developments
  - direct contracting with employers
  - expanding liability concerns

—provider ownership of managed care companies

—regulation of managed care companies and products

Legal Services Relationship

The health care executive should understand the role of lawyers in both preventing legal problems and resolving them. To effectively use legal services, there must be a gatekeeper system that identifies when and how to seek advice. Using lawyers proactively and efficiently can yield advantages. Deciding between the use of in-house counsel and outside counsel, local counsel and national counsel, and generalists and specialists is important. So too is managing legal resources and legal costs. Using ongoing legal audits or profiles can avoid future problems. Ultimately the goal is to coordinate legal work and analysis with business decision making (see Table 27-3).

Similarly, an effective lawyer should understand the role of health care executives in operating a complex, multifunction organization whose constituents often have competing interests and values. Beyond knowing the mission of the organization and its organizational structure, the lawyer should have a sense of its history and relationship with other organizations. For the lawyer to be effective, he or she must have access to accurate information about the problem or question being brought by the manager. In the case of some institutions, particularly larger ones, the lawyer should be a member of the management team.

LEGAL ISSUES IN HEALTH SERVICES MANAGEMENT

In order to use lawyers effectively, health care executives must be able to identify and understand the legal issues that confront health care organizations. With such an understanding, the executives can know when to call in the lawyers and how to work with them to make more effective decisions. Below is a discussion of areas of the law in which executives are likely to face important legal issues.

Corporate Law

Hospitals are unique institutions that are increasingly broadly diversified and integrated both horizontally and vertically (i.e., they are health care conglomerates, not just acute care centers). Hospital corporations now own outpatient surgery centers, skilled nursing facilities, fitness centers, health maintenance organizations (HMOs), substance abuse treatment facilities, home health agencies, and durable medical equipment companies, among other types of ventures.

Corporate restructuring took place in most hospitals in the 1970s and 1980s to accommodate this diversification, but now hospitals are repositioning themselves from a corporate standpoint as we enter the 1990s. Many hospital corporations have found their reorganized structures to be too unwieldy and are seeking to streamline, to reduce the number of boards of directors that need to meet, and to coordinate their various ventures more rationally.

Another important corporate issue relates specifically to the role of hospital trustees in the governance of hospitals, particularly in the community hospital setting, where boards of trustees usually include many "community" members. As competi-

---

Table 27-3 The Health Executive–Legal Counsel Relationship

Health Executive	Legal Counsel
Is generally familiar with laws	Is generally familiar with the institution's mission and operation
Knows when to seek legal advice	Provides updates on legal developments
Uses legal advice in decision making	Provides legal audit of ongoing institutional activities

tion in the health care industry intensifies, the struggle to satisfy both the community service and business goals of health care institutions becomes more and more difficult. Indeed, concern over trustee liability has increased significantly, and a careful examination of the means of identifying trustee liability and insuring trustees against their liability is an important task of any health care organization.

While health care has been around for a long time, the "health care industry," as a discernible, competitive sector of our economy, is relatively new. The regulatory programs of the 1960s and 1970s, coupled with the emphasis on competition in the 1980s, have turned health care into a mature industry in which mergers, acquisitions, and, indeed, failures are commonplace.

Thus, health care executives must become corporate consolidation specialists and master the process of negotiating the purchase or sale of health care companies, including the nuances of an effective due diligence process (with special attention to all of the unique regulatory requirements and restrictions applicable to health care institutions). Once an executive has been involved in a few acquisitions, for example, he or she will understand that there is no effective substitute in acquisition documents, no matter how many representations and warranties by the seller are included, to a thorough due diligence effort. Ultimately, if a buyer wants to own the facility, he or she is going to have to fix the problems one way or another, and, generally speaking, the sooner the buyer knows about them, the better.

Being sufficiently knowledgeable about acquisitions requires at least understanding the differences between the sale of assets, mergers, and stock sale transactions. There is also the structural option of an affiliation between nonprofit institutions where the transaction consists solely of the coming together of two separate institutions under a single nonprofit parent or holding company. An affiliation of this nature generally does not constitute a true change of ownership and hence makes the regulatory requirements associated with the transaction less onerous. Moreover, understanding something

of the federal bankruptcy codes is necessary, since Chapter 7 and Chapter 11 filings by hospitals, HMOs, and other health care companies are becoming increasingly common.

Finally, in the corporate arena, a health care executive has to know how joint ventures and partnerships work. For tax reasons (i.e., to preserve tax-exempt status for a nonprofit system) and other reasons, partnerships are often the chosen form of organization for health care ventures. Moreover, joint ventures, as somewhat nebulous but very flexible vehicles for two or more disparate parties to share risk on a limited basis, remain popular in the health care field. Health care joint ventures, especially where physicians are involved, raise a whole host of legal issues, including corporate, tax, securities, antitrust, reimbursement, and fraud and abuse issues.

Tax Law

Concluding a complex corporate transaction, especially a merger or acquisition, requires an understanding of the tax implications for both parties; indeed, the structure of most health care transactions is ultimately determined by tax and reimbursement considerations. If health care executives do not have an ongoing working understanding of exempt organization tax law, they may run into problems grasping the goals and needs of a significant component of the health care industry—the many hospitals, nursing homes, other health care facilities, HMOs, and trade associations that are tax-exempt organizations.

Most health care provider facilities, as opposed to trade associations, are exempt under section 501(c)(3) of the Internal Revenue Code. Note that there are over 20 different code sections providing exemptions from income tax. Section 501(c)(3), however, is the only one that allows donors to the organization to deduct their donations. To be exempt under Section 501(c)(3), an organization has to engage in a charitable activity that is recognized in the code or in related Internal Revenue Service (IRS) regulations or rulings or court cases.

There are two basic tests established in the code applicable to Section 501(c)(3) organizations: the organizational test and the operational test. The organizational test has to do with the basic purposes of the organization. Fortunately, the "promotion of health" historically has been recognized as exempt under Section 501(c)(3), and therefore the organizational test has been, until now, fairly easy to satisfy for hospitals, nursing homes, and other health care facilities.

HMOs as well as some hospital spinoff activities are not necessarily exempt or may not be viewed by the IRS as exempt, and, in regard to these, careful study of the law and requirements prior to the submission of an application for exemption is advised. In particular, recent IRS General Counsel memoranda have been issued presenting that agency's restrictive view of the applicability of tax exemptions to HMOs.

To pass the operational test, an organization must operate on a charitable basis. Generally speaking, the good news is that once obtained, tax-exempt status is generally not taken away except under relatively egregious circumstances. Thus, while exempt organizations need to be vigilant about how they must operate, in gray areas they generally analyze both how risky they think a proposed activity is and how likely it is to be audited or discovered.

Two key issues of concern for health care exempt entities these days, with regard to the operational test, are private benefit/inurement and unrelated business income. The former issue has to do with the operation of a hospital or other charitable organization in a manner that puts money in the pockets of private individuals. The concern over losing tax-exempt status is most intense where the individual or individuals are "insiders" and have some degree of control over the charitable organization's decision making. Where the private benefit is not to insiders, the IRS supposedly applies a substantiality test to the activity (i.e., the benefit will probably be considered acceptable if it is only an insubstantial part or effect of the charitable organization's activity). Where the private benefit or inurement is to insiders, even one dollar could, in theory, trigger loss of exempt status. A major area of concern for

hospitals is whether any of its myriad physician recruitment and retention programs, including joint ventures with physicians, results in private inurement. Indeed, there is current controversy and speculation as to whether physicians should be considered insiders in connection with hospitals. A number of revenue rulings and other IRS pronouncements deal with this issue.

The unrelated business income issue involves the question of when, if ever, diversification activities become distant enough from the fundamental purpose of a hospital or other charitable organization to constitute unrelated and therefore taxable activities. This issue is behind much of the spinning off of for-profit subsidiaries commonly done by hospitals today, and it is also behind much of the corporate structure planning that accompanies the establishment of joint ventures. Unrelated income analysis focuses both on the question of whether certain activities constitute unrelated business subject to taxation and on the question of whether a particular organization is involved in so much unrelated activity as to jeopardize its exempt status.

Finally, the whole idea of granting tax-exempt status to hospitals is being questioned at the federal, state, and local levels of government. As hospitals have become more "businesslike" in order to respond to market competition, many people in the Congress, at the IRS, and at many state and local taxing agencies are beginning to wonder whether hospitals still provide sufficient public benefit to justify tax exemption.

Labor and Employment Law

Health care organizations are often large employers facing many sensitive employment issues. These include not only issues related to the National Labor Relations Act and collective bargaining with employees but also complex issues related to employment discrimination law as well as employee benefits law. An array of statutes and cases mandate actions and policies to end nondiscrimination in the workplace (the most recent of these is the

Americans with Disabilities Act). Executives must manage their organizations with a clear understanding of these regulations and how to avoid costly litigation over employment discrimination. Where organizations have contracts with the federal government, specific affirmative action requirements may apply.

As employers, health care executives also must understand and manage employee health care, pension, and other benefits costs. Increasingly, health care organizations are participating in managed care programs both as employers and as vendors of services.

The dramatic growth of negligent hiring cases and the erosion of the employment-at-will doctrine also have serious implications for all executives involved in day-to-day management. Finally, health care executives should be aware of legal issues related to substance abuse in the workplace and drug testing.

Medical Staff and Credentialing

Health care executives need to understand the fundamentals of and current trends in hospital–medical staff relations and credentialing and the peer review process as conducted by hospitals, by HMOs, and increasingly by other health care entities.

Every executive should be familiar with a typical set of hospital–medical staff bylaws as a way of understanding how hospitals and their admitting physicians have traditionally dealt with their relationship. A key legal issue is the determination of how much process is due to physicians who are seeking medical staff privileges or whose privileges have been terminated. This issue applies to physicians seeking admission to a managed care provider panel as well. There is a body of case law that can aid hospitals and other organizations in establishing fair credentialing procedures. Good general advice is to establish the procedures, in medical staff bylaws and elsewhere, ahead of time and stick to them—making up the rules along the way often leads to legal difficulties.

To jump ahead a bit, challenges to staff privileges or other credentialing decisions are often based on antitrust theories, and so antitrust law principles must be part of an executive's arsenal of knowledge. A case in point is the analysis of exclusive contracts between hospitals and hospital-based physicians. Generally, these have been upheld, but where the market share of the hospital or the physicians is too great, an exclusive contract can be problematic. Additionally, hospitals need to assess the structure of their credentialing process. Recent cases have suggested that a hospital and its medical staff are more likely to be viewed as coconspirators in an antitrust context if the medical staff has broad, independent decision-making authority in credentialing matters.

A specific area of ongoing current interest is the credentialing of nonphysician practitioners, such as chiropractors, podiatrists, and nurse practitioners. This is a sensitive area, and state nondiscrimination laws as well as the requirements of the Joint Commission on the Accreditation of Healthcare Organizations should be consulted in establishing proper criteria and procedures.

An important factor in credentialing are the laws and cases dealing with the confidentiality and disclosure of peer review data. This is a complex area in which both statutory and common law are involved and in which the law differs significantly from jurisdiction to jurisdiction. Those involved in peer review and credentialing want the data and information to remain confidential and to be held nondiscoverable in court proceedings, and they also want to be protected from being sued themselves in connection with their peer review activities. In fact, the law currently is very uneven in giving such peer review participants what they want.

The Health Care Quality Improvement Act of 1986 speaks to all of these issues and more. Broadly speaking, the act includes the following basic provisions:

- immunity protections for participants in the peer review process
- reporting requirements for certain actions taken by health care facilities that adversely affect the clinical privileges of a physician

- reporting requirements for insurance companies and health care facilities of payments made in settlement or satisfaction of judgments in medical malpractice actions
- a national databank containing information on health practitioners that can be accessed by hospitals as part of the credentialing process
- due process requirements for hospitals in connection with credentialing hearing and appeal procedures

Antitrust Law

At one time, years ago, it was believed that the health care field and its participants generally were not subject to antitrust laws; cases over the past several years and recent enforcement priorities of the federal antitrust enforcement agencies have demonstrated that such is not the case. Indeed, something in the order of 20 percent of all antitrust cases now involve health care issues.

The Sherman Act is the most fundamental and frequently litigated antitrust law. Section 1 prohibits any contract, combination, or conspiracy that unreasonably restrains trade. To establish a violation, it must be demonstrated that multiple parties and a conspiracy are involved. The multiple parties issue can be tricky in the case of parents and subsidiaries and employers and employees. The general principle is that these are not separate entities, but there can be questions where ownership is partial or where the employee has a separate economic interest. Conspiracy can also be found based on patterns of conduct or on statements in meetings or formats other than actual written agreements.

Once the existence of multiple parties and a conspiracy are established, the reasonableness of the conduct in question must be assessed—under rule-of-reason analysis, courts look to both the purpose and effect of the conduct in question. Rule-of-reason analysis is difficult and burdensome to administer. Prosecution and defense of rule-of-reason cases is time consuming and expensive. Thus, certain per se rules have been developed as rules of judicial economy to avoid lengthy and fact-specific

inquiry as to reasonableness. Among the important categories of per se violation are the following.

Agreements as to Price. In the health care arena, this issue has triggered lengthy and continuous litigation regarding provider ownership of HMOs, PPOs, and other managed care programs, beginning with the famous *Maricopa* case in 1982.

Market Allocation among Competitors. This issue can arise if competing hospitals allocate services.

Group Boycotts. This is relevant to staff privilege cases as well as some cases involving alleged provider boycotts of certain payers (e.g., where all the providers in a particular area agree to contract with only one HMO or other managed care plan).

Tie-in Arrangements. In this type of arrangement, a seller ties the sale of a product in one market to the sale of a product in another market. The use of tie-ins has been at issue in the so-called downstream referral cases, in which hospitals have been sued for allegedly requiring patients to use hospital-owned durable medical equipment or other ancillary companies.

In many cases, even where the per se rules apparently apply, the courts have moved to a modified rule of reason, or "quick look" approach, in order to soften the automatic presumption of the per se rule without engaging in a full-blown rule-of-reason analysis.

Section 2 of the Sherman Act prohibits unlawful monopolization or attempts to monopolize. In either case, significant market power by a single actor, coupled with predatory acts, is required. A critical concept in Section 2 analysis and also, in many cases, in Section 1 analysis is market power, even where the per se rules supposedly apply. Thus, health care executives should understand the concept of market power (in terms of its product component and its geographic component) and how it has been defined in the health care context. Of particular relevance in this regard are the recent hospital merger cases. The Department of Justice and the Federal Trade Commission (FTC) have begun to challenge the merger of nonprofit hospitals and are expected to continue such challenges. Understanding how the Department of

Justice and the FTC define hospital markets and what criteria they bring to their analysis of hospital and other health care company mergers, such as mergers of large physician organizations, is essential for health care executives, whether or not they expect to be involved in an antitrust-sensitive transaction.

A related question involves whether or not Section 7 of the Clayton Act, the principal federal antitrust statute used to challenge mergers and acquisitions, is applicable to nonprofit hospitals. Furthermore, as recent hospital merger cases have shown, in addition to market analysis, health care executives should understand the defenses to an antitrust challenge, such as barriers-to-entry analysis and the failing company defense. They should also understand the concept of economic efficiencies and how mergers can be analyzed on a cost-benefit basis to assess the relative economic harm they may cause as compared to the economic benefit they may bring to consumers.

The Hart-Scott-Rodino Premerger Notification Program requires that the Department of Justice and the FTC be notified of mergers, acquisitions, and joint ventures of a certain size prior to their consummation. The health care industry has grown to a size today that many proposed mergers and acquisitions trigger Hart-Scott-Rodino filing requirements.

And finally, joint ventures, which are so common in health care today, are analyzed under the antitrust laws. Both Section 1 of the Sherman Act and Section 7 of the Clayton Act may be applicable. In certain circumstances, joint ventures are viewed as pro-competitive entities—entities that enhance competition. But the degree of risk, if any, shared by the joint venturers, the market power of the joint venturers, and the existence of other restraints on competition created by the joint venture are all factors taken into consideration when determining whether a particular joint venture could be held to violate the antitrust laws.

Patient Care Issues

There is a range of important legal issues relating to the delivery of patient care, including the following:

- Consent-to-treatment issues and issues related to informed consent policies, including exceptions to consent requirements, as in emergencies, and rules regarding consent to treatment for minors.
- Legal issues surrounding the patients' right to discontinue or refuse treatment, including issues of surrogate consent.
- Detention of patients and potential liability for false imprisonment charges in cases where patients allegedly have been held against their will.
- Liability in connection with discharge planning and the importance of appropriate discharge policies and documentation.
- Emergency services (or antidumping) laws. At the federal level and in many states, the consequences of a failure to properly screen or transfer an emergency patient can include fines and termination of a hospital's Medicare participation agreement. In particular, the role of physicians in making emergency services treatment and transfer decisions are very important, as the trend is toward holding hospitals liable for the decisions of their physicians.
- Issues related to AIDS patients and the law, particularly liability for treatment decisions and AIDS infection as well as confidentiality issues and notification of persons exposed to the AIDS virus.
- The unique legal issues related to psychiatric and substance abuse services, including the potential liability of health care facilities as well as the voluntary and involuntary commitment of mental health patients. Confidentiality of mental health records is a particularly sensitive issue.
- State and federal law regarding the confidentiality and retention of medical records and patient information.

Hospital and Professional Liability

Hospitals, physicians, insurance companies, and managed care companies, as well as self-insured employers, are all experiencing greater liability exposure in connection with health care delivery and payment. Liability generally is incurred under one of three broad legal theories: negligence, intentional tort (e.g., defamation, battery), and breach of contract. "Malpractice" usually refers to negligence. The theory used may have important implications for liability insurance coverage, since some policies cover liability for negligence but not for breach of contractual obligations or intentional torts. Common to all liability suits, regardless of the legal theory involved, are these elements: (1) a legal duty owed by the provider or health care company to the patient, (2) a breach of that duty, and (3) injury resulting from the breach.

Starting with hospital cases and moving into the managed care arena, there has been a significant expansion in liability findings by U.S. courts. Liability exposure for health care companies is expanding not only in connection with the acts of employees and independent contractors that are imputed to health care companies, but also in connection with direct corporate negligence, such as the failure of a hospital to supervise treatment properly or the failure of an HMO to operate a utilization management system properly.

An important development is the trend toward tort reform and using alternative ways of resolving disputes, including traditional approaches (e.g., arbitration). Using alternative approaches may be critical to the survival of health care organizations in the coming years. Finally, liability issues must be understood in order to maintain up-to-date and effective risk management programs and thereby reduce liability exposure as much as possible.

Third-Party Reimbursement

For health care providers, an efficient reimbursement system is critical to the success of the organization. Ensuring the efficiency of the system is impossible in the current environment without an understanding of many of the legal and accounting issues related to reimbursement. Staying on top of the constant changes in Part A and Part B reimbursement under Medicare and Medicaid and in the payment schemes of the major indemnity insurance carriers and numerous managed care companies is a full-time job, to say the least.

Executives of insurance and managed care companies need to be aware of the fundamentals of government payment schemes, both as potential participants in programs where the government serves as payer and also in order to compare their own payment mechanisms with government payment methodologies. From a transactional standpoint, the reimbursement implications of any proposed merger, acquisition, or joint venture are often of determinative importance. Also, as part of the entire reimbursement arena, health care executives should be cognizant of the legal issues related to PRO review of Medicare services, how PROs work, and what implications PRO activities may have for their organizations.

Fraud and Abuse

There is a wide array of state and federal laws governing fraud, abuse, and misrepresentation in connection with the payment of medical claims. These laws include federal criminal statutes for violations related to Medicare, such as false statements in connection with claims, illegal remuneration for referrals, or violations of participation agreements. Additionally, there are federal criminal statutes for false representations under the Social Security Act, federal criminal statutes for false statements with respect to Medicare supplemental insurance policies, the False Claims Act, mail fraud statutes, and federal racketeering laws. Noncriminal federal statutes include Medicare civil sanctions and civil monetary penalty laws. Moreover, nearly every state has some laws that could be applied to fraud and abuse situations, including commercial bribery laws, prohibition on payment for patient referrals, fee-splitting prohibitions, and unfair trade practices. Furthermore, there are state and federal laws dealing with false advertising and commercial disparagement as well as state regulation of medical advertising.

The foregoing universe of laws provides for many serious sanctions against health care providers and others who run afoul of their provisions. Moreover, there is currently an aggressive climate of enforcement of these laws not only at the federal level but also at the state level. A particular concern in recent years has been the apparent breadth of the federal Medicare illegal remuneration (or antikickback) law as that law has been interpreted in several court cases and by the Office of Inspector General of the Department of Health and Human Services. Safe harbor regulations interpreting this law were published in July 1991, but many legitimate questions of providers regarding the scope of the antikickback law remain unanswered. Moreover, many states have become more aggressive in their enforcement activities in the fraud and abuse arena. For example, Florida, in response to studies showing that there is a statistically significant relationship between physician ownership in joint ventures and referrals to such ventures, passed legislation in 1991 that prohibits physician referrals to certain kinds of joint ventures in which the physicians have an ownership interest.

Health care executives need to be familiar with the cases and situations in this arena that are applicable to the activities of their organizations. As with certain key concerns in the tax area and in the fraud and abuse area, a clear answer is often not available for many cutting-edge situations and transactions health care executives will be facing. However, understanding the background to the laws, the principal transgressions that regulators are looking for, and the fact patterns that have tended to be troublesome will aid executives, in conjunction with their attorneys, in charting a course that will be both ethical and effective from a business standpoint and reasonably safe from a legal standpoint.

Managed Care

Generally speaking, managed care is a process by which the parties responsible for paying for health care services, either directly or through arrangements with providers or independent managed care service companies, intervene in the health care delivery process in various ways in order to, in theory, reduce the costs and improve or maintain the quality of such care. Managed care is both an industry and a process. Ultimately, managed care is nothing more than a range of activities designed to control to a greater or lesser extent the means by which health care is delivered for cost or quality purposes. The activities within this range can be categorized according to the degree to which they actually manage or intervene in the traditional fee-for-service practice of medicine. At the risk of greatly oversimplifying this area of health care law, the managed care activities or approaches can be divided into three basic categories.

The first category or type of managed care is utilization management. Most indemnity insurers now offer some form of utilization management as part of their indemnity insurance programs. PSROs and PROs spawned a whole private peer review industry as other health care payers, such as indemnity insurers and employers, tried to obtain some of the same kind of cost and quality review sought by Medicare. Numerous companies have been formed locally and nationally to provide private utilization management services. Indeed, there has been so much utilization management activity that health care providers have sometimes felt smothered by requests for medical records and other information to be reviewed. One result of this proliferation of utilization management activity has been legislation in many states, largely promoted by the provider community, to control and regulate private utilization review organizations.

The second broad category of managed care consists of preferred provider arrangements. In this type of arrangement, the ultimate party responsible for payment—typically an insurance company or employer—creates a benefit plan structure for its beneficiaries that includes economic incentives to use certain health care providers in the community over others. The economic incentives are usually in the form of lower copayments and deductibles. On the provider side of the preferred provider equation, the providers designated as preferred agree to accept certain conditions in order to be included in the panel. Typically, these conditions include discounted fees and agreement to participate in a utilization management program. In many cases, the preferred provider panel is put together by a broker or by the providers themselves, and then the panel seeks to contract with various payers. This type of panel is referred to as a preferred provider organization (PPO). In other cases, the payer goes out and puts together the preferred provider plan.

In the typical PPO situation, the payer remains responsible for all medical payments and holds on to all the insurance-type risk involved in the program. Hence, preferred provider arrangements typically do not involve the transfer of the insurance risk from the indemnity insurer or employer to the providers, and the preferred provider panels or networks established in a preferred provider arrangement are not for the most part regulated as insurance companies. However, there are laws in a number of states that govern the establishment of preferred provider panels by insurance companies. In some cases, the insurer or PPO is required to file certain information with the state insurance or health department, but this is a process far less onerous than obtaining a license to engage in the business of insurance. Also, where companies that are not licensed insurers involve themselves in processing the payment of medical claims, whether or not this activity is associated with the preferred provider arrangement, such companies may face regulatory requirements as third-party administrators.

The third major category of managed care comprises health maintenance organizations (HMOs). HMOs generally preceded preferred provider arrangements in time because of the impetus of the 1973 federal HMO law, but they are more invasive than either simple utilization management or a preferred provider arrangement. HMOs are separately licensed and incorporated entities that combine the delivery of care and the payment for such care. They are licensed in every jurisdiction in the country except the District of Columbia. HMOs collect prepayments or premiums from their enrollees and provide or arrange for the provision of all of the medical care covered under their benefit plans. Generally, enrollees of an HMO are required to obtain all of their health care from providers under contract with the HMO. The HMO's rates, its benefits, and the provisions of its contracts with providers are all subject to state regulation.

In recent years, owing to the financial failures of a number of HMOs, state regulatory requirements have become tougher, closer to those for insurance companies. Originally, the federal HMO qualification program and many state HMO laws were geared in part toward encouraging this form of health care payment and delivery. Generally speaking, HMOs aggressively manage care to ensure that it is efficiently provided and of a high quality. Such management of care involves various utilization controls, such as preadmission certification and concurrent review of patient lengths of stay, and it also involves establishing payment arrangements with providers that put the providers, both hospitals and physicians, at some financial risk themselves for the amount of care being provided. (In other words, providers will not be paid all of their fees if the HMO is forced to pay for more care than was projected in a given time period.)

In addition to these three basic categories of managed care, there are a number of hybrid products and services. For instance, some preferred provider arrangements are exclusive in nature, meaning that beneficiaries have to receive their care from a member of the preferred provider panel. As another example, some HMOs are now experimenting with allowing beneficiaries to receive care outside of the HMO panel of providers. Among the most visible innovations are point-of-service products, which allow beneficiaries to opt for an HMO, PPO, or traditional indemnity product at the time he or she seeks to obtain health care services. Health care executives need to understand at a minimum some of the new directions that managed care product development is taking and the regulatory implications of the changes. State laws remain uneven in regard to their overall governance of HMOs, PPOs, and utilization management programs, and as the distinctions between these approaches blur and more hybrid products appear, the regulatory scheme will become more complex.

Many health care providers have moved beyond merely contracting with managed care companies and have sought to develop their own managed care companies or to joint-venture with others to establish some control over managed care products and services. Many hospital corporations now include a managed care company as part of their diversified system. Given the general expectation that the percentage of health care delivered in this country through managed care systems will continue to grow, this trend in provider control, management, and joint-venturing of managed care also can be expected to continue. Therefore, an executive's understanding of the corporate structure of health care companies will need to include an understanding of the strategic role of managed care in diversified health care systems. (For more on managed care, see Chapter 8.)

RESOURCE REQUIREMENTS

Numerous factors affect how legal services are provided in a health care organization: size, setting, history, corporate culture, degree of centralization of management and services, stage of development of the organization, governing board role, and risk financing or liability insurance arrangements.

Nevertheless, the basic options are to use (1) in-house legal counsel, (2) outside legal services, or (3) a combination of in-house counsel and outside legal services (see Figure 27-1).[1]

Choosing a Model

In-house counsel is used by an increasing number of teaching hospitals and large community hospitals or health care systems. National corporations operating or managing hospitals, HMOs, laboratories, or other multisite health care organizations generally have a legal staff at the corporate central office. An in-house attorney, however, may be provided to each individual institution in addition to access to the central office legal staff. In the case of government hospitals and health care agencies, legal services may be provided by the county or municipal attorney or the office of the state attorney general. Again, individual hospitals or agencies may have their own in-house attorneys. In-house lawyers can be full time or part time. Some are members of the management team, whereas others provide staff support.

For many hospitals, a local lawyer or law firm serves as "general counsel" and plays a role analogous to the role of in-house counsel. A member of such a firm often sits on the hospital's board of directors. This kind represents a hybrid of the in-house counsel model and outside legal services model. The larger the local firm, the more areas it can cover and the less additional outside counsel will be needed.

Outside legal services can be obtained by a retainer contract or on a temporary basis for special purposes. For some types of services, a retainer may be indicated, such as providing frequent and routine operational advice to management and the governing board. In cases where the need for specific legal assistance occurs infrequently (e.g., management-labor negotiations, Medicare fraud and abuse investigations, antitrust problems, corporate tax or bond issues, medical malpractice litigation, or certificate-of-need matters), the organization may want to hire a qualified lawyer or law firm on a temporary basis.

Combining inside and outside legal services is increasingly common, since health care organizations face increasingly complex and diverse legal issues. An in-house lawyer or staff of lawyers can handle many of the functions demanding daily attention, such as corporate contracts, personnel matters, and risk management and quality assurance programs. However, for liability lawsuits, collective bargaining problems, corporate restructuring, and complicated reimbursement questions, the in-house lawyer may need to seek assistance or consultation from a law

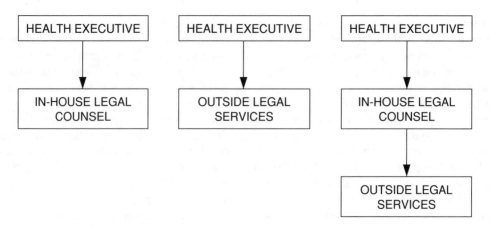

Figure 27-1 Legal Service Arrangements

firm that specializes in those matters. In such situations the in-house counsel can serve as the gatekeeper for legal services and can also monitor the performance of the outside legal services. Combining inside and outside legal services may prove to be the most economical type of arrangement.

A Survey of Hospital Legal Service Arrangements

A national survey conducted in 1984 by a consulting firm in conjunction with two law firms showed that the use of in-house counsel is a widespread phenomenon.[2] Of 675 nongovernment, nonmilitary hospitals with over 50 beds and with a legal staff, more than half did not have in-house counsel prior to 1980. More than a third of the survey respondents said their primary reason for acquiring in-house counsel was better service, and a fifth cited cost savings. The survey found that larger hospitals are more likely to have full-time lawyers, and the average number on staff was 2.6. Part-time staff averaged 1.3 members.

The surveyed hospitals allotted their full-time in-house legal staff an average budget of $148,170, paying the staff director an average salary of $51,130. Less than 10 percent paid salaries over $70,000, 15 percent paid less than $40,000, and 44

percent declined to reveal the salaries. Half had legal staff budgets of less than $98,000, and only 2 percent reported budgets over $500,000.

According to the survey, the typical head of a hospital legal staff was 41 years old and had 9.4 years of outside legal experience. The most common title was *general counsel;* other titles included *legal counsel, vice-president,* and *director of legal affairs.* Sixty-four percent of the directors reported to the hospital CEO, 82 percent maintained outside legal relationships, 80 percent performed services for administrative committees, half attended hospital board meetings, and three-fourths provided services to medical staff committees.

The survey found that one out of five hospitals utilized both in-house counsel and outside legal services, while four out of five used outside services exclusively. At the time of the survey, only 1 percent used in-house counsel exclusively. Perhaps surprisingly, in light of the reported increase in the use of in-house counsel, 85 percent said they would look to outside services for future legal needs.

Controlling Legal Service Costs

One of the continuing goals of health care organizations is to control the cost of legal services while ensuring their high quality. One observer has suggested the following ideas for reducing outside legal fees[3]:

- For certificates of need and other government approval applications, use managerial staff for most of the paperwork, especially for collecting marketing, budgetary, and architectural data.
- For physician contracts, vendor contracts, leases, and so on, fill out "form contracts" prepared by the legal counsel and submit the filled-out contracts to the legal counsel for execution.
- Restrict personal meetings with the legal counsel and communicate primarily by letter and telephone.
- Restrict "teaming" of lawyers by asking the legal counsel to furnish only one lawyer for meetings and projects when possible.
- Require detailed statements of services provided.
- Use different lawyers or firms for different kinds of legal problems.

Although these suggestions may help control the cost of legal services, it is ultimately the responsibility of the health care executive to ensure that these services are appropriate for the organization. The health care executive should periodically review with the inside and outside counsel various ways in which the arrangement can be made more efficient and cost-effective.[4]

Difficult times in the health care industry in the late 1980s and the recession of the early 1990s have created even greater cost pressures on health care corporations. Yet, increasingly, complex regulatory problems, including a step-up in investigations of health care activities by government agencies, require even more legal involvement. There is tremendous current demand for new and creative ways to provide and pay for legal services.

Billing Arrangements with Outside Services

The standard arrangement is to bill on an hourly basis (usually calculated in tenths of an hour) for all services provided, including telephone calls, committee meetings, representation before agencies, and associated travel. Organizations are increasingly careful to scrutinize outside law firm bills to make sure all billings for fees and disbursements are proper. Executives should become familiar with law firm bills and should require law firms to provide specific, detailed information about the nature of work completed and the attorneys involved. Organizations also should be assertive about not paying for work not clearly assigned and discussed in advance. Alternatives to full hourly billing that might be explored include the following:

- The organization and the law firm might establish specific budgets in advance for work assigned.
- The organization might ask for discounts on hourly fees, especially for major projects.
- The organization might try a fixed fee for defined projects or transactions, such as a corporate reorganization or a joint venture.
- The organization could use a "requirements" contract or special retainer to engage a law firm for a defined purpose, such as tax consultation or risk management. Under this arrangement the firm would be paid a fixed amount per month for whatever services were provided during the contract period (e.g., a year).
- If the organization is involved as a plaintiff in litigation, a contingent arrangement might make sense, such as the sharing of a percentage of the recovery of damages (in addition to payment for expenses incurred for witnesses, travel, documents, etc.).

Other ideas include permitting the law firm to use associates and paralegals since the hourly charges are less. However, it is important to retain full and complete access to a responsible partner. Moreover, using less experienced attorneys, while cheaper by the hour, may not result in lower overall costs, since the attorneys might be much less efficient.

One final consideration in developing a relationship with an outside law firm: It is essential that the firm divulge any conflicts of interest. For example, if a member of the law firm currently represents a medical staff member in litigation or sits on the board of another hospital in the community, this should be disclosed, although it might not prevent the establishment of a relationship with the firm. Since large law firms represent a wide range of clients, complete separation from all competitors or associated organizations may not always be feasible, but disclosure is the first requirement in discussing an arrangement.

QUALITY MANAGEMENT AND LEGAL SERVICES

The health care executive is the prime mover in any effort to create a program for promoting continuous quality improvement in an organization. It is well documented that quality depends on the corporate culture, especially as it exists at the top levels of administration. Total quality management of one department is never ultimately successful without organization-wide involvement. Therefore, quality in an organization is not necessarily ensured by having the best available legal services, whether provided by a highly competent in-house counsel or by the best law firm in the community.

Quality in an organization is strongly related, nevertheless, to the effectiveness of its legal resources. An organization that makes decisions based on inadequate or unreliable legal advice is doomed to have to deal with unpleasant problems. At worst, an organization otherwise geared up for pursuing a goal of quality services can stumble by having to confront regulatory delays, medical staff and employee disputes, contractor difficulties, and damaging liability lawsuits. A legal services arrangement that supports the mission of the organization with careful and considered legal guidance will increase the organization's chances of attaining its objectives.

There are several ways that competent legal services can assist an organization that has decided to pursue total quality management. But for the assistance provided to be effective, the management of the organization must

- remain loyal to the organization's charter
- follow an efficient path through the regulatory maze
- be prepared to adapt organizational plans to changes in the legal and political environment
- avoid circumstances that invite litigation
- respond to legal challenges with effective defenses
- have mechanisms for resolving disputes (both external and internal) in a positive and responsible manner
- find ways to merge legal considerations with ethical principles for the furtherance of the aims of both the organization and society

Patients' rights are related to the quality concept of "meeting customer requirements," and clearly the in-house attorney (or the outside legal counsel) can assist in identifying those rights. The attorney can also provide advice about the specific operational and regulatory framework for ensuring they are not infringed. In particular, the attorney can help in developing an organizational statement of patients' rights and responsibilities (a starting point is found in the preamble to the accreditation standards promulgated by the Joint Commission) and in devising systematic procedures for obtaining and documenting patients' authorization and consent to medical services and third-party payment for those services.

Organizational efforts to ensure quality of care and to adhere to risk management principles also require the attorney's participation. Legal involvement is required for (1) maintaining appropriate procedures that ensure the confidentiality of patient and provider information (this may require interpreting federal and state laws relating to peer review, attorney work product, and medical recordkeeping); (2) devising an internal mechanism for identifying and sanctioning unacceptable behavior by health care providers; and (3) reporting admitting privileges limitations and liability settlements or payments to state and national agencies in accordance with state laws and the federal Health Quality Improvement Act of 1986.

Finally, if an organization uses in-house legal staff, they must be included in the quality management training and orientation programs. If the legal services are supplied by an outside firm, the law firm should be consulted as to the best ways to incorporate the relevant legal personnel into the organization's quality efforts.

MANAGING LEGAL RESOURCES IN THE FUTURE

The use of lawyers by institutions in the health care field is changing rapidly as health care companies, after the tremendous expansion and growth of the early to middle 1980s, adjust to a period of slower growth or no growth and to the need to carefully monitor and control expenses in order to survive. As a result, institutional legal budgets are being examined as never before. At the same time, the scope and complexity of legal issues are as great as ever and appear to be increasing. Health care executives face a daunting challenge: responding to the legal demands placed on their organizations while effectively managing legal costs.

Using lawyers effectively requires knowing enough about legal problems to be able to evaluate what lawyers are saying, asking the right questions, involving lawyers at the appropriate time, and knowing when lawyers are not needed (see Exhibit 27-1). The overall strategy for management should be to get the most benefit from using lawyers, not simply to minimize lawyer involvement. Lawyers should not be overutilized (because management does not want to get involved in legal decision making) or underutilized (for cost reasons or because of concern that they will create more problems than they solve). Obviously, it is essential that executives be able to identify lawyers who can provide both effective and efficient assistance. But executives need to know clearly what they are looking for in order to make the best selection.

Health care law is highly interdisciplinary. Specialists in this field need a detailed understanding of the unique attributes of health care and also an un-

Exhibit 27-1 Process for Using Legal Services

1. Identify problem
2. Analyze possible legal considerations
3. Seek legal review
4. Present facts and questions to legal counsel
5. Interact with legal counsel
6. Receive legal advice
7. Utilize legal advice in decision-making process
8. Notify legal counsel of management decision
9. Monitor results
10. Prevent recurrence of problem

derstanding of, or at least a working familiarity with, all of the areas of the law discussed in this chapter. It is extremely difficult—and will probably become more difficult in the future—for any one lawyer to be able to retain a mastery of so many different fields of law as they relate to the health care system. A certain critical mass of attorney knowledge and skills is necessary to handle modern health care law issues. A small in-house staff or a small local law firm simply may not have the necessary resources at their beck and call.

To effectively manage legal services and costs in the future, the executives of any health care institution will need to establish (1) an effective gatekeeper system, whether the gatekeeper is in house, outside in a small firm, or outside in a large firm; (2) a group or groups of lawyers that can handle all of the health care institution's complex legal matters, including litigation; and (3) a cost arrangement that will provide some budget security for the health care institution.

Many health care companies with large legal budgets have begun to implement an array of retainer-type arrangements in order to obtain predictability regarding legal services. Some companies make payments based on estimates, which may or may not be accurate in the long run. Other companies use capitation payment arrangements, which place the law firms at risk if the costs of services are greater than the agreed retainer amounts.

The next decade can be expected to be a period of continued intense competition among health care institutions, featuring increased cost consciousness by payers, including the federal government. Profit margins of many health care companies may continue to fall, money may be difficult to borrow, and there will be less room than ever for a health care executive to make a mistake or begin a program that runs into difficulties, particularly legal difficulties. At the same time, the level of legal scrutiny from federal, state, and local taxing, fraud and abuse, antitrust, and other authorities can be expected to increase. New rules and regulations will continue to be promulgated. Health care executives will have to be more proactive in getting on top of the legal issues that are likely to be part of every project or program on which they embark. It will generally be too risky to leave legal issues unattended until specific problems arise.

Health care executives will need to establish protocols for consulting legal counsel at the appropriate times and to involve counsel in planning processes in order to avoid difficulties down the road. Routine legal audits or reviews of various areas of corporate activity are likely to become increasingly common. The successful executives will be those who make effective decisions and develop workable programs. Making sure such decisions and programs are legally sound from the outset will be essential.

ADDITIONAL RESOURCES

Organizations

American Academy of Hospital Attorneys, 840 North Lake Shore Drive, Chicago, IL 60611. 312\280-6600.

American Society of Law and Medicine, 765 Commonwealth Avenue, Boston, MA 02215. 617\262-4990.

American Society of Risk Management, 840 North Lake Shore Drive, Chicago, IL 60611.

National Health Lawyers Association, 1620 Eye St. NW, Washington, DC 20036. 202\833-1100.

Health Law Forum, American Bar Association, 750 North Lake Shore Drive, Chicago, IL 60611.

Periodicals

American Journal of Law and Medicine,

Business and Health,

Health Advocate, National Health Law Program,

Health Law Digest, National Health Lawyers Association,

HealthSpan, Law and Business, Inc.,

Hospital Risk Management, American Health Consultants, Inc.,

Hospitals (law section), American Hospital Association,

Journal of Health and Hospital Law, American Hospital Association,

Journal of Health Politics, Policy and Law, Duke University Press,

Journal of Legal Medicine, American College of Legal Medicine,

Law, Medicine and Health Care,

Journal of Health Law and Policy, Catholic University of America,

Modern Health Care,

Washington Report on Medicine and Health, McGraw-Hill,

Newsletters are published periodically by many universities, health law firms, state societies of hospital attorneys, health care supply and pharmaceutical companies, and other commercial organizations.

Books

Hall, M.A., and I.M. Ellman. *Healthcare law and ethics.* St. Paul, Minn.: West Publishing Co., 1990.

Hospital law manual. 3 vols. Rev. ed. Gaithersburg, Md.: Aspen Publishers, 1991.

Macdonald, M.G., K.C. Meyer, and B. Essig. *Health care law: A practical guide.* New York: Matthew Bender & Co., 1986.

Miller, R. *Problems in hospital law.* 6th ed. Gaithersburg, Md.: Aspen Publishers, 1990.

National Health Lawyers Association. Annual binders from conferences on various health law topics.

Wing, K.R. *The law and the public's health.* 3d ed. Ann Arbor, Mich.: Health Administration Press, 1990.

NOTES

1. See the discussion of this topic as it relates to corporations generally in The Inside View: Nine Corporate General Counsels Talk about In-House Management and Outside Firms, *The American Lawyer,* June 1991, p. 172.

2. Witt Associates Inc., *Health Care Legal Counsel: Report of a Survey,* reported in *Hospitals,* November 16, 1985, p. 50.

3. Cotora, C. Controlling and Reducing Legal Fees in the Age of Fixed Reimbursement, *Hospital and Health Services Administration,* July-August 1986, pp. 45–54.

4. See the following discussions of controlling legal services costs: R.J. Burdett, Jr. and M.Z. Taylor, Cost Control Should Extend to Legal Services, *Healthcare Financial Management,* March 1991, pp. 68–72; Special Report: Law Firm Billing, *Legal Times,* December 9, 1991, pp. 11–16.

Part V

Health Service Access and Delivery

Stephen J. Williams

Accessing Health Care

28

Purpose: Access to care results from a complex balancing act involving numerous financial, organizational, patient, provider, and societal factors. Ultimately, it is the responsibility of the health care system's managers, working in collaboration with the professional providers of care and the nation's health care policy makers, to structure and operate the system in such a manner as to enhance access and quality while simultaneously controlling costs and increasing efficiency and patient and provider satisfaction.

and control of points of patient access. Access to health care systems and its management by provider organizations is also key to ensuring the efficient provision of services, reducing unnecessary utilization, and managing the financial burdens of providing care.

The increasing role of managed care programs, which rely heavily on managing patient access to services, is an important current trend. Eventual further rationalization of the health care system will require a more aggressive approach to management of patient access and better utilization of patient triage and other mechanisms for channeling patients so that they receive the most appropriate types of care.

INTRODUCTION

This chapter describes the health care continuum of services provided to patients, how patients access those services, and how access to health care services is affected by various environmental, social, and economic factors. It delineates the structure of the health care system, focusing on patient entry points into the system and the role of various provider organizations in facilitating access.

A central aspect of the organization and operation of health services systems is the establishment

This chapter discusses both macro- and micro-characteristics of the health care system and of patient access. It reviews the structure of the health care system in terms of the various major components contributing to the provision of health care and describes personal health services, the delivery of specific health care services to individuals in response to their care-seeking behavior, and public health and other environmental and preventive approaches to ensuring the adequacy of health care.

561

Reliance on therapeutic intervention after the onset of disease or following injury, which has been the traditional strategy of the health care system, is now increasingly recognized to have significant limitations. Society must focus on preventive health services and other population-based efforts to reduce the need for health care in the first place. As a result, access to health care services and the need for health care must also be considered in the context of primary avoidance of disease through widespread society-based prevention efforts and specific preventive behavior and healthier life styles on the part of individuals. Eventual control of health services utilization will be achieved not only through limiting or channeling access to curative services but also through reducing the demand for those services.

This chapter delineates the organization of therapeutic, curative, and other individual health services. Rehabilitative, extended care, and related forms of health care are also brought into the discussion.

The key points of patient entry into the health care system are discussed, particularly as they affect use of services, quality of care, and cost of services. Specific factors subject to organizational control by the managers of health care systems are given particular attention, including methods for managing patient utilization of primary care services, such as the use of physician gatekeepers. Utilization and access can also be influenced by the management of patient scheduling and reimbursement.

This chapter includes specific suggestions for enhancing access. The roles of individual patients, provider organizations, professional providers, management, and society (through government intervention) in affecting, controlling, and ensuring access to care are discussed.

The chapter ends with remarks on how to deal with those who have limited access or no access at all. Each of the key parties involved in providing, organizing, paying for, and utilizing health care services has a role to play in making better use of the existing system and in changing the system to be more responsive to the needs of all consumers while simultaneously meeting the needs of providers and payers.

MEASURING ACCESS

The measurement of the actual use of health care services is achieved through counts of patient visits, hospital use, and other related indicators. Actual utilization of services does not necessarily reflect the true underlying need or demand for care, however.[1] *Demand* is defined as care-seeking behavior that may or may not result in actual utilization, whereas *need* for services connotes either patient or professional provider evaluation of requirements for service, which again may or may not be actually met.[2] And the care-seeking behavior of individuals differs as a result of variations in sociodemographic characteristics, attitudes, and many other factors.

Differentials between actual utilization and need and demand, where measurable through special surveys and other evaluation techniques, reflect deficiencies on the part of the health care system in providing services. Since not all potential utilization that is avoided will lead to adverse outcomes, barriers introduced by system providers to reduce utilization, such as in a managed care environment, can also lead to differences between need, demand, and actual utilization.

Measuring the Utilization of Services

Utilization of physician services is measured by the number of patient visits, the type of visits, and other characteristics; utilization of dental services is measured using the same indicators; and institutional utilization is measured by the number of hospital bed-days and long-term care bed-days.[3] Tables 28-1, 28-2, and 28-3 present typical measures of physician, dentist, and hospital utilization (which reflect access to care) and the current values for each indicator in the United States.

Differential access to health services is reflected in the tables by differences in use among groups in the population. For example, income and other

Table 28-1 Physician Contacts, United States, 1990

		Place of Contact				
Characteristic	Physician Contacts (no. per person)	Doctor's Office (%)	Hospital Outpatient Department[a] (%)	Telephone (%)	Home (%)	Other[b] (%)
Total[c,d]	5.5	59.9	13.7	12.7	2.1	11.6
Age						
Under 15 Years	4.5	60.7	13.6	14.9	0.9	9.9
Under 5 Years	6.9	59.1	14.0	15.9	1.1	9.8
5–14 Years	3.2	62.6	13.1	13.7	0.6	10.0
15–44 Years	4.8	59.4	14.3	12.0	0.6	13.7
45–64 Years	6.4	60.4	14.1	12.2	2.0	11.4
65 Years and Over	9.2	58.7	11.1	9.9	11.8	8.4
65–74 Years	8.5	60.2	13.7	9.7	7.0	9.4
75 Years and Over	10.1	56.8	7.8	10.2	18.1	7.0
Sex[c]						
Male	4.7	57.6	16.1	11.3	2.1	12.9
Female	6.1	61.6	12.2	13.4	2.0	10.9
Race[c]						
White	5.6	61.7	12.3	13.1	1.9	11.0
Black	5.1	48.2	24.3	9.1	2.8	15.6
Family Income[c]						
Less Than $14,000	6.3	48.9	19.9	11.5	3.2	16.4
$14,000–$24,999	5.6	56.9	16.0	11.8	1.7	13.5
$25,000–$34,999	5.2	60.9	13.8	13.2	1.6	10.4
$35,000–$49,999	5.7	62.0	11.5	14.6	1.1	10.9
$50,000 or More	5.6	66.1	8.9	14.1	1.5	9.5
Geographic Region[c]						
Northeast	5.2	62.6	13.0	11.7	1.9	10.8
Midwest	5.3	55.8	14.7	15.4	1.9	12.3
South	5.6	61.1	13.6	11.3	2.6	11.3
West	5.6	60.4	13.6	12.8	1.4	12.0
Residence Location[c]						
Within MSA[e]	5.6	59.6	13.7	13.1	1.9	11.7
Outside MSA	4.9	61.4	14.1	10.7	2.6	11.2

[a]Includes hospital outpatient clinic, emergency room, and other hospital contacts.
[b]Includes clinics or other places outside a hospital.
[c]Age adjusted.
[d]Includes all other races not shown separately and unknown family income.
[e]MSA = Metropolitan Statistical Area
Source: Data from the *National Health Interview Survey* by the Division of Health Interview Statistics, National Center for Health Statistics, 1990.

measures of financial access to the health care system, such as health insurance coverage, are associated with differences in utilization. Individuals with greater financial resources generally have greater access to services and use them more, except for the poor ill (financial resources include patient income and wealth as well as insurance coverage and coverage by entitlement programs).

Other factors that are commonly found to be related to access include age, which is highly associ-

Table 28-2 Dental Visits and Intervals Since Last Visit, United States, 1989

| Characteristic | Dental Visits (no. per person) | Interval Since Last Dental Visit[a] | | |
		Less Than 1 Year (%)	2 Years or More (%)	Never Visited Dentist (%)
Total[b,c]	2.1	57.7	21.4	6.4
Age				
Under 15 Years	2.1	60.5	6.6	19.7
Under 5 Years	0.9	32.1	1.0	55.0
5–14 Years	2.5	69.5	8.4	8.6
15–44 Years	2.0	59.7	22.8	1.4
45–64 Years	2.4	56.8	28.9	0.4
65 Years and Over	2.0	43.2	43.7	0.5
65–74 Years	2.2	47.6	39.7	0.4
75 Years and Over	1.8	36.3	50.0	0.6
Sex[b]				
Male	2.0	55.4	23.2	6.7
Female	2.3	60.0	19.6	6.1
Race[b]				
White	2.3	60.0	20.2	6.1
Black[c]	1.2	44.0	29.5	7.7
Family Income[b]				
Less Than $10,000	1.3	41.9	33.7	9.6
$10,000–$14,999	1.6	49.5	27.5	7.8
$15,000–$19,999	2.2	60.3	20.3	6.3
$20,000–$34,999	2.7	69.7	15.1	4.5
$35,000 or more	3.1	76.1	10.6	3.4
Geographic Region[b]				
Northeast	2.2	61.4	17.9	4.8
Midwest	2.1	62.2	20.1	5.0
South	1.8	52.5	25.4	8.0
West	2.4	58.0	19.7	6.7
Residence Location[b]				
Within MSA[d]	2.2	58.8	20.2	6.2
Outside MSA	1.7	54.2	25.5	6.8

[a]Percentages not shown for the 1–2 year interval.
[b]Age adjusted.
[c]Includes all other races not shown separately and unknown family income.
[d]MSA = Metropolitan Statistical Area
Source: Data from the *National Health Interview Survey* by the Division of Health Interview Statistics, National Center for Health Statistics, 1991.

ated with differences in utilization; sex (women in general utilize more services than men); race; ethnicity; and education. In some instances, the relationship between these variables and utilization is counterintuitive. For example, individuals with less education and, in some instances, lower income or wealth are likely to use hospital services more, at least when they do finally access the health care system, because of the greater severity of their illnesses.

Table 28-4 lists variables associated with utilization differentials and summarizes the effect of each variable on utilization in the United States. To be useful, these results have to be taken in the context of the population specifically being served by the

Table 28-3 Discharges, Days of Care, and Average Lengths of Stay in Short-Stay Hospitals, United States, 1964 and 1989

Characteristic	Discharges (no. per 1,000 pop.)		Days of Care (no. per 1,000 pop.)		Average Length of Stay (no. of days)	
	1964	1989	1964	1989	1964	1989
Total[a,b]	109.1	91.0	970.9	607.1	8.9	6.7
Age						
Under 15 Years	67.6	46.7	405.7	271.3	6.0	5.8
Under 5 Years	94.3	79.9	731.1	496.4	7.8	6.2
5–14 Years	53.1	29.0	229.1	150.8	4.3	5.2
15–44 Years	100.6	62.6	760.7	340.5	7.6	5.4
45–64 Years	146.2	135.7	1,559.3	911.5	10.7	6.7
65 Years and Over	190.0	248.8	2,292.7	2092.4	12.1	8.4
65–74 Years	181.2	215.4	2,150.4	1719.3	11.9	8.0
75 Years and Over	206.7	300.6	2,560.4	2669.9	12.4	8.9
Sex[a]						
Male	103.8	91.0	1,010.2	622.7	9.7	6.8
Female	113.7	91.7	933.4	592.9	8.2	6.5
Race[a]						
White	112.4	89.5	961.4	580.9	8.6	6.5
Black[c]	84.0	112.0	1,062.9	875.9	12.7	7.8
Family Income[a,d]						
Less Than $14,000	102.4	142.2	1,051.2	1141.2	10.3	8.0
$14,000–$24,999	116.4	98.4	1,213.9	594.5	10.4	6.0
$25,000–$34,999	110.7	85.1	939.8	560.6	8.5	6.6
$35,000–$49,999	109.2	73.0	882.6	380.3	8.1	5.2
$50,000 or more	110.7	72.5	918.9	446.2	8.3	6.2
Geographic Region[a]						
Northeast	98.5	84.9	993.8	623.4	10.1	7.3
Midwest	109.2	91.5	944.9	570.8	8.7	6.2
South	117.8	106.4	968.0	713.6	8.2	6.7
West	110.5	70.5	985.9	444.6	8.9	6.3
Residence Location[a]						
Within MSA[e]	107.5	85.9	1,015.4	599.6	9.4	7.0
Outside MSA	113.3	109.5	871.9	636.0	7.7	5.8

Note: Excludes deliveries.

[a]Age adjusted.

[b]Includes all other races not shown separately and unknown family income.

[c]1964 data include all other races.

[d]Family income categories for 1989. Income categories in 1964 are: less than $2,000; $2,000–$3,999; $4,000–$6,999; $7,000–$9,999; and $10,000 or more.

[e]MSA = Metropolitan Statistical Area

Source: Data from the *National Health Interview Survey* by the Division of Health Interview Statistics, National Center for Health Statistics, 1964, 1991.

provider organization. The organizational form of the provider (e.g., managed care) and related factors (e.g., the availability of a usual source of care) will also affect access to care regardless of the un- derlying demographic variables. Thus it is essential for any provider organization to compare and contrast the characteristics of its own population to these national data to determine through analysis

Table 28-4 Selected Factors Associated with Utilization

Variable	Effect
Sociodemographic Factors	
Sex	Women use more care (higher percentage of physician visits; more visits per person).
	Men are less likely to seek care in response to symptoms.
	Women use more dental care.
	Women use more hospital care, partly because of obstetrical needs.
Race	Whites generally use more services than nonwhites; this gap has narrowed in recent years.
	Blacks may have lower utilization rates in comparison to need than whites.
	Blacks are more likely to receive ambulatory care in hospital outpatient departments and emergency rooms than whites.
	Whites are more likely to use dental services than are blacks and to make more dental visits.
	Hospital utilization rates are somewhat higher for blacks than whites; this differential has also narrowed.
	Blacks utilize nursing homes significantly less than whites.
Income	Poor people have higher utilization rates for many types of services than nonpoor people.
	Low-income children and pregnant women use less care than high-income women and children.
	Low-income people may receive less care than high-income people in relation to illness levels.
	Low-income people are more likely than high-income people to use hospital outpatient departments and emergency rooms.
	Low-income people use less dental care than high-income people.
	Hospital utilization is greater for low-income people than for high-income people.
Ethnicity	Hispanics tend to utilize health services less than others.
	Other minorities have varying degrees of access; access is highly dependent on education, income, and other variables.
Education	Education is related to access and utilization.
	Education is an important factor in the use of preventive services.
Residence	Utilization is generally lower for individuals living outside of major metropolitan areas.
	Hospital admission rates are higher for people outside of major metropolitan areas but hospital stays are not longer.
Health Status	
Patients' Perceived Need for Care	Individuals with greater perceived need tend to have higher utilization rates.
Evaluated Need	Utilization generally is associated with professionally evaluated need for services; patients' perceived need and professionally evaluated need frequently do not coincide.
Organization of Services	
Regular Source of Care	Individuals with a regular source of medical care generally have higher utilization rates.
Managed Care Systems	Patients enrolled in prepaid or managed care plans generally have higher ambulatory and lower inpatient utilization rates.
Financial Variables	
Insurance Coverage	Insurance coverage is directly associated with use of services; public and entitlement programs stimulate utilization for people without private insurance coverage.

the likely association between patient characteristics and actual utilization. With an adequate data base and information system and by utilizing statistical techniques, calculations can be performed that will have practical managerial applications.

Models of Use

Health services researchers, in their attempt to explore and understand better how people access the health care system, have applied various analytical methods to develop models of health services utilization, including sociodemographic, sociostructural, sociopsychological, economic, organizational, and systems models. Many of these models lack applicability in an ongoing managerial context owing to limited availability of data and other considerations. But the models do provide an interesting framework for thinking about access to the health care system and the role of consumers and providers in facilitating such access.[4]

The sociodemographic models, which are the most practical, utilize typical and generally measurable variables such as age, race, and sex.

Sociostructural, sociopsychological, and behavioral models apply social class theory and other sociological and psychological approaches, including investigation of individuals' health beliefs, values, and psychological characteristics, to predict use of services.[5] These models require special survey techniques and are generally not appropriate for ongoing application in operating organizations, but they do provide information about the types of patients likely to have greatest difficulty in accessing health care services.

Economic models rely heavily on financial indicators, such as income and wealth, insurance coverage, the price of health care services to the patient, and the density of services available in the community.[6] Again, these models are not generally useful in an operating environment, but they can play a role in the development of national policy.

Organizational models examine the structure of the health care system and its effect on the use of services. For example, they provide insight about differences between access in managed care systems and access in fee-for-service organizational structures.

Finally, the systems model is intended to bring all the multidisciplinary approaches of the other models together into one all-encompassing approach. These models are the least successful and most complex from a practical perspective.

ACCESS AND SYSTEM STRUCTURE

Access to care is heavily dependent on the way the health care system is organized. The types of services offered, how they are tied together, and insurance and payment mechanisms and structures define access for patients and channel care-seeking behavior.

Access and Service Type

Access to services varies by the type of service involved. Access is greatest for inpatient hospital, emergency room, and physician office visits and lowest, as measured by indicators of utilization, for mental health services, nursing home care, and certain other types of specialized services (see Table 28-1). Access to care is dependent on a number of factors, including the availability of health care resources and services in the community, the financial resources of patients, and geographic or system barriers. As noted elsewhere, access to specific types of services is also a function of the organization of the health care delivery system, particularly in the case of managed care programs or government clinics and entitlement programs.

Limitations on access to primary care and similar front-line services can lead to more serious severity of illness or to the self-limiting or self-resolution of problems, depending on the nature of the patient's illness. It is important to ensure that access is available for those services that facilitate more rapid patient problem resolution and alleviate future serious illness.

Individuals requiring health care should also be channeled to the least expensive, most efficient types of services.[7] For example, surgical procedures are increasingly being performed on an ambulatory basis at lower cost and with a shorter recovery time. Recent organizational changes and the proliferation of technological advances, such as fiber optic surgical equipment, will further accelerate this trend.

Access and the Structure of the System

Access to health care services is heavily influenced by the structure of the health care system. The effects of structure on access can be best understood by examining regionalized and centrally controlled health care systems such as the British National Health Service, similar systems in other countries, and some forms of managed care in this country (especially closed-panel HMOs). In these systems, aggressive planning and resource allocation techniques are used to influence patient utilization in a variety of ways aimed at rationalizing consumer use of services and limiting or otherwise controlling such use.

Access in such highly structured systems is characterized by the assignment of patients to primary care physicians who serve in a role analogous to gatekeepers in managed care plans. These primary care providers are responsible for delivering primary care services and controlling access to other levels and types of care, particularly specialty services and care requiring hospitalization or other institutional services. Such control over patients' use of services is beneficial from the perspective of continuity of care, elimination of or reduction in duplication of services, and other quality-enhancing aspects of the care process. On the other hand, as with managed care and other rationing approaches used in the United States, these systems also tend to reduce consumer choice and potentially limit access inappropriately.

Centralized systems seem to provide adequate care to large populations, ensuring access for all citizens and yielding quality of care comparable to that provided in the United States. They achieve this with expenditures for total health care services of approximately 8.5 percent of the gross national product, substantially less than the equivalent expenditure in the United States, which stands at more than 12 percent of the gross national product. The evidence from these other countries, although they face less daunting health care delivery challenges than in the United States, suggests that the control of access to care is critical for controlling the total societal cost of providing services.

Prepayment and Access to Care

Prepaid health care services in the United States have assumed many forms. Prepayment had its origins with closed panel, multispecialty group practices providing care to enrolled populations. Early prepaid health care systems included the Kaiser Foundation health plans and Group Health Cooperative of Puget Sound, a consumer-owned cooperative.

In the mid-1970s, prepayment received a substantial boost with the development of the federal health maintenance organization (HMO) initiative. Prepaid group practices and independent practice associations were two types of HMOs promoted under federal legislation designed to encourage the development of prepaid programs. Federally qualified HMOs had to meet specific criteria regarding services provided and other delivery system characteristics designed to enhance consumer access and to control the costs of health care services.

More recently, prepayment programs have been expanded further under the rubric of managed care to include a variety of insurance plans and programs designed to extract discounts from providers, better channel patients through health care systems, control costs, and enhance the quality of services. These managed care programs include new types of HMOs as well as other contracting and insurance mechanisms, such as preferred provider, exclusive provider, and point-of-service arrangements. (For more on managed care, see Chapter 8.)

Numerous variations on prepaid approaches to health care have been developed during the continuous expansion of managed care services. However, the fundamental purpose of managed care and prepayment remains the same: to control patient access to services through better structuring of the health care system, particularly with regard to entry points for specific services.

From an access perspective, managed care is enhanced through the use of primary care physicians as gatekeepers. The object of having gatekeepers is to control patient utilization, and primary care physicians are in the best position to determine patient needs and judge the appropriateness of referrals for specialty services and other care. Primary care physicians may be given a financial incentive to appropriately control and hopefully reduce utilization. Financial rewards are based on utilization savings achieved by more aggressive patient management.

Use of primary care physicians as gatekeepers is widely assumed to be a successful method of controlling patient utilization. Gatekeepers can reduce excessive utilization resulting from patient-generated but unnecessary demand and aggressive but inappropriate physician-generated demand, particularly by specialists, and they can also control the use of laboratory, x-ray, and other ancillary services. The extent to which such savings are actually achieved by using gatekeepers has not been fully determined empirically. However, gatekeepers do provide patients with assistance in dealing with their health care needs and can enhance the coordination of services and the assessment of the appropriateness of referrals for specialty care. In some respects, gatekeepers are a new version of the old-time general practitioner.

MECHANISMS TO INHIBIT AND ENCOURAGE ACCESS

Health care provider systems employ a variety of mechanisms to affect access to health care explicitly or implicitly (Exhibit 28-1). Implicit inhibitions to access are the result of normal operating procedures

Exhibit 28-1 Typical Access-Inhibiting and -Facilitating Factors

Inhibiting Factors
- Waiting times for appointments
- Use of telephone contact rather than office visits
- Limited appointment availability
- Impersonal or unappealing facilities and staff
- Excessive bureaucracy
- Deposits, prepayments, and other financial hurdles

Facilitating Factors
- Friendly, supportive staff
- Attractive facilities
- No financial barriers or incentives
- Broad appointment availability
- Short waits for appointments

that may limit access to care without such limitation being intended. For example, operating hours may be set that make it inconvenient for a certain segment of the population to patronize the practice.

The Role of Controls on Use

Explicit controls on utilization are those that the practice establishes for purposes of inhibiting, moderating, directing, or otherwise controlling utilization. Explicit procedures may exist to encourage utilization as well, particularly in the fee-for-service arena. These are discussed separately. In managed care provider systems, most controls are used to prioritize utilization and to discourage what the managers may view as unnecessary utilization, such as care-seeking behavior associated with routine viral infections like the common cold.

In most instances, utilization-inhibiting mechanisms are designed so that patients are unaware of the explicit intent to reduce their consumption of services. Consumer satisfaction is likely to be adversely affected if consumers have the perception that the provider system is not receptive to their perceived health care needs. While inhibiting mechanisms perceived to be such can reduce utilization in the short run, in the long run the resulting dissatisfaction can lead to disenrollments and reductions in payments.

Ideally, utilization control mechanisms should be part of a larger patient services management environment that responds to all patient perceptions of need for services, although not necessarily with a resource-consuming office visit. Particularly in prepaid settings, triage and the dispensing of advice over the telephone, as well as the employment of intelligent and consumer-sensitive front-line personnel to interact with patients, can effectively meet patient demands and control utilization of services.

Specific Control Methods

Among the specific procedures used to control utilization are those associated with the patient scheduling and appointments system. These are among the most effective mechanisms for allowing the provider organization to meet consumer needs in an economical manner.

Patient-initiated telephone contact is the most common means of access for primary care and certain specialty services. Management of patient telephone contact is critical to ensuring access and controlling utilization. A patient's telephone call reflects a perceived need for health care services. It is imperative that any provider organization be responsive to such an expression of need for care. Appropriate reactions include giving advice and counseling over the telephone, directing the patient to an alternative source of care, or scheduling an appointment at the facility. Efficient, courteous, and responsive behavior on the part of the staff member is essential for ensuring consumer satisfaction and quality of care. The staff member must also identify the patient's health care needs precisely. Therefore, health system managers should pay special attention to the quality of training received by front-line staff having contact with patients.

Screening can be used at the initial point of contact to determine if the patient has a potentially self-resolvable problem that can be dealt with over the telephone. Some aggressive managed care organizations provide tape-recorded information for patients calling with specific types of easily resolv-able problems, such as the common cold. However, screening may be essential to ensure that a patient's symptoms do not require professional examination to rule out other possibilities.

Scheduling appointments to include a long waiting period is a practice used by some provider organizations. For example, routine or self-resolvable problems might be assessed through the initial telephone contact, and the patient would then be offered an appointment five or six days later in expectation that the problem would be resolved and the patient would cancel. The value of such an approach from a cost-saving perspective, however, has to be weighed against the cost in potential consumer dissatisfaction and the possibility of some illnesses gaining in severity.

Unacceptable constraints on patient access include not answering the telephone at all, answering only after a long period of ringing, or putting the patient on hold. Nonresponsiveness or hostility on the part of staff is also unacceptable. Although consumer-oriented philosophies of management are just beginning to take hold in the health care arena, responding sympathetically and effectively to care-seeking behavior should be standard operating procedure. Increasing competition in the marketplace will require organizations to adopt a totally responsive consumer approach. Managers have the responsibility to wring out any vestiges of the clinical mentality or other forms of insensitivity toward patients.

Queuing is another popular rationing technique, particularly in centrally managed or financed health care systems, both in the United States and abroad. Queuing does effectively ration services, although consumers may be driven to other providers or to seek care outside of the established systems. Queuing, because it limits the availability of needed services, can also result in reduced quality of care, increased morbidity and mortality, and other adverse consequences. It is preferable to assess and triage patients immediately and to ensure that those who do not receive care initially are carefully monitored and serviced appropriately as soon as feasible.

Queuing is achieved through appointment waiting times, long waits between initial contact and scheduled delivery of services (e.g., for elective surgery), patient callback lists, and other mechanisms. Queuing forces increased efficiency and rationalization, but at the same time it limits patient access to potentially needed care. This raises important ethical issues, which are discussed later.

Financial Controls

Financial disincentives also serve to inhibit use. Copayments, exclusions, and limitations are all designed to selectively reduce the use of services, especially when patient initiated. Managed care programs may rely less on these barriers than traditional insurance programs. The key issue in plan design is to differentiate patient needs so that barriers do not unjustly reduce the provision of truly required health care.

ACCESS, INTEGRATION OF SERVICES, FINANCING, AND GOVERNMENT

Access to health services is essential at all levels of care. Initial entry points, including hospital outpatient departments and physician offices, must be effectively integrated with the entire health care system so that needed services, such as secondary and tertiary care services, are adequately provided.

Integrating Mechanisms

Organized health care systems must have effective mechanisms to ensure the integration of their various components. For example, integration can be achieved through effective patient and intrasystem communications; medical record systems, particularly those that are unified and comprehensive; patient referral systems that include a feedback link to the referring or primary care physician; and comprehensive patient needs assessment approaches, such as health risk appraisals, case management of severe illnesses, and other techniques.

Ensuring integration between levels and types of care is primarily the responsibility of the health services delivery system rather than the patient. A well-integrated system with effective communication channels can make a major contribution to the quality and continuity of care and to patient access. Modern communications, computer, and transportation technologies and systems can greatly facilitate the system's role in achieving such integration. It is the responsibility of the administrator to implement these approaches.

Access with Financial Limits

Over 30 million Americans had no coverage for health care services in 1989, either through private insurance plans or entitlement programs. Table 28-5 summarizes health insurance coverage for U.S. citizens under age 65. Table 28-6 presents similar data for the 65-and-above age group, who are generally eligible for Medicare. For this group, it is important to note the limits of Medicare coverage, especially for long-term care services.

It is worth noting that even individuals with insurance often have only partial coverage. Coverage for these individuals is limited by plan benefits that are not complete or comprehensive, various exclusions and limitations of the plans themselves, substantial copayments or deductibles, and by other insurance mechanisms that, in effect, represent barriers to access to health care services. In addition, many policies exclude coverage for care required as a result of congenital abnormalities. Even Medicare covers only about half of the eligible population's total health care expenses—coverage for long-term care is one glaring limitation.

Insurance contracts are designed to provide insurers with significant control over access to care and use of the health care system. Obviously, managed care programs are also intended to allow control of access to health care services; public entitlement programs are increasingly utilizing various forms of managed care to achieve the same goal. Medicaid contracting in various states and Medi-

Table 28-5 Health Care Coverage for Persons under 65 Years of Age, United States, 1989

Characteristic	Private Insurance	Medicaid[a]	Not Covered[b]
Total[c,d]	76.6	6.4	15.7
Age			
Under 15 Years	71.7	11.4	15.9
Under 5 Years	68.1	13.3	17.0
5–14 Years	73.6	10.4	15.3
15–44 Years	76.6	4.4	18.1
45–64 Years	83.3	3.4	10.6
Sex[c]			
Male	76.9	5.2	16.4
Female	76.2	7.6	14.9
Race[c]			
White	79.7	4.5	14.5
Black	59.2	17.1	22.0
Family Income[c]			
Less Than $14,000	34.6	26.6	37.3
$14,000–$24,999	71.4	4.8	21.4
$25,000–$34,999	87.9	1.2	9.3
$35,000–$49,999	92.4	0.8	5.6
$50,000 or More	95.7	0.4	3.2
Geographic Region[c]			
Northeast	83.4	5.8	10.3
Midwest	81.9	7.1	10.7
South	71.8	5.7	20.0
West	72.1	7.2	19.1

Note: Percentages do not add to 100 because the percentage of persons with other types of health insurance (e.g., Medicare, military) are not shown and because persons with both private insurance and Medicaid appear in both columns.
[a]Includes persons receiving Aid to Families with Dependent Children or Supplemental Security Income or those with current Medicaid cards.
[b]Includes persons not covered by private insurance, Medicaid, Medicare, and military plans.
[c]Age adjusted.
[d]Includes all other races not shown separately and unknown family income.
Source: Data from the *National Health Interview Survey* by the Division of Health Interview Statistics and Division of Analysis, National Center for Health Statistics, 1989.

care's capitated plans are examples of entitlement program adoption of typical managed care principles and approaches. This trend is likely to continue in the future, with an increased emphasis on prepaid, contracted, entitlement programs that have a restricted scope of benefits and other governmentally mandated constraints. Frequently in these arrangements, the actual access to care is also controlled by the provider organization rather than by the funding source, with the providers sending entitlement plan patients through access channels that are similar to those used for other managed care patients.

Changes in insurance coverage, especially in Medicaid and other programs for the poor and medically underserved, will alter historical patterns of care. The extent of change in health services utilization, however, is difficult to predict due to uncertainty concerning prior sources of care, patient behaviors, and system constraints.

Access in the Absence of Coverage

For those individuals with no coverage and few out-of-pocket resources, access to care has been

Table 28-6 Health Care Coverage for Persons 65 Years of Age and Over, United States, 1989

Characteristic	Medicare and Private Insurance	Medicare and Medicaid[a]	Medicare Only[b]
Total[c,d]	73.5	5.7	16.8
Age			
65–74 Years	74.2	5.0	15.5
75 Years and Over	72.3	6.8	19.0
75–84 Years	74.1	6.4	17.4
85 Years and Over	64.8	8.5	26.1
Sex[c]			
Male	73.9	4.0	17.2
Female	73.4	6.8	16.4
Race[c]			
White	77.3	4.5	14.7
Black	39.3	16.5	37.9
Family Income[c]			
Less Than $14,000	64.8	11.4	21.5
$14,000–$24,999	81.2	2.6	13.4
$25,000–$34,999	80.0	2.4	12.5
$35,000–$49,999	80.3	1.9	10.2
$50,000 or More	76.5	1.1	12.6
Geographic Region[c]			
Northeast	73.1	4.0	18.0
Midwest	79.6	2.9	14.1
South	70.6	7.7	18.3
West	71.4	7.6	16.0

Note: Persons with Medicare, private insurance, and Medicaid appear in both columns. In 1989, 5.2 percent of all persons 65 years of age and over had no Medicare coverage, but only 0.9 percent were without health insurance.

[a]Includes persons receiving Aid to Families with Dependent Children or Supplemental Security Income or those with current Medicaid cards.

[b]Includes persons not covered by private insurance or Medicaid and a small proportion of persons with other types of coverage, such as CHAMPUS or public assistance.

[c]Age adjusted.

[d]Includes all other races not shown separately and unknown family income.

Source: Data from the *National Health Interview Survey* by the Division of Health Interview Statistics and Division of Analysis, National Center for Health Statistics, 1989.

much more limited. In general, local units of government, by law, are providers of last resort for somatic and mental health services. As such, these government units have a number of options for directly providing or otherwise arranging care for medically indigent individuals not eligible for other entitlement programs. These alternatives include contracting with local providers to accept these patients and provide care on either a prepaid or fee-for-service basis.

A second alternative, more traditional but currently less popular, is for the local government to directly provide services through government hospitals and other facilities (usually county hospitals). A variation of this alternative is for the local government to establish a grant-type program that supports, partially or wholly, local clinics and other providers in return for the provision of care for indigent patients.

Access and Local and State Public Health Services

Public health services represent an important access point for a variety of health care needs. Managers should be aware of the role of public health services in the overall delivery of health care and in the provision of specific services.

Public health services provided in this country are remarkably broad based. In addition to traditional public health department functions, such as monitoring disease incidence, public health agencies, particularly at the local level, provide a wide array of important environmental and preventive services. These services are provided either directly by the agencies or in the private sector through contract arrangements with the agencies. Contracting for specific public health services presents an additional business opportunity for providers. Services that fall under the responsibility of government agencies tend to be oriented toward categorical disease problems of significant magnitude (e.g., epidemics) or toward ensuring access to care for those individuals not covered under other entitlement programs. Targeted programs aimed at specific diseases include care and clinics related to sexually transmitted disease, AIDS, immunization and vaccination, and many other (often challenging) social and health problems.

Prevention of illness, accident, and injury is the first line of defense against the adverse consequences of health problems. Public health agencies have a significant role in providing educational and other preventive services related to numerous social and environmental problems. Examples include reduction of risk from various infectious diseases such as tuberculosis, leprosy, sexually transmitted diseases, and other problems that can be prevented; protection of the food supply; protection of humans from disease transmission from animals and insects; protection of the environment from pollutants; and, to an increasing extent, enhancement of behavior patterns that are protective and preventive.

Access and the Role of Government

Government health care programs include such specialized programs as the Indian Health Service, programs that target the needs of infants and mothers, military health care, and prison health services. Con-

tract opportunities are evolving for private sector providers interested in participating in these programs.

All members of the society benefit from the prevention and health promotion aspects of public health agency activity. Those unable to access services through private, nongovernmental channels or specific entitlement programs benefit from the agencies' role in direct provision of services. The partnership between public and private organizations involved in provision of services will be of immense future importance in protecting our society from illness on the one hand, and ensuring access to needed services for all Americans on the other.

The increasing attention being paid to the uninsured and underinsured is also prompting debate on whether to enhance government and private financing for health services. Initiatives to fill current gaps in coverage are likely to require the cooperation of different levels of government and the private sector.[8] Managers of the nation's health care system need to monitor carefully the evolution of this cooperation to ensure it is part of the solution and does not contribute to the problem.

Government agencies will increasingly stress issues of access, quality, and utilization and cost controls regardless of the specific changes in the nation's financing and delivering mechanisms. The government's role in health policy and planning and in the financial management of health-related resources will increase. The nature of the government's involvement will be substantially different from its ineffectual attempts during the 1960s and 1970s to influence the system through various forms of planning and regulation. The use of financing mechanisms rather than direct control over elements of the system is in all likelihood going to be the preferred method for achieving various social goals related to access, cost, and utilization.

ACCESS: THE POLICY AND MANAGEMENT CONCERNS

This section summarizes the national policy issues associated with access to care and the specific managerial and ethical issues faced by health services administrators on a daily basis. Ultimately, access to care is closely intertwined with the organization, financing, and operation of the health care system and its component parts. At the most basic level, national policy regarding access fundamentally relates to the nature of our health care system and the extent to which we follow through with a commitment to ensure access for all citizens.[9]

International Lessons

Commitment to ensuring widespread access to care is greatest in those nations with national health services, such as the United Kingdom and Sweden. Guaranteed access to care can be more readily implemented when government or quasi-government entities control the operation of the system and the distribution of resources within that system. Control over the design and functioning of the health care system is greatest under conditions of regionalization such as exist internationally through national health services and in the United States through closed systems like the Kaiser and military health care systems.

Under regionalization and centrally controlled systems, resources are allocated to meet the specific needs of all individuals entitled to receive services (either as a result of health plan selection or national identity). In national health care systems that are organized and managed by government entities, access to care is treated as virtually a fundamental right. Lack of ability to pay and other barriers to care that are experienced in the United States by many individuals are alleviated in these national systems, and copayments, deductibles, limitations, exclusions, and other contract terms are generally much less relevant, although the scope of benefits may have some limitations (e.g., elective cosmetic surgery may not be covered). Wealthier individuals who are, for one reason or another, dissatisfied with the national system or who are seeking services not covered by the system may still obtain care privately by using their financial resources.

Regionalization, Financing, and Access in the United States

In the United States, regionalized and centrally managed systems do exist—both under government sponsorship and in the private sector. These systems generally function in a manner somewhat analogous to the national health systems of other countries, and access to care, although controlled through a variety of mechanisms, is at least partially ensured.

At the other extreme is the totally competitive, market-driven approach that has characterized the largest segment of the U.S. health care system in recent years. Under this approach, an individual's access to care is a function of the availability of services and the individual's financial and other resources. Ultimately, individuals who lack such resources become the clients of entitlement programs and of the provider of last resort—the local government. Whereas national health systems in relatively wealthy, developed countries ensure equal access, or nearly equal access, for all citizens, the competitive model is characterized by highly variable access. Many individuals, by design or by chance, will lack adequate access to needed health care services in this configuration.

Resource Limitations in Health Care

In the United States, recognition of the limits on the availability of financial resources and access to health care led, during the 1960s, to the development of national entitlement programs for the elderly and for the medically indigent. Medicare and Medicaid were designed to provide financial resources for individuals to utilize in seeking care through the established health care system. Both of these programs have had tremendous success in enhancing access to care for their eligible populations.

However, these programs, even combined with other government entitlement programs, have left significant gaps in coverage, and as a result many individuals still do not have adequate access to needed health care services. This fact has increasingly gained recognition, and political pressure to address the deficiencies in our health care system is building. However, such pressure and the recognition of the problems have existed for at least 50 years, so that it is premature to conclude that an adequate solution will be found in the near future. Further, the battle lines are increasingly being drawn over the key issue of where the money will come from to provide financial support for individuals with limited access to health care services.

At the same time, limits on the availability of resources and financing, particularly at the state and local government levels, are motivating discussions about the need to ration care and restrict services. Particularly in regard to Medicaid and local government programs, pressures caused by the high cost of health care are leading politicians and policy makers to conclude that ensuring widespread, unlimited access to health care is not feasible. One strategy under consideration would be to allocate funding first to preventive and primary care services and then to secondary and tertiary care services—to the extent that resources remain available. An upper limit would be set that would exclude very expensive and very rare types of care.

Access and National Ethics

The fundamental ethical and moral issues surrounding access to care are tightly interwoven with the broader policy issues related to allocation of health care resources. Whether every citizen has the right to liver transplants or other highly sophisticated and extremely expensive services is an issue that is not readily addressed and resolved by politicians—or by health care professionals. Health care professionals, particularly physicians, see their role as curing and healing and not necessarily as limiting access to services. Further, malpractice considerations and the need to practice defensive medicine; financial incentives for providing more care; patient demands and expectations; and the increasing availability of new, sophisticated, and highly successful technologies complicate the picture.

Access to care is an issue that cannot be easily separated from the many other issues related to quality of care and allocation of resources. A commitment to access is part and parcel of our commitment to our nation's population and its health. It is also connected to our willingness to invest for the future by promoting the health of pregnant women and other key populations and our willingness to provide needed services for our elderly population in recognition of their contributions in building this country.

New initiatives at the federal and state levels and a heightened awareness of national needs and past deficiencies have led the nation to reassess the requirements for health care reform. As this process continues, the national framework for health policy will need to be matched to the operation of frontline delivery organizations. As access is enhanced, competitive and cost pressures will increase the pressure to more efficiently manage the patient and the system's resources.

Management's Role in Influencing Access

In the day-to-day operation of the health care system, pragmatic issues regarding access to care must be addressed. These issues will exist regardless of the status of national health policy.

From a management perspective, ensuring access to care is facilitated by recognizing the consumer-driven nature of health care services and being responsive to the organization's clientele (e.g., by enhancing communication, physical access, and patient follow-up and monitoring). Matching patient-perceived need and professionally assessed need to appropriate, high-quality services is also a key management consideration, again regardless of the direction of national policy.

This chapter has discussed a number of ways in which managers can facilitate access to care for their clientele. Facilitating access makes particular sense for managed care programs, especially HMOs. However, even fee-for-service practices can take a more aggressive and positive stance regarding access (e.g., by monitoring patients more closely to determine their specific health care needs and the resources required to meet those needs). In more complex situations, advanced management approaches such as case management can be very effective in matching resources to patient needs.

Access should be a key consideration in ongoing quality assurance monitoring, in risk assessment, and in other types of evaluation. In the health care system, provider organizations traditionally have assumed a passive role, opening their doors and responding to patient-initiated and physician-generated demand for services. The current evolution of our nation's health care system suggests that managers will have to become much more aggressive in ensuring access to care and in matching patient needs with specific resources. This is likely to be the case for both prepaid and fee-for-service health care.

ACCESS IN THE FUTURE

A variety of important social, economic, and demographic trends are increasingly influencing access to care. Understanding these trends is critical for managers and policy makers.

Among the most important trends is the aging of the nation's population. The percentage of individuals aged 65 and above has been increasing and will continue to increase over the next 30 years as the baby boom generation reaches retirement age.

As shown in Tables 28-1, 28-2, and 28-3, utilization of health services is highly intercorrelated with age. As a result, total national utilization of health services will substantially increase over the next 30 years, assuming that disease patterns and medical interventions remain similar to those current today. Those services that are more heavily utilized by individuals in the higher age brackets, such as long-term care services, will be especially likely to increase.

Managers of course should be cognizant of the sociodemographic patterns in their local service areas and should keep abreast of changes that might affect the future use of services. They should also understand the special needs of the older population as regards geographic and physical access.

The elderly, as a group, are also becoming better educated and will be more sophisticated as consumers. Health care systems, particularly with regard to communication channels and patient-physician interaction, will need to recognize that the elderly population is changing in character.

Public policy deliberations must resolve a number of fundamental conflicts in national goals. Access for individuals who are unable to obtain insurance or eligibility for entitlement programs is dependent on a resolution of national funding priorities. Rationalization of care and efficient channeling of patients into various parts of the system require well-designed integration mechanisms. Ensuring access to adequate personal health care services while reducing waste, duplication, and abuse will require more effective quality assurance, risk management, and rationing methods and better-designed financial incentives.

Finally, changes in national reimbursement policy will also greatly affect access to care. Enhanced funding for preventive services, increased shifting of funding for primary and similar services, such as the Medicare physician reimbursement changes; increased scrutiny by reimbursers and government agencies of the cost-effectiveness and appropriateness of care; and other important reforms will face health services administrators. Since access is so highly correlated with financial variables, including patient wealth and insurance or entitlement program availability, these financing trends will have a major impact on access and on the day-to-day operation of health care organizations.

Ultimately, our nation will have to force greater efficiencies from the health care system. Access will be more tightly controlled. Financial incentives for providers and consumers will promote health, quality care, and cost-effectiveness. Dollars saved will help pay for care for more Americans. And the duty to make all of this happen will fall on the shoulders of the system's managers and providers.

ADDITIONAL RESOURCES

Aday, L.A. Equity of access to medical care: A conceptual and empirical overview. *Medical Care* 19, suppl. (1981): 4–27.

Aday, L.A., and R. Andersen. *Development of indices of access to medical care.* Ann Arbor, Mich.: Health Administration Press, 1975.

Aday, L.A., R. Andersen, and G.V. Fleming. *Health care in the U.S.: Equitable for whom?* Beverly Hills, Calif.: Sage Publications, 1980.

Andersen, R., A. Giachello, and L.A. Aday. Access of Hispanics to health care and cuts in services: A state-of-the-art overview. *Public Health Reports* 101 (1986): 238–252.

Burgess, J.F., Jr., and T. Stefos. Federal provision of health care: Creating access for the underinsured. *Journal of Health Care for the Poor and Underserved* 1 (1991): 364–387.

Fossett, J.W., J.A. Peterson, and M.C. Ring. Public sector primary care and Medicaid: Trading accessibility for mainstreaming. *Journal of Health Politics, Policy and Law* 14 (1989): 309–325.

Jones, K.R. The Florida Health Care Access Act: A blended regulatory/competitive approach to the indigent health care problem. *Journal of Health Politics, Policy and Law* 14 (1989): 261–285.

Maurana, C.A., R.L. Eichhorn, and L.E. Lonnquist. *The use of health services: Indices and correlates: A research bibliography, 1981.* Rockville, Md.: National Center for Health Services Research, 1981.

Mechanic, D. Correlates of physician utilization. Why do major multivariate studies of physician utilization find trivial psychosocial and organizational effects? *Journal of Health and Social Behavior* 20 (1979): 387–396.

National Center for Health Services. *Health indicators for Hispanic, black and white Americans.* Series 10, No. 148. DHHS Pub. No. (PHS) 84-1576. Washington, D.C.: U.S. Government Printing Office, 1984.

National Center for Health Statistics. *Health, United States, 1990.* DHSS Pub. No. (PHS) 91-1232. Washington, D.C.: U.S. Government Printing Office, 1991.

Newhouse, J.P. Geographic access to physician services. *Annual Review of Public Health* 11 (1990): 207–230.

Patrick, D.L., and M. Bergner. Measurement of health status in the 1990s. *Annual Review of Public Health* 11 (1990): 165–183.

Rice, D.P. Ethics and equity in U.S. health care: The data. *International Journal of Health Services* 21 (1991): 637–651.

NOTES

1. S.A. Wartman et al., Impact of Divergent Evaluations by Physicians and Patients of Patients' Complaints. *Public Health Reports* 98 (1983): 141–145.

2. R. Andersen et al., Health Status and Health Care Utilization, *Health Affairs* 5 (1986): 154–172.

3. National Center for Health Statistics, *Health, United States, 1990,* DHHS Pub. No. (PHS) 91-1232 (Washington, D.C.: U.S. Government Printing Office, 1991).

4. C. Muller, Review of Twenty Years of Research on Medical Care Utilization, Part 1, *Health Services Research* 21 (1986): 129–144.

5. M.H. Becker and L.A. Maiman, Models of Health-related Behavior, in *Handbook of Health, Health Care, and the Health Professions,* ed. D. Mechanic (New York: The Free Press, 1983), 539–568.

6. R. Andersen et al., *Ambulatory Care and Insurance Coverage in an Era of Constraint* (Chicago: Pluribus Press, 1987).

7. D. Ermann and J. Gabel. The Changing Face of American Health Care: Multihospital Systems, Emergency Centers, and Surgery Centers, *Medical Care* 23 (1985): 401–420.

8. R.J. Blendon et al., Uncompensated Care by Hospitals or Public Insurance for the Poor, *New England Journal of Medicine* 314 (1986): 1160–1163.

9. L.A. Aday et al., *Access to Medical Care in the U.S.: Who Has It, Who Doesn't* (Chicago: Pluribus Press, 1984).

Frederick J. Wenzel

Primary Care Services

29

Purpose: Primary care often refers to the services provided during the patient's initial contact with the health care system, particularly those services provided by physicians in family practice, general/family practice, general internal medicine, general pediatrics, and internal medicine and pediatric primary care. Viewed from this perspective, primary care appears to be passive and reactive. But there is increasing emphasis upon defining primary care more comprehensively and proactively to incorporate the concepts of health promotion, prevention, early intervention, maximizing accessibility, and assuring continuity of care.

INTRODUCTION

Primary care services can be viewed as the foundation of the health care system—the fundamental base of care supported by secondary and tertiary acute care services, mental health services, chronic care services, and other health services that may be required. In most countries of the world, primary care is strongly emphasized and substantial investments have been made to create networks of community-based primary care centers. In contrast, primary care services in the United States have been over-shadowed by an emphasis on acute care and hospitalization. Historically, primary care services in America were provided by a physician in general practice—often a solo practitioner who provided care to the entire family over a prolonged period. As social and practice patterns changed, resources and attention were drawn away from general practice toward medical specialization and hospital-centered acute care (see Chapter 30 for more on acute care services). In recent years, however, as pressures to constrain the costs of specialty services and hospitalization have mounted, primary care services are being reemphasized as cost-effective methods for delivering quality health care services.

This chapter outlines the key features of primary care and describes the functional components of a primary care system. Primary care's organization and operational characteristics, and its relationship to other components of the health care system, are also described. The resources required by primary care facilities of various size and complexity are outlined and quality management considerations in primary care are presented. Finally, the role that primary care will play in the future is discussed.

Features of Primary Health Care

A central aim of primary care is prevention—intervention to reduce the risk of illness, as when an expectant mother is counseled on the benefits of breast feeding or when a child is immunized. Primary care also aims for early intervention—to intercede when the first symptoms of illness are evident and before the illness has progressed to a point where more acute care is required.

Effective prevention and early intervention require accessibility. One aspect of accessibility is the convenience of location. Many countries that are working to achieve universal access to health care have placed a priority on creating widely dispersed networks of community-based primary care clinics, typically staffed by a primary care physician or, in the absence of a physician, by nurses, nurse practitioners, midwives, or auxiliary health care workers. Unfortunately, all but a few countries have fallen short of their goals because of limited financing and/or strong competition from hospitals for the available resources. In the United States, health care accessibility used to be measured by the convenience of the physician's office location. In some communities, accessibility was reflected by the willingness of the physician to make house calls. Today, accessibility is measured more on the basis of insurance coverage, entitlement, cost, convenient hours, and waiting times (see Chapter 28 for more accessing health care services.)

Primary care also aims to provide continuity in the provision of health services. Successful continuity infers the ongoing involvement of health care professionals who are knowledgeable about the individual patient's family, employment, personal lifestyle, and history of health and disease. Ideally, continuity gives assurance that the patient's needs will be considered in an integrated way and that potential gaps or conflicts in diagnosis, therapy, and personal circumstances will be minimized or eliminated.

Several defining features, or advantages, account for the reemphasis on primary care as the foundation of the health care system:

- Primary care services provide the platform from which to focus on health promotion, prevention, and early intervention, thereby reducing incidence of illness and mitigating complications that can arise when early symptoms are neglected.
- Appropriate primary care reduces the need for specialized acute care and hospitalization and consequently contributes to the reduction of health care costs.
- Primary care implies the involvement of a health care team that enhances the potential for collaboration among medical specialists and other health resources, thus ensuring greater continuity and appropriateness in the services provided.

ORGANIZATION OF PRIMARY CARE SERVICES

In theory, primary care services are provided by physicians in family medicine, general practice, pediatrics, and obstetrics, and by appropriately trained nurses and physician assistants. In reality, however, a significant portion of primary care services are provided by general internists, general surgeons, and, to a lesser but still important degree, by a wide array of medical specialists and subspecialists. The number of solo practitioners is rapidly decreasing and primary care is increasingly provided through medical group practices, hospital ambulatory care centers, and community health centers. Primary care services are now provided in a number of organizational settings: solo practice, single-specialty and multispecialty clinics, community and migrant health centers, hospital ambulatory care centers, and hospital emergency care centers.

Primary Care and the Growth of Group Practice

The single physician practicing alone has been the principal setting for primary care, but is becoming rare. In rural areas medicine is increasingly being provided through rural and migrant health centers, regional health systems, and HMOs.[1] In urban areas, most physicians completing their specialty training find single-specialty and multispecialty groups more attractive than solo practice. Starting a solo practice, whether as a general practitioner or a specialist, requires a substantial investment in facilities, equipment, and supporting staff. A group practice reduces or eliminates the need for a capital investment and provides the benefits of working with colleagues, sharing the work load, and living a less demanding lifestyle.

Single-Specialty and Multispecialty Clinics

Beginning in the early 1960s, patterns of medical practice changed dramatically—shifting from solo practice and modes of practice that emphasized primary care, toward greater specialization. During the period 1965–1988, for example, the number of multispecialty and single-specialty clinics increased four-fold, from 4,289 to 16,579 (Table 29-1).

A single-specialty clinic is a medical group practice involving physicians in one specialty or subspecialty area such as internal medicine, orthopaedics, or proctology. The inconvenience of referral for consultation is lessened to a degree in "medical arts" arrangements in which several single-

specialty clinics have office suites in the same building. For patients presenting a number of diagnoses, however, the provision and coordination of care is not as efficient as in multispecialty clinics.

A multispecialty clinic is a medical group practice composed of physicians representing several specialties. Most multispecialty clinics and large single-specialty clinics are organized to facilitate primary, secondary, and tertiary care. Services are coordinated to make effective use of advanced technology and operational efficiencies.

Community Health Centers

Community health centers are found in larger communities and are supported through federal funds and local governments. These clinics target their services to the medically indigent. Some public health clinics focus on immunization or on screening for communicable diseases (such as screening immigrants for tuberculosis or sexually transmitted diseases). The largest primary care-based public health system in the United States is the Indian Health Service.

Hospital Ambulatory Care Centers

As acute care hospital diagnostic and treatment capabilities increased during the 1940s through the

Table 29-1 Number of Groups and Group Physicians and Percentage Change from Previous Census Year, 1965–1988

Year	Number of Groups	Percentage Change from Previous Census Year	Group Physicians	Percentage Change from Previous Census Year
1965[a]	4,289	—	28,381	—
1969	6,371	48.5	40,093	41.3
1975	8,483	33.2	66,842	66.7
1980	10,762	26.9	88,290	32.1
1984	15,485	43.9	140,392[b]	59.0
1988	16,579	7.1	155,628[b]	10.8

[a]Medical groups were defined in terms of full-time physicians.

[b]These figures represent physician positions. They were obtained by asking groups to report the number of physicians in their groups. Because physicians may practice in more than one group, some physicians may be counted more than once. Thus, these figures may overestimate the number of group physicians.

1960s, many primary care services were drawn into the hospital setting with strong economic incentives. A physician might decide, for example, to perform a physical examination in the hospital because insurance reimbursement favored the hospital over the medical office. While primary care was still practiced in the medical office, physicians increasingly chose to provide more services in the hospital. In many community hospitals, primary care services were simply an extension of inpatient services—a preadmission physical or a postadmission follow-up visit. This trend began to reverse in the 1970s with the growth of health maintenance organizations (HMOs), which promoted preventive and ambulatory care in preference to inpatient services. The trend toward ambulatory services was further stimulated when, in 1983, the Federal government introduced the diagnostic related group (DRG) system for paying hospitals for services provided to Medicare patients. Economic pressures and controls on inpatient services, emanating from government and a growing number of managed care plans, encouraged hospitals to shift services into the ambulatory care setting, thus breaking away from the hospital's traditional acute care role and perspective. As a result, ambulatory services expanded, enhancing the base of primary care.

Medical Training and Primary Care

The 1910 Flexner Report emphasized hospital-based medical training and encouraged an educational environment more conducive to pursuing specialization than general practice. The doubling of medical school graduates in the 1960s was intended to restrain the costs of physician services through competition and increase the likelihood that physicians would choose to locate in rural and underserved areas, thereby providing access to primary care. Unfortunately, the expanded medical workforce remained oriented to specialty practice, costs continued to escalate, and there was little movement to underserved areas.

Recently, residency training programs have begun to change. Zones and Shroeder discovered there were major changes in ambulatory training requirements from 1961 to 1988 (see Table 29-2).[2] They found increased ambulatory training requirements in internal medicine as well as requirements under consideration in two of the other major specialties. They suggest that there will be a major shift in postgraduate training toward the ambulatory care setting—a trend that should support the expansion of primary care.

Creating more primary care physicians, or even more specialists who are sensitive to primary care approaches, will be difficult. Even schools that stress the preparation of primary care physicians find it difficult to maintain students' commitment to primary care. While in school, a majority of students may express a strong preference toward one of the primary care modes of practice. By the time they finish residency training, however, only a minority still elect to pursue a primary care practice. Until the incentives favoring specialization are altered, primary care will not attract practitioners in significant numbers.

PRIMARY CARE GROUP PRACTICE CLINICS

Staffing

In addition to those who provide direct patient care, the typical staffing of a primary care center, medical group practice, or community health center includes personnel who can deal with appointment scheduling, registration, billing and insurance, purchasing, maintenance, and accounting. Diagnostic support, laboratory, radiology, electrocardiography, and other ancillary services must be available and staffed by certified personnel.

The makeup of the medical staff will largely depend on the size of the clinic. In the case of a single-specialty clinical group practice, all the physicians should be able to substitute for one another except in highly subspecialized areas. A multispecialty group clinic, on the other hand, usually is divided into departments composed of physicians sharing

Table 29-2 Evolving Residency Requirements for Ambulatory Care Training for Five Specialties, 1961–1989

Specialty	Year	Specified Recommendations and Requirements
Internal Medicine	1961	No mention is made of ambulatory care.
	1971	Training should include experience in social, ambulatory, preventive, and rehabilitative aspects of medicine; no specifics mentioned.
	1980	Residents should spend at least 1 half-day per week in ambulatory care.
	1989	Ambulatory experience in each year of training, with at least 25% of the 3 years in an ambulatory care setting; continuity care in at least 2 and preferably 3 years.
Pediatrics	1961	Clinical training should be obtained in outpatient clinics.
	1978	There must be an equivalent of at least 6 months in ambulatory pediatrics during the 3 years; it is recommended that at least a portion of ambulatory experience consist of continuing care.
	1980	There should be weekly or biweekly assignment to a continuity clinic for at least 2 years.
	1985	Continuity requirement increased to 3 years; patient populations specified to include children with variety of chronic diseases.
Family Practice	1969	Residents should be responsible for comprehensive and continuing care to a select group of patients.
	1979	Residents to have opportunity to provide continuing care for a specified panel of patients over at least 2 years.
	1983	Assignment to family practice center specified as at least 1 half-day per week during the first year of residency, 2 to 4 half-days the second year, and 3 to 5 half-days the third year.
General Surgery	1961	Valuable experience may be obtained from outpatient services.
	1979	Adequate outpatient services considered necessary.
	1983	Active participation in outpatient services is essential.
Obstetrics and Gynecology	1961	Outpatient facility is essential.
	1982	Ambulatory training is essential, with a ratio of outpatient visits to admissions documenting this emphasis.

similar backgrounds and training (e.g., family medicine, general internal medicine, obstetrics and gynecology, general surgery, and pediatrics).

Leadership and Administration

Physician leadership is a principal resource requirement for all primary care organizations. Those organizations that fail or do not do well generally have not had the strong physician leadership necessary for guidance and direction. Although a very small group practice may not have a great need for strong physician leadership, by the time the group grows beyond eight or ten physicians, such leadership is absolutely essential. In hospital-associated primary care settings, physician leadership is a frequently overlooked resource, and hospitals are developing strong physician leadership.

Large physician groups will have a medical director responsible for the medical affairs of the staff. The medical director is responsible for recruiting clinicians, new service development, and quality improvement. The group may also have a president elected from its physician membership. In contrast to the medical director, the president is responsible for guiding policy development. The president is generally responsible to a board of directors made up of physicians within the group. In the case of community health centers, nonprofit centers, or hospitals, boards are usually primarily composed of community representatives with some physician participation.

The administration of a primary care center is usually under the direction of an administrator. That person often holds a bachelor's or master's degree in business or health services administration. Staff reporting directly to the administrator include the clinical managers, the business office, and the heads of finance, accounting, marketing, public relations, legal services, information systems, facilities management, and other functional support departments.

Information Systems

All primary care organizations have substantial information management needs. An information system is required that will serve both the business and clinical needs of the organization. Ideally, the information system is especially adapted for ambulatory care or group practice and begins developing the record for each patient at the time the first appointment is made.[3] Information from the appointment system should be coordinated with the clinical encounter and the billing process. There are now information systems specifically designed for smaller facilities. It is exceptional, however, to find a commercial system that will work well in a large multispecialty group or community health center. Many large and complex organizations will need to adapt existing software or develop their own.

Where a primary care program and a hospital are closely associated, the information system should be integrated. Integration facilitates the use of a common medical record and joint laboratory and radiology facilities. Great care must be taken, however, to develop both clinical and management information systems specifically to fit the function of the primary care organization, because there are markedly different requirements for hospital inpatient and community-based ambulatory services.

Technology and Primary Care

Technology has played an important role—first in moving primary care into the hospital and more recently in moving primary care services out to free-standing ambulatory care and primary care settings. Many of the technological advances of the last 25 years were originally available only in the hospital. The original CAT scan units were a hospital-based device, but the CT and MRI scanners of today are principally found in ambulatory settings. Nuclear imaging and echo scanning have followed the same pattern. In addition, ambulatory patients are now monitored for cardiac arrhythmias and esophageal PH, administered dosages of chemotherapeutic drugs, or automatically administered medications to control pain. Additional technologies for primary and ambulatory care are being rapidly introduced. An essential element of primary care organization management is monitoring the development of technologies that may substantially change the scope of staffing, space needs, or costs of the services provided (see Chapter 23 for more on technology assessment).

QUALITY MANAGEMENT

Continuous quality improvement is emerging as fundamental to the organization of primary care services in all kinds of facilities. A great deal has been written about the quality of primary care in the ambulatory setting. Emphasis is placed on the need for a quality assurance committee and an ongoing commitment from the organization's leadership for continuous quality improvement. The processes followed are similar to those used in hospitals. They include problem identification, criterion development, quality assessment, decision making and feedback, problem solution, and evaluation and restudy. The deficiencies most often noted in primary care quality management programs are lack of or ineffective feedback to the provider and a failure to restudy the problems identified.

Palmer suggests three distinct dimensions of quality that can be measured in the ambulatory setting: (1) accessibility, the equitable and timely provision of health care; (2) acceptability, the degree to which care satisfies the patient; and (3) technical competence, the coordination of knowledge, skill, and judgment in delivering appropriate technology to improve the health of the patient.[4]

Benson and Townes describe a generic model for evaluating quality based on a two-phase process. The first phase is monitoring and evaluation and the second phase is problem resolution.[5] The model includes the following steps:

1. Determine the focus of responsibility of organizational quality assurance activity.

2. Determine the scope of services being generated by the organization.

3. Select significant aspects of care for the organization to track routinely.

4. Choose specific indicators of quality to monitor, those that directly relate to the important aspects of care that have been chosen.

5. Develop performance criteria and establish related measurement standards.

6. Systematically monitor and evaluate the indicators of quality, through collection and analysis of appropriate data.

7. Take appropriate action to resolve the problem when the organization's performance standard has not been met.

8. Track resulting corrective actions to be sure they are continually effective.

9. Create a permanent record of all quality assurance activities, ensuring that all relevant information is fully integrated into the organization.[6]

As in acute settings, evaluating and improving quality in primary care suffers from the lack of a clear definition of quality. In many cases, ambulatory care must base its assessment of patient needs on brief and intermittent encounters. A key objective of primary health care is the establishment of a broader, longer relationship with the patient that provides the basis for a more comprehensive record and process of evaluating service quality.

Whatever other measures of quality are ultimately developed, attention must be paid to the patients' perceptions of quality as they move through the system. Patients often base their assessments of quality on the ambience of the setting and on the professional and caring attitude of the staff. It is not unusual for a patient to rate the quality of care as high because "the nurse was kind to me and the doctor spent time with me and answered my questions."

Figure 29-1 illustrates a management model that is useful for examining and improving patient satisfaction during ambulatory clinic and medical group encounters.[7] Patient waiting times in various areas, along with execution times, are noted and measured. These measures are used by management to enhance the efficiency of the system. The patient should access the system at the earliest practical date, be given a quick but thorough examination, and then be provided with as much feedback as possible during the visit, including the results of any diagnostic tests.

THE FUTURE OF PRIMARY CARE

Primary care services will play an increasingly important role in the health system, with group practices, community health centers, and ambulatory care centers the principal locus of providing such services. Some of these centers will be freestanding, but many will be associated with inpatient facilities and other health care providers. The most successful will be part of integrated comprehensive arrangements involving a full array of provider organizations. Among group practices, the Mayo Clinic in Rochester, Minnesota, and the Park-Nicollet Clinic in Minneapolis are examples encompassing urban multispecialty clinics, regional rural clinic networks, hospitals, managed care plans, and related hotels and medical schools. Integrated collaborative organizations, with multispecialty clinics at the center, are likely to develop extensively over the next several years.[8]

Group practice HMOs, such as Kaiser-Permanente, have demonstrated a capability to serve broad geographic areas. Primary care centers, inpatient facilities, and prepayment are combined into a single organization. Many smaller practices and single-specialty groups will eventually become part

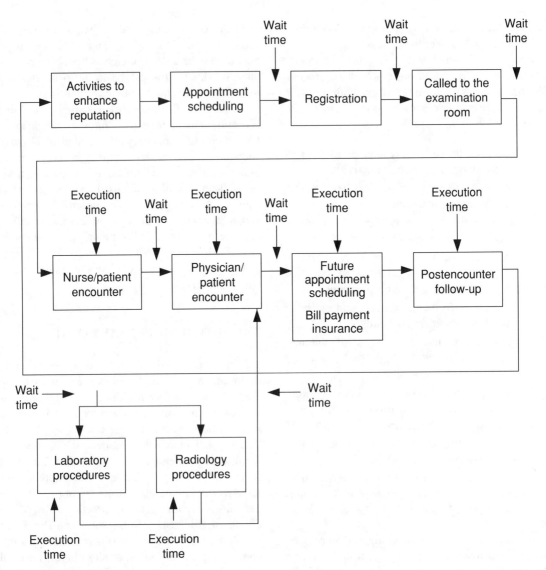

Figure 29-1 Flow Patterns in an Ambulatory Care Center. *Source:* Reprinted from *Journal of Ambulatory Care Management,* Vol. 12, No. 3, p. 41, Aspen Publishers, Inc., © 1989.

of such large regional multispecialty group-centered systems.

The dramatic growth in multispecialty group practices was mentioned earlier. Although the number of large groups has not grown appreciably, the number of physicians in them has. The total number of group practices may in fact decline as more mergers and acquisitions occur. As primary care and multispecialty groups increase in size, there is a tendency to departmentalize. Care must be taken to avoid creating barriers to the overall effectiveness of the organization.

Payment for primary care and ambulatory services remains problematic. It was believed for a long time that HMOs, particularly those associated with group practices, would flourish and become the model for payment systems of the future. Growth in HMOs, however, has slowed dramatically in the last several years. Much of the change in payment systems now occurring is due to government reforms in physician payments that began in 1992, when ambulatory visit groupings (DVGs) were introduced.[9] These innovations make it difficult to predict what kind of payment system will prevail in the future. Based on the work done on physician payment reform, the Medicare fee schedule, and the volume performance standards, it appears that capitation is likely to become the prevailing payment system of the future. This will make the primary care delivered in the ambulatory setting even more important, since payment will be made on a per-person/per-month basis rather than per-procedure. Prevention, early detection, and shifting diagnostic and treatment modalities from inpatient to outpatient settings will become more important. As Medicare adopts these new approaches, commercial insurers will follow. The future role of third-party insurance carriers remains unclear, although a mandated package of basic health coverage seems likely.

Information management and data collection will also become increasingly important. As both government and private payers increase the emphasis on containing costs and increasing physician productivity, the information system will emerge as the cornerstone of the primary care practice. The automated medical record will provide data instantaneously on previous and current visits, tests, and treatments. Patient satisfaction with particular providers will be used as a management tool for discipline and quality improvement.

The use of nonphysician providers in primary care will increase as well. The primary care center is an excellent setting for the creative use of nurse practitioners, physician assistants, and other primary health care workers. The legal system may be adjusted to accommodate expanded scopes of practice but it is likely that professional and legal domain issues will clash if physicians are subject to suit because of their responsibility for the work being done by nonphysicians.[10]

The supply of primary care physicians will continue to be an issue of great importance during the next decade. There is a serious shortage of primary care physicians. Recent changes in Medicare reimbursement that favor primary physicians over specialists over some years will help to level the economic playing field for primary care physicians. In the meantime, the shortage will continue to constrain the expansion of primary care services.

The group practice setting provides high level satisfaction for many physicians. Group practice, because of the collegial relationship among members of the group, offers the physician the opportunity to participate directly in the management of the organization and to take responsibility for the cost and quality of care. A fully capitated system will change the physician's approach to practice. The result could be increased emphasis on controlling costs and promoting continuous quality improvement in the primary care setting. The growing interest in applying Deming's 14 Principles[11] to primary care organizations is therefore very timely.

Insufficient emphasis has been placed on the need for physician leadership and management in primary care and group practice settings. Physician-managers must have the authority to actively manage their peers as primary care organizations grow larger and more complex. Training in management will become essential to organizational effectiveness. The Medical Group Management Association and the American College of Physician Executives are making available for physicians appropriate training in management.

CONCLUSION

As the health system evolves, the manager of primary care services would do well to bear in mind the following points:

- Coordination of inpatient, outpatient, home care, and community health and social services is an essential component of primary care.

- Proximity of primary and ambulatory care facilities to an inpatient facility is desirable.
- An appointment system providing timely access for urgent, routine, or follow-up care promotes the efficient use of primary care services.
- An integrated information system is essential. On-line medical records and results reporting will increase the efficiency of the primary care system.
- Management of primary care services requires continual development of managerial skills at all levels and for all professions.
- Physicians must have a meaningful role in the leadership and the management of the primary care organization.
- Proper incentives must be provided professionals to encourage productivity.

ADDITIONAL RESOURCES

Organizations

American College of Medical Group Administrators, 104 Inverness Terrace East, Englewood, CO 80112-5306.

Medical Group Management Association, 104 Inverness Terrace East, Englewood, CO 80112-5306.

Periodicals

College Review of the American College of Medical Group Administrators, American College of Medical Group Administrators, 104 Inverness Terrace East, Englewood, CO 80112-5306.

Group Practice Journal, American Group Practice Association, 1422 Duke Street, Alexandria, VA 22314-3420.

Journal of Ambulatory Care Management, Aspen Publishers, Inc., 200 Orchard Ridge Drive, Gaithersburg, MD 20878.

Journal of Medical Practice Management, Williams & Wilkins, 428 Preston Street, Baltimore, MD 21202.

Medical Group Practice Journal, Medical Group Management Association, 104 Inverness Terrace East, Englewood, CO 80112-5306.

Books

Benson, D.S., and P.G. Townes. *Excellence in ambulatory care.* San Francisco: Jossey-Bass, 1990.

Brown, B.J., and A. Ross. *Integration of clinical and financial information systems.* Gaithersburg, Md.: Aspen Publishers, 1989.

Hillestad, S.G., and E.N. Berkowitz. *Health care marketing plans.* 2d ed. Gaithersburg, Md.: Aspen Publishers, 1991.

Howard, D.M. *New business development in ambulatory care.* Chicago: American Hospital Publishing, 1988.

Organizing, designing and building ambulatory healthcare facilities. Madison, Wis.: Marshall Erdman and Associates, 1990.

Palmer, H.R. *Ambulatory health care evaluation principles and practices.* Chicago: American Hospital Publishing, 1983.

Portnoy, S., et al. *Acquiring and enhancing physicians' practices.* Chicago: American Hospital Publishing, 1988.

Rising, E.J. *Ambulatory Care Systems.* Vol. 1, *Design and Improved Patient Flow.* Lexington, Mass.: Lexington Books, 1977.

Shouldice, R.G. *Introduction to managed care.* Arlington, Va.: Information Resource Press, 1991.

NOTES

1. J.B. Christiansen, Alternative Delivery Systems in Rural Areas, *Health Service Research* 23 (1989): 849–889.

2. J.S. Zones and S.A. Shroeder, Evolving Residency Requirements for Ambulatory Care Training for Five Medical Specialties, 1961 to 1989, *Western Journal of Medicine,* 151 (1989): 676–678.

3. C.D. Olson, Clinical Records on Computer for Ambulatory Patients, *Journal of the American Osteopathic Association* 88 (1988): 1509–1515.

4. H.R. Palmer, The Challenges and Prospects for Quality Assessment and Assurance in Ambulatory Care, *Academic Medicine* Spring (1989): 522–527.

5. D.S. Benson and P.G. Townes, *Excellence in Ambulatory Care* (San Francisco: Jossey-Bass, 1990).

6. Ibid.

7. K.D. Bopp, Value-Added Ambulatory Encounters: A Conceptual Framework, *Journal of Ambulatory Care Management* 12, no. 3 (1989): 36–44.

8. J.D. Beckman, Group Advantage, *Healthcare Forum Journal,* September–October (1990): 35–40.

9. M. Gold, Common Sense on Extending DRG Concepts to Pay for Ambulatory Care, *Inquiry* 25 (1988): 281–289.

10. S.B. Goldsmith, Ambulatory Care: Emerging Legal Issues, *The Medical Staff Counselor* 2, no. 1 (1988): 41–45.

11. G. Brooks and J.R. Linklater, Statistical Thinking and W. Edwards Deming's Teaching in the Administrative Environment, *National Productivity Review* 5 (1986): 271–280.

John H. Westerman
Robert J. Taylor

Acute Care Services

30

Purpose: The principal focus of acute care is to serve patients who are in that stage of illness or injury when symptoms are most severe and life or well-being is at greatest risk. Typically, acute care covers a wide array of services from emergency trauma services to subspecialized medical services. Acute services are commonly equated with hospital services but, as the result of technological, economic, and social pressures, patterns of delivering acute care are changing.

INTRODUCTION

Acute care, as provided in the hospital setting, has been the primary focus of health care services in much of the world since early in the twentieth century. Bolstered by their diagnostic and therapeutic capabilities, hospitals prospered and grew to dominate the health care system—assembling a critical mass of professional, technological, and financial resources geared to addressing acute conditions. Almost in reverence, society bestowed on hospitals great riches, granting them wide latitude in pursuing missions of service and encouraging them to pursue increasing levels of medical and technologi-

cal sophistication. As a result, in most western societies hospitals became citadels of acute medical care, promising and providing dramatically successful diagnostic procedures and treatment interventions for both common and esoteric diseases.

As they became more successful, hospitals also became more expensive and began to compete for increasingly scarce resources. As costs continued to escalate, reverence for hospitals waned, and economic and political pressures grew. Pressure mounted for improved economies in hospital operations, for greater control over hospitals for perceived abuses of the public trust, and for less costly alternatives to hospitalization.

Today, hospitals are still, and will remain, the dominant force in the provision of acute care services, but their role is changing rapidly. The financial and social forces that have favored acute care services, and that provided the incentives for the growth and dominance of hospitals, are being rethought. The health care system is being reshaped to place a greater emphasis on prevention and primary health care and to encourage the provision of acute care in noninstitutional settings. Acute care hospitals are being challenged to redefine their place in the larger health care system. In one dimension, they are becoming the focus for increasingly intensive levels of sophisticated and costly health services for the most severely ill and injured. In another dimension, they are being held more accountable for addressing a broad range of health needs in their communities, requiring the development of collaborative arrangements with other health service providers and related organizations. In both dimensions, hospitals need to demonstrate their commitment to community service and their effectiveness in producing quality outcomes at a reasonable cost.

As the provision of acute care services and the role of hospitals are reconfigured, the following principles should be considered:

1. The economic incentives that have stimulated the growth and development of acute care are being mitigated, placing a greater priority on primary health care services. As a result, hospital-centered acute care services will decline in volume but increase in severity. The growth of hospital-centered acute care will stabilize at a new level in proportion to alternative forms of health care delivery.

2. As the level of acute service hospitals provide becomes increasingly intensive, they will be obligated to operate efficiently and effectively. Hospitals will embrace the concept of continuous quality improvement to create an organizational culture committed to meeting the health needs of the community in the most accessible, efficient, and economical means possible.

3. Hospitals will acknowledge their place as part of a larger continuum of health care services, entering into collaborative organizational arrangements with physicians embracing components of preventive, primary health care, acute care, and continuing care.

FOUNDATIONS OF ACUTE CARE*

Acute care has been traditionally reactive and episodic—interceding when a person displays overt, and often severe, symptoms of illness or injury. As a result, acute care has developed around two obvious but fundamental concepts: diagnosis and treatment. A *diagnosis* is a conclusion, either tentative or final, about a patient's condition or problem based on a complex of symptoms, signs, and findings. *Treatment* is any or all of the activities and interventions applied for the correction or relief of the patient's condition or problem.[1] While simple in concept, diagnosis and treatment have been powerful forces in shaping the way acute care services are organized and provided.

Primary care, rather than acute care, has been the foundation of health care services since early human history when virtually every primitive society had its equivalent of the shaman or medicine woman, observing symptoms and interceding with a carefully selected ritual, herb, or poultice. For a significant portion of the world's population "traditional healers" are still the most readily available, and even preferred, source of health care services. One might argue that these earlier interventions were the advent of acute care, but primitive societies did, and still do, little to address health issues except on a primary basis. Acute care in primitive societies was, and is, more often an artful show than substantive cure, although not without at least a perceived, sometimes real benefit. Even in Hippocrates' time, medical practice was more art than science.

It was not until very recently that medical care became a true science. Just over 100 years ago Louis Pasteur argued that microscopic life played an important role in the diseases of humans. At about the same time, Wilhelm Roentgen discovered x-rays. Their discoveries were important advances and led to a better understanding of the causes of diseases, to improved sanitation, and to improved techniques of diagnosis. Even more recently, Joseph Lester founded antiseptic surgery which, in

---

*Adapted from R. Taylor, Economic, Social, and Political Changes and the Maturing of the Health Care System, *Topics in Health Record Management* 8(4) (1988): pp. 1–8, Aspen Publishers, Inc.

combination with the discovery of effective anesthesia, led to safer and less painful surgical treatments. In the 1930s, with the introduction of sulfanilamide and similar medications, doctors discovered the full power of active treatment and intervention in the disease process, and the era of modern medicine and modern hospitals began.[2]

Hospital-Centered Acute Care

Hospitals proved to be the ideal environment for nurturing further advances in medical diagnosis and treatment. In the hospital environment medical science made enormous strides, developing wonders of diagnostic capability and life-saving treatments. With their concentration of professional talent, hospitals were able to assemble the resources necessary to establish and nurture internal diagnostic capabilities, especially in laboratory medicine and radiology. Advances in pharmacology, surgical technique, and anesthesiology led to similar developments in therapeutic interventions. Ultimately, a whole array of hospital-based specialty medical services developed (see Chapter 31 for more on medical specialty services). As a product of their success, hospitals were able to attract highly qualified nurses, technicians, and professional staff and ever more sophisticated levels of technology.

By the 1960s it seemed possible, at least in the United States, that everyone could be provided any hospital-centered acute care services they might need. The success of hospitals and physicians created an aura of invincibility and a society of reverent followers. Society's infatuation with physicians, and with hospitals as their workshops, led to strong political support. In the United States, the Hill-Burton program helped to build hundreds of hospitals nationwide during the late 1940s and well into the 1960s. During that same period there were dramatic increases in the number of medical schools and a doubling of medical school students.[3] These new students were trained in hospitals (the preferred mode of medical training since early in the century), and most became enamored with the professional satisfactions of working among highly trained colleagues with ready access to advanced technologic support. This new crop of doctors gravitated toward careers of narrow specialization—even further stimulating the development and concentration of more advanced diagnostic and treatment capabilities in acute care hospitals.

Furthermore, and most importantly, throughout those years virtually all insurance companies and other payers reimbursed hospitals on the basis of cost per procedure—a strong expression of public endorsement and an open checkbook for hospital expansion and technological innovation. The incentives were all geared toward increasing the number of procedures, both diagnostic and therapeutic, with little emphasis on the costs incurred.

Most hospitals thrived, evolving to the veritable pinnacle of the health services hierarchy. By the late 1960s nearly every township of any size in the United States could boast of having its own or a nearby hospital providing the basic four medical services: general medicine, general surgery, pediatrics, and obstetrics/gynecology. Even the smallest hospitals were well equipped with laboratory, radiology, and surgical capabilities. Most community hospitals were nonprofit organizations, founded and financed by groups of civic-minded citizens or members of religious orders, many with the assistance of Hill-Burton grants. Some were founded and financed by local governments. In larger communities, in bouts of community exuberance and optimism, two or more hospitals were sometimes constructed. These community-based hospitals were often referred to as secondary hospitals—a term more commonly used outside of the United States. Secondary hospitals were intended to provide convenient access to basic acute hospital services, with the expectation that complex cases would be referred to more specialized, tertiary hospitals.

At major universities with academic health centers, hospitals of considerable sophistication developed around the research and teaching interests of their medical faculties. These tertiary (highly specialized) centers drew patient referrals for complex medical problems that could not be handled adequately at local community (secondary) hospitals. Their dual role as tertiary centers and as teaching hospitals strongly influenced the career choices of their medical students. Technical sophistication and specialization were valued while primary care roles received little attention and were devalued by inference.

Specialization was also an economically favored career choice. As these medical specialists moved out into practice they strongly influenced the community hospitals where they settled to increase the breadth of the services they provided and to raise the level of their technological investments. Secondary hospitals expanded and increased their diagnostic and treatment capabilities and some aspired to become tertiary centers in their own right. A surprising number were successful in fulfilling their ambitions, especially those in larger metropolitan areas. Increasingly, physicians were able to establish practices in very specialized fields, competing successfully with traditional academic tertiary centers. Except for rural hospitals, where specialists had a more difficult time establishing a practice, the stratification between secondary and tertiary hospitals became blurred.

Pressures for Change in Acute Care Delivery

Even as hospitals were realizing great success, economic, political, and demographic pressures for change in the way health services were organized and delivered were mounting. These dynamics are discussed in detail in other chapters (see especially Chapter 6), but the major forces affecting acute care include the following:

Rising Costs of Acute Care

Health care expenditures in the United States have increased dramatically, due in large part to the unbounding success of hospitals. With rising hospital and physician costs have come increased public attention, a request for restraint, efforts for greater control, and a demand for new approaches to managing and financing acute care services.

Institutional Disenchantment

People have become disenchanted with institutions of all kinds and are beginning to see that high technology cannot provide for all human needs. Springing from the growing discontent with institutions and technology has been a growing sense of personal responsibility for health.[4] By the early 1980s about half the people in the United States were involved in some type of ongoing effort to maintain their own health. With increased personal responsibility also came a less passive and more demanding and critical health care consumer. Today, consumers are asking the hospitals and physicians for more objective measures of quality, more convenience and accessibility, more sensitivity and humanity, and more accountability and affordability.

Erosion of Political Clout

With rising costs and social disenchantment came an erosion in the health care system's political clout, both in the business and government sectors. Physicians and hospitals no longer have the stature and influence they once enjoyed. The power in health care has shifted to those who pay the bills—managed care organizations, government, and business.

The Growth of Managed Care

Employers have been inclined to shop around for less costly health coverage. A variety of managed care systems responded to the growth demand for more economical health plans. (See Chapter 8 for more on managed care organizations.) Managed care systems control costs and the premiums they charge to their clients by controlling the use of hospitals and physicians.

Government Controls Increased

Hospitals are under growing pressure from government. Both federal and state governments, along with business, began complaining about rising costs and backed up those complaints with a progression of legislated efforts aimed at bringing hospital and physician costs under control. As a result, hospital admissions and average length of stay dropped markedly. Hospitals began to experience reduced cash flow resulting from lower utilization, discounted payments from HMOs, and declining reimbursement, and began to experience an erosion of working capital and decreased access to long-term financing. For the first time, hospitals throughout the country were facing a serious, in some cases life-threatening, financial crisis.

Changing Population Demographics

American society is changing in composition as well as attitude and is making different demands on acute care providers. The population is growing older, due in part to the health system's ability to save people from early death. For hospitals, an aging population is a double-edged sword. The aged use medical services more frequently than younger people and are hospitalized about twice as often. But almost 70 percent of their bills are paid through government programs through which utilization and reimbursement are increasingly restrictive. While the elderly have a preponderance of chronic health problems that are more suitably cared for in nonacute settings, they often incur substantial hospital bills in their final few days as heroic, expensive, and futile efforts are made to prolong life. Hospitals need to rethink how they can better serve this aging population.

Medically Disenfranchised

Another burgeoning population group includes the medically indigent and the uninsured. There are now in excess of 35 million people in the United States who have no health insurance and another 35 million who are underinsured. A key question of debate is: Whose responsibility is it to care for these people? The United States is one of the few countries in the world that has not formally adopted a national policy on universal accessibility, relying instead on local governments, market forces, and individual initiative to ensure access (see Chapter 28 for more on accessing health care).

In the absence of federal policy, local governments and public hospitals have picked up much of the responsibility for providing acute services to the medically disenfranchised. Private hospitals too, are sharing the responsibility of serving the poor, but with shrinking financial resources they are less able to handle the charity load. To turn their backs on people who cannot afford medical care, however, would run counter to the very principles on which public acute care hospitals, and most private hospitals, were founded.

IMPACT ON ACUTE CARE AND HOSPITALS

The impact of the nation's changing economic and political climate on acute care has been severe, and hospitals especially, are seeking new ways to organize and support their services. The character of the hospital business is changing markedly. Some of the key changes are described below.

Only the Most Severely Ill Are Hospitalized

Hospitals have become a focal point for the most intensely ill and injured patients—those who require the most complex array of diagnostic and treatment interventions, those who need to be watched most closely, and those with the most life-threatening conditions.

After years of continued growth, acute hospital use peaked in 1981 and has been slipping ever since. Average length of patient stay (ALOS) has been dropping, down to 7.4 days in 1984 after a decade of stability at about 7.8 days, and is now down to about 6.1 days.[5] Additional declines in the ALOS can be expected. Preadmission screening, during which the need for a patient's hospitalization is verified by someone other than the admitting doctor, is now commonplace. Complex diagnostic and treatment procedures, once the exclusive domain of acute hospitals, are increasingly being performed in outpatient settings (see Chapter 29 on primary care services). The result is that those patients who do become hospitalized are more severely ill than in the past.

Hospital Services Have Become More Intensive

More severely ill patients require more intensive care. There is greater urgency for diagnostic support, patients require more aggressive and complex treatments, and many patients require continuous attention or close monitoring. Intensive care units and coronary care units, where patients can be closely observed and their vital signs can be electronically monitored, have grown in numbers and size. Additional intensive units have been created around even more narrowly defined patient populations—neonatology and burns are two prominent examples. The personnel who staff these units have also become extremely proficient in caring for patients in critical conditions, creating a new and growing complement of professional intensivists (see Chapter 31 for more on medical specialty services).

Hospitals Will Adopt Disciplined Management Methods

The combination of severely ill patients and constrained payment systems make it incumbent upon hospitals to operate efficiently. Even minor delays in completing diagnostic procedures, or in reporting their results, can result in costly extensions to a patient's stay. In critical situations, the unavailability of any of a number of essential resources (e.g., staff, equipment, blood products, or medications) can be life threatening.

To address these challenges, hospitals will adopt more rigorous disciplined management methods. One such strategy widely adopted by hospitals has been to become more business oriented, putting greater emphasis on marketing, productivity, and diversification. Early efforts in this direction, however, adopted more of the vernacular of business and less of the substance. Too often, community in-formation (advertising) campaigns were not backed up by substantive improvements in the services promoted. More recent efforts by hospitals to adopt the principles of continuous quality improvement, proven successful in the business world, hold promise for more substantive changes in hospital culture, efficiency, and performance.

Information Must Be Immediate and Interactive

In the high intensity environment of today's hospital, a whole host of complex resources and inputs needs to be scheduled and coordinated. It is no longer adequate to track information on individual components of the system, such as drugs, medical supplies, or nursing hours. Increasingly, the interdependency of hospital resources and activities is being recognized and more sophisticated information systems are being developed to help manage them. Health professionals need "real time" information from numerous sources that can be used immediately to manage a patient's care (see Chapters 13, 14, and 15 for more on information systems management).

Technology Assessment and Management Is More Critical

Technology is essential in providing acute care in today's hospital. Laboratory and radiologic diagnostic tests are now faster, safer, and more accurate than ever before. Surgery is being performed using less invasive laparoscopic techniques. Drug incompatibilities can be automatically flagged by computer. A patient's heart rate, blood gases, and other parameters can be monitored electronically, in some cases while the patient is ambulatory.

Technological advances in acute care will continue, although the pace of new developments may slow because of financial constraints. Hospitals will need to have greater assurance that a proposed new technology will pay off as an investment. Technology assessment will take on increasing importance as will managing existing technology to ensure that its full value is obtained (see Chapter 23 for more on technology assessment and management and Chapter 16 for more on financing capital investments).

THE FUTURE OF ACUTE CARE

In light of a changing economic and social climate, fundamental changes are occurring in the way acute care services are organized and managed. Hospitals especially, are beginning to redefine what they are, their role in the health care continuum, and how they will conduct their business in the future.

Incentives for Acute Care Will Diminish

Hospital-centered acute care grew, to quote Willy Sutton when asked why he robbed banks, "Because that's where the money is." As managed care's influence on the market increases, so will its influence upon when and where patients receive acute care and how much doctors and hospitals will be paid for providing such services. While it is hard to imagine that the array of acute services currently available in the hospital will diminish significantly, the future availability of such services will be more constrained. It might also be argued that, without the financial incentives of the past, acute care innovations and new technologies will develop and proliferate more slowly. The tendency to relocate high volume acute care services in low overhead nonhospital environments will also accelerate (see Chapter 29 for more on primary care alternatives to acute care).

Hospitals Will Be Fewer, But Costs Will Continue To Increase

The trend is already clear. As acute patients decline in number or are diverted to nonhospital settings, and as the ALOS declines, some hospitals will close or be converted to other uses. The patients who remain in hospitals will be more severely ill. While hospital costs as a proportion of total health expenditures may be constrained, the aver-

age cost per hospitalized patient is likely to continue to increase. In fact, increases in the average cost per day or stay may reflect, at least in part, the success of efforts to define the hospital's role more narrowly.

Hospitals Will Collaborate and Diversify

As their role in acute care becomes more narrowly focused on treating the severely ill, hospitals will seriously examine the kind of business they are in. It seems likely that many hospitals will simply concentrate on serving severely ill patients, but all hospitals will need to do this aspect of their job very well. Some hospitals will seek to define themselves more broadly as community-service health care institutions. These hospitals will enter into complex collaborative arrangements—sometimes called regionally integrated systems—with other hospitals and with multispecialty medical groups, regional networks of primary care clinics serving rural areas, home care systems, and managed care plans.[6] Hospitals will become the acute care core of a comprehensive health care system (see Chapter 9 for more on multiunit systems).

QUALITY MANAGEMENT

Quality management in health services delivery has historically focused on acute care and the hospital. Until recently, most quality-oriented efforts stressed the monitoring of health service resources and processes. Over the years hospitals acquired considerable experience in physician credentialing, retrospective reviews, utilization review, and quality assurance. It is only recently that a concerted effort to examine outcomes has been initiated (see Chapter 3 for more on the history of quality management).

A major force shaping the delivery of acute care in the future will be the drive to define and measure health service outcomes. Traditionally, medical practitioners have developed diagnostic and treatment protocols that detail recommended processes for specific diseases and conditions. Too often, however, the ideal process was determined more by consensus among peers rather than through scientific inquiry. Protocols typically ignored the cost implications of recommended processes.

Most recent efforts to define outcomes are pursuing two different concepts: (1) that a critical mass of volume is necessary to assure quality outcomes, and (2) that cost/benefit ratios can help judge the relative effectiveness of various diagnostic and treatment approaches. The critical mass approach aims to concentrate certain specialty procedures, such as open heart surgery, in a few high-volume centers. The cost/benefit approach aims to identify effective and economical protocols rather than ideal protocols.

The cost/benefit approach, while controversial, holds interesting possibilities. For example, we may discover that for an expenditure of $1,000, 98 percent of the patients who present certain symptoms can be successfully diagnosed and treated. But to successfully treat the remaining 2 percent will require an additional investment of $10,000. What choice do we make? What do we decide if the cost ratio is 1:100 instead of 1:10, or the benefit ratio is 80:20 instead of 98:2? Serious ethical considerations arise when we have unlimited capability but limited resources.

Even though the concepts of quality review and quality assurance have been practiced in hospitals for decades, continuous quality improvement is relatively new to the health care industry. (The concepts and essential knowledge underlying continuous improvement are discussed in detail in Chapter 4.) Continuous quality improvement is a disciplined management method and requires fundamental changes in a hospital's culture in order to be successful. Without informed, sincere, and active commitment from hospital leadership, efforts in continuous quality improvement can be less than successful. Yet continuous quality improvement offers the best opportunity for hospitals to advance their capabilities significantly to provide acute services in an efficient and cost-effective manner.

Hospitals have some hard work ahead as they learn to manage their increasingly intense environment and as they reassess their role in the larger health care system. As hospitals change, acute care services will change as well. Acute care will probably not be favored with the economic support it received in the past, nor will it recede into the background. Rather, acute care will find a new place in the larger continuum of health care services.

ADDITIONAL RESOURCES

Organizations

American Hospital Association, 840 North Lake Shore Drive, Chicago, IL, 60611. 312\280-6000.

Books and Periodicals

Griffith, J.R., *The Well-Managed Community Hospital,* Ann Arbor: Health Administration Press, 1987.

Hospitals, American Hospital Association, Chicago: American Hospital Publishing, Inc., published twice monthly.

Roland, H.S., and B. Roland, *Hospital Management: A Guide to Departments,* Gaithersburg, MD: Aspen Publishers, 1984.

Rosenberg, C.E., *The Care of Strangers: The Rise of America's Hospital System,* New York: Basic Books, 1987.

Stevens, R., *In Sickness and in Wealth: American Hospitals in the Twentieth Century,* New York: Basic Books, 1989.

NOTES

1. V.N. Slee and D.A. Slee, *Health Care Terms,* 2nd ed. (St. Paul: Tringa Press, 1991).

2. L. Thomas, *The Youngest Science: Notes of a Medicine-Watcher* (New York: Viking Press, 1983).

3. Department of Teaching Hospitals, *Toward a More Contemporary Public Understanding of the Teaching Hospital* (Washington, D.C.: Association of American Medical Colleges, 1981).

4. J. Naisbitt, *Megatrends* (New York: Warner Books, 1982), 145.

5. American Hospital Association, *Hospital Statistics* (Chicago: American Hospital Association, 1992).

6. H.J. Anderson, Hospitals Seek New Ways To Integrate Health Care, *Hospitals* 66, no. 7 (1992): 26–36.

Michael B. Shirk

31

Specialty Diagnostic and Therapeutic Services

Purpose: The purpose of specialty diagnostic and therapeutic services is to provide health care practitioners with information that assists them in reaching diagnostic conclusions regarding their patients and in applying appropriate treatment interventions. Specialty diagnostic and therapeutic services typically include the departments of anesthesiology, radiology, and laboratory, and may include rehabilitation, cardiology, neurology, nephrology, and radiation oncology, and numerous others.

INTRODUCTION

Specialty diagnostic and therapeutic services are a core distinguishing feature of the contemporary acute care hospital and they will become increasingly important as hospitals focus on caring for the most severely ill and injured. These specialty services rely heavily on highly trained professional staffs and advanced technologies, and the operation of the entire hospital is dependent on their performance. They pose unique managerial challenges and opportunities and special understandings, techniques, and skills are required in their direction and

coordination. As a starting place, in order to comprehend how specialty services fit into the overall patient care process, the manager needs to understand

- the motivation of the employees who work in specialty service
- the expectations of the physicians involved in these services
- the expectations of the physicians ordering tests or procedures
- the impact of technology assessment
- the efficient use of resources
- the quality of performance of special services as it relates to the cost

In reaching an increased understanding of specialty services, the manager should keep in mind the following principles:

1. Employees who staff specialty services often have more loyalty to their profession than to their employer. Their technical knowledge obtained through a unique curriculum provides career security, a level of expected ben-

efits, and a recognized status within the health care community. Employees in nonprofessional or nondegreed jobs have employment security that is more employer dependent. Managers of specialty services rarely direct the actions of their professional employees. Rather, they work to create an atmosphere supportive of professional excellence, stressing a consensus on goals and work processes.

2. Each specialty service department must become an integrated contributor to overall institutional goals. The hospital must ensure that the physicians involved in providing services understand how they can assist the manager in achieving the hospital's stated mission. Employees of specialty departments can easily become isolated from patients and other hospital services. They must become as comfortable on the patient units as they are within the confines of their department.

3. The role of the physician director of a specialty service must be clearly delineated by establishing measurable, objective goals in terms of output and outcome. The relationship between the physicians and the hospital cannot be based on number of referrals, number of tests ordered, or revenue generated. It must be based on the exchange of real effort toward documented outcomes in return for defined payment.

4. The manager of a specialty department has to assume responsibility for ensuring the department works efficiently and effectively to provide services necessary to support patient care. The patient care team and specialty service employees have to reach agreement as to the level of service provided by the specialty department. The manager's role includes defining expectations within the care team and monitoring performance. The department's success must be quantifiable in terms of beneficial outcomes to patients and not in terms of work outputs.

5. Continuing communication among management and the specialty services is essential. Professionals want to understand the purposes and intentions of the organization and want to be kept informed on its progress toward meeting its goals. The manager of a specialty department must communicate as much information as possible if departmental staff are to appreciate their contribution toward overall organizational efforts. Collaboration among management, specialty service staff, and other hospital personnel is dependent upon the knowledge and understanding everyone has of each other's needs and importance.

6. The technology needed to support the activities of special services must be carefully assessed. Specialty services are characterized by large investments in instrumentation. In a time of scarce resources and increasing costs, the manager must be able to assess current technological capability and to predict future technological needs. Management must develop a strategic technology acquisition plan in order to maximize return on investment as measured by positive impact on the institution overall, rather than exclusively on the desires of the individual department.

THE ORGANIZATIONAL ROLE OF SPECIALTY SERVICES

As described in Chapter 30, beginning early this century, acute care hospitals provided the ideal environment for the development of specialized diagnostic and therapeutic services. Originally, specialty services emanated from the research or teaching interests of one physician who might be asked to provide consulting advice to another physician. As the demands for consulting support increased, small cadres of technical experts clustered around these consultants to assist them in their work. Eventually these cadres evolved to the highly sophisticated, functionally separate, specialty departments found in today's hospitals. In recent years, hospital managers have faced the challenge of breaking down the barriers that have separated these functional departments. Managers are attempting to create organizational cultures where communication, coordination, and teamwork are rewarded.

Development of Departments

Clinical specialists came into their own early in this century as advances in medical science burgeoned. As medical specialists developed, technicians and nurses began to assist them, relieving them of repetitive or routine tasks. As knowledge increased regarding the evaluation and measurement of chemicals, blood cells, and bacteria in the body fluids, time was also spent analyzing the resulting data. Increased knowledge required increased training, and technicians and nurses who had provided assistance became experts in their own right. More and new technical positions were added as the volume of work grew and additional technologies were developed. Still, physicians continued to be seen as the primary source of specialty consultative advice, but with a growing array of professional support and technological resources to draw on for assistance.

As physicians became more specialized, evolving from general practitioners into surgeons, pathologists, and radiologists, their need for hands-on assistance increased. Pathologists began to train technicians to conduct tests, to operate laboratory instruments, and to perform a growing array of laboratory procedures. Radiologists taught technicians radiology theory and the proper positioning of patients for examination. Similar changes occurred in physical therapy, surgery, anesthesiology, and nursing. For example, respiratory therapy was originally provided by nurses under medical supervision, but eventually was turned over to technicians who evolved into respiratory therapists, a professional group now quite separate from its nursing roots.

Acute patients began to congregate in hospitals because of their growing diagnostic and therapeutic capabilities. Attendants, who had been employed previously in physician's offices, began to find work in the hospital setting where they could staff the instruments necessary to get accurate diagnoses and provide care to patients after surgery.

Almost all medical crises as well as medical mysteries were handled on an inpatient basis. Hospitals became more segregated by training and function, leading to the development of separate departments in each of the specialized services. This trend continues today, and physicians, for example, more skilled in the manipulation of catheters have specially trained nurses and radiology technicians to assist them with cardiac catheterization and laparoscopic procedures.

The evolution of the services into specialty requiring different education and training departments. Specialization was further formalized when state governments passed laws that designated certain functions as the province of specific professions. States, utilizing their police powers in an effort to protect the public and ensure the highest quality of care, granted monopolies to these professions (in the same way they had granted monopolies to physicians, pharmacists, and nurses). Only individuals passing a specific examination or showing evidence of specific schooling would be licensed to practice in a given discipline. Licensing and certification requirements have bolstered the continuing demand for qualified personnel, and in light of continuing shortages have resulted in relatively high levels of compensation.

The schooling for each technical discipline has become more standardized, with essentially the same curricula offered throughout the country in various colleges, universities, and technical schools. Strong professional identity and loyalty is often created among those who share these common training experiences. These feelings of professional identity and loyalty tend to be reinforced once they begin employment in the hospital where they are placed in departments that are functionally separate and distinct. Other health care employees, especially nonskilled or nonprofessional workers, tend to be more dependent on their employer for symbols of status, recognition, and levels of pay. Their lack of a defined body of knowledge also makes them more vulnerable to discipline or replacement. As a result, nonskilled workers have relied more than technicians and professionals on unions and labor laws to protect their interests. For technicians, limited school slots and long training times have tended to keep the supply of graduates low, giving them greater leverage in mandating their own work rules. As a result, the formation of bargaining units among technicians and professionals has been much less common than among nonprofessionals.

A uniform and distinct knowledge base for each profession reinforced the natural evolution toward specialty diagnostic and therapeutic departments in hospitals. These departments were characterized by expensive instrumentation; the provision of intermittent care; and focus on specific processes or organs, rather than on the entire person. Specialty departments provided data to the caregivers and became important sources of revenue to the institution.

In many hospitals, in recognition of their common characteristics, specialty departments are administratively brought together in organizational divisions although, even then, individual departments tend to remain quite separate, operationally. Specialty services define their services by maintaining exclusive control over specific procedures and tests. They compete with each other and other departments for the allocation of hospital resources.

As the knowledge base expands, sections within each specialty service tend to become themselves more specialized and autonomous. For example, clinical laboratories are commonly divided into a blood bank, hematology, microbiology, and chemistry sections. Each section tends toward a separate identity from the overall department and even to require a separate credentialing process for its personnel. The expanded knowledge base, and increased specialization, tend to foster fragmentation within the health care process. Hospital management is challenged to create an environment in which these disparate specialty functions are linked together in a common effort to serve the health needs of the community.

Evolving Role of the Medical Director

Physicians have always been, and will remain, the essential diagnostic and therapeutic resource upon which other physicians rely for consultive assistance. The complexity of medical technology and the amount of knowledge necessary to perform most procedures require physicians to be directly in the operation of the specialty services. Since the fundamental purpose of each specialty service is to provide clinical information to the practitioner who ordered the exams, the medical director of the specialty service is viewed as the person most responsible for the accuracy of the service's output. Although the management could attest to the efficiency of operations, the training of the employees, and the other environmental aspects of a specialty service, the practicing physicians continue to demand that a medically qualified individual endorse the results of all tests and procedures. Therefore, hospitals designate medical directors for their specialty services, typically compensating them on the basis of a percentage of revenue, a fee per test, or a straight salary. However, medical directors have sought alternative methods of compensation, stimulated perhaps by the level of their incomes compared to that of physicians in private practice, pressures from professional societies, or their perceived status among their peers. Over time, many medical directors have switched to separate billing so that their incomes are no longer derived from hospital revenue but are viewed as patient driven. The evolution away from the use of salaried or contracted physicians again raises issues of loyalty. Medical specialty leaders and the technical employees may be motivated by their desire to be independent practitioners, treating patients directly, and by their professional loyalties, and may identify only indirectly to the organization.

Current Organization of Specialty Services

The evolution of specialty services has resulted, in the present era, in the establishment of separate and independent departments, each essentially a fiefdom headed by a medical director overseeing professionally oriented employees utilizing instrumentation and technology little understood outside the department. The separations between the specialty services, the hospital, and the other departments has intensified, with a certain amount of mystery surrounding each department's activities, relationships, and reason for existing. The patient care process has become more and more fragmented, with institutions divided into small units, each clamoring for a larger share of the economic pie.

Managers faced with these issues in the 1980s and with changes in reimbursement methods had to develop ways to combine the special service professionals and non-specialty-service staff to create a more unified service delivery process with the ultimate goal of providing high-quality care. They explored new organizational forms (see Chapter 7 for alternative organizational designs), and ultimately resorted to renegotiating contractual agreements with the medical directors specifying their expected involvement in the overall patient care process. Managers confronted by a scarcity of resources also have to worry about acquiring technology at lowest cost. The rest of this chapter reviews how today's managers struggle with these issues.

MANAGING HUMAN RESOURCES

Managers of a specialty diagnostic or therapeutic service are seldom able to lead their departments by dictate. Rather, they seek to gain a consensus on shared goals. One of those goals is for health care professionals to focus more on outcomes and less on outputs. Increasingly, the main criterion for success in health care is the amount of benefit the patient receives as a result of the service provided. Managers of specialty services must lead their departments in identifying where to place the focus for improvements in quality and service, to mobilize the department's resources in a continuing effort to address these priorities, and to help integrate the department's efforts with those of other departments.

Motivating Employees to a Common Mission

A manager of a specialty service cannot allow the department to be isolated or walled off from other hospital services. Isolation perpetuates the tendency toward professional and department loyalty. If the manager is able to bring the service technicians into the mainstream of the caring process, then technicians can gain fulfillment from the accomplishments of the entire health care team not just from what they contribute as individuals. In order for this kind of integration to occur, technicians must be recognized not so much for what they know or for their professional orientation but for how they contribute to the patient's overall diagnosis and treatment. In other words, the specialty service department must be viewed not as a functionally separate unit but as a link in the chain of a comprehensive patient care process. As stated earlier, employee stress and dissatisfaction, even labor unrest, are often directly related to employees' sense of separation from the mission and main purpose of the organization.

Emphasizing Outcome, Not Output

The entire health care industry is facing serious financial constraints, and specialty departments must be able to justify the resources they consume in terms of the contribution they make to improved patient care. Traditionally, departmental performance focused on inputs (e.g., technology, human resources, and supplies) and resulting outputs (e.g., test results and number of procedures). If inputs were turned into outputs efficiently, and the costs incurred were adequately covered by revenue, the consumption of resources and the continuing existence of the service were considered justified. Today, specialty services are being held accountable for outcomes as well as outputs. Specialty services managers are more comfortable with input-output ratios because they are easily defined, easily measured, and are minimally subjective in nature. Outcome measures are not easily defined or measured and often their link to input is unclear.

Outcomes are results. They range from death and disease, to emotional health and patient satisfaction. Outcomes measurement in medical care is the assessment of these results to evaluate the effectiveness of care. Most outcome measures are comparative. Patients' disease states at the end of a course of treatment are compared with their beginning conditions; the death rate for a particular category of disease is compared with the expected rate.[1]

Today's specialty services managers need to be comfortable discussing input-outcome ratios as well as input-output ratios. In the past, managers have allowed non-outcome-related factors, such as protection from malpractice, concerns about adequate reimbursements, and the convenience of standing orders, to be utilized as justification for the use of specialty services. Today, however, with ever increasing financial constraints, specialty departments need to demonstrate where their services logically fit into the overall care process. This means educating the practitioners about the prudent use of tests and procedures and how to define and measure the resulting outcomes.

Integrating Specialty Services into the Patient Care Process

Specialty departments cannot isolate themselves from other departments and the patient care process. They cannot maximize their contribution to patient care by limiting their relationships with other members of the health care team by what comes through their in-box and out-box. In the past many specialty departments felt it was acceptable to passively await the receipt of requisitions or orders from an outside source, perform the requested tests or procedures, and then report the results back via the out-box or its equivalent. Health care services can no longer been as functionally segmented and departmentalized; rather, they need to be viewed and organized as a continuum, with patient outcomes being of paramount concern for everyone involved. A specialty department's main goal cannot be simply to pass accreditation or inspections, as by the Joint Commission on Accreditation of

Healthcare Organizations, but to contribute to the care and cure of the hospital's patients.

The team approach to care provision is reinforced if the manager of a specialty service accepts responsibility for all segments of the relevant work process. A simplified workflow diagram, illustrating the main segments in ordering, performing, and reviewing laboratory tests is shown in Figure 31-1. Often, the laboratory manager confines his or her attention to the work that occurs between the time a specimen reaches the laboratory and the time the results leave the department. However, if the manager assumes responsibility for ensuring that laboratory tests maximally benefit the patient, he or she would be involved in all phases of the workflow and would review all critical links of the process to assess their impact on patient outcomes. With a more comprehensive perspective, the manager might consider questions such as these:

- Do the physicians have sufficient knowledge to order the appropriate tests?
- Are orders recorded or transcribed correctly?
- When is verification of orders necessary and when is it unnecessary?
- How are specimens collected and by whom?
- How fast and in what condition do specimens reach the laboratory?
- Are the tests performed correctly and expediently?
- Are results posted promptly, correctly, and in the right patient record?
- Do the physicians know how to interpret the results?

In order to address these questions the laboratory manager would need to involve each member of the department as well as the managers of other departments. When all managers assume responsibility for every aspect of the care process, then successful outcomes can be more easily achieved.

Quality Management

Focusing on the interaction between the specialty personnel and the other staff provides an opportu-

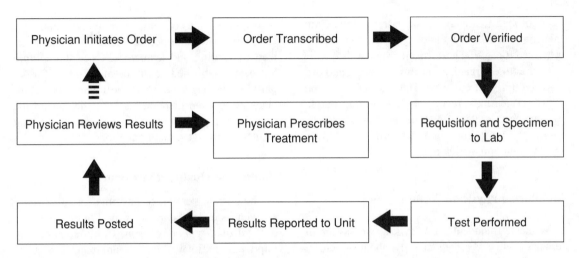

Figure 31-1 Simplified Workflow for Laboratory Testing

nity for analyzing the expectations each person in the care process has regarding the other providers. Satisfaction with service equals reality minus expectations. If expectations are greater than reality, then the quality of service would be considered inadequate or even poor. In order to set quality expectations, managers must be able to indicate how quality will be measured and to reach agreement on the level of quality currently achieved. Quality indicators must be understandable, objective, and agreed to by all involved.

Often specialty department managers attempt to delegate quality or outcome improvement to others in the organization. In their zeal to meet departmental quality control standards, whether self-imposed or imposed by a specialty accrediting agency, they become focused on the performance of their departments. What is forgotten is how each department contributes to the overall quality of the institution. How important is it that the standards of the Society of Nuclear Medicine Technologists are met if the performance of nuclear medicine tests increases lengths of stay because of inefficiency in getting patients to the department? Is it more important to meet the quality control standards of urinalysis or to ensure that the urine specimen does not sit out at room temperature on the nursing unit for extended periods of time?

How does the manager of the blood bank balance having American Association of Blood Banks accreditation and ensuring that nurses know how to identify the proper unit to give to a patient?

The manager of a specialty department cannot concentrate solely on departmental quality issues while delegating patient care quality issues to a quality assurance department. The process used by a quality assurance or quality control department involves reaching agreement on quality parameters and then indicating where an organization is in terms of those parameters. Quality assurance does not encompass the development of processes or technologies to achieve quality goals. The development of such processes and technologies is the responsibility of management. The manager of the specialty department must reach agreement, contractual where appropriate, with the professionals in the department as to what standards of performance support quality outcomes without being overly costly for the amount of benefit they provide. These performance standards must meet three criteria: (1) They must be realistic, (2) they must be agreed to, and (3) they must impact patient outcomes positively.

Performance standards should be set to increase the likelihood that patients will be better off as a result of their treatment. In the past, the Joint Commission and other regulatory agencies have been criticized for setting performance standards dealing with structure, organization, environment, and process but not with outcome. The manager of a specialty service must recognize that existing regulatory agency standards must be met but that, in the future, the more important standards are likely to involve outcome indicators.

Monitoring Physician Performance

Medicare fraud and abuse laws, as well as the Internal Revenue Service's concern about private inurement through public funds, require that job descriptions for physicians associated with hospitals, in particular, with specialty services, clearly outline expected duties and responsibilities. The manager should review each contract to ensure that it clearly specifies the amount of effort the job requires and contains an outline of educational, procedural, and outcome goals. If a physician is being contracted to be medical director of a specialty service, the contract must specifically outline how the physician is expected to relate to his or her peers and what type of education or training the physician is expected to provide department staff. The role of specialists in setting performance standards should include developing outcome parameters and medical criteria for ordering procedures and tests. Efficiency requires that physicians in specialty departments replace the question that used to be asked—Why are all tests ordered STAT?—with a new question: Why are these tests being ordered at all? Managing a specialty department requires identifying how the specialty service fits into the continuum of care and how the specialty service physicians can optimize utilization of the service. The manager and the physicians accept a twofold responsibility: (1) to ensure the proper utilization of resources, both human and material; and (2) to develop mechanisms to ensure the utilization results in positive patient outcomes.

Specialty department medical directors and physicians, by interacting routinely with the other medical staff in a cooperative, nonjudgmental way, can help create an organizational culture characterized by sharing and teamwork. Once this culture has been established, it will be much easier for department managers to shift the loyalty of technicians away from their professions and toward the organization's mission: providing superior care that results in positive patient outcomes.

Continuous Quality Improvement

The current version of customer-oriented management is called *continuous quality improvement* or *total quality management.* Continuous quality improvement fits well into a team management approach. The object of quality improvement is to increase the efficiency and effectiveness of the patient care process.

The use of teams of employees to look at the total process helps to break down departmental and professional barriers. Integration is achieved by bringing together individuals who have different backgrounds and levels of authority but who all play a role in ensuring better outcomes for patients. Each team member feels a sense of fulfillment and accomplishment by sharing in the improvement process. The team, which includes specialty and nonspecialty staff and managers, analyzes the patient care process from the physician's, the nurse's, and the technician's point of view. Universal goals are then set by the specialty and nonspecialty managers on the team. In the past, the tendency was to minimize error but to accept what was considered reasonable error. Currently, the strategy is to acknowledge error as a contributor to learning and continuous improvement. Identifying deviations from perfection constitutes the basis for learning how to improve the process. When deviations are uncovered, the burden in placed on individuals to come up with solutions. "The key to both the productivity of the knowledge worker and his achievement is to demand responsibility from him. Direction of the knowledge worker toward contribution is the first job of the manager. Perhaps the most important thing is to enable the knowledge workers to do what they are being paid for."[2]

MANAGEMENT OF TECHNOLOGICAL RESOURCES

Assessing and acquiring technological equipment is an important part of the management of specialty services. Just as managers are always seeking new ways to improve the effectiveness of employees, so must they always be alert for possible technologies that may improve the services being provided. However, it is critical to avoid purchasing technology just for the sake of owning technology. Equipment acquisition needs to be considered in light of the facility's mission and resources.

Technology Appraisal

Improving quality requires managers of specialty services not only to be experts in the utilization of professionals and supplies but to have some familiarity with the ever-expanding field of medical technology. These managers have to know something about magnetic energy, laser technology, and ultrasonography, to name just a few topics, as well as something about the traditional fields of radiology, laboratory medicine, anesthesiology, and oxygen therapy. In the old environment of cost reimbursement, managers could invest in technology in a more haphazard way, with the motto "more is better." Today, faced with a shrinking resource pool and a high rate of technological obsolescence, managers must be skilled in technological assessment and be able to negotiate a purchase package that protects the facility now and several years hence. Possibly one of the major weaknesses of most specialty department managers is their lack of understanding of how to appraise technology.

Acquiring appropriate technology has several benefits. Technology not only contributes to the achievement of positive patient outcomes but also gives the institution a competitive advantage, since the public will tend to view the institution as the provider of choice. Selecting appropriate technology, however, is becoming a more demanding task. First, people are becoming more sophisticated in their knowledge of what technology can do, and they expect technological treatments that are painless, inexpensive, and convenient. Second, at the same time that the public's acceptance of technology is growing, health care experts are questioning where technology is headed and are divided over what its real impact on patient outcomes is.

Technology Acquisition

More now that ever before, managers need to collaborate with physicians and other health care professionals to determine which technologies to invest in. There are three important categories of technology acquisition: (1) some technologies are acquired to meet mandatory guidelines, (2) some are acquired to provide a market advantage, and (3) some are acquired in an attempt on the part of the institution to become a dominant, cutting-edge provider in a certain area of medicine.

Acquisition of mandatory technologies requires shrewd purchase agreements followed by careful maintenance. In the purchase of each technology, the manager needs to negotiate with the manufacturers to obtain the technology at a good price and ensure maintenance and the ability to upgrade the equipment at a guaranteed cost base. It is important for the manager to negotiate with at least two manufacturers of the technology. If the manager allows the medical staff to indicate covertly to a specific manufacturer that it is the only manufacturer being considered, then there will be little room for negotiation. The immediate benefits of having a piece of equipment or a technology creates only a partial advantage. Full advantage is achieved if the manager is able to negotiate low maintenance costs and a guaranteed minimum amount of downtime. "Although price is still a prime consideration, executives are aggressively negotiating the fine print on imaging contracts."[3] There is a trend toward inclusion of the following provisions:

- comparison matrices (acquisition costs, installation costs, operating costs, life-cycle costs)

- installation and deinstallation
- detailed service contracts with an emphasis on predictability
- guarantee of uptime of 98 percent or better
- protection against early obsolescence
- discounts on future upgrades

Acquiring technologies to create market advantage is more risky, since the manager must rely on the intuition of the medical staff, other members of the health care continuum, and marketing experts. Being first in the marketplace does not necessarily guarantee that a certain technology will benefit the health care institution. The manager needs to pick technologies the institution has the ability to utilize. For example, some hospitals were rushed into purchasing surgical lasers without understanding the need to have a strong biomedical department and to have physicians recently schooled in the application of lasers. In many cases, the lasers sat unused because of poor repair or because the medical staff did not feel comfortable using them. As this shows, the manager should consult with the entire medical staff of the institution and even outside physicians and health care experts to ensure the institution is capable of supporting a technology being considered for acquisition. A 1990 survey of 524 health care CEOs ranked the importance of physician opinion and other criteria in technological acquisition. The results are summarized in Tables 31-1 and 31-2.

Acquiring cutting-edge technologies is the riskiest kind of investment, yet it can be the most rewarding. In a typical situation, a manager, working with the medical staff, might look into the future, assess the institution's strengths, and decide to invest scarce resources to maximize the institution's capability in an area of treatment. (The manager must often have broad support and at least one physician champion who shares the manager's belief in the institution's ability to utilize the innovative technology effectively.) The investment could allow the institution to gain the reputation of being a technological leader.

In such a case, the purpose of acquisition is to dominate, not just to expand. A hospital that seeks to dominate its market needs to develop the confidence that, when better technologies are developed, it will be among the first institutions to acquire and implement them. Keeping ahead of the competition requires an institutional commitment and technological assessment far above the average, and the manager must be able to motivate many professionals to commit themselves to new projects enthusiastically.

Hospitals that truly dominate their markets are characterized by managers who look at today's technology as commonplace and expect their institutions to lead the way into the future. Some managers of specialty services are prone to become satisfied with the status quo and shy away from innovation. Yet, just as a commitment to continuous quality improvement is essential, so is a com-

Table 31-1 Ranking of Recommendations Regarding New Technologies

	Very Important (%)	Somewhat Important (%)	Not Important (%)
Medical Staff	96.0	4.0	—
Department Heads	83.7	16.3	—
Senior Management	76.0	23.6	0.4
Vendors	11.2	66.1	22.6

Source: Reprinted from *Hospitals*, Vol. 65, No. 21, p. 30, by permission. November 5, 1991. Copyright 1991 by American Hospital Publishing, Inc.

Table 31-2 Ranking of Criteria Used in Technology Acquisition Decisions

	Very Important (%)	Somewhat Important (%)	Not Important (%)
Ability to Establish or Expand Services	84.9	14.5	0.6
Return on Investment	70.8	28.6	0.6
Ability to Reduce Operating Costs	66.7	32.7	0.6
Enhanced Image of Hospital	46.5	49.5	4.0
Medical Staff Pressures	42.7	55.3	2.0

Source: Reprinted from *Hospitals,* Vol. 65, No. 21, p. 30, by permission. November 5, 1991. Copyright 1991 by American Hospital Publishing, Inc.

mitment to continuous technological improvement. (For more on assessing and acquiring technology, see Chapter 23.)

THE FUTURE OF SPECIALTY SERVICES

The end of the twentieth century will witness the continued rapid expansion of medical needs and capabilities. Managers will have access to more data than can be communicated. Technology will continue to expand. Events will happen so quickly and situations will become so complex that the environment will become more unstable and uncertain. Individuals will increasingly work in self-directed teams, and problem solving will occur without traditional management authorization.

Physician Partnerships

The team approach established by managers of specialty services will provide a foundation for meeting the challenges and taking advantage of the opportunities presented during the rest of this decade and well into the next century. As government fraud and abuse regulations and IRS diligence, in looking at the use of public dollars for private inurement, restrain the creation of so-called sweetheart deals, managers will have to form defined and measurable relationships with the physicians running the specialty services as well as the physicians referring to the services. The ability of managers to indirectly reward physicians for referrals or to augment the incomes of specialty physicians for encouraging other physicians to refer patients will be curtailed.

> The Medicare and Medicaid Patient and Program Protection Act of 1987 directed the Office of Inspector General (OIG) to HHS to promulgate regulation identifying payment practices protected from criminal prosecution or civil sanctions. . . . On July 29, 1991, the Department of Health and Human Services (HHS) issued long-awaited regulations designating "safe harbors" from civil sanctions or criminal prosecution under the Medicare and Medicaid anti-kickback statutes.[4]

The anti-kickback statutes are founded on the belief that physicians should be paid only for real effort, defined objectively and measurably. In joint ventures, health care managers must no longer be the active partners and physician-investors the passive partners. The new environment calls for equal risk sharing, equal investment, and equal participation. The philosophy of paying a physician for a defined outcome or output has been formalized by the federal government. In January 1992, the Medicare Program replaced the payment system based on physician charges with a fee schedule designed to reflect the resources used in providing services to patients. We are moving into an atmosphere of mutual trust in order to obtain mutual gain, and away from the previous environment of the customer versus provider, them versus us, and the health care professionals favoring the manager who gave them the most "toys." The three points of the health care dilemma described earlier—access, quality, and cost—will shift in the years ahead from having accessible quality at the risk of higher cost to quality at low cost with some restrictions on access.

With the simultaneous reduction of reimbursements by all payers to both facilities and physicians, managers are faced with the choice of increased maneuvering for ever-decreasing health care dollars or working together to obtain the best possible outcomes for the patients while seeking to keep costs low. At the same time, managers of specialty services and health care professionals have to realize that, by providing low-cost, high-quality care, they will inevitably curtail their ability to serve everyone equally. This fact will put increasing pressure on managers and physicians to prioritize services on the basis of outcome, efficiency, and cost. (For example, the services with the highest ranking will be those that produce good outcomes in a reasonable period of time at a reasonable cost.)

In the years ahead, all health care professionals will recognize the need to implement continuous quality improvement and to define quality. The agreed definition of quality will include appropriate provision of services, appropriate use of resources, and appropriate application of technology.

There will also be a trend toward rewarding care that meets the expectations of patients and other clients. Joint ventures will be viewed not as a way to increase income for facilities and individuals, but as a way to provide needed health care services—with each partner sharing in risk and reward and each committed to the establishment of outcome parameters.

Technology Acquisition

Probably no other challenge in the next decade is going to be as difficult as the selection of the right technologies. The ability of manufacturers to create new diagnostic equipment in a short period of time is greater than ever. The advent of the DNA restructuring and the ability to harvest and enhance stem cells will create a new approach to the treatment of disease.

With the effort to identify all human genes underway, managers of specialty services are facing challenges and opportunities never before presented.

During this same time, information systems technology has given managers the ability to communicate data instantly to all members of the health care team. Information is becoming the property of everyone. Managers who seek to stifle the dissemination of information to other team members only ensure failure. The likelihood there will soon be a completely automated medical record that can be transmitted anywhere in the facility and also to outlying referral centers requires managers to consider cutting back on investment in diagnostic capabilities and devoting more resources to communication. In the years ahead, managers must become more comfortable communicating and networking, since the massive amount of knowledge available is more than one individual can master. The need for managerial networking and communicating have led many to suggest that the female managers will have increasing success since men are prone to allow competitiveness to interfere with open communication.

The specialty services will be the first to feel the full impact of the human genome project and the almost complete decline of major traumatic interventional surgery as nonradiologic imaging and endoscopic laser surgery replace the scalpel and the large incision. Those managers who have traditionally seen technology as a way to establish market domination will be comfortable with the fast-paced changes that medicine will undergo. They will be in the best position to take advantage of new developments in immunology, genetic engineering, computer technology, and other up-and-coming technologies.

Dismantling the Hierarchies

Employees in the health care facility of the future, like employees in the typical Walmart, will become associates of the management team. As they become more involved in day-to-day problem solving and quality improvement, their traditional loyalty to their professions will slowly be replaced by a commitment to solving patient problems. Attending this shift will be an increased acceptance of job sharing and occupation swapping. Employees will readily agree to cross-training modalities and to the establishment of a reward system that recompenses the entire health care team for the achievement of beneficial patient outcomes. Managers of specialty departments will recognize that the walls of each department must be taken down and that employees across departments must be willing to share knowledge and in some cases even share each other's jobs. It is clear that enthusiasm for teamwork increases when cross-training is instituted. The list of skill combinations in Table 31-3 indicates that eight out of the top twelve involve traditional specialty departments.

Management has not yet developed a system to reward those employees who want to work in a cross-training modality and are willing to become

members of a multifunctional team. "It's almost easier to move a graveyard than to change a practice act. Experts warn that cross-training won't become commonplace until the health care industry changes age-old compensation practices and more facilities regard people who become multiskilled."[5] As stated earlier, evaluations must focus on how the team does and how individuals perform within the team.

Management must encourage employees to become partners and to view the operations and processes of the facility as a joint venture that requires them to share information and, when necessary, even share job duties. Each employee will have one special set of skills or body of knowledge, but each must be willing to help other health care professionals to achieve the desired outcomes.

While managers focus on integrating specialty services into the patient care process, they will also have to deal with a contradictory change. Owing to the inevitable curtailment of access to hospitals

Table 31-3 The Most Frequently Mentioned Skill Combinations for Multiskilled Health Practitioners

Combination	Percentage of Total Skill Combinations
Respiratory Therapist or Technician and ECG and/or EEG	9.0
Radiologic Technologist and Ultrasound	6.4
Laboratory Technologist/Technician and Radiography	3.4
Radiologic Technologist and Special Procedures (e.g., CT, MRI, and other imaging)	2.9
Radiologic Technologist and Mammography	2.6
Multiple Business Office Functions (e.g., Payroll, Purchasing)	2.4
Laboratory Technologist/Technician and ECG	2.1
Registered Nurse and Respiratory Therapy	2.1
Registered Nurse and Quality Assurance/Utilization Reviewer	2.1
Registered Nurse and Discharge Planning	1.7
Manager Multiple Support Departments (e.g., Housekeeping, Laundry, Maintenance)	1.7
Radiologic Technologist and Laboratory	1.5
Other[a]	62.1
Total	**100.0**

Note: Combinations based on 137 hospitals with cross-trained workers.
[a]Each of the other mentioned skill combinations comprised less than 1 percent of the total.
Source: Reprinted from L. Perry, Staff Cross-Training Caught in Cross-Fire, *Modern Healthcare,* May 6, 1991, with permission of Crain Communications, Inc., © 1991.

caused by changes in the reimbursement structure, hospital inpatient units will downsize to become high-severity, small-volume intensive care units. Traditional specialty services will primarily be provided in free-standing facilities connected to but not within hospitals. In 1990 total outpatient visits increased by 6.0 percent, compared with 4.3 percent in 1989. Diagnostic imaging was up 8.1 percent in 1990, the greatest increase of any hospital service. "The overall movement of free-standing facilities will likely favor multi-dimensional services over those which emphasize a single specialty orientation."[6]

Trust, Communication, and Participation

Guiding specialty services in the future will require a strong commitment to participation and consensus by managers. The knowledge worker responsible for using highly complex technology will continue to be an anomaly, and standard management principles will only partially apply. At the same time, physicians will remain autonomous collaborators in the health delivery process. In order to manage these individuals and their interaction, the specialty department manager must try to create agreement on institutional goals. Individuals become teams if common goals are established.

Managers in the future, due to the amount of data available and the speed at which events change, will not be able to control or direct significant parts of the work process. The members of patient care teams will become more self-directed, and the managers' role will be to provide the teams with data on the progress toward the achievement of goals and to evaluate the resource needs of the teams.

Managers, employees, and physicians will have to develop trust based on the acceptance of a common purpose. Participation and effective communication will be twin foundations of this trust.

ADDITIONAL RESOURCES

Periodicals

Administrative Radiology, Glendale Publishing Corporation, 1305 Glenoaks Boulevard, Glendale, CA 91201.

Decisions in Imaging Economics, GE Medical Systems (in conjunction with Curant Communications), 1849 Sawtelle Boulevard, Suite 770, Los Angeles, CA 90025.

Harvard Business Review, Graduate School of Business Administration, Harvard University, Boston, MA.

Healthcare Forum Journal, Healthcare Forum, 830 Market Street, San Francisco, CA 94102.

Hospital and Health Services Administration, Health Administration Press, 1021 E. Huron Street, Ann Arbor, MI 48104-9990.

Laboratory Medicine, American Society of Clinical Pathologists, 2100 W. Harrison Street, Chicago, IL 60612.

Books

Griffith, J.R. *The well-managed community hospital.* Ann Arbor, Mich.: Health Administration Press, 1987.

Rowland, H. S. *Hospital management: A guide to departments.* Gaithersburg, Md.: Aspen Publishers, 1984.

Sanderson, E. *Effective hospital material management.* Gaithersburg, Md.: Aspen Publishers, 1985.

Wolper, L.F. *Health care administration: Principles and practice.* Gaithersburg, Md.: Aspen Publishers, 1987.

NOTES

1. P. Hilsenrath et al., Assessing Hospital Productivity, *Administrative Radiology,* August 1991, p. 61.
2. P. Drucker, The New Productivity Challenge, *Harvard Business Review,* November-December 1991, p. 71.
3. M. Burke, Technology Acquisition: Trends in Imaging, *Hospitals,* November 5, 1991, p. 26.
4. D.M. Mancino, Safe Harbors: Developments Affecting Physician-Imaging Center Relationships, *Decisions in Imaging Economics,* 4, no. 4 (1991):21.
5. L. Perry, Staff Cross-Training Caught in Cross-Fire, *Modern Healthcare,* May 6, 1991, p. 26.
6. T. Matson, Deployment of Outpatient Technologies, *Administrative Radiology,* September 1991, p. 30.

Saul Feldman
Eric N. Goplerud

Mental Health Services

32

Purpose: Mental health services help people with psychiatric and/or substance abuse disorders to attain the highest possible level of functioning and independent living. The services should be provided in the most supportive, least restrictive environment consistent with the nature and intensity of the disorder. Mental health services include outpatient counseling for problems in everyday living, intervention for those in crisis where there may be a danger to self or others, and long-term care for persistent or chronic disorders that require continuing psychological, vocational, and residential support.

INTRODUCTION

Prevalence of Mental Disorders

Disorders such as schizophrenia, affective disorders (e.g., depression), and alcohol and drug dependence are described in a widely used psychiatric diagnostic manual, the *Diagnostic and Statistical*

A portion of this chapter has been adapted from Saul Feldman, *The Administration of Mental Health Services,* 1980, courtesy of Charles C Thomas, Publisher, Springfield, Illinois.

Manual of Mental Disorders, third edition (DSM III-R). The manual, which is in the process of revision, defines a mental disorder as "a clinically significant behavioral or psychological syndrome . . . that is associated with present distress (a painful symptom) or disability (impairment in one or more important areas of functioning) or with a significantly increased risk of suffering death, pain, disability, or an important loss of freedom."[1] In this chapter, *mental disorder* should be taken to include substance abuse unless specified otherwise.

A significant number of people in the United States suffer from a mental disorder at any given time. Current estimates, based on large samples of carefully interviewed adults, indicate that 19 percent of adults have some type of mental disorder during any six-month period. This is roughly equivalent to the combined adult population of California, New York, and Texas. Severe anxiety or panic disorders, for example, affect 8.3 percent, 6.0 percent suffer from affective disorders, and 6.4 percent are addicted to alcohol or drugs. Additionally, 1 percent suffer from schizophrenia, 1 percent have severe cognitive impairment, and .9 percent have diagnosable antisocial personality problems.

Comorbidity, the presence of both mental and substance abuse disorders, is common. A study of mental disorders in patients seeking assistance for alcohol and other drug problems, for example, found that 78 percent had a history of psychiatric disorders in addition to substance abuse and 65 percent had a current mental disorder.[2]

Children and adolescents are also susceptible. It is estimated that nearly 12 percent of children under age 18 are clinically maladjusted. About 1 in 20 (three million children and adolescents) has a serious emotional disturbance. At any point in time, as many as 600,000 children and adolescents have emotional problems of such severity as to require hospital treatment, and another 400,000 need treatment for alcohol or other drug problems.[3]

Treatment Settings

It is more difficult to describe the places in which mental health services are provided than it may first appear. People with mental disorders are not always seen in mental health facilities. Nor does everyone entering such a facility have a primary mental disorder. Studies show that at least one person in ten seeking psychiatric treatment suffers from an undiagnosed physical illness that is the sole cause of the psychological symptoms. Another one in three has a major physical illness (also generally not recognized) with symptoms requiring medical treatment.

Further, people with mental disorders are more likely to receive treatment within the general health care sector than the mental health sector. In a typical year, less than 25 percent of those treated for a mental disorder are seen in a mental health program.[4] The other 75 percent are seen either in general health or social service settings. Kiesler and Sibulkin found that twice as many general hospital patients with DSM III-R diagnoses are treated outside of rather than in the psychiatric units.[5] Even more impressive is the amount of care provided to persons with mental disorders in nursing homes and other intermediate care facilities. The National Nursing Home Survey found that, in 1985, 65 per-

cent of all nursing home residents—nearly 975,000 people—had at least one condition that could be classified as a major mental disorder.[6] Nearly half (47 percent) of nursing home residents had an organic brain syndrome, 24 percent were schizophrenic or depressed, 4 percent had alcohol or drug abuse disorders, and 11 percent had anxiety disorders. Since the mid-1970s, the nursing home has replaced the state (or county) psychiatric hospital as the main provider of institutional care for people with mental disorders.[7]

Further blurring the boundaries of the mental health sector is the large number of people with mental disorders who are seen in other than medical or mental health settings. Correctional facilities are an example. A study of the Michigan prison system found that 3 percent of the prisoners were schizophrenic and 9 percent had a major affective disorder. Nearly 47 percent were diagnosed with either alcohol abuse or alcohol dependence and 50 percent as antisocial personalities.[8] The National Coalition for Jail Reform estimates that 700,000 mentally ill persons are incarcerated annually in local and county jails.[9] A very small proportion of these receive professional help for their problems. The Institute of Medicine, for example, estimated that only about 40,000 (about 6 percent) prisoners at any time are being treated for their alcohol or drug problems.[10]

Finally, there are many people with mental disorders who receive no treatment, anywhere. About half of the more than 29 million Americans who suffer from some type of mental disorder during any six-month period do not seek any treatment. The likelihood of pursuing such treatment is less for minorities, the aged, and the poor.

Regier and his colleagues describe a de facto mental health services system that encompasses general health services, specialty mental health services, and other human services. The general health sector includes facilities and practitioners that offer treatment for persons with mental disorders within their regular health care programs or practices (i.e., primary care practitioners, general hospitals, nursing homes, and other related intermediate care facilities). The mental health sector includes those practitioners and facilities that offer treatment for mental disorders as the primary focus of their regular programs or practices. The non-mental-health human services sector includes social services, correctional facilities, and educational programs in which efforts are made to work with clients with mental problems.

Implications for the Health Administrator

This distribution of people with mental disorders, far beyond the boundaries of the organizations typically associated with the mental health field, is an important element in the administration of general health care. Many people in the general health care system have mental disorders, and this fact has substantial clinical, financial, administrative, and legal implications. Patients with mental disorders (often unrecognized and undiagnosed) in the general health care system increase the likelihood that they will be inappropriately treated. Missed diagnoses, ineffective treatment, and "difficult" patients can lengthen stays, increase a hospital's legal liability, and complicate the lives of staff. There are reimbursement implications as well when patients with significant mental disorders are not diagnosed correctly. The diagnosis-related group (DRG) system rewards hospitals that treat people with psychiatric disorders in separate units. DRGs exempt such units from capped reimbursement. Patients with psychiatric diagnoses treated elsewhere in the hospital are not so exempt. Reimbursement rates are higher and average lengths of stay are longer for patients with psychiatric diagnoses hospitalized in specialty mental health rather than in general medical-surgical units.

Whether or not a general health care facility includes a discrete mental health service, it is likely that, as a matter of fact, it is in the mental health business and is serving patients with significant mental disorders. While this can complicate the life of the health administrator, it can also be an opportunity. There is now a substantial body of research

demonstrating that behavioral interventions significantly affect the clinical care of patients with primary medical disorders. Counseling, presurgery coaching and information, and psychological support after surgery or after a heart attack, for example, can help patients cope with medical crises better. Psychological interventions have been shown, for example, to significantly reduce length of hospitalization post-surgery or post–heart attack.[11]

Mental Health Services

Changes over the last 30 years have had a major effect on the way mental health services are provided. The introduction of psychotropic drugs has helped control many of the most disruptive symptoms of mental disorders, making it possible for most patients to function outside of the hospital. Dissatisfaction with the state mental hospitals fueled public support for a restructuring of mental health services, and treatment in one's own community became a national goal. Over 700 community mental health centers were started with federal funding to provide comprehensive outpatient and inpatient treatment for geographic catchment areas. As a result of public interest litigation, the courts extended to those in mental hospitals the "right to treatment," requiring states to provide hospitalized patients with treatment for their mental disorders or release them, and the right to refuse treatment. The courts also mandated that treatment occur in the least restrictive environment consistent with effectiveness and community protection. Medicare and social security programs allowed states to reduce their treatment costs by shifting either a part or all of them to the federal government. Finally, there was a dramatic expansion in the availability of employer-sponsored mental health insurance. By 1990, 96 percent of employer health benefit plans covered at least inpatient mental health treatment.

In the 1980s, there was a rapid expansion of inpatient services, corresponding to the increased availability of third-party payments and of psychiatric beds. Dowart has chronicled the explosive growth of free-standing for-profit psychiatric hospitals through the early and mid-1980s and the conversion of general hospital beds into psychiatric and substance abuse units.[12]

While these changes increased the availability of mental health services, they also increased the costs, putting an end to the era of expansion. In the past several years, benefits have been reduced both for inpatient and outpatient care. These reductions have largely been in response to rapidly growing expenditures, which have increased at a rate far greater than in general medical care. The increase in costs, attended by no perceived increase in value, has fueled the interest in controlling costs through such approaches as managed care. Managed mental health programs are now growing rapidly. Initially focused primarily on the private sector, they are now being expanded to the public sector as well, particularly Medicaid.

Expenditures

Mental health care spending has risen by more than 15 percent per year since 1985 and now constitutes as much as 25 percent of all health care expenditures.[13] There are a number of reasons for the rapid increase in costs. Mental health and substance abuse treatment in hospitals was exempted from the DRG system in 1983. Expenses continue to be reimbursed under inflationary cost-based formulas. Coverage for mental health and substance abuse services are mandated by most states, increasing subsidized access to treatment. Currently 29 states require group health plans to cover mental health, 41 states mandate coverage for alcohol abuse, and 27 states mandate coverage for drug abuse.

Another factor increasing inflationary pressure is the broadening popular acceptance of treatment for mental disorders and the lessening of the shame ordinarily associated with it.[14] Inappropriate benefit designs also result in unnecessary and costly treatments. Many benefit designs are tilted toward utilization of inpatient care and have strong disincentives for outpatient care through high copayments and limitations on the number of treatments or epi-

sodes. Such benefit designs contributed to a sharp increase during the 1980s in the number of psychiatric hospital beds owned by for-profit chains.

To control costs, employers are limiting mental health benefits, increasing copayments and deductibles, providing incentives to use alternatives to inpatient treatment, contracting with managed mental health firms to control utilization, and implementing employee assistance programs.

INPATIENT MENTAL HEALTH SERVICES

Inpatient care (24-hour care provided in a hospital) is the most intensive form of treatment. Inpatient care can be roughly divided into long-term care (over 30 days) and shorter term care. Extended inpatient treatment for mental disorders is primarily provided in state and county psychiatric hospitals. A limited amount of long-term inpatient care also takes place in Veterans Administration psychiatric units. The number of state and county hospitals went from 310 in 1970 to 286 in 1988. From a high of nearly 600,000 beds in 1955, there was a drop to about 400,000 in 1970 and to 107,163 in 1988.

Long-term care facilities account for 45 percent of all inpatient psychiatric beds but treat only 20 percent of all inpatient psychiatric episodes due to their relatively long average length of stay. The average facility has 375 beds. The state and county mental hospitals employ 180,226 full-time equivalent (FTE) staff, about 65 percent of whom are involved in direct clinical care. In 1988, state and county long-term hospitals accounted for $6.99 billion in expenditures, over 30 percent of all spending on mental health treatment in that year.

These hospitals were primarily set up in rural areas where, it was thought, the "insane" could recover through work, contemplation, and rational discussion. Shortly after the hospitals were founded, problems developed. Fewer people recovered than were expected. Among the immigrants who came to America in the early 1900s were many who were or became mentally ill due to poverty and deprivation. Severe economic cycles throughout the late nineteenth and early twentieth centuries undermined the ability and willingness of states to provide consistent support for the hospitals. The hospitals grew very large, few patients were discharged, and the quality of care deteriorated badly.

Despite the decline in their numbers, however, state mental hospitals continue to be an important part of the mental health services system, particularly for the care of the indigent and aged. The hospitals continue to have the primary financial and legal responsibility for those who cannot afford private care. State funds account for three-fourths of all revenues received by these hospitals. As large institutions, many of which are located in rural areas, the hospitals often are the largest employers in town and play an important role in the local economy. It is not surprising that efforts to close many of them, while ultimately successful, caused major conflict and political turmoil.

State hospitals in their early days were generally headed by physicians. In the past decade, this has changed dramatically. By and large, physicians have been replaced by nonmedical mental health professionals and by trained administrators.[15] Clinical care is generally provided by a team of professionals, headed by a psychiatrist. Team members include psychologists, social workers, nurses, and aides. Disorders are generally considered illnesses or syndromes, the causes of which are considered to be primarily biochemical or neurophysiological. The primary treatment of choice is medication.

Free-standing private psychiatric hospitals increased from 150 in 1970 to 444 in 1988, nearly tripling the number of inpatient beds during that time (from 14,295 to 42,255). These private facilities average 95 beds. Two-thirds of all private psychiatric hospitals are operated by multihospital chains. The explosive growth of the 1980s appears to have stabilized. Annual revenue of private psychiatric hospitals was $4.6 billion in 1988, two-thirds of which came from patient fees.

Private psychiatric hospitals have fewer beds and higher staff-to-patient ratios. Funding for the treatment they provide comes primarily from third-party payers and patient fees. The availability of health insurance coverage for inpatient treatment produced a rapid expansion of beds in general hospitals and private psychiatric hospitals, particularly those owned by the national chains. Nongovernment psychiatric inpatient beds in private facilities increased from 7 percent of the total in 1970 to 35 percent in 1987. Between 1970 and 1986, the proportion of nonfederal psychiatric inpatient beds under corporate for-profit auspices grew from about 1 percent to 15 percent. Privatization has become a "megatrend" in mental health economics. The number of beds operated by psychiatric hospital systems increased by 5.4 percent in 1988 (to 34,546), by 12 percent in 1987, by 21.9 percent in 1986, and by 41.2 percent in 1985.

In 1988, there was a total of 1,484 nonfederal general hospitals with 48,421 beds in separate psychiatric services, more than double the number of psychiatric beds in 1970. In the average general hospital with a short-stay psychiatric unit, there are 33 beds in the unit. Psychiatric units generated revenues of $3.6 billion in 1988, 41 percent of which came from patient fees and 41 percent from federal sources. Cost remains the major reimbursement basis for inpatient psychiatric services, while the rest of hospital care is shifting to prospective payment. Inpatient psychiatric services are less regulated than are other forms of inpatient care; they are also less capital intensive (fewer expensive machines, operating rooms, and the like). As a result, psychiatric services have been profitable, yielding returns on investment of about 30 percent annually. A significant portion of the 1,484 psychiatric units in general hospitals nationwide are owned, leased, or managed by multifacility systems.

Distinct chemical dependency units were reported in 1,351 general hospitals and specialty psychiatric hospitals. These units treated approximately 90,000 patients in 1989.[16] The primary sources of payment for treatment in chemical dependency units were private health insurance (44 percent), self-payment (7 percent), Medicaid and Medicare (16 percent), and other public support (17 percent).

Short-term inpatient treatment is provided in specially designated psychiatric and substance abuse units in general hospitals and free-standing facilities. Some treatment units use an admitting physician model, in which an MD is assigned to each patient and orders all treatment for that patient. Most of the units, however, use a staff model, in which patients are admitted into a structured interdisciplinary treatment program.

ALTERNATIVES TO INPATIENT TREATMENT

Next in intensity are alternatives to inpatient care. Although there are a number of alternative settings, three types predominate: residential nonhospital care in conjunction with intensive day treatment and partial hospitalization and outpatient services provided on either an individual or group basis. Least intensive are self-help programs that can be undertaken individually or as a member of a group.

People with mental disorders or substance abuse problems often have functional deficits that require supportive and rehabilitative services as well. Supportive services can include supervised or unsupervised residential supports such as halfway houses, group homes, and cooperative apartments. They can also include educational and vocational supports, such as sheltered workshops and job preparation groups, socialization and recreation programs, and self-care training and assistance.

Partial Hospitalization

Partial hospitalization programs are a rapidly expanding alternative to inpatient care. These programs offer time-limited, ambulatory treatment in controlled environments, often in hospitals or extended day treatment settings. Patients receive the treatment they need but can interact with family and community. Partial hospitalization programs may operate days, evenings, nights, or weekends. Typically they provide at least 20 hours of scheduled programming extended over at least five days per week.

In 1988, there were 2,161 organizations providing partial hospitalization services, accounting for 518,442 episodes of care. The American Association of Partial Hospitalization estimates that the number of partial hospitalization programs has been growing at a rate of 10 percent per year.[17] Presently there are no accreditation standards. Staffing is typically based on a multidisciplinary clinical team model, with psychiatric services available. The staff-to-patient ratio depends on function; it ranges from 1:4 in crisis stabilization programs to between 1:6 and 1:8 in intermediate term programs. With the growth of managed mental health and its emphasis on cost-effective alternatives to inpatient care, such programs as day care, partial hospitalization programs, and structured outpatient care are likely to become increasingly important.

Community Support Programs

Community support generally includes a loose grouping of programs that operate three or more hours per day, providing structured ambulatory care for patients with severe and persistent mental disorders. These programs are built on a set of guiding principles enunciated by the National Institute of Mental Health (NIMH). In essence, a community support program is "an organized network of caring and responsible people committed to assisting a vulnerable population meeting their needs and developing their potentials without being unnecessarily isolated or excluded from the community."[18] The overall goal of the model is to improve the quality of life of persons with long-term, severe psychiatric disabilities by assisting them to assume responsibility for their own lives and to function as actively and independently in society as possible. The programs provide a package of services—social, recreational, vocational, residential, and educational. All services are directed at helping people to develop skills and at providing the environmental supports they need to function within the community. They tend to be staffed by social workers, nurses, rehabilitation counselors, and a variety of paraprofessionals who have specific vocational and training skills. A 1986 study done by the NIMH found that 133,194 people were under care in such programs; 47 percent had a primary diagnosis of schizophrenia and 17 percent had affective disorders. The average length of stay was 115 days.

Substance Abuse

The treatment approach used by the vast majority of hospital substance abuse programs is generally referred to as either the Minnesota Model or the chemical dependency approach.[19] The approach, developed in Minnesota during the 1950s, blends diagnostic and therapeutic activities used in psychiatric inpatient programs with the self-help program of Alcoholics Anonymous (AA).

Substance abuse services developed much later than mental health services. Because of their reliance on self-help and their use of recovering addicts as counselors, they require a smaller funding commitment. In 1989, states spent one billion dollars for all forms of substance abuse treatment, about one-seventh the amount they spent for treatment of mental disorders.

The roots of substance abuse treatment are in the self-help program used by AA. Founded in 1935, AA has profoundly affected the system of alcohol and drug treatment in the United States. Presently there are over 800,000 members nationwide. AA insists on complete abstinence from alcohol, reinforced by mutual help and support. The lifelong process of "recovery" from alcohol addiction, according to AA, requires ongoing participation in group meetings that can be found most nights in almost every city and town in the country. The basis of AA is "working the twelve steps." The 12 steps are guides to a process of personal change. At meetings, members share the history of their alcohol-related problem and their experiences in maintaining sobriety. They view their problems with alcohol as "alcoholism," an illness that prevents those afflicted with it from controlling their drinking. The use of AA principles and techniques has become an integral part of the majority of treatment programs for alcohol abuse in this country.[20] This is true despite the paucity of clinical research on the effectiveness of AA as a treatment or an adjunct to treatment.[21]

Residential Substance Abuse Treatment: Therapeutic Communities

Therapeutic communities are long-term (6- to 24-month) residential treatment programs for addictions that are designed to get patients to face the fact that they are addicted and then to foster personality and behavioral changes so that they can live without drugs and alcohol. Costs range from $1,200 to $2,500 per month. Of the 1,914 residential programs, about half (960) are run by private for-profit firms, and a third (801) are run by nonprofit organizations. Nearly 80 percent of their revenue comes from private health insurance or patient self-pay. The public sector accounts for only about 8 percent of all residential programs.

Substitution of Services

A controversial issue in mental health and substance abuse treatment is the degree to which less expensive and intensive treatments can be substituted for hospital and residential services. Rapidly rising costs have increased the pressure on payers to find acceptable lower cost alternatives to inpatient treatment.

Studies such as those by McClellan and colleagues[22] as well as others reviewed by the Institute of Medicine[23] and Marlatt[24] show that treatment outcomes improve when patients are matched to the treatment regimen best suited to their particular psychological, behavioral, and cognitive needs. A number of studies have found equivalent and even superior outcomes for alternatives to inpatient care. Longabaugh and colleagues, for example, found that addicted patients who were treated in a partial hospitalization program functioned as well as or better than randomly assigned inpatient controls.[25]

Similarly, Harrison and Hoffman found that there were no differences in outcome for patients assigned to a four-week intensive outpatient alcohol counseling program compared with those receiving four weeks of inpatient treatment.[26] Kiesler concluded from his extensive review of studies comparing alternatives such as day hospitalization and inpatient care for mental illness that "alternative care always is as good [as] or better than hospitalization regarding outcomes, and almost always is less expensive."[27]

The sharp increase in the cost of mental health and substance abuse services during the past few years, minus any apparent increase in value, has led to the rapid growth of managed mental health organizations emphasizing the use of alternatives to inpatient care wherever possible. In many instances, they can apply mental health benefits flexibly (i.e., using inpatient dollars to pay for structured outpatient care where appropriate).

PERSONNEL

There are four primary disciplines staffing mental health services: psychiatry, psychology, psychiatric social work, and psychiatric nursing. Other associated professionals that are frequently employed include vocational and rehabilitation counselors, occupational therapists, marriage and family counselors, and addiction counselors.

Psychiatrists are physicians with specialized training in the diagnosis and treatment of persons with mental disorders. Psychiatric training builds on basic medical education and includes a postgraduate psychiatric residency of four years. Psychiatrists work in hospital and private practice settings, where they provide direct services, including diagnosis, treatment planning, medications management, and psychotherapy. A survey of practicing psychiatrists conducted by the American Psychiatric Association found that 45 percent of psychiatrists reported private practice as their primary work setting.[28] Of the remaining psychiatrists who are based in various organized settings (e.g.,

hospitals, community mental health agencies, health maintenance organizations, and medical schools), about one-third (35 percent) reported part-time private practice as a secondary work setting.

Between 1970 and 1990, the number of actively practicing psychiatrists in the United States increased by nearly 50 percent, from 21,146 in 1970 to 39,506 in 1990. Psychiatrists (and other mental health professionals) are spread unevenly across the country, with major concentrations in urban areas on the two coasts.

Clinical psychologists generally receive a doctorate requiring four years of graduate training in psychological theory and clinical practice and one year of supervised clinical internship. Clinical psychology emerged as one of the core mental health treatment disciplines in the aftermath of World War II. Psychologists do diagnostic assessments, devise treatment plans, and engage in psychotherapy. There were 57,000 doctoral level psychologists in 1989, the large majority involved in clinical practice. The geographic distribution of psychologists mirrors that of psychiatry (i.e., they are concentrated in urban areas). About two out of five psychologists are primarily in private practice working with outpatients.

Psychiatric social workers work in mental health organizations and in private practice. Social work training generally involves a three-year postgraduate degree focusing on counseling, family and systems intervention, case work, and program administration. A six-month supervised practicum is also required for licensure. The field first emerged in the 1920s from the settlement houses and the child guidance centers. Social work continues to be primarily associated with outpatient care. A survey in 1989 identified 81,737 social workers in clinical settings. About one in eight psychiatric social workers is in private practice.

Psychiatric nurses generally work in hospitals with chronic and severely disturbed patients. The majority of nurses working in mental health settings are generalists—they have either an associate degree (two years), a diploma (three years), or a bachelor of science in nursing degree (four years).

There were 10,567 nurses with specialized psychiatric master's degrees working in clinical psychiatric settings in 1988.

Addiction counselors are the most numerous professional group treating patients in specialized substance abuse treatment settings. These settings are far more likely than mental health facilities to employ lay people, such as addiction counselors, whose major qualification is personal experience with the drug. Although most states credential addiction counselors, there is no national competency-based credentialing system. Recovering alcoholics and addicts provide the human resources for most of the addiction treatment programs that have evolved in the United States. There are approximately 20,000 addiction counselors.

CHARACTERISTICS OF MENTAL HEALTH ADMINISTRATION

The characteristics of the particular field or setting in which administrators work have a profound and too frequently unrecognized effect on what they do (or should do) and how they do it. In this sense, generic administration and the setting in which it is applied are inseparable and interdependent. Mental health administration is essentially the adaptation of generic administrative concepts to the environment of the mental health field and the organizations within it.

The kinds of people who work in and are served by these organizations, the nature of the services provided, and the knowledge base of the mental health field have (or should have) a profound effect on the work of the administrator. The inability to recognize this and the assumption too frequently made that all administration is basically the same are not infrequent causes of failure. This does not mean that all mental health administrators, to be successful, must be clinically trained. Rather, it means that effectiveness in mental health administration is, in good measure, dependent on an understanding of the characteristics of the mental health field, particularly those that differentiate it in kind or magnitude from other fields, even those that are closely related.

Mental health practitioners, for example, have different treatment styles and technologies than those common to other health services. There is considerable overlap in training and competence. Unlike in most health care, the physician (psychiatrist) is not automatically the leader of the treatment team or the unquestioned authority when it comes to making treatment decisions.

The typical staff in a mental health organization is multidisciplinary, professional, and highly autonomous—a bit like a navy with more admirals than ships. Disciplinary rivalries and conflicts over status and salary add to the mental health administrator's task. Further, staff members of a mental health organization tend to view its policies as subordinate to their own professional standards. In the event of a real or imagined conflict between the two, their allegiance would likely be with the standards. This attitude is, of course, not uncommon among physicians in general.

Mental health professionals work in treatment settings that operate under unique legal restrictions. Other health professionals might find it difficult to imagine, for example, what it would be like to work in a system where 40 percent of the patients are mandated to undergo treatment against their will. Yet the courts commonly require people convicted of driving while intoxicated to receive (and pay for) substance abuse treatment. People who are judged a danger to themselves or others can be involuntarily hospitalized for observation and diagnosis. Because intention, a psychological state of mind, is a fundamental factor in determining guilt or innocence in criminal proceedings, mental health facilities have a unique forensic evaluation and treatment function. Courts can request psychiatric evaluations to determine capacity to stand trial. They can also remand to treatment patients who are found not guilty of a crime by reason of insanity.

Legal decisions emanating from class action lawsuits have enunciated a right to treatment for those who are detained in psychiatric hospitals, a right to refuse treatment, and a requirement that care take place in the least restrictive setting consistent with proper treatment and community protection.

The interaction between the practitioner and patient is highly private and intimate in mental health—more so than in most other helping professions. It is, therefore, difficult for the organization to collaborate with or intrude in the process, even when warranted. It is not unusual for the patient and therapist to enter into an alliance, not always conscious, in which the organization is viewed as the enemy, particularly regarding such unpleasantries as fee charging and decisions to terminate treatment.

Mental health organizations frequently deal with a different and more difficult patient population than do other health services. Some 30 years ago, the Joint Commission on Mental Illness and Health strongly disagreed with what had become the conventional wisdom—that people with severe emotional problems or mental illness are really no different from those who are physically ill. The commission pointed out that the compassion and understanding with which society views victims of physical illness are frequently replaced by anger, annoyance, and fear of the mentally disabled.

Mental health professionals, well trained as they may be, are not immune from such feelings of anger, alienation, and fear. One of the participants in a seminar on mental health policy and administration described a situation in which he, as the director of a state mental health department, had been strongly and publicly critical of what he considered the overuse of tranquilizers in the state mental hospitals. Under his leadership, a new state policy to reduce the use of such medication was implemented. Some time later and for other reasons, the state hospital employees went on strike, and he as well as other administrators from the central office went into the hospitals to help staff them. Shortly thereafter the new policy was revoked.

In another seminar with directors of community mental health centers, all but 1 or 2 of the 30 participants reported that at some time in the past threats had been made against them by patients. They acknowledged that fear and anger, not always conscious, were ongoing if unwelcome components of their jobs. Much less clear than the presence of such feelings but certainly no less important is their effect on administrative behavior.

In mental health, the process and the product are intangible, and success is difficult to determine and measure. It is, therefore, very difficult for the mental health administrator to evaluate the effectiveness of the organization, or even of individual staff members for that matter. These difficulties also exist for outside groups and organizations attempting to evaluate the utility of mental health programs.

The boundaries of mental health services are very difficult to define, and it is no simple task to arrive at a generally agreed operational definition of mental health. While the ambiguity regarding boundaries and objectives has some obvious advantages, particularly for the administrator who wishes to avoid accountability, it permits the mental health organization to be seen as the vehicle for meeting a wide variety of frequently divergent needs and may encourage unreal expectations. The discrepancy between these expectations and the actual services provided has been responsible for many conflicts in community mental health programs, particularly in large urban areas.

The poor public image of mental health services, the enduring stigma associated with their use, and the problems posed by confidentiality add significant complications to administering a mental health organization.

While a great deal of progress has been made in recent years, the diagnosis of mental disorders is generally based on syndrome rather than cause. There remains considerable disagreement both between and within the professional disciplines about diagnoses, causes, and treatments. Although general medicine is not without such disagreements, the variability is considerably less. Not only does this create difficulties for an administrator interested in developing quality assurance mechanisms, it is also a source of conflict between professional staff members, many of whom subscribe to different treatment orientations.

Due to the high proportion of patients who have difficulty functioning without a variety of support services, mental health programs often include a much broader array of services than does medical care. These services range from self-help and outpatient treatment, to community support programs, therapeutic communities and partial hospitalization, to inpatient and 24-hour nursing care. Typically there is little vertical service integration, which makes case management of patients crossing levels of care difficult. Close working relationships are also required with a number of community agencies (e.g., schools, social services, and probation programs).

Financing for mental health is not the same as for other health services. In mental health, there are two major and highly contrasting sources of funds—one public, the other private. State governments, the traditional source of funds for public mental health services, continue to pay for the care of people who have severe and persistent mental disorders and are poor. State governments are also a major source of funds for private nonprofit community mental health centers. Through block grants to the states, the federal government also funds these centers.

This dependence on public funds means that mental health programs are frequently subject to a high degree of government regulation. Mental health administrators must therefore understand the political process and be able to work closely with government at all levels. While the degree of involvement varies between political jurisdictions, both the constraints and opportunities inherent in close ties to government are omnipresent in mental health administration.

Third-party payments for mental health services are much more limited than for general medical care, and they are especially limited for substance abuse services. Coverage for outpatient services has declined substantially during the past five years and is now difficult to find. Although more widely covered, inpatient care is often limited to 30 days per year or less. Most health benefit plans also impose annual and/or lifetime limits on expenditures for mental health services, limits that are far lower than for general medical care. Substance abuse services are often limited to one or two episodes of care within an overall dollar maximum.

The characteristics of the mental health setting, the impact of these characteristics on the administration of mental health organizations, the ways in which they affect the behavior of mental health administrators, and their implications for training represent the core of knowledge on which the theory and practice of mental health administration is built. If these factors are not taken into account, intuition and experience become substitutes for rather than components of knowledge, and training programs will almost certainly qualify for Einstein's definition of education as "that which remains when one has forgotten everything he's learned in school."

ADDITIONAL RESOURCES

Organizations

American College of Mental Health Administration, 225 West Swissvale Avenue, Pittsburgh, PA 15218-1632.

Journals

Administration and Policy in Mental Health, 850 California Street, San Francisco, CA 94108 (published by Human Sciences Press).

Books

Austin, M.J., and W.E. Hershey. *Handbook on mental health administration.* San Francisco: Jossey-Bass, 1982.

Barton, W.E., and G.M. Barton. *Mental health administration: Principles and practice.* New York: Human Sciences Press, 1983.

Brooks, A.D. *Law, psychiatry and the mental health system.* Boston: Little, Brown, 1974.

Feldman, S. *The administration of mental health services.* 2d ed. Springfield, Ill.: Charles C Thomas, 1980.

Feldman, S. *Managed mental health services.* Springfield, Ill.: Charles C Thomas, 1992.

Greenblatt, M., and P. Rodenhauser. *Anatomy of psychiatric administration: The organization in health and disease.* New York: Plenum Press, 1992.

Grob, G.N. *From asylum to community: Mental health policy in modern America.* Princeton, N.J.: Princeton University Press, 1991.

Talbott, J.A., and S.R. Kaplan. *Psychiatric administration: A comprehensive text for the clinician-executive.* New York: Grune & Stratton, 1983.

NOTES

1. American Psychiatric Association, *Diagnostic and Statistical Manual of Mental Disorders,* 3d ed. (Washington, D.C.: American Psychiatric Association, 1987).

2. H.E. Ross et al., The Prevalence of Psychiatric Disorders in Patients with Alcohol and Other Drug Problems, *Archives of General Psychiatry* 45 (1988): 1023–1031.

3. Institute of Medicine, *Broadening the Base of Treatment for Alcohol Problems* (Washington, D.C.: National Academy Press, 1990).

4. D. Regier et al., The De Facto U.S. Mental Health Services System, *Archives of General Psychiatry* 35 (1978): 685–693.

5. C.A. Kiesler and A.E. Sibulkin, Proportion of Inpatient Days for Mental Disorders, 1969–1978, *Hospital and Community Psychiatry* 34 (1982): 606–611.

6. G.W. Strahan, Prevalence of Selected Mental Disorders in Nursing and Related Care Homes, in *Mental Health, United States 1990,* eds. R.W. Manderscheid and M.A. Sonnenschein, DHSS Pub. No. (ADM) 90-1708 (Washington, D.C.: U.S. Government Printing Office, 1990).

7. Comptroller General of the United States, *Returning the Mentally Disabled to the Community: Government Needs To Do More,* DHEW Pub. No. (HRD) 76–152 (Washington, D.C.: U.S. Government Printing Office, 1977).

8. R. Jemelka et al., The Mentally Ill in Prisons: A Review, *Hospital and Community Psychiatry* 40 (1989): 481–491.

9. H.H. Goldman and R.W. Manderscheid, *Mental Health United States 1987,* U.S. Department of Health and Human Services, Public Health Services, National Institute of Mental Health: Division of Biometry and Applied Sciences, 1987.

10. Institute of Medicine, *Broadening the Base of Treatment.*

11. E. Mumford et al., The Effects of Psychological Intervention on Recovery from Surgery and Heart Attacks: An Analysis of the Literature, *American Journal of Public Health* 72 (1982): 141–151.

12. R.A. Dowart and M. Schlesinger, Privatization of Psychiatric Services, *American Journal of Psychiatry* 145 (1989): 543–553.

13. S. George-Perry, Easing the Costs of Mental Health Benefits, *Personnel Administrator* 33 (1988): 62–67.

14. S. Minter, A Healing Hand for the Troubled Employee, *Occupational Hazards* 53 (1990): 55–58.

15. S. Feldman, *The Administration of Mental Health Services,* 2d ed. (Springfield, Ill.: Charles C Thomas, 1980).

16. National Institute on Drug Abuse, *National Drug and Alcoholism Treatment Unit Survey: 1989 Main Findings Report* (Washington, D.C.: U.S. Government Printing Office, 1990).

17. Knight, personal communication, September 1991.

18. B.A. Stroul, *Models of Community Support Services: Approaches to Helping Persons with Long-term Mental Illness* (Boston: Boston University, Center for Psychiatric Rehabilitation, 1986).

19. Institute of Medicine, *Broadening the Base of Treatment.*

20. Ibid.

21. W.R. Miller and R.K. Hester, The Effectiveness of Alcoholism Treatment: What Research Reveals, in *Treating Addictive Behaviors: Process of Change,* eds. W.R. Miller and N. Hester (New York: Plenum Press, 1988).

22. A.T. McClellan et al., Increased Effectiveness of Substance Abuse Treatment: A Prospective Study of Patient-Treatment Matching, *Journal of Nervous and Mental Diseases* 171 (1983): 597–605.

23. Institute of Medicine, *Broadening the Base of Treatment.*

24. G.A. Marlatt, Matching Clients to Treatment: Treatment Models and Stages of Change, in *Assessment of Addictive Behaviors,* eds. D.M. Donovan and G.A. Marlatt (New York: Guilford Press, 1988).

25. Longabaugh et al., Cost Effectiveness of Alcoholism Treatment in Partial versus Inpatient Settings: Six Month Outcomes, *Journal of Studies on Alcoholism* 44 (1983): 1049–1071.

26. P.A. Harrison and N.G. Hoffman, *Chemical Dependency Inpatients and Outpatients: Intake Characteristics and Treatment Outcome,* prepared for the Minnesota State Department of Human Services, Chemical Dependency Program Division (St. Paul: St. Paul-Ramsey Foundation, 1986).

27. C.A. Kiesler, Public and Professional Myths about Mental Hospitalization: An Empirical Reassessment of Policy-related Beliefs, *American Psychologist* 35 (1982): 1327.

28. American Psychiatric Association, A National Study of Psychiatrists' Professional Activities, *American Journal of Psychiatry,* 1987.

Kenneth D. Bopp
Gordon D. Brown
Robert H. Daugherty

Continuum of Care

33

Purpose: Chronic illness management requires both new managerial approaches and improved management techniques in the health care delivery field. Chronic illness is managed primarily by the individuals and their families, supported by a dynamic network composed of a variety of health service organizations.

INTRODUCTION

It is fitting that this chapter comes at the end of the manual, for it addresses how the health care system in the United States will need to be managed in the nineties and beyond if it is to meet the needs of its aging population. This will require an understanding by managers of the nature, scope, and effects of chronic illness. It will further require changes in management concepts, abilities, and techniques that may go beyond what most managers and executives are currently equipped to handle.

The intent of this chapter is (1) to clearly explicate, from a management point of view, the impact that chronic illness has and will continue to have on our health care system and (2) to present a different

managerial framework that we believe more appropriate for health care delivery in both today's and tomorrow's environment. To begin to establish such a framework, we propose several management principles that will be discussed later.

MANAGEMENT PRINCIPLES

- Chronic illness affects all aspects of one's life and requires a continuous and comprehensive biopsychosocial approach that focuses on the person rather than the disease.
- The chronically ill person and/or the family must function as competent service coproducers if the treatment of illness is to be effective.
- The continuum of care to address chronic illness must be broadened beyond traditional diagnosis and treatment types of services. The continuum of care must include (1) information and educational services that transfer know-how to patients and families to make them effective coproducers, (2) brokering services to mediate linkages between patients and

families and the wide array of social and support services they need, and (3) systems that assist patients and families in organizing and managing daily living.

- The broad continuum of care needed by the chronically ill requires network organizational forms of governance to coordinate services across specialties and organizations.

- A critical management function in a network is brokering—linking and managing horizontally across specialties and organizations rather than through hierarchical structures. The brokering function, which includes architect, lead operator, and caretaker roles, serves as the operating mechanism through which administrators at the organization-to-organization level and health care providers at the care coordination level exchange trust, information, and resources.

- Network organization and management requires teamwork by patients, family members, and health and social service specialists, including multidisciplinary problem analysis and problem solving.

- An information system that is updated continuously and allows information to be accessed at any time by members of the network is essential to the functioning of the network organization.

- Case-based financial arrangements must be developed that cover the continuum of care and allow participating network organizations to be paid in accordance with the value of the services they render to the chronically ill.

- Managing diverse professions in a teamlike context requires an understanding of the subcultures of the various professions as well as how they interact to form the culture of the service delivery organizations within which they operate.

- The primary responsibility of the general manager in health care is the creation of an organizational climate in which patient-centered care will be provided by an interdisciplinary health care professional team.

- Patient-centered service requires a management strategy that not only meaningfully involves patients in their health care but places them in the prime decision-making role with regard to their health care.

THE CHANGING CONTEXT OF ILLNESS

Chronic Illness

Medicine, like everything in society, is culturally driven. What we choose to consider as illness, as well as the techniques we use to treat such conditions, is culturally derived. As a practical matter, U.S. health care practitioners have tended to view illness narrowly, in a disease and clinical context.[1] The predominant focus in U.S. medical care has been on science-based diagnosis and treatment of disease. In the so-called medical model, disease is seen as an alien threat that suddenly intrudes on a person's pre-existing condition of health and well-being. As Parsons pointed out some time ago, to deal with the threat, a sick person seeks out a health care provider and enlists the provider and his or her medical knowledge, skill, and technology in defending against and attacking the disease.[2] The goal of medicine has therefore been the restoration of the person to his or her pre-existing state of health. While the medical model has been reasonably efficacious in the treatment and elimination of infectious diseases and other acute illnesses, its application to chronic illness has been less than totally successful.[3]

Parsons has posited a sociological paradigm for articulating illness that incorporates the total human being in the context of society.[4] It is to this context of illness that health care managers must return if they are to create an interorganizational environment that successfully addresses the management of chronic illness.

Chronic illness and chronic disease are distinct from one another. Chronic diseases, such as arthritis, cancer, dementia, diabetes, epilepsy, heart disease, respiratory disease, and kidney disease, may be characterized as disturbances in structure or function of any part, organ, or system of the body. Illness, on the other hand, afflicts all aspects of the person's life. Chronic illness has been defined as "the irreversible presence, accumulation, or latency of disease states or impairments that involve the total human environment for supportive care and self-care, maintenance of function, and prevention of further disability."[5] The medical model focuses on controlling disease processes but, for the most part, ignores the psychosocial aspect of chronic illness.

Chronic illness, unlike acute illness, is progressive, is inherent in the aging process, and is a global threat to the individual (encompassing all aspects of the individual's life). Chronic illness is a threat in that it disrupts a person's life with periods of restricted activity and mobility and unwanted dependence. It often interferes with the ability to work, which threatens the person's basic livelihood and economic security, to say nothing of more ambitious future life plans. Chronic illness and disability often have a negative impact on the ill person's dignity and self-respect and cause stigmatization, fear, and misunderstanding that disrupt relationships with others. Moreover, it may stress intimate and family relations by placing new burdens on both the person needing special care and the family caregivers whose own lives and hopes are drastically changed to accommodate the ill person's needs. Consequently, the chronically ill not only suffer the pain and disabling effects of the disease but often experience a sense of powerlessness, helplessness, and hopelessness; a loss of life's meaning; a sense of betrayal; a feeling of isolation; and unremitting fear.[6]

Implications for Health Care Delivery

Our contemporary health care system, which focuses on the disease rather than the sick person, tends to ignore chronic illness until it reaches a stage where the person suffers severe functional impairment and/or the disease has become life threatening. Then legions of resources are employed to pull the patient through the life-threaten-ing episode—and provide care for the person if he or she has become functionally incompetent. Although these heroic medical interventions may extend the person's life, they fail to deal with the psychosocial ramifications and associated suffering of the chronic illness. And often the medical intervention results in the patient suffering from the treatment as well as his or her disease.[7]

Strauss and Corbin argue that health care professionals and the health care system have not yet developed an adequate way of addressing chronic illness, primarily because they focus on disease rather than take a holistic, biopsychosocial view of the sick person.[8] Strauss and Corbin articulate a different paradigm of chronic illness treatment and management. They suggest that the primary obligation of chronic health care is not to cure the chronic disease, which is impossible. Rather it is to (1) detect the onset of chronic illness early enough to slow the trajectory of the disease toward its debilitating and life-threatening manifestations; (2) assist the person in reorganizing and managing his or her daily living, including work, home life, and other functions of day-to-day existence; and (3) help the person to reconcile the psychosocial and personal identity struggles associated with chronic illness and thereby relieve the suffering caused by the illness. It is their contention that each of these tasks must be attended to and integrated with the others if the health care system is to successfully deal with chronic illness.

The chronic illness management paradigm suggested above has significant implications for the organization and management of the health care system as well as the production and delivery of health services. First, health care professionals and patients must accept the reality that health care professionals do not treat chronic illness. The chronically ill treat themselves, with the help of family and health care providers. Although providers play a role in the treatment process, patients, for the most part, are in charge of managing their illness (often with the help of family members). Patients determine their own food and activities, whether or not to take their medication, whether to visit the doctor, and most of the details of their medical treatment. Furthermore, a chronically ill person's personality, character, intelligence, store of knowledge, previous experience, goals, relationship to his or her own body, relationship to society and others, socioeconomic status, and living circumstances all influence the nature, content, and adequacy of treatment. Consequently, the chronically ill person and/or family members must function as competent coproducers if the treatment of illness is to be effective.

Second, the chronic care service concept must be broadened if the service production and delivery system is to meet the needs of the chronically ill. The service concept determines the benefits offered to the patient (i.e., what the chronically ill person is going to receive, experience, or be helped to accomplish by using the services of the health care system). The existing health care system has primarily offered the chronically ill its capacity to diagnose and treat disease. Pursuant to the medical model, health care providers concentrate their knowledge, expertise, and technology on diagnosing the patient's disease and carrying out or prescribing a therapeutic intervention directed at the disease process. While this kind of treatment, with the patient's cooperation, may be effective in slowing the course of the disease and deflecting life-threatening manifestations, it does not help the patient take charge of the illness. If the health care system is to effectively meet the needs of the chronically ill, three other ingredients need to be added to the service concept: transfer of know-how, brokering linkages and social relations, and systems and techniques for organizing and managing daily living.

In chronic illness, a medical intervention directed at a disease process without the active mediation of the ill person and the family will be ineffective.[9] The ultimate efficacy of chronic illness management rests with the ill person and the family, who must take charge. Since the chronically ill person and the family, not health professionals and biomedical institutions, provide most of the care, the ill person and the family must be empowered with information and know-how that will allow them to perform as effective coproducers. For example, the ill person and the

family need information and know-how that allows them to perform disease management–related work (i.e., regimen work, crisis prevention and management, symptoms management, and diagnostic-related work). In addition to the daily, sometimes hourly, work of managing the disease, the ill person and the family must deal with normal household activities and their employment responsibilities and also maintain the ill person's psychosocial stability.[10] The integration of the ongoing work of managing chronic illness into the context of daily life often is a major challenge for the ill person and the family. To assist them in coping with the instability and disruption that chronic illness has brought to their lives, providers must supply them with management systems and techniques to coordinate the work of managing illness with their other responsibilities.

Historically, the treatment of chronic disease has focused on the acute (and sometimes dying) phase, in which diseases are treated in the hospital, and the severe disability phase, in which the ill are cared for in a nursing home owing to the severity of their illness and/or their lack of support. A holistic, biopsychosocial approach to chronic illness treatment and management will result in a shift away from the tardy treatment of chronic illness in the acute and severely disabled phases toward proactive early detection and management of all phases of the illness. During all but the acute and severely disabled phases, it is the ill and their families who do the major work of managing the illness, with supplemental assistance from health and social service providers. A holistic approach to chronic illness treatment and management will require the integration of psychosocial services with traditional medical services and an increased emphasis on delivering the services to the patient in the home and the residential community instead of the hospital or nursing home.[11]

ORGANIZATION AND MANAGEMENT IMPLICATIONS

The biopsychosocial approach to chronic illness has important health services management implications. To meet the needs of the chronically ill, a continuum of care must be available to them. A continuum of care is a comprehensive array of health, mental health, and social services that span all levels of intensity and are coordinated and integrated into a system of care (see Exhibit 33-1). Although many communities have most of the component parts of a continuum, some services, particularly those needed to supplement and facilitate the work done in the home, may need to be developed.

Most communities have a fragmented collection of functionally specialized service providers. These providers operate within the boundaries of their functional specialties and organizations and lack coordination and integration. A holistic approach to managing chronic illness requires that functional specialties be coordinated horizontally across specialties to meet the needs of ill persons and their families. Moreover, the broad range of health and social services required to meet the needs of the chronically ill makes it infeasible for all the needed

Exhibit 33-1 Continuum of Care Services

Extended	High-technology home therapy
Skilled nursing care	Durable medical equipment
Intermediate care	Home visitors
Swing beds	Home-delivered meals
Nursing home follow-up	Homemaker and personal care
Respite care	
	Outreach
Acute	Screening
Medical/surgical	Information and referral
Psychiatric	Telephone contact
Rehabilitation	Emergency response system
Comprehensive geriatric assessment	Transportation
Geriatric consultation services	
	Wellness
Ambulatory	Educational programs
Physician care	Exercise programs
Outpatient clinics	Recreational and social groups
Geriatric assessment clinics	Senior volunteers
Day hospitals	Congregate meals
Adult day care	Wellness clinics
Mental health clinics	Respite relief
Satellite clinics	Support groups
Psychosocial counseling	
Alcohol and substance abuse services	**Housing**
	Retirement communities
Home Care	Senior housing
Home health—Medicare	Congregate care facilities
Home health—private	Adult family homes
Hospice	Short-term housing/hotels

Source: Reprinted from *Health Progress,* Vol. 70, No. 5, pp. 36–39, with permission of the Catholic Health Association of the United States, © 1989.

services to be offered by a single organization. Therefore, traditional organizational approaches that operate within vertical hierarchies will not provide the needed coordination. In terms of continuum of care and multiorganizational service delivery, no such hierarchical structures exist. Rather, market mechanisms and contractual agreements hold the different functions of the system together. In the words of Snow, Miles, and Coleman, "In industry after industry, multilevel hierarchies have given way to clusters of business units coordinated by market mechanisms rather than layers of middle-management planners and schedulers."[12]

Dynamic Network Organization

What is required is an organizational approach that synthesizes service activities across functional and organizational boundaries. One evolving organizational form that makes possible horizonal coordination and integration across functional specialties and organizations is the dynamic network organization.

Miles and Snow suggest that dynamic network organizations have four characteristics.[13] First, they are vertically disaggregated, with member organizations performing specialized functions. The current health and social services system clearly is vertically disaggregated. Second, there is virtually no formalized hierarchy. Instead, governance is achieved through a set of marketlike contractual relations. Such marketlike governance mechanisms already have been introduced to health care by the managed care movement. However, the application of such governance mechanisms to health care has centered on acute illness, with the exception of a few social HMO demonstration projects. Third, a strategy maker who plays the role of broker identifies, assembles, and links functional specialists and organizations together. The brokering role is not necessarily an independent function. The role may be played by any one of the players who takes the lead in putting all or part of the network together. However, the brokering role is the key role in the

network. Fourth, broad-access information systems substitute for coordination built on trust or hierarchical relationships.

Brokering Role

A central management task of the network organization is to link the components together through brokering. Brokers are key managers who operate across the network's many functions rather than up and down within individual functional areas, as managers in the traditional hierarchical structure do. Lawless and Moore have described the broker as a single strategy maker who "promotes integration by acting as the link needed to bring member agencies together, and get them committed to the overall system."[14]

Three types of brokers are essential to the success of network organizations: architects, lead operators, and caretakers.[15] Architects focus on the health system functions and design. They facilitate the emergence of the network by formulating a business concept that visualizes how the specialized components may be linked together to produce and deliver the continuum of services to be offered by the network.

The role of the lead operators is to link the providers together formally into an operating network. Their main task is to negotiate agreements that link together providers in more or less permanent alliances so that all the components are available to provide the continuum of care services. The management focus of lead operators is on creating alliances that benefit all participants.

Networks require continual monitoring, maintenance, and enhancement if they are to operate smoothly and effectively. Therefore, an essential brokering role is the role of caretaker. Caretakers are concerned with the development of a sense of trust and community among the autonomous members of the network. Trust may be viewed as confidence in the continuation of a mutually satisfying relationship and awareness by the respective network members of what this requires in terms of their performance. Trust is based on reputations and, more importantly, on past performance. It is also built on personal friendships and social bonds established in day-to-day interactions. Community is based on shared values and unifying ideas that transcend individual and organizational interests and boundaries.

In network management, coordination must occur at two levels: the organization-to-organization relationship level and the professional-to-professional care coordination level. The main brokering responsibility at the interorganizational level is to negotiate contracts with functional specialists and/ or organizations to link them together in the network. At the care coordination level, brokering is used to mediate the linkage between the chronically ill and the health and social service resources they need to solve their problems. At each of these levels, there must be some individuals who assume the roles of architect, lead operator, and caretaker.

Network Management: Interorganizational Coordination

The availability of an integrated continuum of care to serve the chronically ill and their families through a network organization is dependent on the establishment of organization-to-organization relationship agreements. These agreements are often formalized in contracts. These contracts are necessarily incomplete, in that it is impossible to specify every possible eventuality and what the obligations of each party would be under future conditions. However, they do provide an infrastructure to guide interorganizational interactions and resource exchanges. As indicated above, the task of building and maintaining these agreements is a brokering function. This task is carried out jointly by the three types of brokers discussed above.

The role of the architect, at the organization-to-organization level, is to develop a business or service vision that transcends the parochial interests of potential network members and provides them with a goal that may only be achieved through joint collaboration.[16] The architect's work is entrepreneurial

in nature and requires (1) marketing research to understand the needs and behavior of the chronically ill and their families, (2) the development of a service concept, (3) the design of the service production and delivery value chain, and (4) the development of a communication and promotion plan. (*Value chain* is a term from microeconomics used to describe the discrete activities constituting the assembly, production, and delivery of the services that are relevant to the ill person's and the family members' needs, perceptions of value, and satisfaction.) Also, the architect must be aware of the network's financial requirements, since his or her responsibilities often include arranging the finances for the integrated system. The overall results of the architect's efforts are: (1) the specification of the bundle of services that are needed to fulfill the needs of the chronically ill and their families, (2) the development of a blueprint of the chain of value-adding activities that will constitute the services, and (3) the identification of the array of resources that are required to produce and deliver services needed by the chronically ill and their families.

The two other brokering roles identified by Snow, Miles, and Coleman are those of lead operator and caretaker. Lead operators are responsible for putting the service concept, envisioned by the architects, into operation by negotiating agreements that will produce benefits for all network participants. Lead operators must have excellent negotiating and contracting skills in order to forge the alliances among the different specialized functions and organizations included in the network.

For the network to operate effectively, members must voluntarily give up some of their autonomy, adjust their own objectives, and commit to the common objectives of the network. Individual entities will sometimes willingly become part of a network and share objectives and rewards if (1) they need resources the network can provide or (2) they are interested in a goal, opportunity, or challenge that may only be achieved through collaboration.[17] Attracting members thus can require the network's management to develop a goal that is mutually ap-

pealing and create a "network culture" that transcends organizational interests and boundaries.

Caretakers concentrate on maintaining and enhancing relationships among the participating entities in the network. Because network development
and maintenance requires ongoing attention and
work, the caretaker role is crucial to both the day-
to-day and long-term effectiveness of the network.
This multifaceted role includes monitoring relationships of participating organizations, disseminating information about the well-being of the network, and nurturing and disciplining the various
members of the network when necessary.

Network Management: Care Coordination

As we have shown, at the macroinstitutional
level, the network management system is designed
to ensure that there is optimal coordination among
health of care resources; at the microlevel, care coordination focuses upon the efficacious movement
of clients through the system. This care coordination is often referred to in the literature as case management, although there are many forms and definitions of case management.[18] Most agree, however,
that the overall goal of case management or care coordination is to make sure that patients receive appropriate, high-quality, cost-effective services
(even as their health care needs change).

Evashwick suggests that there are five steps involved in this coordination mechanism:

1. interdisciplinary assessment
2. care planning
3. service arrangement
4. monitoring
5. follow-up and reassessment

Weil and colleagues posit an eight-step model that
encompasses:

1. client identification and outreach
2. individual assessment and diagnosis
3. service planning and resource identification
4. linking client to services
5. service implementation and coordination
6. monitoring
7. acting client advocate
8. evaluation and service decision making

The Evashwick approach implies that the role of
the case manager is almost strictly facilitative and organizational in nature; the primary task is to ensure
that the client is moving through the system as
planned. This "medical model" approach assumes
there exists a scientific, rational process in which the
patient moves through the designed system with dispatch, convenience (mainly convenience for the providers), and maximum time- and cost-efficiency.

The Weil model, on the other hand, adopts a
more biopsychosocial approach and assumes a
more proactive role for the case manager, who is
expected to help clients through a system that may
or may not always meet their needs or act in their
interests. By emphasizing the outreach and client
identification function (step 1), the proactive linking of clients to services (step 5), and the advocacy
function (step 7), Weil acknowledges that no matter
how well the system may be internally designed,
the case manager's role in the brokering of services
includes making sure that prospective clients know
about available services and that the services are
delivered appropriately and expeditiously to each
client. The biopsychosocial model expands the context of illness and ultimately the involvement of the
patient in the health care process. The patient is not
simply an object on a conveyor belt moving efficiently through the service system but an active participant in the service delivery process from beginning to end.

Recent research into hospital-based case management programs seems to indicate that the assumptions underlying the model proposed by Weil
are closer to reality.[19] In most of the programs studied, for example, there was miscommunication,
unclarity of roles and functions, turf battles, problems with access, and competitive behavior on the

part of the providers and services involved.[20] Physicians, for example, have found it difficult to view other health care practitioners as professionals in their own right and have not always communicated with them in a timely manner. The control of discharge planning is often a tug of war between the social services department and nursing rather than a collaborative effort.

To date, case management programs have not paid enough attention to planning and design. Case management has often operated at the service delivery level without the benefit of organization-to-organization agreements that provide an infrastructure to guide interorganizational interactions and resource exchanges. Moreover, case planning has consisted of ad hoc assembly of more or less congruent service components for each case rather than a carefully planned and designed "critical pathway" that links and coordinates service components in a congruent manner.

Illness, as we have seen earlier, is not simply a physiological disease process but a condition that affects the person's whole life. The health care network is not simply an efficiently designed and well-oiled rational system but a configuration of people providing highly technical and personal service in an atmosphere of anxiety, tension, and uncertainty, where, for all of the high-tech trappings, there often is a lack of consensus among providers regarding the efficacy of alternative diagnostic and therapeutic interventions. In short, things go wrong, people make mistakes, emotions run high, and the system breaks down. In this context, the case management function demands individuals who act as architects, lead operators, and caretakers at the microlevel in much the same way that other individuals assume these brokering roles at the organizational level.[21]

The role of the architect is to design the patient flow, interorganizationally and intraorganizationally, within each agency setting. The goal is to devise critical paths of services that will address the myriad illness states and service needs of the patients seen by the network. This requires more than the usual protocols that are developed within clinical departments. It calls for the development of pathways and linkages across organizations and individual units and departments that facilitate the meshing of the various services and procedures necessary not only for the diagnosis and treatment of disease but for the maintenance of the total well-being of the patient.

The linkage of service across functions and organizations is illustrated in Figure 33-1. In this example, the broker, as architect, pulls together a team of functional specialists from organizations that have been assembled through the organization-to-organization brokering efforts described in the previous section. The architect's role, at the care coordination level, is to convene functional specialists to hammer out clinical pathways for common chronic illnesses. Each critical pathway charts a general care plan and delineates the responsibilities of the health care organizations and professionals and the ill person and his or her family. A critical pathway merely provides a general guide and of course may be adjusted to meet the specific needs of the patient.

The negotiation of the critical pathways is perhaps the most challenging task of the entire brokering process, because it requires mutual adjustment by the parties involved and agreement on how the health care work is done, the relative importance of functions, the rationale for the techniques used, and the sets of problem-solving processes and techniques to be employed. In short, it requires a new way of thinking about health care delivery—one that is client (patient) focused rather than provider or institution focused. Difficulty in reaching agreement on a critical pathway often stems from the lack of consensus among health care professionals regarding what is appropriate and necessary care. Different medical specialties often have dissimilar opinions regarding the nature of a person's illness and may suggest divergent treatment approaches. For example, a person with a diagnosis of cancer consulting different oncology specialists for treatment may be advised that he or she needs alternative therapeutic interventions—surgery, chemotherapy, or radiation therapy—depending upon the training and experience of the specialist. Moreover, nurses may be especially con-

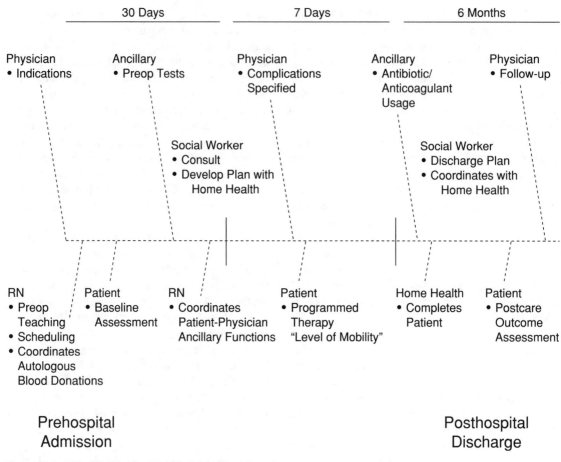

Figure 33-1 Critical Pathway for Total Hip Replacement Procedure

cerned about the care and comfort aspects of the illness. Social workers will focus on the effects of the illness upon the patient's psychosocial functioning and on the patient's ability to cope with the illness. Physical and occupational therapists will address how the patient is able to physically and cognitively overcome the effects of the illness. Each discipline has much to contribute to the diagnosis, treatment, and management of the patient's chronic illness; thus the management and coordination of the interdisciplinary team is critical to the day-to-day delivery of care. This management and coordination depends upon establishing a consensus among health care professionals at the outset regarding the process and components of the critical pathway.

Once the critical pathway is agreed upon, the person acting as lead operator develops and maintains effective relationships and linkages among the various service subsystems and front-line personnel that make up each organization's service constellation. The lead operator's role is (1) to build the systems that allow the patients to flow through the continuum of care and (2) to facilitate the interface and exchange of information and the other resources that the functional specialists need in order to perform their roles effectively.

Those individuals in the caretaker role focus on maintaining the day-to-day effectiveness of the coordination of care. These case managers become the front-line articulators of the relationships between the service providers and between the patients and service providers as the patients move through the health service process.

Kane has argued that case management is often a role that is simply assumed by a health care provider, such as a primary care physician or a hospital discharge planner.[22] Thus, case management is often invoked by the professional who believes that what he or she is doing is appropriate. However, the degree to which the function is actually being effectively performed is another matter. And beyond that is the issue of exactly in whose interests the case manager is acting. Striking a balance between the patient's needs, desires, and understanding and the organization's services and competencies is a crucial case management responsibility.

In addition, there are philosophical issues often unacknowledged by health professionals, including the proper extent of patient autonomy to make quality-of-life decisions that are contrary to professional judgments. There also are questions concerning the benefits and costs of multidiscipline assessment and critical pathway planning and implementation versus specialization and fragmentation of decision making. Those in the caretaker role must strive to reconcile these philosophical differences focusing on strengthening relationships between functional specialists at the service production and delivery level and building trust and commonality of purpose.

NETWORK COORDINATION AND FINANCING

Network organizations cannot operate effectively unless member organizations have the ability to communicate quickly and accurately from any point in the network to any other point in the network. Traditional health services management concepts and practices are significant impediments to developing and sustaining networks. Traditional health services management approaches have rewarded a specialist orientation, fragmented responsibility, emphasized analysis rather than synthesis, and dictated downward and upward information and communication flows within organizations, all of which create significant barriers to networking.

In a network, functional specialists must be team players. To encourage teamwork among functional specialists, network managers must reward specialists, not only for their expert contribution to the network's services but also for participating, communicating, and acting as reliable team players. In a network, fragmented responsibility must be replaced with cross-functional responsibility for helping to solve the client problems. Traditional management relies on single-specialty problem analysis and problem solving; networks, on the other hand, require multifunctional synthesis. Participation in a network involves extensive exchange of information, the identification of different points of view, and the resolution of differences in order to come up with a sound plan of action. Finally, networking calls for lateral coordination rather than the vertical coordination of traditional management. Instead of emphasizing the narrow analysis of problems within functional boundaries, managers must ask employees to coordinate with other functions, work together, and take multifunctional or multidisciplinary approaches to meet the needs of the chronically ill.

Broad-Access Information Systems

Miles and Snow indicate that a broad-access, computerized information system is essential to the effective functioning of network organization-to-organization relationships.[23] They indicate that the participants in the network must agree on a general structure of payment for value added through interorganizational contracts and then link themselves together in a continuously updated information system so that contributions can mutually and instantaneously be verified.

Given the ambiguity of quality in health care and the limited rationality of the negotiators, it is impossible to write a comprehensive contract that specifies every future eventuality and what the future obligations of each party would be under future conditions. Therefore, a contract will succeed only if the parties can trust each other not to be opportunistic. In order to maintain an effective and fair relationship and protect themselves from opportunism, participants in a network can be expected to go to considerable expense to negotiate safeguards and monitor and enforce the performance of their partners in the network. Miles and Snow suggest that the monitoring and control system must be a broad-access information system that is continuously updated and allows the parties to monitor and verify each other's contributions to the network continuously. In other words, the broad-access information system becomes a substitute for hierarchical control or lengthy trust-building processes.

Evashwick indicates that an integrative information system is also essential for the effective functioning of a network at the care coordination level.[24] Information must flow horizontally across departments within the individual organizations as well as between the member organizations for the network to succeed.[25] The information system must be updated continuously and allow information to be accessed at any point in the service delivery system. It is crucial for the information system to contain clinical, financial, and administrative information. Without such a system in place, tracking of patient experience and resources used across service providers cannot occur.[26]

Case-based Financing

It is generally agreed that, like the health care system itself, the financing of health care is fragmented and uncoordinated and is not consistent with the network model. System coordination takes resources that, at present, are unreimbursed by the current third-party payer system,[27] although several states and the National Long-Term Care Channel-

ing Demonstration project have attempted to demonstrate the efficacy of various case management models over the last ten years or so. While focusing upon the case management aspect of the network, the models have sought to demonstrate that improved coordination of services reduces acute care lengths of stay, reduces readmissions for chronic illness, and prevents premature long-term care institutionalization.[28] While there is no doubt that the projects have sought to improve quality and access to care, the driving force behind them was the demonstration of cost containment. And as Kane notes, cost containment and appropriateness of utilization have traditionally been the concern of payers attempting to use case management as a method of limiting the amount of and access to services.

The demonstration projects fall into three categories, which are useful points of departure for a discussion of finance. The National Long-Term Care Channeling project focused upon those medical and personal or social services that would maintain persons in their homes and thus obviate the need for costly long-term care institutionalization. Social health maintenance organizations (S/HMOs) provide a range of both social and mental health services and have as their focus the reduction of acute care service usage. The Robert Wood Johnson hospital initiatives program sought to determine how case management in the hospital setting could facilitate the transition of frail elderly from the acute hospital setting to community-based services after discharge.

Linking case management with direct financial savings, however, has been less than totally successful. In fact, there is some indication that even payers, whose primary concern is cost containment, emphasize increased quality of services while acknowledging that cost reduction is not the only goal in all cases.[29]

The National Long-Term Care Channeling Demonstration project used Medicare and Medicaid waivers, used a capitation system of reimbursement, and was carried out at several sites throughout the country. Its goal was to demonstrate alternatives to nursing home care for the frail elderly. A report from the Miami Channeling Project indicated that its cost per client was a little over $500 per month, as opposed to $1,600 per month average cost per client for nursing home care.[30]

Social health maintenance organizations (S/HMOs) operate on a strict capitation basis. Their experience has shown that, because enrollment is voluntary and the capitation fee is partially paid by the beneficiary, extensive marketing is necessary to make the program financially feasible. Financial feasibility appears to require between 2,000 and 5,000 enrollees, depending on the maturity of the sponsoring HMO (more mature organizations can break even with fewer enrollees). On balance, there is not much indication of the extent of their cost-effectiveness, but some evidence exists that S/HMOs improve access, increase appropriate linkage to services, and decrease acute care utilization.[31]

The results from the Robert Wood Johnson hospital initiatives program indicated that, while case management seemed to provide better coordination and focus, its ability to impact cost and access varied over the 24 demonstration sites. The major problem was access, with almost all projects reporting that enabling clients to avail themselves of community long-term care resources was a universal difficulty. Moreover, it was clear that the cost of case management services had to be absorbed within the existing financial reimbursement structure in those projects that chose to continue after the demonstration period.

Several key financing issues have emerged from such demonstration projects. When the costs of case management and coordination are isolated under a fee-based arrangement, very few clients are willing to pay for, and presumably see little value in, such services.[32] Further, the demonstration projects conducted so far have addressed limited and specific goals—reduction of long-term care institutionalization and acute care cost containment—and there has been little attempt to determine care coordination costs and benefits in the context of a total community health care network. It seems clear, then, that from a financial standpoint,

case management and care coordination costs will need to be financed as indirect costs of the total health care system, much like administrative costs. Cost-benefit analyses will, therefore, need to measure both the efficiency of the coordination function in terms of its ability to contain costs appropriately and the quality and appropriateness of services from the clinical and patient satisfaction points of view.

THE CONTINUUM OF CARE IN THE FUTURE

Paradigm Shift

Managing the broad continuum of care needed by the chronically ill is a complex undertaking. It requires a shift from the current biomedical model to a biopsychosocial model. It requires replacement of provider-centered care by patient-centered care, where the ill person and family function as partners of health care professionals in specifying health care needs and assembling, producing, and delivering health care services. It requires collaboration among service providers who are accustomed to functioning independently. It requires the implementation of integrative mechanisms at the top management level of the organizations participating in the network and at the front lines, where the services are produced and delivered to the chronically ill and their families. It requires health care professionals, across organizations, agreeing on critical pathways—on how the health and social service work is done, on the relative importance of functions, and on the sets of problem-solving processes and techniques to be employed. Finally, it requires the development of financial arrangements that cover the continuum of care and allow participating providers to be paid in accordance with the value of the services they render to the chronically ill and their families. Although these are large managerial challenges, they are essential if the needs of the chronically ill are to be adequately met.

Managing the Network Organization

The network organization appears to be an effective organizational form for managing chronic illness. It uses existing community resources rather than building capabilities from the ground up. It allows for effective use of scarce resources that historically have been accumulated, allocated, and maintained by each individual organization. It can provide a broader array of services needed by the chronically ill than any single organization. It offers the opportunity for each member entity to pursue its particular specialty or distinctive competence within the context of a unified framework and to jointly solve the problems of the chronically ill. However, the management of a network is radically different than management of a hierarchical organization. In the network model of resource allocation and control, transactions occur neither through discrete exchanges nor by administrative fiat but through participating organizations and individuals engaging in reciprocal, preferential, mutually supportive actions.[33]

As indicated earlier in this chapter, many of the managerial functions in networks are performed by brokers, who assemble, locate, build relationships, and subcontract for specific services. The focus of the broker in network management is on developing among the members of the network a commitment to the goals of the network (e.g., better service to the chronically ill) and a mutual orientation. The broker must build a shared vision that gives network members a sense of purpose that transcends their parochial interests and creates alignment. Furthermore, the development of a mutual orientation requires sufficient commitment of time and resources to develop among partners a knowledge of each other's business and a respect for each other's interests through a learning and adaptation process. Although formal contracts are important in providing a legal framework for network relationships, the social architecture is crucial to the formation and maintenance of the network.[34] Larson indicates that personal relationships and prospective partners' knowledge of each other's reputation are critical in

the creation of a network.[35] The key function of the broker is to establish, maintain, and enhance relationships. This involves

- bringing organizational members together and getting them to commit to an overall vision
- introducing members to each other and serving as a focal source of information about each other
- redirecting individual perspectives to encompass both the goals of the network and each organization's goals through joint planning and coordination of routines
- mutually reinforcing trust through social processes
- providing feedback to the members regarding the equity of payment to members for their value-added contributions to the network

Although nurturing relationships between organizations is critical in network management, absolute harmony will not be obtained. Consequently, a very important broker role in network management is ongoing mediation and conflict resolution.

Service Integration across the Continuum of Care

The shift in thinking about health care delivery outlined in the previous section requires a concomitant change in managerial strategies, methods, and techniques at the care coordination level. Health care has been mired in a functionally organized service delivery system with strict divisions of labor among organizations as well as among departments and specialists within organizations. Although patients and families have been burdened with the responsibility of coordinating care services provided by diverse organizations, within hierarchical organizations there is an obdurate belief that sufficient coordination occurs by virtue of management fiat. Organizational research has proved otherwise,[36] and researchers have identified the extent to which patients are harmed by the fragmentation of health care delivery coupled with an overreliance on biophysiological science technology, even within a single institution.[37]

The education and training process for health care professionals in the United States produces technicians who typically focus only on their specialty. Overcoming this socialization and getting health care professionals to work as a team across organizations, functions, and specialties is one of the most difficult challenges faced by the manager at the care coordination level. While it is impossible to address at length the management changes that are endemic to chronic illness management, we will identify the most significant.

Of primary concern will be the development of knowledge and abilities to effectively manage a team of diverse professionals with their own distinct ideologies regarding how care should be rendered. Networking requires coordination with other disciplines and functions, working together to identify and frame problems, as well as developing proposals for the resolution of problems. In this context, networking means bridging vocabulary differences, learning new frames of reference, and meeting with different people. It means listening to people who see the world differently and whose near-term goals may be different. It also means going outside one's area of expertise.

In a hierarchical organization, individuals focus on the goals of the organization or their unit, not the goals of the network. This fragmentation leaves few individuals feeling responsible for the success of the whole network. Without a compelling reason to coordinate activities, each department or specialty will go its own way. For the network to function effectively at the frontlines, coordination must become a part of each provider's job rather than a responsibility of a few designated individuals. By making coordination everyone's responsibility, the network ensures that a lateral structure exists across all functions and specialties.

The social psychology literature indicates there are two important strategies that help create a climate in which a diverse team can be effective in coordinating and working together on problem-solving tasks. The first is the strategy of superordinate goal setting—the setting of goals in such a way that it becomes clear to the work group that the goals cannot be achieved without the talents and cooperation of all.[38] By changing the context of the expected outcomes from absence of disease to the ability of patients to effectively cope with illness, management can widen the goals to the point where interdisciplinary teamwork is required if the goals are to be achieved.

This shift in goals must be re-enforced by a networkwide patient-oriented culture. A patient-oriented culture will only emerge if "patient-centeredness" becomes a relentless pursuit of management in both the structure and processes within the organization.[39] Structural congruence with patient-centeredness comes about when the organization's systems and procedures are designed with patient values as their driving force. Process congruence is facilitated when management's interaction patterns with affiliated individuals are marked by a conspicuous and consistent focus upon patient values and patient and family satisfaction as the prevailing criteria for successful quality service.

The second strategy is to institute a team-oriented organizational reward system. Traditional management approaches are specialist oriented, fragment responsibility, and dictate downward and upward information and communication flows within organizations, all of which create significant barriers preventing continuity of care. In a network, the emphasis is on multidisciplinary synthesis, and thus specialists should be rewarded for their contribution to the team's effort in meeting the needs of the chronically ill person and the family. The specialists' demonstrations of technical competence in a network environment are important not only for accomplishing team tasks but also for establishing and maintaining their credibility as reliable members of the network.

In managing the continuum of care, managers are almost always going to encounter work groups in which power and status are unequal. For example, physicians are always considered as having the highest status in health care. Yet a physician's contribution, albeit critical, is only part of the total group effort to help a person deal with his or her illness. Physicians, however, traditionally have the expectation that their contribution is both the prevailing and controlling one. It is incumbent upon management to structure the organization's rewards in such a way that individual success is based upon group success. Only in this way can there be any real migration of the power and privilege that professional status confers.[40]

Financing the Continuum of Care

As indicated earlier in the chapter, the health care system has been organized around acute illness—a life-threatening act of God. Pursuant to this acute care model, we have used a casualty model of health insurance, premised on the fundamental unpredictability of disease, to finance health care.[41] Just as the medical model does not fit the needs of the chronically ill, neither does the casualty model of health insurance. Chronic illness is correlated closely with the aging process and is predictable. Advances in genetics and immunology are converging to make it possible to predict chronic disease risks in many persons before symptoms emerge so that steps may be taken to modify the risks and the disease trajectory.[42] Thus, the onset and progression of chronic illness are not fortuitous, and a casualty-based insurance model cannot be expected to finance a biopsychosocial approach to the management of chronic illness.

To fully implement the chronic illness management paradigm, we must shift from a sole reliance on the casualty model of insurance to finance the services for the chronically ill. Although unforeseen health care problems may be covered by casualty-based insurance plans, different approaches must be developed to underwrite predictable chronic illness. The increased ability to predict chronic illness and to initiate early stage management to modify risk factors has significant implications for patients, families, and society in terms of both avoidance and financing of chronic illness. Individuals, families, and society will have increased responsibility for managing the environmental and behavioral risk factors that accelerate the onset and progression of chronic illnesses. Individuals and families have a responsibility to avoid or manage illness by ameliorating risk factors, and they should be financially liable if they, having known the risks, did nothing to reduce them. Moreover, ways must be found to balance individual and family obligations and societal obligations for promoting good health and financing needed services when unavoidable chronic illness must be managed. For the chronic illness management paradigm to be completely financially underwritten, casualty-based health care insurance plans must be supplemented with chronic care, IRA-type plans that allow individuals with known risk of chronic illness to begin saving early in life to pay for the biopsychosocial care they may need at the onset of chronic illness later in life. Individual and or family investment in such plans should be encouraged by government policy.

In addition to the development of new mechanisms to finance the broad range of services needed by the chronically ill, mechanisms also must be developed to distribute payment to participating providers in accordance with the value of the services they render to the chronically ill and their families. The current trend in health care reimbursement is to bundle payment in a diagnosis-related group (DRG) or capitation fee. For a network comprising multiple organizations to be established, maintained, and enhanced, participating providers must perceive that their exchanges within the network are equitable and mutually beneficial. Financial arrangements that allow participating providers to be paid in accordance with the value they add and information systems that allow participating providers to mutually verify each other's contributions are critical to the development and maintenance of the network.

ADDITIONAL RESOURCES

Bush, J.B., and A.C. Frohman. Communication in a network organization. *Organizational Dynamics* 20, no. 2 (1992): 23–36.

Cassell, E.J. *The nature of suffering and the goals of medicine.* New York: Oxford University Press, 1991.

Curtin, M., and I. Lubkin. What is chronicity? In *Chronic illness: impact and interventions,* ed. I. Lubkin. Boston: Jones and Bartlett, 1986.

Evashwick, C.J. Creating a continuum. *Health Progress* 70, no. 5 (1989): 36–39, 56.

Goldsmith, J. A radical prescription for hospitals. *Harvard Business Review* 67, no. 3 (1989): 104–111.

Goldsmith, J.C. The reshaping of health care. *Healthcare Forum Journal* 35, no. 3 (1992): 19–27.

Kane, R.A. Case management: Ethical pitfalls on the road to high quality managed care. *Quality Review Bulletin* 14, no. 5 (1988): 161–166.

Kane, R.A. Case management in health care settings. In *Case management in human service practice,* eds. M. Weil and J. Karls. San Francisco: Jossey-Bass, 1985.

Larson, A. Network dyads in entrepreneurial settings: A study of the governance of exchange relationships. *Administrative Science Quarterly* 37, no. 1 (1992): 76–104.

Lawless, M.W., and R.A. Moore. Interorganizational systems in public service delivery: A new application of the dynamic network framework. *Human Relations* 42 (1989): 1167–1184.

Leutz W., et al. *Financial Performance of the Social HMO.* Unpublished working paper from the Social HMO Consortium, Brandeis University, Waltham, Mass. 1989.

MacAdam, M., et al. Case management for frail elders: The Robert Wood Johnson Foundation's Program for Hospital Initiatives in Long Term Care. *The Gerontologist* 29 (1989): 737–744.

Miles, R.E., and C.C. Snow. Organizations: New concepts for new forms. *California Management Review* 28, no. 3 (1986): 62–73.

Powell, W.W. Hybrid organizational arrangements: New form or transitional development. *California Management Review* 30, no. 1 (1987): 68–87.

Snow, C.C., et al. Managing 21st century network organizations. *Organizational Dynamics* 20, no. 3 (1992): 5–20.

Strauss, A.J., and J. Corbin. *Shaping a new health care system: The explosion of chronic illness as a catalyst for change.* San Francisco: Jossey-Bass, 1988.

Weil, M., et al. Historical origins and recent developments. In *Case Management in Human Service Practice,* ed. M. Weil and J. Karls. San Francisco: Jossey-Bass, 1985.

NOTES

1. E.J. Cassell, *The Nature of Suffering and the Goals of Medicine* (New York: Oxford University Press, 1991).

2. T. Parsons, *The Social System* (New York: The Free Press, 1951).

3. A. Strauss and J. Corbin, *Shaping a New Health Care System: The Explosion of Chronic Illness as a Catalyst for Change* (San Francisco: Jossey-Bass, 1988).

4. Parsons, *The Social System;* T. Parsons, Definitions of Health and Illness in Light of American Values and Social Structure, in *Patients, Physicians, and Illness,* ed. E. Gartly Jao (New York: The Free Press, 1972); T. Parsons, The Sick Role and the Role of the Physician Reconsidered, *Milbank Memorial Fund Quarterly* 53 (1975): 257–278.

5. M. Curtin and I. Lubkin, What Is Chronicity? in *Chronic Illness: Impact and Interventions,* ed. I. Lubkin (Boston: Jones and Bartlett, 1986).

6. Cassell, *Nature of Suffering,* 44.

7. Ibid., 32.

8. Strauss and Corbin, *Shaping a New Health Care System.*

9. Cassell, *Nature of Suffering.*

10. Strauss and Corbin, *Shaping,* 48.

11. J. Goldsmith, A Radical Prescription for Hospitals, *Harvard Business Review* 67, no. 3 (1989): 104–111.

12. C.C. Snow, R.E. Miles, and H.J. Coleman, Managing 21st Century Network Organizations, *Organizational Dynamics* 20, no. 3 (1992): 5–20.

13. R.E. Miles and C.C. Snow, Organizations: New Concepts for New Forms, *California Management Review* 28, no. 3 (1986): 62–73.

14. M.W. Lawless and R.A. Moore, Interorganizational Systems in Public Service Delivery: A New Application of the Dynamic Network Framework, *Human Relations* 42 (1989): 1167–1184.

15. Snow, Miles, and Coleman, Managing 21st Century Network Organizations.

16. A.H. Van De Ven and D.L. Ferry, *Measuring and Assessing Organizations* (New York: Wiley, 1980).

17. Ibid.

18. Joint Commission on Accreditation of Healthcare Organizations, *Case Management: Guiding Patients through the Healthcare Maze* (Chicago: Joint Commission on Accreditation of Healthcare Organizations, 1988), 5–6.

19. M. McAdam et al., Case Management for Frail Elders: The Robert Wood Johnson Foundation's Program for Hospital Initiatives in Long Term Care, *The Gerontologist* 29 (1989): 737–744.

20. Ibid., 740–741.

21. Snow, Miles, and Coleman, Managing 21st Century Network Organizations.

22. R.A. Kane, Case Management in Health Care Settings, in *Case Management in Human Service Practice,* eds. M. Weil and J. Karls (San Francisco: Jossey-Bass, 1985).

23. Miles and Snow, Organizations.

24. C.J. Evashwick, Creating a Continuum, *Health Progress* 70, no. 5 (1989): 36–39, 56.

25. J.B. Bush and A.C. Frohman, Communication in a Network Organization, *Organizational Dynamics* (1992): 23–36.

26. Evashwick, Creating a Continuum.

27. MacAdam et al., Case Management for Frail Elders, 743.

28. Kane, Case Management in Health Care Settings; MacAdam et al., Case Management for Frail Elders.

29. M. Henderson and A. Collard, Measuring Quality in Medical Case Management Programs, *Quality Review Bulletin* 14, no. 2 (1988).

30. D. Humphries et al., The Miami Channeling Program: Case Management and Cost Control, *Quality Review Bulletin* 14, no. 5 (1988): 154–160.

31. W. Leutz et al., *Financial Performance of the Social HMO* (Unpublished working paper from the Social HMO Consortium, Brandeis University, Waltham, Mass., 1989).

32. MacAdam et al., Case Management for Frail Elders, 743.

33. W.W. Powell, Hybrid Organizational Arrangements: New Form or Transitional Development, *California Management Review* 30, no. 1 (1987): 68–87.

34. A. Larson, Network Dyads in Entrepreneurial Settings: A Study of the Governance of Exchange Relationships, *Administrative Science Quarterly* 37, no. 1 (1992): 76–104.

35. Ibid.

36. C. Perrow, *Complex Organizations: A Critical Essay* (New York: McGraw-Hill, 1986).

37. A. Bursztajn et al., *Medical Choice, Medical Chances* (New York: Routledge, Chapman, Hall, 1990); MacAdam et al., Case Management for Frail Elders; A. Strauss et al., *The Social Organization of Medical Work* (Chicago: University of Chicago Press, 1985).

38. M. Sherif et al., *Intergroup Conflict and Cooperation: The Robbers' Cave Experiment* (Norma, Okla.: University of Oklahoma Institute of Group Relations, 1961).

39. E. Schein, *Organizational Culture and Leadership* (San Francisco: Jossey-Bass, 1989).

40. L. Meese et al., But Some Animals Are More Equal Than Others, in *Group Process and Productivity,* eds. S. Worchel et al. (Newbury Park, Calif.: Sage Publications, 1992).

41. J.C. Goldsmith, The Reshaping of Health Care, *Healthcare Forum Journal* 35, no. 3 (1992): 19–27.

42. Ibid.

Index

A

Access to health care
  controls on use, 569–571
  deterrents to, 569
  ethical/moral issues, 576
  future view of, 577
  and governmental role, 574–575
  and health insurance, 571–572
  and lack of health insurance, 572–573
  managerial role in, 576–577
  measurement of, 562–567
  models of use, 567
  and prepayment, 568–569
  and public health services, 573–574
  resource limitation aspects, 575–576
  and structure of system, 568
  and type of service, 567–568
Accountability of health care institutions, 268–271
  and comparison of institutions, 270
  and government regulation, 269
  historical view, 268–269
  institutional accountability, 270
  and public expectations, 269–270
  and public sanctions, 271

Accounts receivable
  accounts receivable reports, 295
  management of, 304
Accreditation, quality program, 57
Accrediting Commission on Education for Health Services Administration, criteria of, 18
Acute care services
  features of, 590–591
  forces affecting services, 592–593
  future view of, 595
  and hospital business, 593–595
  hospital-centered care, 591
  quality management, 595–596
Addiction counselors, 619
AIDS testing, release of information, 264
Alternative work arrangements, 340
Ambulatory care services, 581–582
American Hospital Association Policy, on restructuring health care delivery, 12–13
Americans with Disabilities Act, 348, 546–547
Antitrust law, and health care industry, 548–549
Appropriation budget, 292
Artificial intelligence, 249–250

Assessment
  information systems performance, 248
  of organizational learning, 78–79
  quality program, 54–55, 115
Audits
  financial, 304–305
  technology audits, 484–485
Authority, definition of, 27–28
Automobile liability insurance, 533
Average length of patient stay, 593–594
Average rate of return method, 307, 309
Avoidance, conflict from, 37–38

B

Balance sheet, 295
Benefits
  future view, 345
  government interest in, 345
  types of benefit programs, 344–345
Bidding, 368–369
  in facilities development, 454
  process of, 369–370
  situations for, 369–370

Biotechnological drugs, 402
Blue Cross/Blue Shield, 285
Boiler/machinery insurance, 533
Bridging, in facilities development, 456
Brokering, continuum of care services, 628–629
Budgeting, 290–294
    appropriation budget, 292
    capital budget, 305–306
    classification of expenses, 294
    fixed forecast budget, 292
    flexible budget, 292
    preparation of budget, 292–294
    purpose of, 292
Bureaucratic approach
    decision making, 30–31
    managed care, 130, 133

C

Cafeteria plans, 293, 344–345
Canada, health care system, 13
Capital equipment purchasing, 367–368
Capital investment, 305–308
    capital analysis techniques, 306–308, 309
    capital budget, 305–306
    financing acquisitions, 308
Capitation, 99
    features of, 139
    strengths/weaknesses of, 187
Career ladders, 340
Case-based financing
    continuum of care services, 634–635
    future view of, 635–638
    service integration in, 636–638
Case method, nursing, 216
Cash reports, 295
Catalog of Electronic Data Products, 273
Central supply supervisor, 380
Certified nurse anesthetists, 208
Charismatic power, 28
Chief executive officer
    financial role of, 289–290

relationship with governing board, 166, 168–169
    and risk management, 538
Chief information officer, 236–237
Chronic illness
    continuum of care services, 626–638
    and health care delivery, 625–626
    management principles related to, 623–624
    nature of, 624–625
    See also Continuum of care services
Civil Rights Act of 1964, 348
Clayton Act, 549
Clinical data systems
    applications for, 259–260
    clinical/administrative data, 257
    data elements in, 259
    department-specific data, 257, 259
    disease registries, 257
    ethical issues related to, 264
    future view of, 264–265
    historical view, 253–254
    importance of clinical information, 254–255
    information related to, 253
    information requirements, 255–256
    legal issues related to, 261–264
    location of, 256
    medical literature information, 259
    patient-carried records, 259
    patient medical records, 257
    personnel for, 256
    quality management, 260–261
Clinical nurse specialist, 208
Clinical psychologists, 618
Coalitional decision making, 30–31
Coercive power, 28
Collaboration
    conflict resolution, 38
    and nurses, 205, 212–213
Communication, 31–32
    horizontal communication, 31
    physician/hospital, 201
    vertical communication, 31, 32
Community
    community health centers, 581

community support programs, mental health, 616–617
    and governing board, 171
Compensation
    administration of pay programs, 341–342
    design of pay programs, 341
    group compensation, 343–344
    incentive compensation, 343
    pay/benefits related to, 349–350
    pay ranges, 342
    performance compensation, 343
Comprehensive health organizations (CHOs), 13
Comprehensive Omnibus Budget and Reconciliation Act, 349
Compromise, conflict resolution, 38
Computerized systems
    continuum of care services, 633–634
    facilities design/drafting, 451
    food/nutrition services, 428–429
    pharmacy, 393, 398
    safety, 510
    See also Clinical data systems; Information systems
Concurrent review, 143
Confidentiality, 275–278
    AMA ethical guidelines, 276–277
    breach of, 278
    and privacy rights, 263–264, 276–278
    and proprietary rights, 278
    release of information, 263–264
Conflict
    affective conflict, 36
    avoidance, 37–38
    cognitive conflict, 36
    goal conflict, 36
    and health care organizations, 34–35
    horizontal conflict, 37
    line-staff conflict, 37
    organizational conflict, 36
    positive/negative conflict, 35–36
    role conflict, 37
    vertical conflict, 37
Conflict resolution, 38–39
    accommodating, 38

bargaining power, sources of, 39, 40
collaborating, 38
compromising, 38–39
forcing, 38
Consignment buying, 367
Construction documents, in facilities development, 451–454
Construction management, 455
Contingency theory of leadership, 23, 24–25
Continuous quality improvement, 114–115
Continuum of care services, 626–638
brokering role in, 628–629
care coordination, 630–633
case-based financing, 634–635
computerized system, 633–634
financing needs, 638
interorganizational coordination in, 629–630
organizational approach to, 628
types of, 627
Contracting methods, in facilities development, 454–456
Contracts, labor, 346–348
Contractual security programs, 517
Control, 376–378
as management function, 23–24
of materials, 376–378
Coordinated care. *See* Managed care
Corporate law, in health care industry, 544–545
Cost plus fee with guarantee, 455
Cost plus fee with guaranteed maximum price, 454–455
Cost-plus pricing method, 299
Costs
direct and indirect costs, 301
job order costing system, 301
management of inefficiency, 302–303
process costing, 302
product line costing, 301
responsibility costs, 301
standard costs, 302
Credentialing, legal aspects, 547–548
Crime
in hospital setting, 511–512

See also Security
Crime insurance, 534
types of policies, 534

D

Databases, of medical information, 272–273
Data management, nursing, 217–219
Data recovery, information systems, 244–245
Data systems, quality program, 52–53
Decentralization, management, 33, 42
Decision making, 30–31
bureaucratic approach, 30–31
centralized, 209
in coalitions, 30–31
group, 110
managerial role in, 21
nurses, 209
participatory, 209
shared, 209
Decision-styles theory, of management, 25, 26
Design, of facilities, 448–451
Design-build method, 455–456
Diagnosis-related groups, 187, 288, 613
advantages/disadvantages, 187
Dietary services. *See* Food/nutrition services
Directing, as management function, 22–23
Directors and officers liability insurance, 532
Direct productive full-time equivalent, 214–215
Discipline, 115–116
Disease registries, 257
Dispatcher, 380
Disposable materials, advantages of, 374–375
Distribution, 373–374
exchange cart system, 373–374
posting charges, 374
requisitioning, 373

stock replenishment, 373
Distribution manager, 380
Divisional design, organizational, 108–110
Dynamic network structure
characteristics of, 127
managed care, 127, 130

E

Employee development, 350–353
entry-level training, 352–353
leadership development, 353
and nature of work force, 351–352
for retention of employees, 353
Employee Retirement Income Security Act, 349, 535
Equipment. *See* Technology assessment/management
Ethics, 275–278
and access to health care, 576
and clinical data systems, 264
confidentiality issue, 275–278
and governing board, 176–177
and nursing, 223
Exchange cart system, 373–374
Expenditures, types in health system, 96–98
Expenditure targets, 99
Expert power, 28
Expert systems, 249–250
External environment, management principles related to, 88
External information management
cost/benefit analysis, 279–280
data, characteristics of good data, 278–280
data requirements, 271–272
data sources, 272–275
computerized databases, 272
National Center for Health Statistics information, 273
National Practitioner Data Bank, 273–274
ethical issues related to, 275–278
future view, 280–281
management principles related to, 268

and public accountability, 268–271
quality management, 278–280

F

Facilities planning, 319
commissioning/startup of project,
459–463
computer-assisted tasks, 451
construction documents, 451–454
contracting methods, 454–459
design process, 448–451
management principles related to,
434–435
master plan development, 438–442
postoccupancy evaluation, 463–
468
programming, 442–448
quality management, 463–468
as sequential process, 433–434
success factors in, 435–436
trends in, 436–437
zoning, 449
Fair Labor Standards Act, 349
False Claim Act, 550
Federal Drug Free Workplace Act,
350
Fee-for-service, 137–138, 187, 301
strengths/weaknesses of, 187
Fidelity bonds, 534–535
types of, 534–535
Fiduciary liability insurance, 535
Figurehead, manager as, 20–21
Finance functions
accounts receivable, 304
audit function, 304–305
budgeting, 290–294
capital investments, 305–308
cost management, 301–302
financial reporting/analysis, 294–
295
inventories, 304
management of inefficiency, 302–
303
management of working capital,
303–304
organization of, 289–290
revenue generation, 295, 298–301

Financial reporting/analysis, 294–295
accounts receivable reports, 295
balance sheet, 295
cash reports, 295
financial ratios, 297–298
flow reports, 294–295
inventory reports, 295
profit and loss statement, 294–295
statement of cash flows, 303–304
stock reports, 294–295
Financing of health system, 96–100
financial constraints, limitations
imposed by, 99–100
future view, 100–101, 308–310
governing board role in, 171
history of, 284–289
insurance. See Health insurance
management principles related to,
283–284
program budgeting, 114
setting prices in hospitals, methods
of, 299–300
sources of resources, 98–99
types of expenditures, 96–98
See also Finance functions
Fire insurance, 529–530
Fixed forecast budget, 292
Flexible budget, 292
Flexner report, 46, 47, 89–90, 184,
582
Flow reports, 294–295
Food/nutrition services
budgeting, 422, 424
computerized system, 428–429
educational/research activities,
418–419
facility operated versus contract
food services, 426–427
feeding staff/employees/public,
412–413
food production systems, 410, 412
functions of, 406
future view of, 425–429
historical view, 407
management principles related to,
406–407
nutritional assessment devices, 429
nutritional assessment of patients,
414

nutrition committees, 416
nutrition counseling/education,
416–418
organization of, 407–410
patient feeding service, 413–414
personnel, 420–421, 429
productivity aspects, 427–428
quality management, 424–425
revenue generation, methods of,
419–420
space requirements, 422, 423, 424
specialized nutrition support, 414,
416
Fraud, of health care providers, 550–
551
Fulfillment process, 325–326
Functional design, organizational,
107–108

G

Gainsharing, 343–344
Gaming, in facilities planning, 451
Governing board
board/CEO relationship, 166, 168–
169
board/interboard relationship, 166–
167
board/medical staff relationship,
166
chairperson, role of, 176
changing role of board, 163–164
and community, 171
compensation of members, 175–
176
composition of board, 165
ethical issues, 176–177
financial oversight function, 171
future view of, 178–179
historical view, 160–163
legal responsibilities of board,
167–168
liability of, 177–178
medical staff relations, 170–171
member selection, 174–175
mission statement development,
169
quality management functions,
172–174

self-evaluation, 173–174
size of board, 165
strategic planning activity, 169–170
structure of, 171
terms of officers, 165–166
Government
and access to health care, 574–575
and acute care services, 592–593
regulation, and public accountability, 268–271
Group compensation, 343–344
Group models, managed care, 121–122
Group practices, 580–582
community health centers, 581
multispecialty group practices, 185, 581
single-specialty groups, 185, 581
Group purchasing, 367

H

Hardware, for information systems, 246, 249
Hart-Scott-Rodino Premerger Notification Program, 549
Hazardous materials programs, 507–508
Hazardous waste. *See* Waste management
Health, definition of, 5
Health Care Quality Improvement Act, 547
Health insurance
and access to care, 571–572
Blue Cross/Blue Shield, 285
commercial insurance plans, 285
cost containment methods, 287–288
direct service plans, 285–286
health maintenance organizations (HMOs), 288
Medicare/Medicaid, 286–288
preferred provider organizations (PPOs), 288
Health maintenance organizations (HMOs), 125, 552–553, 587

closed panel type, 125
direct contracts model, 123
independent practice association models, 122–123
open plans, 125
for special populations, 125–126
Health services, versus medical care, 5–6
Health services management
challenges to leadership/management, 14–15
communication in, 31–32
complexity in, 27
conflict and conflict resolution, 34–39
decision making in, 30–31
leadership in, 39–42
lines of authority in, 29–30
management structure in, 32–34
managerial decisions in, 4
power/authority in, 27–29
tasks for future, 3–4, 42–43
Health system
characteristics of, 7
components of system, 92–95
economic factors related to, 95–96
evolution of, 6–7
financing of, 96–100
historical view, 88–92
need for restructuring of, 11–14, 16–17
primary care system, 8–10
Hippocratic Oath, 277
Horizontal communication, 31
Hospital-based practices, physicians, 185–186
Hourly rate pricing method, 299
Housekeeping
equipment for, 494–495
functions of, 487–488
future view of, 496–499
historical view, 488–489
hospital cleanliness standards, 497
infection control, 488–489
interior maintenance, 492
management principles related to, 488
quality management, 496
staff, 492–494

standards, 489–490
supplies for, 495–496
training, 499
waste management, 491–492, 498
Human resource management
budgeting, 213
contractual management, 345–348
employee development, 350–353
functions of, 335–336
future view, 358–359
human resource department, role of, 336–338
labor shortages, 354–355
legal compliance tasks, 348–350
management principles related to, 336
payment/benefits administration, 341–345
personnel related functions, 338–339
quality management, 356–358
resource requirements, 355–356

I

Immigration Reform and Control Act, 348
Incentive compensation, 343
Incompetent patients, release of information, 264
Indemnity plans, 124–125
managed, 125
Independent practice association models, 122–124
coordination in, 130
created entities, 123
direct contracts model, 123
risk sharing in, 139
Independent practice organizations, 124
Independent solo practices, physicians, 184–185
Indirect productive full-time equivalents, 215
Infection control, 488–489
Information management, external. *See* External information management

Information ownership, 262
Information systems
    as aid to management functions,
        229–230
    assessment of, 248
    centralized versus decentralized
        systems, 233–235
    chief information officer, 236–237
    clinical applications, 238
    commercial versus internally
        developed software, 232
    data recovery plan, 244–245
    decision support systems, 238–239
    facilities for, 247–248
    financial applications, 237–238
    future view of, 249–250
    hardware components, 246, 249
    historical view, 231–232
    in-house versus shared-service
        processing, 233
    management principles related to,
        230–231
    master plan for, 232
    multiple-versus-single vendor
        supplied software systems, 233
    new technologies, 249–250
    organizational policies related to,
        232–235
    primary care services, 584
    security, 243–245
    staffing, 246–247
    and total quality management,
        248–249
    vendors
        consultants and vendor
            selection, 243
        contract/performance
            requirements, 241–242
        cost-benefit analysis, 243
        legal counsel in dealing with,
            242–243
        selection of, 239–241
Informed consent, 261–262
    and liability, 526
Inpatient services, mental health,
    614–616
Insurance
    boiler/machinery insurance, 533
    crime insurance, 534
    fidelity bonds, 534–535

fiduciary liability insurance, 535
fire insurance, 529–530
liability insurance, 530–533
limiting services covered by, 100
multiperil insurance, 533
workers' compensation insurance,
    533–534
See also Health insurance
Internal small business units, 33–34
Inventory
    inventory management, 371–373
    inventory reports, 295
    management of, 304
    statistical methods related to, 372–
        373
    See also Materials management

J

Job order costing system, 301
Joint Commission on Accreditation
    of Healthcare Organizations, 186,
    220–222, 547
    history of, 46–48

K

Knowledge, in quality improvement,
    60–61, 64–68

L

Labor contracts, 345–348
Labor law, and health care industry,
    546–547
Labor relations
    administration of labor contract,
        347–348
    decertification, 348
    human resource role, 346
    laws related to, 349
    negotiation of labor contract, 346–
        347
    strikes, 347
    union status in health care, 345–
        346
Labor shortages, 354–355
Leadership, 39–42

commitment to public benefit, 42
commitment to others in, 40–41
development of, 353
education for, 17–18
needs of health services
    management, 14–15
problem solving and, 41–42
quality program, 50, 56–57, 63–64,
    68–71
succession planning, 82–83
values of, 41
vision in, 40
Legal compliance, laws related to,
    348–350
Legal services
    antitrust law, 548–549
    billing for outside services, 555–
        556
    corporate law, 544–545
    cost control for, 554–555
    and credentialing, 547–548
    and fraud, 550–551
    future view of, 557–558
    historical view, 542
    labor law, 546–547
    liability cases, 549–550
    and managed care, 551–553
    management principles related to,
        540–541
    patient care issues, 549
    quality management, 556–557
    relationship to health executive,
        544
    tax law, 545–546
    and third-party reimbursement,
        550
    trends in health law, 543–544
    types of arrangements, 553–554
Legitimate power, 28, 29
Liability, 549–550
    bases for claims, 526, 550
    elements of professional liability,
        525
    theories of, 550
Liability insurance, 530–533
    automobile policy, 533
    characteristics of, 530–531
    directors and officers insurance,
        532
    fiduciary liability insurance, 535

general liability insurance, 532
umbrella policy, 533
Licensed vocational/practical nurse,
207
Line-staff conflict, 37
Locality rule, and liability, 526
Lump sum bidding, in facilities
development, 454

M

Macro-assessment, technology
assessment, 472, 473
Managed care
bureaucratic structure, 130, 133
control aspects, 135–136
dynamic network framework, 127,
130
foundation of, 118–119
future view for, 146–147
group models, 121–122
health maintenance organizations
(HMOs), 125, 552–553
history of, 119–121
indemnity plans, 124–125
independent practice association
models, 122–124
independent practice organizations,
124
physician compensation methods,
137–139
and physician productivity, 140
preferred provider organizations
(PPOs), 125, 551–552
quality management, 145–146
risk sharing function, 139
services offered to health care
organizations, 126
single-specialty companies, 126
staff models, 121
systems differentiation in, 126–127
utilization management, 140–145,
551
value structure, 133, 135
Managed fee schedules, 137–138
Management
effectiveness, elements of, 19
managerial roles in
decisional role, 21

informational role, 20
interpersonal role, 20
See also Health services
management
Management functions
controlling, 23–24
directing, 22–23
organizing, 22
planning, 21–22
staffing, 22
Management styles, 24–26
contingency theory, 23
decision-styles theory, 25, 26
path-goal model, 25–26
situational factors, 25–27
Marketing
external communications tasks,
324–325
fulfillment function, 325–326
future view, 328–330
management functions related to,
314
market research, 322
program design, 323–324
quality management, 327–328
relationship to strategic planning,
311–313
strategic marketing analysis, 322–
323
tasks in, 313
Master plan, in facilities planning,
438–442
Materials management
acquisition planning, 377
centralization/decentralization of,
378–379
control, 376–378
distribution, 373–374
equipment for, 381
facilities for, 381
functions of, 361–362
future view, 384
management principles related to,
362–363
monitoring/security of materials,
377–378
organization of, 378–379
personnel for, 379–380
policies/procedures, 376–377
processing, 374–376

purchasing, 363–370
quality management, 382–384
receiving, 370–373
resource requirements, 380–382
Materials safety data sheet, 507–508
Matrix organization, 111
Medicaid, characteristics of, 287
Medical care, versus health services,
5–6
Medical staff
credentialing, 173, 192–193
future view for, 194–202
managed care
compensation methods, 137–
139
productivity of physician, 140
strengths/weaknesses, 187–188
organizations in hospitals, 186,
188
quality management, 192–194
and quality program, 50–51, 55
relationship to governing board,
170–171
role of, 29
structural integration with
hospitals, 195–199
See also Nursing; Physicians
Medicare
characteristics of, 286–288
diagnosis related groups, 288
physician reimbursement, 289
prospective payment system, 287–
288
resource-based relative value
system, 289
Mental disorders, prevalence of, 611–
612
Mental health records, release of
information, 264
Mental health services
community support programs,
616–617
expenditures for, 614
and health administrator, 613
inpatient services, 614–616
mental health administration,
elements of, 619–621
partial hospitalization, 616
staff, types of, 618–619
substance abuse programs, 617

substitution of services, 617–618
therapeutic communities, 617
treatment settings, 612–613
trends related to, 613–614
Micro-assessment, technology
assessment, 472, 473
Minors, release of information, 264
Mission statement
characteristics of, 317–318
and governing board, 169
Motivation, extrinsic motivation, 67–
68
Multiperil insurance, 533
Multispecialty group practices, 185,
581
Multiunit systems
and asset maximization, 157–159
development of, 150–153, 155–
157
leveraging of, 153–155
organizational focus needs, 156–
157

N

National Center for Health Statistics,
information from, 273
National Labor Relations Act, 345–
346, 349, 546
National Labor Relations Board, 349,
350
National Long-Term Care
Channeling project, 634
*National Practitioner Data Bank
Guidebook,* 273
Negotiations, purchasing, 369
Net present value, 307, 309
Nonproductive full-time equivalents,
215
Nurse executive, role of, 210, 212
Nurse manager, role of, 212
Nurse midwives, 208
Nurse practitioners, 208
Nurses, role of, 29–30
Nursing
and ancillary/support departments,
213
case method, 216

collaboration in, 212–213
data management, 217–219
decision making, 209
definition of, 222
ethical decision making, 223
expanded nurse roles, 208
historical view, 205–206
knowledge of patient
characteristics, 213–214
levels of personnel, 207
management functions related to,
205
nurse executive, 210, 212
nurse manager, 212
nursing education, 210
nursing process
aspects of, 204
steps in, 206
and patient care management, 212
practice acts, 207–208
practice settings, 206–207
primary nurse, 217
quality management, 219–222
regulation of nursing, 222–223
research, 210
salary budget for, 214–215
standards, 208–209, 219–220
Nutrition services. *See* Food/nutrition
services

O

Occupational Safety and Health
Administration (OSHA), 349–350
standards, 503
Optical storage systems, 249
Organizational design
definition of, 103
determinants of, 104–106
divisional design, 108–110
functional design, 107–108
and individual functioning, 107
integration in, 110
management principles related to,
104
matrix organization, 111
program management, 111–116
review of, 106–107

Organizational learning
equipment needs, 80
evaluation of programs, 78–79
functions of education department,
79–80
future view for, 81–83
history of, 75–76
implementation of programs, 78
management principles related to,
74–75
needs assessment in, 77–78
program design, 78
quality program, 80–81
staffing, 80
structure of department for, 79
training outcomes, 79
types of programs in, 76–77
Organizing, as management function,
22
Outcome assessment, 15, 54–55

P

Paid-time-off programs, 345
Path-goal model, management style,
25–26
Patient classification system, 214
Patient education, nutritional
education, 416–418
Pay. *See* Compensation
Payback method, 307, 309
Performance evaluation procedure
audits, 48
Personnel, 338–339
alternative work arrangements, 340
career ladders, 340
promotion/transfers, 339–340
recruitment, 339
staffing planning, 339
supplemental staffing, 340
See also Staffing
Pharmacy
clinical pharmacy services, 396–
397
computerized system, 393, 398
distribution process, 393–396
drug information task, 388, 390–
392

future view of, 400–402
management principles related to, 386–387
organizational functions, 387–388
performance indicators, 398–400
quality management, 398–399
receiving, 393
resource requirements, 397–398
teaching/research tasks, 397
Physicians
ambulatory care services, 581–582
group practices, 580–582
hospital-based practices, 185–186
independent solo practices, 184–185
management principles related to, 183
mission of, 183–184
physician-hospital teams, 199–202
preparation/training, 190
supply of, 190–191
support services for, 191–192
Planning, 21–22
and nurses, 204
See also Strategic planning
Policies/procedures
materials management, 376–377
of quality program, 52, 53–54
Power
charismatic power, 28
coercive power, 28
definition of, 28
expert power, 28
legitimate power, 28, 29
and professional in health care system, 29–30
representative power, 28
reward power, 28
Practice standards, 115
Preferred provider organizations (PPOs), 125, 288, 551–552
Prepayment programs, 568–569
Pricing methods, for hospitals, 299–300
Primary care services
administration of, 583–584
features of, 580
future view of, 585–587
and group practices, 580–582

information management, 584
and medical training, 582
quality management, 584–585
staffing, 582–583
technology in, 584
Primary care system
characteristics of, 8–10
definition of, 9
Primary nurse, role of, 217
Privacy, release of information, 263–264, 276–278
Problem solving
creativity in, 83
leadership role, 41–42
Process costing, 302
Processing materials, 374–376
cleaning/sterilization, 375–376
disposables, advantages of, 374–375
disposal, 376
preparation of materials, 375
Process measures, 54–55
Product line costing, 301
Product organizations, 32
Product research, 363–364
Professionalization, of health care enterprises, 27
Professional standards review organizations, 47–48
Profit and loss statement, 294–295
Program development, 319–321
Program management, 111–116
characteristics of, 111–113
impact of, 113–115
professional issues related to, 115–116
Programming, in facilities planning, 442–448
Project groups, 110
Promotions, 339–340
Proprietary security programs, 516–517
Prospective payment system, 99, 287–288
Prospective review, 142–143
Psychiatric nurses, 618
Psychiatric social workers, 618
Psychiatrists, 618
Purchase agreement, 369–370

Purchasing, 363–370
bidding process, 368–369
capital equipment purchasing, 367–368
consignment buying, 367
group purchasing, 367
negotiations, 369
product research, 363–364
product standardization, 366–367
purchase agreement, 369–370
quotations, 369
specifications documents, 364–365
stockless purchasing, 367
supplier selection, 365–366
tasks of, 363
Purchasing assistant, 380
Purchasing manager, 380

Q

Quality
basic assumptions about, 45–46
characteristics important to consumers, 62
history of quality assurance, 46–49
management focus on, 43
and medical staff, 192–194
relationship to knowledge, 60–61, 64–68
Quality management
clinical data systems, 260–261
external information management, 278–280
facilities planning, 463–468
food/nutrition services, 424–425
and governing board, 172–174
housekeeping, 496
human resource management, 356–358
legal services, 556–557
marketing, 327–328
materials management, 382–384
nursing, 219–222
pharmacy, 398–399
primary care services, 584–585
risk management, 535–537
security, 519–520
specialty services, 602–604

strategic planning, 327–328
Quality program
    accreditation, 57
    assessment of, 54–55, 115
    continuous quality improvement,
        114–115
    data systems, 52–53
    and education department, 80–81
    future view of, 57–58
    goals of, 49–50
    governance of, 55
    infrastructure, construction of, 70–
        71
    initial activities in, 69–70
    investments in quality, 64
    leadership, 56–57, 63–64, 68–71
    management of, 55–56
    participants in, 50–52, 55
    policies of, 53–54
    program structure in, 50
    staffing, 52
    strategic planning in, 56
    training, 53
Queuing, 570–571
Quotations, purchasing, 369

R

Ratios, financial, 297–298
Receiver, 380
Receiving, 370–373
    inventory management, 371–373
    pharmacy, 393
    staff functions, 370
    tasks related to, 370
    warehousing, 370–371
Records
    preservation of, 262
    See also Clinical data systems;
        Information systems
Recruitment, personnel, 339
Registered nurse, 207
Regulatory planning, 321
Release of information
    confidentiality/privacy, 263–264
    type of, 263
Representative power, 28
Requisitioning, 373

Research
    food/nutrition services, 418–419
    market research, 322
    nursing, 210
    pharmacy, 397
    product research, 363–364
Resource-based relative value
    system, 289
Responsibility costs, 301
Retrospective review, 143–144
Reward power, 28
Risk
    and managed care, 139
    scope of, 524
Risk management
    and chief executive officer, 538
    and clinical records evaluation,
        537–538
    and contractual relations, 538
    future view, 538
    litigation
        bases of, 526
        implications for health services
            delivery, 526–527
    management principles related to,
        524–525
    preventive measures, 528–529
    quality management, 535–537
    risk elimination in, 527–528
    risk evaluation in, 527
    risk identification in, 527
    risk reduction in, 528
    risk transfer in, 528
Role conflict, 37

S

Safety
    computers, use of, 510
    corrective action, 506
    future issues, 503–504
    hazardous materials programs,
        507–508
    hazardous waste programs, 508
    historical view, 502
    monitoring of program, 508–509
    monitoring safety activities, 506–
        507

    quarterly reports on, 505
    safety committee, 504–505
    safety cycle, steps in, 505–507
    safety department, 504
    safety officer, 504
    staff, 509–510
    training, 503–504
    trends related to, 502–503
Salaries
    managed care compensation, 138
    nurses, 214–216
    See also Compensation
Security
    contractual security programs,
        517
    equipment used for, 518–519
    future view of, 521–522
    goal of, 510
    information systems, 243–245
    law enforcement officers, use of,
        517–518
    materials, 377–378
    organizational role, 510–511
    programs, structure of, 512–515
    proprietary security programs,
        516–517
    quality management, 519–520
    security devices, 519
    shared services programs, 518
    staff, 515–516
Service contracts, for equipment,
    482–483
Service line management, 34
Shared services programs, security,
    518
Sherman Act, 548, 549
Single-specialty groups, physicians,
    185, 581
Social Health Maintenance
    Organizations, 126
Space
    facilities planning, 319
    food/nutrition services, 422, 423,
        424
    for materials, 381
    pharmacy, 397
    See also Facilities planning
Specialty services
    current organization of, 600–601

development of departments, 599–
600
future view of, 607–610
integration into patient care
process, 602
management principles related to,
597–598
medical director, role of, 600
physician performance, monitoring
of, 604
quality management, 602–604
technology resources, 605–607,
608
Specifications, for products, 364–365
Staffing
alternative work arrangements, 340
education department, 80
food/nutrition services, 420–421,
429
housekeeping, 492–494
for information systems, 246–247
as management function, 22
for materials management, 379–
380
planning for, 339
primary care services, 582–583
quality program, 52
safety staff, 509–510
security, 515–516
supplemental staffing, 340
utilization management, 141
See also Personnel
Staff models, managed care, 121
Standard costs, 302
Standards
housekeeping, 489–490
nursing, 208–209, 219–220
Statement of cash flows, 303–304
Sterilization, 375–376
Stockless purchasing, 367
Stock replenishment system, 373
Stock reports, 294–295
Strategic planning, 327–328
future view, 328–330
governing board, 169–170
information gathering tasks, 316–
317
management functions related to,
314

organizational role/planning, 314–
316
planning activities, 316–322
program development/project
review, 319, 321
quality program, 56
regulatory planning, 321
relationship to marketing, 311–313
space/facilities planning, 319
strategic technology planning,
474–476
tasks in, 313
Strict liability, 526
Strikes, 347
written plan for, 347
Structure
managerial, types of, 32–34
quality program, 50
Substance abuse programs, 617
Suppliers, selection of, 365–366
Supplies. *See* Inventory; Materials
management

T

Task forces, 110
Tax law, and health care industry,
545–546
Tax Reform Act of 1986, 349
Technology assessment/management
and acute care, 594
audits, 484–485
clinical engineering departments,
477, 479
definition of, 471–472
equipment control system, 479–
481
equipment inspection/repair, 482
future view of, 485
hazard/recall information, 483–484
macro-assessment, 472, 473
micro-assessment, 472, 473
service contracts, 482–483
strategic technology planning,
474–476
technology acquisition, 476, 481–
482
technology management, 476–484

training/education functions,
484
Theory X, 23
Theory Y, 23
Therapeutic communities, 617
Third-party reimbursement, and legal
services, 550
Time-adjusted return method, 308,
309
Total quality management, 15, 303
and information systems, 248–249
Training
by pharmacists, 397
housekeeping, 499
nursing education, 210
quality program, 53
safety, 503–504
technology assessment/
management, 484
See also Employee development;
Organizational learning

U

Umbrella liability insurance, 533
Unlicensed assistive personnel, 207
Utilization management, 140–145,
551
concurrent review, 143
educational programs, 144
functions of, 141
and organizational culture, 144–
145
prospective review, 142–143
retrospective review, 143–144
staffing, 141
structural aspects, 141–142
use of term, 140
Utilization review, use of term, 140

V

Value structure, managed care, 133,
135
Vendors, comparison of, 382–383
Vertical communication, 31, 32

Vietnam Era Veterans Readjustment
    Assistance Act, 348
Voice recognition systems, 249

W

Warehousing, 370–371
Waste management, 491–492, 503
    hazardous waste, types of, 498,
        508

hazardous waste programs, 508
waste disposal, 376
Weighted value pricing method, 299,
    300
Worker Adjustment and Retraining
    Notification Act, 350
Workers' compensation cases,
    release of information, 264
Workers' compensation insurance,
    533–534

Workforce. *See* Human resource
    management
Workplace safety, laws related to,
    349–350

Z

Zoning, master zoning plan, 449